W9-APP-004

Magale Library
Southern Arkansas University
Magnolia, AR 71753

SALEM HEALTH
CANCER

Magale Library
Southern Arkansas University
Magnolia, AR 71753

SALEM HEALTH
CANCER

Second Edition

Volume III

Cancer Biology
Carcinogens and Suspected Carcinogens
Chemotherapy and Other Drugs
Complementary and Alternative Therapies
Lifestyle and Prevention

Editors

Michael A. Buratovich, Ph.D.
Spring Arbor University

Laurie Jackson-Grusby, Ph.D.
Children's Hospital Boston, Harvard Medical School

Editor, first edition

Jeffrey A. Knight
Mount Holyoke College

SALEM PRESS
A Division of EBSCO Information Services, Inc.
Ipswich, Massachusetts

GREY HOUSE PUBLISHING

Magale Library
Southern Arkansas University
Magnolia, AR 71753

Copyright © 2016 by Salem Press, A Division of EBSCO Information Services, Inc., and Grey House Publishing, Inc.

All rights in this book are reserved. No part of this work may be used or reproduced in any manner whatso ever or transmitted in any form or by any means, electronic or mechanical, including photocopy, recording, or any information storage and retrieval system, without written permission from the copyright owner except in the case of brief quotations embodied in critical articles and reviews or in the copying of images deemed to be freely licensed or in the public domain. For information contact Grey House Publishing/Salem Press, 4919 Route 22, PO Box 56, Amenia, NY 12501.

∞ The paper used in these volumes conforms to the American National Standard for Permanence of Paper for Printed Library Materials, Z39.48-1992 (R2009).

Note to Readers

The material presented in *Salem Health: Cancer* is intended for broad informational and educational purposes. Readers who suspect that they or someone whom they know or provide caregiving for suffers from cancer or any other physical or psychological disorder, disease, or condition described in this set should contact a physician without delay; this work should not be used as a substitute for professional medical diagnosis or staging. Readers who are undergoing or about to undergo any treatment or procedure described in this set should refer to their physicians and other health care team members for guidance concerning preparation and possible effects. This set is not to be considered definitive on the covered topics, and readers should remember that the field of health care is characterized by a diversity of medical opinions and constant expansion in knowledge and understanding.

Library of Congress Cataloging-in-Publication Data

Publisher's Cataloging-In-Publication Data
(Prepared by The Donohue Group, Inc.)

Names: Buratovich, Michael A., editor. | Jackson-Grusby, Laurie, editor.
Title: Cancer / editors, Michael A. Buratovich, Ph.D., Spring Arbor University, Laurie Jackson-Grusby, Ph.D., Children's Hospital Boston, Harvard Medical School.
Other Titles: Salem health (Pasadena, Calif.)
Description: Second edition. | Ipswich, Massachusetts: Salem Press, a division of EBSCO Information Services, Inc.; Amenia, NY: Grey House Publishing, [2016] | Editor, first edition, Jeffrey A. Knight, Mount Holyoke College. | Includes bibliographical references and index. | Volume I. Diseases, Symptoms and Conditions: Achlorhydria – Ovarian epithelial cancer – Volume II. Diseases, Symptoms and Conditions: Paget disease of bone – Zollinger-Ellison syndrome, Medical Specialties, Organizations, Social and Personal Issues – Volume III. Cancer Biology, Carcinogens and Suspected Carcinogens, Chemotherapy and Other Drugs, Complementary and Alternative Therapies, Lifestyle and Prevention – Volume IV. Procedures.
Identifiers: ISBN 978-1-61925-950-8 (set) | ISBN 978-1-68217-230-8 (vol. 1) | ISBN 978-1-68217-231-5 (vol. 2) | ISBN 978-1-68217-232-2 (vol. 3) | ISBN 978-1-68217-233-9 (vol. 4)
Subjects: LCSH: Cancer.
Classification: LCC RC265 .C336 2016 | DDC 616.99/4–dc23

First Printing

PRINTED IN THE UNITED STATES OF AMERICA

▶ Contents

Complete List of Contents ix

Cancer Biology

Angiogenesis 761
B-lymphocytes 762
BRAF gene 765
BRCA1 and *BRCA2* genes 766
Cancer biology 768
Cancer epigenetics 771
Cell cycle control 774
Cell death 777
Chromatin 779
Chromosomes and cancer 781
Circulating tumor cells 783
Cyclin-dependent kinase inhibitor-2A (*CDKN2A*) 785
Cytokines 786
DNA methylation 787
DNA repair 788
DNMT3A 791
Epidemiology of cancer 791
Estrogen Receptor Downregulator (ERD) 795
Exosomes 795
Genetics of cancer 797
Genomics of cancer 801
Histone acetylation/deacetylation 803
Histone methylation/demethylation 805
Human Chorionic Gonadotropin (HCG) 806
IDH1 807
Immune response to cancer 808
Lysine Histone Demethylases (KDMs) 810
Menopause and cancer 811
Mesenchymal stem cells and cancer 813
Mitochondrial DNA mutations 814
MLH1 gene 816
MSH genes 817
Mutagenesis and cancer 817
MYC oncogene 819
Myeloid-derived suppressor cells 820
NK cells 821
Oncogenes 823
Personalized medicine/whole genome sequencing 826
Placental Alkaline Phosphatase (PALP) 827
PMS genes 828
Proteasome 829
Proteomics and cancer research 830
Proto-oncogenes and carcinogenesis 832
RB1 gene 833
Regulatory T-cells 834
RhoGDI2 gene 835
SCLC1 gene 836
Telomerase 837
T-lymphocytes 838
TP53 protein 840
Tumor biomarkers 842
Tumor Necrosis Factor (TNF) 844
Tumor-suppressor genes 845

Carcinogens and Suspected Carcinogens

Acrylamides 847
Aflatoxins 848
Agent Orange 850
Air pollution 850
Alcohol, alcoholism, and cancer 853
4-Aminobiphenyl 854
Arsenic compounds 855
Asbestos 857
Azathioprine 858
Bacteria as causes of cancer 859
Benzene 860
Benzidine and dyes metabolized to benzidine 861
Beryllium and beryllium compounds 863
Birth control pills and cancer 864
Bis(chloromethyl) ether and technical-grade chloromethyl methyl ether 866
Bisphenol A (BPA) 867
1,3-Butadiene 868
1,4-Butanediol dimethanesulfonate 869
Cadmium and cadmium compounds 870
Caffeine 871
Carcinogens, known 872
Carcinogens, reasonably anticipated 876
Cell phones 879
Chewing tobacco 880
Chlorambucil 882
1-(2-Chloroethyl)-3-(4-methylcyclohexyl)-1-nitrosourea (MeCCNU) 882
Chromium hexavalent compounds 883
Cigarettes and cigars 884
Coal tars and coal tar pitches 885
Coke oven emissions 886

Cyclophosphamide 887
Cyclosporin A 888
Di(2-ethylhexyl) phthalate (DEHP) 889
Diethanolamine (DEA) 890
Diethylstilbestrol (DES) 891
Dioxins 891
Electromagnetic radiation 893
Epstein-Barr Virus 894
Erionite 896
Ethylene oxide 896
Fertility drugs and cancer 897
Formaldehyde 899
Free radicals 899
Hair dye 901
Helicobacter pylori infection 901
Hepatitis B virus (HBV) 905
Hepatitis C Virus (HCV) 906
Herpes simplex virus 907
Herpes zoster virus 909
HER2/neu protein 910
HIV/AIDS-related cancers 911
Hormone Replacement Therapy (HRT) 914
Human growth factors and tumor growth 916
Human Papillomavirus (HPV) 917
Human T-cell Leukemia Virus (HTLV) 918
Ionizing radiation 919
Melphalan 920
Mineral oils 921
Mustard gas 921
2-Naphthylamine 922
Nickel compounds and metallic nickel 923
Oncogenic viruses 924
Organochlorines (OCs) 925
Pesticides and the food chain 927
Phenacetin 929
Plasticizers 930
Polycyclic aromatic hydrocarbons 931
Radon 932
Report on Carcinogens (RoC) 933
Silica, crystalline 933
Simian virus 40 934
Sunlamps 935
Thiotepa 936
Ultraviolet radiation and related exposures 937
Vinyl chloride 938
Wood dust 938

Chemotherapy and Other Drugs

Abiraterone acetate (Zytiga) 941
Adenoviruses 942
Alkylating agents in chemotherapy 943
Androgen drugs 945
Angiogenesis inhibitors 945
Anthraquinones 947
Antiandrogens 948
Antidiarrheal agents 949
Antifungal therapies 951
Antimetabolites in chemotherapy 953
Antinausea medications 956
Antineoplastics in chemotherapy 958
Antiviral therapies 960
Bacillus Calmette Guérin (BCG) 963
BCR-ABL kinase and inhibitors 963
Benzodiazepines 965
BET inhibitors 966
Biological therapy 967
Bisphosphonates 971
Bortezomib (Velcade) 972
Brompton cocktail 973
Capecitabine 974
Cetuximab 974
Chemotherapy 975
Chimeric Antigen Receptor T-cell treatment 978
Colony-Stimulating Factors (CSFs) 980
Corticosteroids 982
Cycloastragenol 983
Cyclooxygenase 2 (COX-2) inhibitors 984
Chemoprevention 985
Decitabine/5-Azacytidine 987
Delta-9-tetrahydrocannabinol 989
Doxorubicin 990
Drug Resistance and Multidrug Resistance (MDR) 992
Erlotinib (Tarceva) 995
Glutamine 996
Hepatitis C drug treatments 996
Histamine 2 receptor antagonists 998
Histone deacetylase inhibitors 999
Hormonal therapies 1000
IDH1 inhibitor AG-120 1002
Imetelstat 1003
Immunotherapy 1004
Interferon 1006
Interleukins 1007

Laxatives 1008
Lenalidomide (Revlimid) 1009
Matrix metalloproteinase inhibitors 1010
Monoclonal antibodies 1010
Nonsteroidal Anti-Inflammatory Drugs (NSAIDs) 1013
Opioids 1014
Oxaliplatin (Eloxatin) 1015
Pain Management 1016
Palliative treatment 1019
Pegfilgrastim (Neulasta) 1022
Pemetrexed (Alimta) 1023
Photodynamic Therapy (PDT) 1024
Plant alkaloids and cancer 1024
Plant alkaloids and terpenoids in chemotherapy 1026
Platinum-based anticancer drugs 1029
Proteasome inhibitors 1030
Radiopharmaceuticals 1031
Ranibizumab (Lucentis) 1032
Rituximab 1033
Romidepsin 1034
Ruthenium based anticancer drug 1035
Stem cell cancer treatments 1036
Texaphyrins 1037
Topoisomerase inhibitors 1038
Trastuzumab (Herceptin) 1040
Tyrosine kinase inhibitors 1041
Vaccines, preventive 1043
Vaccines, therapeutic 1044
Vorinostat 1046

Complementary and Alternative Therapies

Antioxidants 1047
Chinese medicine and cancer 1049
Coenzyme Q10 1051
Complementary and Alternative Therapies 1051
Curcumin 1054
Dietary supplements 1055
Electroporation therapy 1058
Gerson therapy 1058
Ginseng 1059
Green tea 1060
Herbs as antioxidants 1061
Integrative oncology 1063
Mistletoe 1064
Motion sickness devices 1065
PC-SPES 1066
Phenolics 1067
Saw palmetto 1067
Sun's soup 1068

Lifestyle and Prevention

Artificial sweeteners 1071
Beta-carotene 1072
Bioflavonoids 1073
Calcium 1073
Cancer vaccines 1074
Carotenoids 1075
Coffee and cancer 1076
Cruciferous vegetables 1077
Esophageal speech 1078
Exercise and cancer 1079
Fiber 1082
Folic acid 1083
Fruits 1084
Garlic and allicin 1085
Indoles 1086
Isoflavones 1087
Lutein 1088
Lycopene 1089
Nutrition and cancer prevention 1090
Nutrition and cancer treatment 1092
Omega-3 fatty acids 1096
Phytoestrogens 1096
Prevention 1098
Resveratrol 1100
Risks for cancer 1101
Screening for cancer 1104
Smoking cessation 1107
Soy foods 1110
Sunscreens 1112
Wine and cancer 1113

▶ Complete List of Contents

Volume 1

Publisher's Note . . . ix
About the Editors . . . xi
Contributors . . . xiii
Complete List of Contents . . . xv

Diseases, Symptoms, and Conditions

Achlorhydria . . . 1
Acoustic neuromas . . . 1
Acute Lymphocytic Leukemia (ALL) . . . 3
Acute Myelocytic Leukemia (AML) . . . 6
Adenocarcinomas . . . 8
Adenoid Cystic Carcinoma (ACC) . . . 10
Adenomatoid tumors . . . 10
Adenomatous polyps . . . 11
Adrenal gland cancers . . . 12
Adrenocortical cancer . . . 14
Aleukemia . . . 15
Alopecia . . . 15
Alveolar soft-part sarcomas . . . 17
Amenorrhea . . . 18
Anal cancer . . . 20
Anemia . . . 21
Angiosarcomas . . . 23
Aplastic anemia . . . 24
Appendix cancer . . . 25
Appetite loss . . . 27
Ascites . . . 28
Astrocytomas . . . 30
Ataxia Telangiectasia (AT) . . . 32
Barrett esophagus . . . 33
Basal cell carcinomas . . . 35
Beckwith-Wiedemann Syndrome (BWS) . . . 37
Benign Prostatic Hyperplasia (BPH) . . . 38
Benign tumors . . . 39
Bile duct cancer . . . 40
Birt-Hogg-Dubé Syndrome (BHDS) . . . 42
Bladder cancer . . . 44
Blood cancers . . . 46
Bone cancers . . . 50
Bone pain . . . 53
Bowen disease . . . 53
Brain and central nervous system cancers . . . 55
Breakthrough pain . . . 58
Breast cancers . . . 59
Breast cancer in children and adolescents . . . 63
Breast cancer in men . . . 64
Breast cancer in pregnant women . . . 66
Bronchial adenomas . . . 67
Bronchoalveolar lung cancer . . . 68
Burkitt lymphoma . . . 69
Cachexia . . . 72
Calcifications of the breast . . . 72
Cancer syndromes resulting from DNA repair defects . . . 73
Candidiasis . . . 75
Carcinoid tumors and carcinoid syndrome . . . 76
Carcinoma of Unknown Primary origin (CUP) . . . 78
Carcinomas . . . 80
Carcinomatosis . . . 81
Carcinomatous meningitis . . . 83
Carcinosarcomas . . . 84
Cardiomyopathy in cancer patients . . . 85
Carney complex . . . 86
Castleman disease . . . 87
Cervical cancer . . . 88
Childhood cancers . . . 90
Chordomas . . . 94
Choriocarcinomas . . . 95
Chronic Lymphocytic Leukemia (CLL) . . . 97
Chronic Myeloid Leukemia (CML) . . . 99
Cold nodule . . . 101
Colon polyps . . . 102
Colorectal cancer . . . 103
Comedo carcinomas . . . 107
Cowden syndrome . . . 108
Craniopharyngiomas . . . 109
Craniosynostosis . . . 111
Crohn's disease . . . 113
Cushing syndrome and cancer . . . 116
Cutaneous breast cancer . . . 117
Cutaneous T-Cell Lymphoma (CTCL) . . . 118
Denys-Drash syndrome and cancer . . . 120
Depression . . . 120
Dermatofibrosarcoma Protuberans (DFSP) . . . 123
Desmoid tumors . . . 125
Desmoplastic Small Round Cell Tumor (DSRCT) . . 126

Diarrhea. 126
Disseminated Intravascular Coagulation (DIC) 128
Diverticulosis and diverticulitis 129
Down syndrome and leukemia 131
Dry mouth 132
Duct ectasia. 134
Ductal Carcinoma In Situ (DCIS). 134
Duodenal carcinomas 136
Dysplastic nevus syndrome. 136
Edema 137
Embryonal cell cancer. 139
Endocrine cancers. 139
Endometrial cancer 143
Endometrial hyperplasia 145
Endotheliomas. 147
Enteritis. 148
Eosinophilic leukemia. 150
Ependymomas. 150
Epidermoid cancers of mucous membranes 152
Erythroplakia. 153
Esophageal cancer. 154
Esophagitis 156
Estrogen-receptor-sensitive breast cancer. 158
Ewing sarcoma 160
Eye cancers 162
Eyelid cancer. 165
Fallopian tube cancer 166
Fanconi anemia. 168
Fatigue. 169
Fever 171
Fibroadenomas 173
Fibrocystic breast changes 174
Fibrosarcomas, soft-tissue. 176
5Q minus syndrome 178
Gallbladder cancer 179
Gardner syndrome. 181
Gastric polyps 183
Gastrinomas 184
Gastrointestinal cancers 185
Gastrointestinal complications of cancer
treatment. 189
Gastrointestinal Stromal Tumors (GISTs) 191
Germ-cell tumors 193
Gestational Trophoblastic Tumors (GTTs). 194
Giant Cell Tumors (GCTs) 197
Glioblastomas 198
Gliomas. 200
Glomus tumors 202
Graft-Versus-Host Disease (GVHD). 202
Granulosa cell tumors 204
Gynecologic cancers. 204
Hairy cell leukemia. 208
Hand-Foot Syndrome (HFS). 210
Head and neck cancers 211
Hemangioblastomas 214
Hemangiopericytomas 215
Hemangiosarcomas. 216
Hematemesis. 216
Hematuria 217
Hemochromatosis 218
Hemolytic anemia. 219
Hemoptysis 219
Hepatomegaly 220
Hereditary diffuse gastric cancer 222
Hereditary Leiomyomatosis and
Renal Cell Cancer (HLRCC) 223
Hereditary mixed polyposis syndrome 225
Hereditary Non-Polyposis Colorectal
Cancer (HNPCC) 225
Hereditary non-VHL clear cell renal
cell carcinomas. 229
Hereditary pancreatitis 230
Hereditary papillary renal cell carcinomas. 230
Hereditary polyposis syndromes. 231
Histiocytosis X 233
Hodgkin disease 235
Horner syndrome 238
Hydatidiform mole 239
Hypercalcemia 240
Hypercoagulation disorders 242
Hypopharyngeal cancer 243
Infection and sepsis. 244
Infectious cancers 247
Infertility and cancer. 249
Inflammatory bowel disease 251
Invasive cancer 252
Invasive ductal carcinomas 252
Invasive lobular carcinomas 253
Islet cell tumors. 254
Juvenile polyposis syndrome 256
Kaposi sarcoma. 256
Keratosis 259
Kidney cancer 260
Klinefelter syndrome and cancer 263
Krukenberg tumors 263
Lacrimal gland tumors 264

Lambert-Eaton Myasthenic Syndrome (LEMS) 265
Laryngeal cancer 266
Laryngeal nerve palsy 268
Leiomyomas 270
Leiomyosarcomas 272
Leptomeningeal carcinomas 274
Leukemias 275
Leukoencephalopathy 279
Leukopenia 281
Leukoplakia 281
Leydig cell tumors 282
Li-Fraumeni Syndrome (LFS) 283
Lip cancers 284
Liposarcomas 286
Liver cancers 288
Lobular Carcinoma In Situ (LCIS) 291
Lumps 292
Lung cancers 293
Lymphangiosarcomas 297
Lymphedema 298
Lymphocytosis 299
Lymphomas 300
Malignant Fibrous Histiocytoma (MFH) 303
Malignant rhabdoid tumor of the kidney 304
Malignant tumors 304
Mantle Cell Lymphoma (MCL) 305
Mastocytomas 307
Mediastinal tumors 307
Medullary carcinoma of the breast 309
Medulloblastomas 310
Melanomas 311
Meningeal carcinomatosis 314
Meningiomas 315
Merkel Cell Carcinomas (MCC) 316
Mesenchymomas, malignant 318
Mesothelioma 319
Metastasis 321
Metastatic squamous neck cancer with occult primary 323
Microcalcifications 324
Moles 324
Mucinous carcinomas 326
Mucosa-Associated Lymphoid Tissue (MALT) lymphomas 327
Mucositis 329
Multiple endocrine neoplasia 330
Multiple myeloma 332
Myasthenia gravis 334
Mycosis fungoides 336
Myelodysplastic syndromes 338
Myelofibrosis 339
Myeloma 341
Myeloproliferative disorders 341
Myelosuppression 344
Nasal cavity and paranasal sinus cancers 345
Nausea and vomiting 347
Nephroblastomas 350
Neuroblastomas 351
Neuroectodermal tumors 352
Neuroendocrine tumors 354
Neurofibromatosis type 1 (NF1) 356
Neutropenia 357
Night sweats 359
Nijmegen breakage syndrome 360
Nipple discharge 361
Non-Hodgkin lymphoma 362
Obesity-associated cancers 365
Oligodendrogliomas 369
Oral and oropharyngeal cancers 371
Orbit tumors 374
Organ transplantation and cancer 375
Ovarian cancers 377
Ovarian cysts 379
Ovarian epithelial cancer 380

Volume 2

Diseases, Symptoms, and Conditions

Paget disease of bone 383
Pancolitis 385
Pancreatic cancers 386
Pancreatitis 389
Paraneoplastic syndromes 390
Parathyroid cancer 392
Penile cancer 394
Pericardial effusion 396
Peutz-Jeghers Syndrome (PJS) 398
Pheochromocytomas 400
Phyllodes tumors 401
Pineoblastomas 403
Pituitary tumors 404

Pleural effusion 407
Pleuropulmonary blastomas 409
Pneumonia. 409
Polycythemia vera. 411
Polyps 412
Premalignancies 414
Primary central nervous system lymphomas 417
Prostate cancer 417
Prostatitis. 419
Rectal cancer. 420
Recurrence 422
Renal pelvis tumors. 422
Retinoblastomas 424
Rhabdomyosarcomas 425
Richter syndrome 427
Rothmund-Thomson syndrome 429
Salivary gland cancer 430
Sarcomas, soft-tissue. 433
Schwannoma tumors. 436
Sertoli cell tumors. 436
Sézary syndrome. 437
Side effects 440
Sjögren syndrome 444
Skin cancers 446
Small intestine cancer. 448
Spermatocytomas 450
Spinal axis tumors. 450
Spinal cord compression. 452
Squamous cell carcinomas 453
Sterility 456
Stomach cancers 457
Stomatitis 460
Superior vena cava syndrome 460
Symptoms and cancer. 462
Syndrome of Inappropriate Antidiuretic Hormone production (SIADH) 465
Synovial sarcomas 466
Taste alteration 468
Teratocarcinomas 469
Teratomas 470
Testicular cancer. 471
Throat cancer 473
Thrombocytopenia 475
Thymomas. 477
Thymus cancer 478
Thyroid cancer 480
Tobacco-related cancers 483
Transitional cell carcinomas 483
Trichilemmal carcinomas 485
Tuberous sclerosis. 486
Tubular carcinomas. 486
Tumor flare 487
Tumor lysis syndrome. 488
Turcot syndrome 489
Urethral cancer 491
Urinary system cancers. 492
Uterine cancer. 496
Vaginal cancer. 498
Virus-related cancers. 501
Von Hippel-Lindau (VHL) disease 504
Vulvar cancer 506
Waldenström Macroglobulinemia (WM) 508
Weight loss 510
Wilms' tumor 512
Wilms' tumor Aniridia-Genitourinary anomalies-mental Retardation (WAGR) syndrome and cancer. 515
Xeroderma pigmentosa. 516
Yolk sac carcinomas 517
Young adult cancers 518
Zollinger-Ellison syndrome 522

Medical Specialties

Cancer care team. 525
Cancer education. 527
Clinical trials. 529
Cytogenetics 532
Cytology 533
Dermatology oncology 536
Endocrinology oncology. 538
Family history and risk assessment. 541
Gastrointestinal oncology 545
Genetic counseling 547
Gynecologic oncology 549
Hematologic oncology 551
Immunocytochemistry and immunohistochemistry. 553
Medical oncology 555
Molecular oncology 558
Neurologic oncology. 559
Occupational therapy 561
Oncology. 564
Oncology clinical nurse specialist 566
Oncology social worker 569
Ophthalmic oncology 569
Orthopedic surgery 572

Otolaryngology . . . 573
Pathology . . . 575
Pediatric oncology and hematology . . . 577
Pharmacy oncology . . . 580
Primary care physician . . . 583
Psycho-oncology . . . 585
Radiation oncology . . . 587
Surgical oncology . . . 589
Urologic oncology . . . 591
Veterinary oncology . . . 594
Viral oncology . . . 596

Organizations

American Association for Cancer Research (AACR) . . . 599
American Cancer Society (ACS) . . . 600
American Institute for Cancer Research (AICR) . . . 601
Bristol-Myers Squibb . . . 603
Dana-Farber Cancer Institute . . . 604
Duke Comprehensive Cancer Center . . . 605
Eli Lilly . . . 607
Fox Chase Cancer Center . . . 608
Fred Hutchinson Cancer Research Center . . . 609
Genentech, Inc. . . . 611
Geron Corporation . . . 612
Jonsson Comprehensive Cancer Center (JCCC) . . . 613
M. D. Anderson Cancer Center . . . 615
Mayo Clinic Cancer Center . . . 616
Memorial Sloan-Kettering Cancer Center . . . 618
Merck & Co. . . . 619
National Cancer Institute (NCI) . . . 620
National Science Foundation (NSF) . . . 622
Prevent Cancer Foundation . . . 623
Roche . . . 625
Sanofi-Aventis . . . 626
Stand Up To Cancer . . . 628
Takeda Pharmaceutical Co. . . . 630

Social and Personal Issues

Advance directives . . . 633
African Americans and cancer . . . 635
Africans and cancer . . . 637
Aging and cancer . . . 639
Aids and devices for cancer patients . . . 641
Antiperspirants and breast cancer . . . 643
Anxiety . . . 644
Asian Americans and cancer . . . 646
Ashkenazi Jews and cancer . . . 649
Cancer clusters . . . 651
Cancer survival support groups . . . 653
Caregivers and caregiving . . . 654
Case management . . . 657
Childbirth and cancer . . . 659
Cognitive effects of cancer and chemotherapy . . . 660
Cost of cancer drugs . . . 662
Counseling for cancer patients and survivors . . . 663
Developing nations and cancer . . . 666
Do-Not-Resuscitate (DNR) order . . . 668
Elderly and cancer . . . 669
Electrolarynx . . . 672
End-of-life care . . . 672
Ethnicity and cancer . . . 675
Fertility issues . . . 678
Financial issues . . . 680
Geography and cancer . . . 683
Grief and bereavement . . . 686
Hereditary cancer syndromes . . . 688
Home health services . . . 690
Hospice care . . . 693
Informed consent . . . 695
Insurance . . . 697
Journaling . . . 700
Karnofsky Performance Status (KPS) . . . 700
Latinos/Hispanics and cancer . . . 701
Living will . . . 703
Living with cancer . . . 704
Long-distance caregiving . . . 707
Managed care . . . 709
Medical marijuana . . . 711
Medicare and cancer . . . 713
Native North Americans and cancer . . . 715
Occupational exposures and cancer . . . 717
Overtreatment . . . 719
Physical therapy and cancer . . . 720
Poverty and cancer . . . 722
Prayer and cancer support . . . 724
Preferred Provider Organizations (PPOs) . . . 725
Pregnancy and cancer . . . 727
Psychosocial aspects of cancer . . . 730
Relationships . . . 732
Second opinions . . . 734
Self-image and body image . . . 735
Sephardic Jews and cancer risk . . . 737

Sexuality and cancer 738
Singlehood and cancer 741
Social Security Disability Insurance (SSDI) 742
Statistics of cancer 743
Stress management 746
Support groups 748
Survival rates. 752
Survivorship issues 754
Transitional care 756
Watchful waiting. 757
Yoga and Cancer. 758

Volume 3

Cancer Biology

Angiogenesis. 761
B-lymphocytes 762
BRAF gene 765
BRCA1 and *BRCA2* genes 766
Cancer biology 768
Cancer epigenetics 771
Cell cycle control 774
Cell death 777
Chromatin 779
Chromosomes and cancer 781
Circulating tumor cells 783
Cyclin-dependent kinase inhibitor-2A (*CDKN2A*) 785
Cytokines 786
DNA methylation 787
DNA repair 788
DNMT3A 791
Epidemiology of cancer 791
Estrogen Receptor Downregulator (ERD) 795
Exosomes 795
Genetics of cancer. 797
Genomics of cancer. 801
Histone acetylation/deacetylation. 803
Histone methylation/demethylation 805
Human Chorionic Gonadotropin (HCG) 806
IDH1 807
Immune response to cancer 808
Lysine Histone Demethylases (KDMs) 810
Menopause and cancer 811
Mesenchymal stem cells and cancer. 813
Mitochondrial DNA mutations 814
MLH1 gene 816
MSH genes 817
Mutagenesis and cancer 817
MYC oncogene 819
Myeloid-derived suppressor cells 820
NK cells 821
Oncogenes. 823
Personalized medicine/whole genome sequencing 826
Placental Alkaline Phosphatase (PALP) 827
PMS genes 828
Proteasome 829
Proteomics and cancer research 830
Proto-oncogenes and carcinogenesis 832
RB1 gene 833
Regulatory T-cells. 834
RhoGDI2 gene 835
SCLC1 gene 836
Telomerase 837
T-lymphocytes. 838
TP53 protein 840
Tumor biomarkers. 842
Tumor Necrosis Factor (TNF) 844
Tumor-suppressor genes 845

Carcinogens and Suspected Carcinogens

Acrylamides 847
Aflatoxins 848
Agent Orange 850
Air pollution 850
Alcohol, alcoholism, and cancer. 853
4-Aminobiphenyl 854
Arsenic compounds. 855
Asbestos 857
Azathioprine 858
Bacteria as causes of cancer 859
Benzene. 860
Benzidine and dyes metabolized to benzidine 861
Beryllium and beryllium compounds 863
Birth control pills and cancer 864
Bis(chloromethyl) ether and technical-grade chloromethyl methyl ether 866

Bisphenol A (BPA) 867
1,3-Butadiene 868
1,4-Butanediol dimethanesulfonate 869
Cadmium and cadmium compounds. 870
Caffeine. 871
Carcinogens, known 872
Carcinogens, reasonably anticipated. 876
Cell phones 879
Chewing tobacco. 880
Chlorambucil. 882
1-(2-Chloroethyl)-3-(4-methylcyclohexyl)-
1-nitrosourea (MeCCNU) 882
Chromium hexavalent compounds 883
Cigarettes and cigars. 884
Coal tars and coal tar pitches 885
Coke oven emissions. 886
Cyclophosphamide 887
Cyclosporin A 888
Di(2-ethylhexyl) phthalate (DEHP) 889
Diethanolamine (DEA). 890
Diethylstilbestrol (DES) 891
Dioxins 891
Electromagnetic radiation. 893
Epstein-Barr Virus. 894
Erionite 896
Ethylene oxide 896
Fertility drugs and cancer 897
Formaldehyde 899
Free radicals 899
Hair dye. 901
Helicobacter pylori infection 901
Hepatitis B virus (HBV) 905
Hepatitis C Virus (HCV). 906
Herpes simplex virus. 907
Herpes zoster virus 909
HER2/neu protein 910
HIV/AIDS related cancers 911
Hormone Replacement Therapy (HRT) 914
Human growth factors and tumor growth. 916
Human Papillomavirus (HPV) 917
Human T-cell Leukemia Virus (HTLV) 918
Ionizing radiation 919
Melphalan 920
Mineral oils. 921
Mustard gas. 921
2-Naphthylamine. 922
Nickel compounds and metallic nickel. 923
Oncogenic viruses. 924
Organochlorines (OCs). 925
Pesticides and the food chain 927
Phenacetin. 929
Plasticizers 930
Polycyclic aromatic hydrocarbons 931
Radon 932
Report on Carcinogens (RoC). 933
Silica, crystalline. 933
Simian virus 40. 934
Sunlamps. 935
Thiotepa 936
Ultraviolet radiation and related
exposures 937
Vinyl chloride 938
Wood dust 938

Chemotherapy and Other Drugs

Abiraterone acetate (Zytiga) 941
Adenoviruses. 942
Alkylating agents in chemotherapy. 943
Androgen drugs. 945
Angiogenesis inhibitors 945
Anthraquinones. 947
Antiandrogens. 948
Antidiarrheal agents 949
Antifungal therapies 951
Antimetabolites in chemotherapy 953
Antinausea medications 956
Antineoplastics in chemotherapy 958
Antiviral therapies. 960
Bacillus Calmette Guérin (BCG) 963
BCR-ABL kinase and inhibitors. 963
Benzodiazepines 965
BET inhibitors. 966
Biological therapy. 967
Bisphosphonates 971
Bortezomib (Velcade) 972
Brompton cocktail. 973
Capecitabine 974
Cetuximab 974
Chemotherapy. 975
Chimeric Antigen Receptor
T-cell treatment 978
Colony-Stimulating Factors (CSFs) 980
Corticosteroids 982
Cycloastragenol. 983

Cyclooxygenase 2 (COX-2) inhibitors . . . 984
Chemoprevention . . . 985
Decitabine/5-Azacytidine . . . 987
Delta-9-tetrahydrocannabinol . . . 989
Doxorubicin . . . 990
Drug Resistance and Multidrug Resistance (MDR) . . . 992
Erlotinib (Tarceva) . . . 995
Glutamine . . . 996
Hepatitis C drug treatments . . . 996
Histamine 2 receptor antagonists . . . 998
Histone deacetylase inhibitors . . . 999
Hormonal therapies . . . 1000
IDH1 inhibitor AG-120 . . . 1002
Imetelstat . . . 1003
Immunotherapy . . . 1004
Interferon . . . 1006
Interleukins . . . 1007
Laxatives . . . 1008
Lenalidomide (Revlimid) . . . 1009
Matrix metalloproteinase inhibitors . . . 1010
Monoclonal antibodies . . . 1010
Nonsteroidal Anti-Inflammatory Drugs (NSAIDs) . . . 1013
Opioids . . . 1014
Oxaliplatin (Eloxatin) . . . 1015
Pain Management . . . 1016
Palliative treatment . . . 1019
Pegfilgrastim (Neulasta) . . . 1022
Pemetrexed (Alimta) . . . 1023
Photodynamic Therapy (PDT) . . . 1024
Plant alkaloids and cancer . . . 1024
Plant alkaloids and terpenoids in chemotherapy . . . 1026
Platinum-based anticancer drugs . . . 1029
Proteasome inhibitors . . . 1030
Radiopharmaceuticals . . . 1031
Ranibizumab (Lucentis) . . . 1032
Rituximab . . . 1033
Romidepsin . . . 1034
Ruthenium based anticancer drug . . . 1035
Stem cell cancer treatments . . . 1036
Texaphyrins . . . 1037
Topoisomerase inhibitors . . . 1038
Trastuzumab (Herceptin) . . . 1040
Tyrosine kinase inhibitors . . . 1041
Vaccines, preventive . . . 1043
Vaccines, therapeutic . . . 1044
Vorinostat . . . 1046

Complementary and Alternative Therapies

Antioxidants . . . 1047
Chinese medicine and cancer . . . 1049
Coenzyme Q10 . . . 1051
Complementary and Alternative Therapies . . . 1051
Curcumin . . . 1054
Dietary supplements . . . 1055
Electroporation therapy . . . 1058
Gerson therapy . . . 1058
Ginseng . . . 1059
Green tea . . . 1060
Herbs as antioxidants . . . 1061
Integrative oncology . . . 1063
Mistletoe . . . 1064
Motion sickness devices . . . 1065
PC-SPES . . . 1066
Phenolics . . . 1067
Saw palmetto . . . 1067
Sun's soup . . . 1068

Lifestyle and Prevention

Artificial sweeteners . . . 1071
Beta-carotene . . . 1072
Bioflavonoids . . . 1073
Calcium . . . 1073
Cancer vaccines . . . 1074
Carotenoids . . . 1075
Coffee and cancer . . . 1076
Cruciferous vegetables . . . 1077
Esophageal speech . . . 1078
Exercise and cancer . . . 1079
Fiber . . . 1082
Folic acid . . . 1083
Fruits . . . 1084
Garlic and allicin . . . 1085
Indoles . . . 1086
Isoflavones . . . 1087
Lutein . . . 1088
Lycopene . . . 1089
Nutrition and cancer prevention . . . 1090
Nutrition and cancer treatment . . . 1092
Omega-3 fatty acids . . . 1096

Phytoestrogens ... 1096
Prevention ... 1098
Resveratrol ... 1100
Risks for cancer ... 1101
Screening for cancer ... 1104
Smoking cessation ... 1107
Soy foods ... 1110
Sunscreens ... 1112
Wine and cancer ... 1113

Volume 4

Procedures

ABCD ... 1115
Abdominoperineal Resection (APR) ... 1115
Accelerated Partial Breast Irradiation (APBI) ... 1117
Acupuncture and acupressure for cancer patients ... 1118
Adjuvant therapy ... 1120
Afterloading radiation therapy ... 1121
Alkaline Phosphatase Test (ALP) ... 1123
Alpha-Fetoprotein (AFP) levels ... 1123
Amputation ... 1124
Angiography ... 1126
Anoscopy ... 1127
APC gene testing ... 1128
Arterial embolization ... 1128
Autologous blood transfusion ... 1129
Axillary dissection ... 1130
Barium enema ... 1130
Barium swallow ... 1132
Bethesda criteria ... 1133
Bilobectomy ... 1134
Biopsy ... 1134
Bone marrow aspiration and biopsy ... 1137
Bone Marrow Transplantation (BMT) ... 1138
Bone scan ... 1141
Boron Neutron Capture Therapy (BNCT) ... 1142
Brachytherapy ... 1143
Brain scan ... 1145
Breast implants ... 1146
Breast reconstruction ... 1147
Breast Self-Examination (BSE) ... 1149
Breast ultrasound ... 1150
Breslow's staging ... 1152
Brief Pain Inventory (BPI) ... 1152
Bronchography ... 1153
Bronchoscopy ... 1154
CA 15-3 test ... 1155
CA 19-9 test ... 1155
CA 27-29 test ... 1156
CA 125 test ... 1157
Carcinoembryonic Antigen Antibody (CEA) test ... 1157
Cardiopulmonary Resuscitation (CPR) ... 1158
Chemoembolization ... 1160
Clinical Breast Exam (CBE) ... 1161
Cobalt 60 radiation ... 1164
Colectomy ... 1164
Coloanal anastomosis ... 1166
Colonoscopy and virtual colonoscopy ... 1167
Colorectal cancer screening ... 1168
Colostomy ... 1170
Colposcopy ... 1172
Complete Blood Count (CBC) ... 1173
Computed Tomography (CT)-guided biopsy ... 1174
Computed Tomography (CT) scan ... 1176
Conization ... 1177
Continuous Hyperthermic Peritoneal Perfusion (CHPP) ... 1178
Cordectomy ... 1179
Cordotomy ... 1179
Core needle biopsy ... 1181
Craniotomy ... 1182
Cryoablation ... 1183
Culdoscopy ... 1184
Cystography ... 1185
Cystoscopy ... 1186
Digital Rectal Exam (DRE) ... 1186
Dilation and Curettage (D&C) ... 1187
DPC4 gene testing ... 1188
Ductal lavage ... 1189
Ductogram ... 1189
Dukes' classification ... 1190
Electrosurgery ... 1191
Embolization ... 1192
Endorectal ultrasound ... 1193

Endoscopic Retrograde Cholangiopancreatography (ERCP) . . . 1194
Endoscopy . . . 1195
Enterostomal therapy . . . 1197
Esophagectomy . . . 1199
Exenteration . . . 1200
External Beam Radiation Therapy (EBRT) . . . 1202
Fecal Occult Blood Test (FOBT) . . . 1202
Flow cytometry . . . 1204
Gallium scan . . . 1205
Gamma Knife . . . 1207
Gene therapy . . . 1207
Genetic testing . . . 1210
Gleason grading system . . . 1213
Glossectomy . . . 1214
Gonioscopy . . . 1215
Grading of tumors . . . 1215
Hepatic Arterial Infusion (HAI) . . . 1216
Hormone receptor tests . . . 1217
HRAS gene testing . . . 1218
5-Hydroxyindoleacetic Acid (5HIAA) test . . . 1219
Hyperthermia therapy . . . 1219
Hyperthermic perfusion . . . 1220
Hysterectomy . . . 1221
Hysterography . . . 1223
Hystero-oophorectomy . . . 1224
Hysteroscopy . . . 1225
Ileostomy . . . 1226
Imaging contrast dyes . . . 1227
Imaging tests . . . 1229
Immunochemical Fecal Occult Blood Test (iFOBT) . . . 1232
Immunoelectrophoresis (IEP) . . . 1233
Infusion therapies . . . 1234
Intensity-Modulated Radiation Therapy (IMRT) . . . 1235
Iridium seeds . . . 1236
Ki67 test . . . 1237
Lactate Dehydrogenase (LDH) test . . . 1237
Laparoscopy and laparoscopic surgery . . . 1238
Laryngectomy . . . 1240
Laryngoscopy . . . 1241
Laser therapies . . . 1242
Leukapharesis . . . 1243
Limb salvage . . . 1244
Linear accelerator . . . 1245
Liver biopsy . . . 1246
Lobectomy . . . 1247
Loop Electrosurgical Excisional Procedure (LEEP) . . . 1248
Lumbar puncture . . . 1249
Lumpectomy . . . 1251
Lymphadenectomy . . . 1252
Lymphangiography . . . 1253
Magnetic Resonance Imaging (MRI) . . . 1254
Mammography . . . 1257
Mastectomy . . . 1260
Mediastinoscopy . . . 1262
Microwave hyperthermia therapy . . . 1262
Mohs surgery . . . 1263
Needle localization . . . 1264
Nephrostomy . . . 1264
Nuclear medicine scan . . . 1266
Ommaya reservoir . . . 1268
Oophorectomy . . . 1268
Oral and maxillofacial surgery . . . 1270
Orchiectomy . . . 1271
Palpation . . . 1272
Pancreatectomy . . . 1273
Pap test . . . 1274
Paracentesis . . . 1276
Pelvic examination . . . 1277
Percutaneous Transhepatic Cholangiography (PTHC) . . . 1278
Pericardiocentesis . . . 1279
Peritoneovenous shunts . . . 1279
Pheresis . . . 1280
Pleural biopsy . . . 1281
Pleurodesis . . . 1282
Pneumonectomy . . . 1282
Polypectomy . . . 1284
Positron Emission Tomography (PET) . . . 1285
Progesterone receptor assay . . . 1287
Prostate-Specific Antigen (PSA) test . . . 1288
Prostatectomy . . . 1289
Protein electrophoresis . . . 1290
Proton beam therapy . . . 1291
Radiation therapies . . . 1293
Radical neck dissection . . . 1296
Radiofrequency ablation . . . 1296
Radionuclide scan . . . 1299
Receptor analysis . . . 1299
Reconstructive surgery . . . 1301
Rehabilitation . . . 1303

Salpingectomy and salpingo-oophorectomy...... 1305
Sentinel Lymph Node (SLN) biopsy and mapping ... 1306
Sigmoidoscopy ... 1307
Splenectomy ... 1308
Sputum cytology ... 1310
Staging of cancer ... 1310
Stent therapy ... 1313
Stereotactic needle biopsy ... 1315
Stereotactic Radiosurgery (SRS) ... 1315
Surgical biopsies ... 1317
Technetium isotopes ... 1319
Testicular Self-Examination (TSE) ... 1320
Thermal imaging ... 1321
Thoracentesis ... 1322
Thoracoscopy ... 1323
Thoracotomy ... 1324
Thyroid nuclear medicine scan ... 1324
TNM staging ... 1326
Tracheostomy ... 1327
Transfusion therapy ... 1329
Transrectal ultrasound ... 1331
Transvaginal ultrasound ... 1331
Tumor markers ... 1332
Ultrasound tests ... 1334
Umbilical cord blood transplantation ... 1336
Upper Gastrointestinal (GI) endoscopy ... 1338
Upper Gastrointestinal (GI) series ... 1339
Urinalysis ... 1341
Urography ... 1343
Urostomy ... 1344
Vascular access tubes ... 1345
Vasectomy and cancer ... 1346
Wire localization ... 1346
X-ray tests ... 1347

Appendixes

Drugs Classified by Drug Classes/Trade Names .. 1353
Associations and Agencies ... 1374
Cancer Centers and Hospitals ... 1379
Cancer Support Groups ... 1384
Carcinogens ... 1389
Glossary ... 1411
Bibliography ... 1429
Index ... 1505

▶ Angiogenesis

Category: Cancer Biology
Also known as: Blood vessel formation

Definition: The formation of new blood vessels from pre-existing blood vessels is angiogenesis. After vasculogenesis produces the first vessels in a developing embryo, angiogenesis drives most or all subsequent blood-vessel growth. Angiogenesis is a perfectly normal process in a developing or growing body, and, during a woman's reproductive years, it enables the menses and pregnancy. In addition, angiogenesis maintains health by developing a new blood supply in injured tissue, controlling inflammation, and even healing fractures of the bone.

When the body requires production of blood vessels it employs proteins called growth factors, including and not limited to vascular-endothelial growth factor (VEGF), which with its receptors comprises a powerful family of angiogenic agents; platelet-derived growth factor (PDGF); fibroblast growth factor (FGF); and tissue growth factor (TGF). Our primary focus will be VEGF (pronounced Veg-F).

Angiogenesis occurs in one of two ways.

Intussusceptive Angiogenesis: Also known as splitting angiogenesis, intussusceptive angiogenesis refers to creating a new blood vessel by dividing an existing one. This happens as the capillary wall of one vessel extends into the lumen of the second, splitting it. Although either type of angiogenesis can occur at any time from before birth until death, intussusceptive angiogenesis is useful for embryos, as it rearranges existing cells to enable a sharp increase in the number of capillaries without need for much increase in the number of cells.

Sprouting Angiogenesis: In sprouting angiogenesis, signals called angiogenic growth factors engage receptors on the endothelial cells that line blood vessels. Activation causes the endothelial cells to release proteases (enzymes) that degrade the vessel wall. The endothelial cells then migrate through the vessel wall into the extracellular matrix, noncellular material that surrounds any tissue rather like a honeycomb enveloping honey. Using proteins and enzymes to digest the extracellular matrix, the endothelial cells grow across gaps in the vasculature and expand into new territory, heading toward the angiogenic signals that began the process. Paired by adhesion molecules known as integrins, endothelial cells lengthen and loop as they migrate, forming the lumen (interior) of the new vessel.

Relation of Angiogenesis to Cancer: For survival, any bodily structure requires the continuous supply of oxygen and nutrients and removal of wastes. Cancerous tumors differ from normal tissue in that they tend to metastasize (spread) without regard to borders between such differing tissues as skin, muscle, connective tissue, and bone. For tumor growth to occur, there must be blood supply; in its absence, the tumor stops growing and may even die. To obtain its blood supply, the cancer must induce the body to build vessels to and throughout the tumor, which seems counterintuitive. Although the body contains defenses against this, as cancer develops, these defenses are short-circuited.

Tumor Angiogenesis: A tumor fools its host into cooperation through subterfuge—with a protein used in healthy angiogenesis but coopted by the tumor. In mimicry of its mission in health, VEGF released from tumor cells binds to endothelial cells lining blood vessels, sparking a chemical cascade that culminates in the sprouting of new vessels lured to their source, the tumor that begat them.

Known Angiogenic Growth Factors

- Angiogenin
- Angiopoietin-1
- Del-1
- Fibroblast growth factors: acidic (aFGF) and basic (bFGF)
- Follistatin
- Granulocyte colony-stimulating factor (G-CSF)
- Hepatocyte growth factor (HGF) /scatter factor (SF)
- Interleukin-8 (IL-8)
- Leptin
- Midkine
- Placental growth factor
- Platelet-derived endothelial cell growth factor (PD-ECGF)
- Platelet-derived growth factor-BB (PDGF-BB)
- Pleiotrophin (PTN)
- Progranulin
- Proliferin
- Transforming growth factor-alpha (TGF-alpha)
- Transforming growth factor-beta (TGF-beta)
- Tumor necrosis factor-alpha (TNF-alpha)
- Vascular endothelial growth factor (VEGF)/vascular permeability factor (VPF)

Source: The Angiogenesis Foundation

Preventing Cancer-Related Angiogenesis: If tumors require angiogenesis to survive and spread, impairing angiogenesis should deter tumor growth. Certainly targeting only vessels developed to serve tumors is preferable to the general aim in chemotherapy of killing every rapidly dividing cell. Methods to impair angiogenesis have historically intercepted one growth factor, VEGF. Experience, however, has revealed adverse or unexpected effects of impairing VEGF, some of which stem from the very absence of the targeted growth factor. While anti-angiogenesis sounds like a good way to inhibit cancerous growth, concerns remain as to its treatment efficacy, in part because of the complexity and diversity of the tumors themselves. What works for one tumor may not work for another. Of more concern is the observation that, after initially shrinking tumors, anti-angiogenesis may promote subsequent, more aggressive tumor growth. While it is true that most tumor-supplying vessels rely on VEGF signaling, increasingly we find that angiogenesis can proceed when VEGF signaling is blocked. Growth factors other than VEGF exist, and, when VEGF is blocked, these alternative growth factors compensate for, and sometimes accelerate angiogenesis in its absence.

Expanded Directions: Researchers are increasingly aware of the perils of over-reliance on VEGF-signal blockade. Combining conventional VEGF blockade with blockade of alternate vessel-developing growth factors has had early successes in suppressing tumors.

This is encouraging not only for treating solid tumors but also as potential therapy for leukemia, which in its chronic form requires extensive blood-vessel support in bone marrow.

Overcoming the primal threat of malignancy hinges on apprehending the range of subterfuges through which a tumor elicits the support of its host. As our understanding is perfected, methods will be found to circumvent both VEGF and compensatory vessel-producing pathways so that tumors will be deprived of blood.

Jackie Dial, PhD

For Further Information

Adair, Thomas H., & Montani, Jean-Pierre. (2010). *Angiogenesis*. San Rafael (CA): Morgan & Claypool Life Sciences. Available at: http://www.ncbi.nlm.nih.gov/books/NBK53238.

Cooke, Robert. (2001). *Dr. Folkman's War*. New York: Random House, Inc.

Figg, William, & Folkman, Judah. (Eds.). (2008). *Angiogenesis: An Integrative Approach from Science to Medicine*. New York: Springer.

Forough, Reza. (Ed.). (2006). *New Frontiers in Angiogenesis*. Dordrecht, The Netherlands: Springer.

Rakhimov, Artour. (2013). *Doctors Who Cure Cancer: Anticancer Biography and New Way of Life to Treat the Emperor of All Maladies*. Ontario: Artour Rakhimov.

Other Resources

Angiogenesis Foundation. "About Angiogenesis." http://www.angio.org/understanding/understanding.html

Cancer.org. "From Mind to Brain to Cancer Cell: A Systemic Approach to Cancer Progression." Susan K. Lutgendorf, PhD. http://www.cancer.org/acs/groups/content/@behavioral-researchcenter/documents/document/acspc-036209.pdf

HHMI BioInteractive. "Angiogenesis." Part of "Learning from Patients: The Science of Medicine." http://www.hhmi.org/biointeractive/angiogenesis

Nishida, Nayoy, et al. "Angiogenesis in Cancer." Vasc Health Risk Manag 2(3); 2006. http://www.ncbi.nlm.nih.gov/pmc/articles/PMC1993983

See also: Angiogenesis inhibitors; Bioflavonoids; Biological therapy; BRAF gene; Bronchoalveolar lung cancer; Cancer biology; Cartilage supplements; Chemotherapy; Gene therapy; Genetics of cancer; Hereditary Leiomyomatosis and Renal Cell Cancer (HLRCC); HIV/AIDS-related cancers; Human growth factors and tumor growth; Immunotherapy; Kidney cancer; Matrix metalloproteinase inhibitors; Oral and oropharyngeal cancers; Phenolics; Sarcomas, soft-tissue

▶ B-lymphocytes

Category: Cancer Biology
Also known as: B-cells

Definition: B-lymphocytes are white blood cells of the adaptive immune system that differentiate into plasma cells and memory B-lymphocytes. Plasma cells secrete antibodies to fight infection and destroy abnormal cells such as cancer cells. Memory B-lymphocytes are activated by contracting a disease or by vaccination. They confer long-lasting immunity to a specific disease. One subset of B-lymphocytes can also infiltrate cancer tumors.

Function: Some background on the immune system is necessary to understand how B-lymphocytes function and the role they play in fighting cancer. The immune system is a complex of tissues, cells, and the chemicals these cells produce that is spread throughout the body. Its function is to rid the body of foreign microbes and damaged or abnormal body cells. The major organs of the immune system are the bone marrow, lymph nodes, thymus, and spleen. Immune system cells and a clear fluid called lymph move throughout the body in a series of channels called lymphatic vessels that are separate from the circulatory system.

The immune system has 2 divisions: the innate immune system and the adaptive immune system. The innate system consists of white blood cells (leukocytes) that respond rapidly to a wide range of microbes but cannot confer immunity against disease. The adaptive system has cells that respond more slowly to disease but can create long-lasting immunity. While cells in the innate system can attack many different microbes, each cell of the adaptive system recognizes and attacks only 1 type of microbe or damaged cell. B-lymphocytes and T-lymphocytes (see separate entry) are the main cells of the adaptive immune system.

All cells have specific marker molecules on their surfaces that identify them as "self-cells" or "non-self-cells." Each B-lymphocyte and T-lymphocyte interacts with only one particular type of surface marker molecule that is displayed on the surfaces of microbes or abnormal cells and identifies them as non-self-cells. These marker molecules (often proteins) that elicit a reaction from B-lymphocytes are called antigens.

Development: B-lymphocytes develop from hematopoietic stem cells. These cells in the bone marrow have the ability to divide and differentiate into many different types of blood cells. As B-lymphocytes mature, each cell develops a unique receptor on its surface that will bind only to a single, specific antigen on a foreign microbe or an abnormal body cell such as a cancer cell. Scientists believe the body can make over one billion unique B-lymphocytes. Any B-lymphocytes that develop receptors that will bind with marker molecules on healthy self-cells are eliminated while still in the bone marrow so as not to harm the body.

Once B-lymphocytes leave the bone marrow, they migrate to lymph nodes. Lymph nodes are places in the lymphatic system, such as in the neck, under the arms, and in the groin, where foreign and abnormal cells are filtered out of lymph. When a B-lymphocyte meets an antigen that matches its specific receptor, the lymphocyte is activated and clones itself, producing massive numbers of identical cells. Most of these clone cells become plasma cells that secrete antibodies. Antibodies are large proteins ten times smaller than a virus particle. They bind with any antigen identical to the one that activated the B-lymphocyte. An activated B-lymphocyte can produce 2000 antibodies per second for up to five days. These antibodies enter the lymphatic and circulatory systems where they attach to the surface of the abnormal cell or invading microbe. This either inactivates the target, causes it to clump with similar cells and be destroyed, or flags the target for destruction by another type of immune system cell. Producing enough antibodies to combat disease takes 10 to 17 days to reach maximal effectiveness, and during that time the individual will show symptoms of the illness.

Not all B-lymphocytes become plasma cells. A few B-lymphocytes, under stimulation by chemicals secreted by helper T-lymphocytes, become memory B-lymphocytes, or memory B-cells. These cells remain in the body for a long time (years to decades). If the same microbe is encountered again, memory B-lymphocytes can ramp up antibody production in2 to 5 days, destroying the invading microbe before it can make a person sick. This is the basis for long-term immunity to disease. Vaccines work by introducing a weakened or partial form of a microbe that does not make the individual sick but stimulates production plasma cells and memory B-lymphocytes.

Another subset of B-lymphocytes called tumor-infiltrating B-lymphocytes (TIL-Bs) appears to migrate to solid cancer tumors and secrete tumor-specific antibodies. Tumor-infiltrating T-lymphocytes (TIL-Ts) are also found in solid tumors, and more is known about how they work. TILs have been associated with substantial remission in metastatic melanoma. Experimentally, the presence of TILs also correlates with improved outcomes in ovarian, breast, colorectal and non-small cell lung cancers.

Why, if the immune system is so effective in preventing illness, does it not wipe out cancer cells and keep the individual cancer-free? One reason is that cancer cells start out as normal body cells. At some point, they are transformed because certain genes are inappropriately turned off or on, or are mutated. When this happens, the transformed cell still has many of the surface marker molecules that originally identified it as a self-cell. B-lymphocytes that have receptors that would interact with healthy self-cell antigens are killed before they leave the bone marrow in order to prevent autoimmune diseases. In many cases, transformed cancer cells still look enough like self-cells that B-lymphocytes do not recognize them as abnormal and do not mark them for destruction. If B-lymphocytes do respond to a transformed cell, the response may not be strong enough to be effective since the growth of cancer cells is not limited the way it is in healthy cells. In addition, some cancer cells make chemicals that inactivate or disrupt the functioning of immune system cells.

Treatment: The properties of the adaptive immune system can be manipulated in ways to prevent and treat cancer by using vaccines and monoclonal antibodies. Some cancers are primarily caused by viruses. By making a vaccine against the causative virus, it will be rapidly destroyed and the cancer can be prevented. As of 2015, 2 cancer prevention vaccines have been approved.

Many strains of human papillomavirus (HPV) are known to cause cervical, vulvar, anal, penile, and mouth cancers. The virus is transmitted through sexual activity. Vaccination before puberty against the most common strains of HPV stimulates the adaptive immune system and creates memory B-lymphocytes that provide long-term immunity. As of 2015, 3 HPV vaccines have been approved by the US Food and Drug Administration (FDA). Their use has and has substantially reduced the rate of HPV-caused cancers.

Hepatitis B is a viral infection that can cause liver cancer. Current recommendations in the United States call for children to receive a hepatitis B vaccine at birth. Research is underway to develop vaccines against other microbe-triggered cancers, including various lymphomas (Epstein Barr virus) and stomach cancer (*Helicobacter pylori* bacterium).

Research is also underway to design treatment vaccines to use in individuals with active cancers. As of 2015, only one treatment vaccine has been approved by the FDA. This vaccine, sipuleucel-T, can extend the life of men with metastatic prostate cancer, but does not cure the disease.

Another B-lymphocyte-related treatment is the use of targeted monoclonal antibodies (mAbs). Scientists first isolate B-lymphocytes from laboratory mice that were vaccinated with a specific antigen and fuse them to cancer cells (myelomas). The resultant hybrid cells or "hybridomas" can successfully grow in culture, but also produce a specific type of antibody. After the hybridoma lines are screened to identify which cells produce the antibody of interest, which is a very labor-intensive process, those lines that make the desired antibody are grown in culture. Then the genes that encode the desired antibodies are transferred to a cell line that grows well in culture (eg, Chinese Hamster Ovary cells) to make small antibody-producing factories. These antibodies are then purified and injected into the body where they attack or mark cancer cells. The effect is short-lived, since no memory B cells are created.

More than a dozen monoclonal antibody biologics have been approved by the FDA to be used in conjunction with other cancer treatments. The mAb drugs can be recognized because their generic name ends in "mab" (eg, alemtuzumab, trastuzumab). Some mAbs, called conjugated mAbs, have a chemotherapy drug or radioactive isotope attached to the antibody to increase its effectiveness (eg, brentuximab vedotin, ibritumomab tiuxetan). Although mAbs have side effects, these are less harsh than those of chemotherapy drugs.

Tish Davidson, AM

For Further Information

Finn, O. J. (2012). Immuno-oncology: Understanding the function and dysfunction of the immune system in cancer. *Annals of Oncology* 23(suppl 8): iiv6-iiv9. http://annonc.oxfordjournals.org/content/23/suppl_8/viii6.full

Melero, I., Gaudemack, G., Gerritsen, W., Huber, C., Parmiani, G., Scholl, S., … Mellstedt, H. (2014). Therapeutic vaccines for cancer: An overview of clinical trials. *Nature Reviews Clinical Oncology* 11: 509–524.

Scott, Andrew M., Wolchok, Jedd D., & Old, Lloyd J. (2012). Antibody therapy of cancer. *Nature Reviews Cancer* 12: 278-287. http://www.nature.com/nrc/journal/v12/n4/full/nrc3236.html

Other Resources

American Cancer Society

What's New in Cancer Immunotherapy Research?
http://www.cancer.org/treatment/treatmentsandsideeffects/treatmenttypes/immunotherapy/immunotherapy-whats-new-immuno-res

National Cancer Institute

Immunotherapy: Using the Immune System to Treat Cancer.
http://www.cancer.gov/research/areas/treatment/immunotherapy-using-immune-system

Clinical Trials – For information on experimental cancer treatment vaccines can be found at
http://www.clinicaltrials.gov

MimAbs –For information on making monoclonal antibodies
http://www.mimabs.org/en/science-technologies/monoclonal-antibodies/

See also: T-lymphocytes; Chemotherapy

▶ *BRAF* gene

Category: Cancer Biology
Also known as: *BRAF1*, *RAFB1*, v-raf murine sarcoma viral oncogene homolog B1

Definition: *BRAF* is an internal part of a cellular signaling pathway. This signaling pathway results in cell growth when the correct chemical message is sent. The mutated form of the *BRAF* gene has a single base (letter) of deoxyribonucleic acid (DNA) changed; this changes the activity of the *BRAF* protein. This mutant *BRAF* protein is broken and is continuously on, sending growth signals even when there are no chemical messages and causing runaway growth of cells. The result is like a broken light switch that will not turn off.

Etiology and symptoms of associated cancers: The BRAF protein is central to causing many types of cancer, including melanoma, colon cancer, ovarian cancer, thyroid cancer, and gliomas. Knowledge of the *BRAF* gene, which was first described as a proto-oncogene in 2002, is useful in diagnosing cancer and deciding what type of treatment to use. The advanced state of knowledge in modern biology and medicine makes it likely that drugs that attack cancers with *BRAF* mutations will be quickly developed.

Tumors are called benign (not harmful) or malignant (harmful). Benign tumors can acquire mutations that change them into malignant cancers. Experts believe that cancer requires multiple steps to form. Many normal functions of cells need to be damaged to create a malignant cancer. Cellular functions typically damaged are cell growth (unregulated cell growth), telomere maintenance (cell aging), apoptosis (cell death), angiogenesis (the ability to grow blood vessels), and metastasis (the ability of cells to detach from one part of the body and migrate to another).

BRAF mutations primarily affect the first of these functions, cell growth. When *BRAF* is mutated in a cell, the cell receives a continuous signal to grow and divide. This signal from *BRAF* also has a smaller effect of reducing the probability of cells dying by apoptosis, an effect promoting metastasis, and effects promoting angiogenesis. *BRAF* mutations are often found in benign growths.

Mutations of other genes are needed to destroy the remaining cell functions and make a growth malignant. For example, the destruction of the *TP53* gene (also known as *p53*) will help the cancer overcome cell aging (which normally slows down the overgrowing cells) and apoptosis (which normally kills off some of the overgrowing cells). For comparison, *TP53* mutations are rarely found in benign growths and are almost always found as secondary changes in cancers.

Because *BRAF* mutations are found in benign and malignant growths, many people believe *BRAF* is an early change that eventually leads to malignant cancers. Cancers that seem to begin with *BRAF* mutations also seem to end up being among the most malignant. Even though *BRAF* is associated with the worst types of malignancies, the silver lining is that since *BRAF* mutations happen early, while the tumors are still benign, the *BRAF* mutation can serve as an early warning.

BRAF mutation is not found in all cancer but only in cancers of certain tissues. Most of these tissues are what doctors call adenoid tissues. Specifically, *BRAF* mutation has been found in melanoma (skin), glioma (nerve), thyroid, ovarian, and colon cancer.

Researchers have shown that 80 percent of the benign nevi (moles) studied carried the *BRAF* mutation and that 66 percent of malignant melanomas studied carried the *BRAF* mutation. In benign gliomas, *BRAF* mutation is rarely observed, but in malignant gliomas, the *BRAF* mutation was almost always observed.

Testing and treatment: Standard tests of DNA can be done on blood or tumor tissue samples to detect the *BRAF* mutation. While these tests are very reliable, the knowledge of the *BRAF* gene mutation and the tests for it are new and are not yet widely available. *BRAF* mutation tests will help doctors determine the exact type of cancer, how dangerous it is, and what types of treatment to use.

One drug in testing is BAY 43-9006. This drug seems to reverse the effect of *BRAF* mutation and stop the growth of cells. It also seems to kill the cancer cells by restoring normal cell death (apoptosis). Although only laboratory experiments have been done, some researchers expect that actual tests in people with cancers will show that the drug will not only stop the growth of the cancers but may kill the cancers entirely.

History: The discovery of the *BRAF* mutation is a direct result of the Human Genome Project. In the 1990's the Human Genome Project sequenced the human genome and described the complete set of about 30,000 human genes, the instructions for the body. In the 2000's the Cancer Genome Project started examining all 30,000 genes in cancers to find broken genes. One result was the discovery of the *BRAF* gene mutation in 2002.

Christopher Pung, B.S., C.L.Sp. (CG)

For Further Information

Begley, Sharon. "Science Journal: Nature's Quirks Limit DNA-Based Drug Possibilities." *Pittsburg Post-Gazette*, November 11, 2005.

Davies, H., et al. "Mutations of the *BRAF* Gene in Human Cancer." *Nature* 417 (2002): 949-954. Shaw, Gina. "BRAF Mutations Predict Tumor Response." *Drug Discovery and Development* 8 (2005): 8.

Other Resources

Atlas of Genetics and Cytogenetics in Oncology and Haematology

BRAF

http://atlasgeneticsoncology.org/Genes/ BRAFID828.html

The Human Genome

Melanoma and the *BRAF* Gene

http://genome.wellcome.ac.uk/doc_WTD020812.html

See also: Genetics of cancer

▶ *BRCA1* and *BRCA2* genes

Category: Cancer Biology

Also known as: Breast cancer susceptibility genes; breast cancer 1, breast cancer 2, early onset

Definition: BRCA stands for *br*east *ca*ncer susceptibility. *BRCA1*, the first breast cancer susceptibility gene, was identified and cloned in 1994. A second breast cancer susceptibility gene, *BRCA2*, was discovered soon after. Identification of *BRCA1* and *BRCA2* as breast cancer susceptibility genes has had a profound impact on understanding the disease. The immediate clinical use of their discovery for both diagnosis and accurate assessment of increased risk through screening has been one of the foremost success stories in the fight against cancer.

Familial disease: Less than 5 percent of breast cancers are hereditary, but more than 90 percent of hereditary breast cancers are caused by mutations in either *BRCA1* or *BRCA2*. Each year approximately 200,000 women in the United States are diagnosed with breast cancer, and about 5 to 10 percent of these women have an inherited mutant *BRCA1* or *BRCA2* gene. The mutations can be inherited from either the maternal or the paternal side of the family.

Mutations in *BRCA1* and *BRCA2* increase a woman's lifetime risk of not only breast cancer but also ovarian, colon, and Fallopian tube cancers. Women with an inherited alteration in one of these genes have an increased risk of developing these cancers before the menopause. Altered *BRCA2* poses a greater risk in men than altered *BRCA1*. Men with altered *BRCA2* are at a higher risk of breast cancer and prostate cancer. Alterations in the *BRCA2* gene have also been associated with increased risks of lymphoma, melanoma, and cancers of the pancreas, gallbladder, bile duct, and stomach in both men and women.

Risks and incidence: Estimates of lifetime risks suggest that approximately 12.9 percent of women in the general population will develop breast cancer, as compared with estimates of 78 percent of women with an altered *BRCA1* or *BRCA2* gene. The ovarian cancer risk is 49.4 percent in carriers versus 1.7 percent in the general population.

Among men, the breast cancer risk is 5.8 percent for carriers versus 0.01 percent in the general population. In carriers, risks for colon, pancreatic, and stomach cancers are also elevated twofold, threefold, and fourfold, respectively, with no increase in prostate cancer risk. Additionally, in *BRCA1* mutation carriers, the lifetime risk of developing cancer of the breast can be as high as 85 percent and that of developing ovarian cancer as much as 42 to 63 percent. In *BRCA2* carriers, the lifetime risk of developing breast cancer is as high as 86 percent and that of developing ovarian cancer about 27 percent.

The likelihood that breast or ovarian cancer is linked with *BRCA1* or *BRCA2* mutations is highest in families with a history of multiple cases of breast and ovarian cancer, particularly involving a mother, sister, or daughter; diagnosis of breast cancer before the age of thirty-five; presence of male breast cancer in the family; two or more primary cancers such as breast and ovarian cancers or bilateral breast cancer (separate cancers in each breast) in an individual; other multiple cancers in the family, especially prostate cancer; and an Ashkenazi (central and eastern European Jewish) background. It is important to note that not every woman with this sort of background will carry a defective *BRCA1* or *BRCA2*, and not every cancer that occurs in such families will be due to a *BRCA1* or *BRCA2* defect. Additionally not all women who carry a *BRCA1* or *BRCA2* mutation will develop breast or ovarian cancer.

Mutations in *BRCA1* account for breast or ovarian cancers in 45 percent of families with a history of breast cancer and up to 90 percent in families with a history of both breast and ovarian cancers. *BRCA2* mutations account for breast cancer in about 35 percent of families with a history of breast cancer. Studies suggest that women who develop breast cancer before the age of fifty have a one in four chance of carrying a *BRCA1* or *BRCA2* mutation if they have any relative who also develops the disease before the age of fifty. There is a 50 percent chance that mutant carriers will transmit the mutated gene to their offspring.

BRCA1-related breast cancer appears to be more aggressive than other types of breast cancer and has a poorer prognosis, and most *BRCA1*-related ovarian cancers are of the invasive type. Some characteristics of hereditary breast cancer, such as how it occurs at an earlier age, more often affects both breasts, and is associated with other cancers, make it clinically distinct from sporadic cancer.

BRCA1 and *BRCA2* were identified by linkage analysis of families with multiple cases of early-onset breast and ovarian cancer. *BRCA1* is 5,592 kilobases long with 24 exons, and *BRCA2* is twice as long with 10,254 kilobases and 27 exons. More than one hundred different alterations scattered throughout *BRCA1* and *BRCA2* have been identified. These alterations tend to be distinct, and in general, most families have a unique alteration. Mutations anywhere along either gene are associated with an increased risk of breast cancer. Some evidence suggests that mutations in the 5′ end of *BRCA1* and mutations in exon 11 of *BRCA2* might be associated with ovarian cancer. Alterations in certain regions of the *BRCA2* gene are known to predispose individuals to a greater risk of ovarian cancer in women and prostrate cancer in men, as compared with alterations in other parts of the gene. This suggests differences in patterns of cancer between individuals with a *BRCA1* mutation versus a *BRCA2* mutation.

Of the more than one hundred alterations identified in each gene (*BRCA1* and *BRCA2*), three alterations have been identified in Ashkenazi Jewish families with a history of breast cancer. These alterations are 185delAG and 5382insC (*BRCA1*) and 6174delT (*BRCA2*). The estimated frequencies of the three alterations in the general Ashkenazi population are 1.0 percent, 0.1 percent, and 1.4 percent, respectively.

Cellular function: *BRCA1* and *BRCA2* are tumor-suppressor genes, and the BRCA proteins are involved in a multitude of key cellular processes. Research has demonstrated the involvement of BRCA1 and BRCA2 proteins in complexes that activate repair of double-strand breaks and initiate homologous recombination, suggesting a key role of BRCA proteins in maintaining genome stability and integrity. In response to deoxyribonucleic acid (DNA) damage, BRCA1 is engaged in the transcriptional regulation of several genes such as *P21* (*CDKN1A*) and *GADD45*, which activate cell-cycle check-point induced replication arrest to allow for repair. It is unclear why a defect in *BRCA* predisposes predominantly to cancer of the breast and ovary, even though the known functions of BRCA proteins are essential to all cell types.

Whether estrogen, a known promoter of sporadic breast cancer, affects the risk of *BRCA1*-and *BRCA2*-related breast cancers is not clear. Given that factors that contribute to enhanced exposure to estrogen, such as early onset of menarche and late menopause, correlate with a higher incidence of breast cancer and that premenopausal oophorectomy (the surgical removal of the ovaries) exerts a preventive effect, an association is suggested between *BRCA1* and *BRCA2* and estrogen receptor alpha (ERα).

Prevention: The best opportunity to reduce mortality is through early detection. Preventive mastectomy and preventive oophorectomy to reduce the risk of breast cancer and ovarian cancer respectively are possible options. Although oophorectomies are usually performed to reduce ovarian cancer risk, having an oophorectomy before menoBRCA1 *and* BRCA2 genes pause also reduces the risk of breast cancer. Removal of ovaries is associated with a decrease in the production of the hormones estrogen and progesterone, which play a major role in breast cancer progression.

For a premenopausal woman with a *BRCA* mutation, oophorectomy reduces the risk of breast cancer by about 50 percent, and it reduces the risk of ovarian cancer by 80 percent, irrespective of the menopausal status. However, it is important to note that prophylactic surgery reduces but does not eliminate the risk of cancer and carries additional risks related to surgery. Behaviors that can reduce breast cancer risk include regular exercising, decreased alcohol consumption, early childbirth, and breast-feeding for more than twelve months—although effects of these on *BRCA* mutation carriers are yet unknown.

Even though tamoxifen is known to reduce the risk of invasive breast cancer by 49 percent in patients with an increased risk of developing the disease, limited data are available regarding the use of tamoxifen for chemoprevention in women with *BRCA1* and *BRCA2* alterations. Existing data suggest that use of tamoxifen reduces the risk of breast cancer in *BRCA* carriers and is recommended for chemoprevention.

Banalata Sen, Ph.D.

For Further Information

Bishop, D. T. "*BRCA1* and *BRCA2* and Breast Cancer Incidence: A Review." *Annals of Oncology* 10, suppl. 6 (1999): S113-S119.

Venkitaraman, A. R. "Cancer Susceptibility and the Functions of *BRCA1* and *BRCA2*: A Review." *Cell* 108, no. 2 (2002): 171-182.

Other Resources

Genetics Home Reference
http://ghr.nlm.nih.gov

HUGO Gene Nomenclature Committee
Symbol Report: BRCA1
http://www.genenames.org/data/hgnc_data.php?hgnc_id=1100

National Cancer Institute
Genetics of Breast and Ovarian Cancer
http://www.cancer.gov/cancertopics/pdq/genetics/breast and-ovarian

National Human Genome Research Institute
http://www.genome.gov

See also: Ashkenazi Jews and cancer; Breast cancer in men; Breast cancer in pregnant women; Breast cancers; Carcinomatosis; Clinical Breast Exam (CBE); Ductal Carcinoma In Situ (DCIS); Estrogen-receptor-sensitive breast cancer; Family history and risk assessment; Genetic testing; Genetics of cancer; Hereditary cancer syndromes; Hormonal therapies; Invasive ductal carcinomas; Invasive lobular carcinomas; Lobular Carcinoma In Situ (LCIS); Medullary carcinoma of the breast; Molecular oncology; Mutagenesis and cancer; Oophorectomy; Ovarian cancers; Ovarian epithelial cancer; Pancreatic cancers; Risks for cancer; Salpingectomy and salpingo-oophorectomy; Tumor markers

▶ Cancer biology

Category: Cancer Biology

Definition: The transformation of a normal cell into a cancerous one is a complicated process consisting of multiple steps and many changes to the cell and its normal control mechanisms. The fact that most human cancers develop later in life reflects the time required for these changes to occur. These changes include the activation of oncogenes, the inactivation of tumor-suppressor genes, and acquisition of cellular immortality, the ability to invade new tissues at distant locations, and induce the formation of new blood vessels.

Characteristics of human cancers: Mutations that are present in the germ cells (egg and sperm) can be passed to the next generation. Somatic mutations occur in the remaining body cells and may affect the cell or tissue in which they occur, but they will not be passed to the next generation. Both germ-line and somatic mutations can cause cancer; it is estimated that approximately 10 percent of cancers are caused by germ-line, or inherited, mutations.

Tumors can be either benign (those that remain localized and noninvasive), malignant (those that invade the basement membrane and underlying tissue), or metastatic (those that shed cells that seed tumors in other locations of the body). Progressive degrees of abnormality are observed in benign, malignant, and metastatic tumors, suggesting that cancer develops in a stepwise process.

Cancers can arise in almost all tissue types in the body, although approximately 80 percent of human cancers arise from epithelial cells. Epithelial cells cover internal and external surfaces of the body, including the linings of internal organs and glands.

The incidence of many types of cancer varies worldwide, and epidemiologic studies show that environment is the largest factor in variations in cancer incidence from country to country. Indeed, a number of environment and lifestyle elements, tobacco smoking being the most obvious, are known to be strongly correlated with the incidence of certain types of cancer. In 1975, it was shown that many chemicals that are capable of causing mutations in deoxyribonucleic acid (DNA) also cause cancer in laboratory animals. Later research showed, however, that not all chemicals that cause cancer also cause mutations. Therefore, other mechanisms besides DNA mutation must be involved in at least some cancers.

Gene expression and signaling pathways: For the cells of an organism's various tissues (e.g., lung and bone) to display complex, tissue-specific characteristics, large groups of genes must be coordinately expressed while other genes must be repressed. Specialized proteins known as transcription factors are responsible for achieving this coordinated expression. Transcription factors bind to specific DNA sequences in the control region of each gene. The transcription of most genes is controlled by the binding of several distinct transcription factors in the gene's control region. A single transcription factor can affect the expression of multiple genes that contain its binding sequence in their control regions. In cancer cells, a defective transcription factor may affect the expression of multiple genes, the end result of which is to create a cancer cell from a normal cell. For example, the MYC oncogene encodes a transcription factor that directs the expression of a host of genes that drive cell proliferation. Inappropriately high levels of the MYC protein play integral roles in cancers of the prostate, breast, gastrointestinal tract, lungs, brain, blood cells, and skin.

Cancer-specific aberrations in gene expression may arise without alterations in transcription factors. Some proteins influence genes expression without directly binding to DNA. Inside cells, DNA is packaged into a compact structure called "chromatin." A group of proteins regulates the assembly and disassembly of chromatin. Such proteins include histone acetylases, decacetylases, methylases, demethylases, and chromatin remodeling proteins. Epigenetics (the prefix "epi" is of Greek origin and means "upon," "near," "over," "before," or "after") refers to factors that regulate or affect DNA transcription but are not a part of the DNA sequence (genome). Instead, epigenetic factors chemically modify the nucleotides that comprise various genes or the histone proteins that package that DNA into chromatin. For example, cancer cells display profound alterations in their DNA methylation patterns. Likewise, histone methylation influences gene expression, and changes in histone methylation may decrease the expression of cancer regulatory genes and tumor suppressor genes and have a significant role in the onset of cellular cancerous states. As an example, the histone methylase EZH2 is part of a larger complex known as the "Polycomb Repressive Complex 2" (PRC2). Aberrant regulation of PRC2 promotes cancer progression and EZH2 is overexpressed in a wide variety of aggressive cancers.

Normal cells within tissues and within an organism communicate with each other in a regulated fashion through a multitude of chemical signals and pathways. Disruption of these normal signaling pathways is an important component of the formation of cancer. In normal cells, signals are transmitted through the various pathways in a number of ways: by a change in the level of activity of signaling molecules by noncovalent modifications, changes in the concentration of a signaling molecule inside a cell, or the direction of signaling molecules to particular locations within the cell.

Oncogenes: Normal cells contain a class of genes involved in the regulation of growth and division called proto-oncogenes. A proto-oncogene can mutate into a version that is permanently activated and causes uncontrolled cell division, one of the hallmarks of a cancer cell. The transformation of a proto-oncogene into an oncogene may involve a change to the structure of the protein itself or an increase in its expression. A change involving the structure of the protein itself may require only very small changes; in some cases a single base pair mutation is sufficient. A change involving an increase in expression often occurs through increasing the number of copies of the gene in the DNA. There are several ways that amplification of a gene can occur: by enhanced replication of a chromosome segment that carries its DNA or by the breaking away of such a chromosome segment to form a small chromosome-like particle that is capable of replicating independently.

Scientists have identified more than one hundred oncogenes. They include growth factors, proteins that signal a cell to divide; growth factor receptors, proteins on the cell surface to which growth factors bind; signal transducers, proteins that make up the signaling pathways between the growth factor receptor and the cell nucleus; and transcription factors.

Tumor-suppressor genes: The class of tumor-suppressor genes includes a large number of genes whose protein products are involved in a multitude of normal cellular functions that in some way regulate a cell's division and reduce the chance that the cell will become cancerous. Tumor-suppressor genes in cancer cells are often inactivated through mutation or other mechanisms. An inherited increased risk of developing a specific type of cancer in some families is often the result of the presence of a defective tumor-suppressor gene. It is the loss of function of tumor-suppressor genes that can lead to cancer, in contrast to oncogenes, which have gained functions or lost the ability to be controlled in their mutant form.

The protein product of a particularly important tumor-suppressor gene, called TP53, causes cessation of cell division and even programmed cell death (apoptosis) in normal cells if the process of cell division malfunctions. In this way, the cell's well-being is monitored, protecting the organism from the effects of runaway division of wayward cells by activating the apoptotic pathway in such cells. Apoptosis is an orderly process in which the DNA of a cell is degraded and the cell itself fragmented into smaller pieces that are taken up by nearby white blood cells whose job is to clean up such debris. Loss of the ability to undergo apoptosis allows cancer cells to survive a variety of environmental stresses and signaling imbalances. The TP53 gene in the DNA of cancer cells often carries mutations that cause it to malfunction; more than 90 percent of small-cell lung cancers and more than 50 percent of breast and colon cancers have been shown to be associated with mutant forms of TP53.

Normal cells throughout the body grow and divide to generate two daughter cells in a highly organized and controlled series of events called the cell cycle. A subclass of tumor-suppressor genes controls cell-cycle events in normal cells. Control mechanisms at various steps of the cell cycle function to ensure that a preceding step is completed before the next step can begin. These control mechanisms are inactivated in many types of cancer cells, allowing them to divide in an unregulated fashion. A particularly important tumor-suppressor gene in this class is the retinoblastoma (RB1) gene. The protein encoded by the RB1 gene, pRb, is affected in most if not all types of human cancer cells. Loss of normal regulation of the signaling pathway of which pRb is a component leads to unrestrained cell proliferation.

Cell immortalization: The ability of a cell to divide indefinitely (cell immortalization) is a characteristic of all cancer cells. This ability is related to the structures of the ends of chromosomes, called telomeres, which are composed of several thousand repeats of a six-base-pair sequence element (TTAGGG). Every time a cell replicates its DNA, the telomeres are shortened by 50 to 100 base pairs. Consequently, cells can only divide a limited number of times before the very act of dividing deletes vital genetic material from the ends of their chromosomes. However, the ability to indefinitely maintain telomere length has been observed in virtually all types of cancer cells. The majority of these cells accomplish this by increasing the expression of the enzyme telomerase, which synthesizes telomeres, and gradually disappears from normal human cells as they age.

Angiogenesis: All cells depend on the availability of oxygen and nutrients for their growth and survival. Virtually all cells in a tissue must be located close to a capillary blood vessel that can deliver nutrients and take away metabolic waste products. For a cancer cell to progress to a macroscopic tumor, it must acquire the ability to induce the formation of new blood vessels, a process called angiogenesis. In normal cells, various negative and positive signaling pathways control the angiogenic process. Cancer cells appear to induce angiogenesis in a number of steps that change the balance of angiogenesis inducers and inhibitors during tumor development.

Metastasis: Most types of human cancer will at some point undergo metastasis, the process whereby new tumors are seeded at distant sites from the primary tumor. Metastases are responsible for approximately 90 percent of all cancer deaths. Metastasis involves tumor cells leaving the primary tumor, invading adjacent tissues, and from there traveling to sites where they are able to settle and start the growth of new tumors. The primary route of metastasis is through the circulatory system, although metastatic cancer cells may also spread through lymph ducts to lymph nodes. Sometimes, cancer cells traveling through the circulation form small obstructions that lodge in the arterioles and capillaries of various tissues. Complex interactions between the metastasizing cell and the microenvironment of the host tissue in which it lands govern the process of invasion into the tissue and colonization to form a metastasis in a process that is not well understood.

Cancer cells that metastasize do not appear to have undergone major changes in their DNA compared with other cells in the original tumor. However, cancer cells that possess metastatic potential have alterations in several classes of proteins involved in the attachment of cells to their surroundings in a tissue, which render them less able to form such attachments. Cancer cells with metastatic potential may also have an increased ability to degrade proteins in their immediate environment. Metastasizing cells from various types of cancers tend to spread preferentially to some organs; for instance, prostate and breast cancers have a strong tendency to metastasize to the bone marrow, and colon cancer has a strong tendency to metastasize to the liver. The reason for this phenomenon is not well understood.

Genomic instability: It has been estimated that multiple genetic changes, perhaps five to seven, are needed for the development of a full-fledged human cancer. A normal cell has numerous control and repair mechanisms that ensure the fidelity of DNA replication and, therefore, that the occurrence of mutations is rare. Malfunctioning of components of these control and repair mechanisms, such as TP53, leads to the observed chromosomal instability and variability of cancer cells. Genetic instability is pervasive in human cancer cells, which commonly exhibit various types of aberrantly structured chromosomes: the loss of entire chromosomes, the presence of extra copies of chromosomes, or the fusion of part of one chromosome with part of another. These chromosomal abnormalities disrupt normal DNA sequence and arrangement and probably help explain how precancerous cells acquire the necessary mutations to render them cancerous.

Jill Ferguson, Ph.D.
Updated by: Richard P. Capriccioso, M.D.

For Further Information

Hanahan, D., & Weinberg, R. A. (2011). Hallmarks of cancer: The next generation. *Cell*, 144(5), 646–674.

Gerald, K., Iwasa, J., & Marshall, W. (2015). *Karp's cell and molecular biology* (8th ed.). New York City, NY: John Wiley.

Weinberg, Robert A. (2013). *The biology of cancer* (2nd ed.). New York City, NY: Garland Science.

Other Resources

Emory University
CancerQuest: Important Tumor Suppressors.
http://www.cancerquest.org/index.cfm?page=52

Inside Cancer
http://www.insidecancer.org

National Cancer Institute
Cancer Topics.
http://www.cancer.gov/cancertopics

See also: Angiogenesis; BRAF gene; BRCA1 and BRCA2 genes; Carcinogens, known; Carcinogens, reasonably anticipated; Cyclin-dependent kinase inhibitor-2A (CDKN2A); Cytokines; Epidemiology of cancer; Estrogen Receptor Downregulator (ERD); Genetics of cancer; Human Chorionic Gonadotropin (HCG); Immune response to cancer; Mitochondrial DNA mutations; MLH1 gene; MSH genes; Mutagenesis and cancer; MYC oncogene; Oncogenes; Placental alkaline phosphatase (PALP); PMS genes; Proteomics and cancer research; RB1 gene; RhoGD12 gene; SCLC1 gene; TP53 protein; Tumor necrosis factor (TNF); Tumor-suppressor genes

▶ Cancer epigenetics

Category: Cancer Biology

Definition: Cancer is a disease characterized by uncontrolled cell growth and proliferation. Normal cell growth and division processes are tightly regulated to ensure error-free DNA replication and repair. Cells with DNA errors that cannot be repaired undergo programmed cell death. Disruption of these normal cellular growth and repair processes leads to cancer.

The notion that genetic changes occur only through alterations in the DNA sequence no longer holds true. Scientists have discovered a second mechanism—epigenetic changes—through which genetic changes can occur without alterations to the DNA sequence. The term "epigenetics" was originally coined by Conrad Waddington in 1940 to describe changes in cellular phenotype without associated changes in cellular genotype. In simpler terms, epigenetics literally means "above the genome," and is characterized by modifications of DNA and chromatin structure that affect gene expression, and ultimately the functioning of normal cellular processes.

Cancer, traditionally seen as a genetic disease, is now recognized to involve both genetic and epigenetic alterations.

Epigenetics: Some epigenetic changes are part of normal development and aging, but external factors like environmental exposures to chemicals/drugs and diet have now been identified to also play a role in causing epigenetic changes.

During cell division, DNA becomes highly organized into tightly condensed chromatin structures, the smallest unit of this structure is the nucleosome which is made up of distinct histone proteins around which the DNA is wrapped. The compaction of the chromatin structure greatly influences the ability of genes to be activated or silenced. Epigenetic mechanisms alter transcriptional regulation of the tightly-packaged chromatin by modifications of the DNA and modification or rearrangement of nucleosomes.

Basic epigenetic mechanisms include DNA methylation, histone modifications, nucleosome remodeling and RNA mediated targeting. Methylation of DNA and modification of histone proteins by acetylation have the ability to alter basic DNA-based processes, including transcription, repair, and replication. Dysregulation of these basic cellular processes can lead to aberrant cell growth, a hallmark of cancer.

DNA methylation—the most studied epigenetic mechanism—involves the attachment of a methyl ($-CH_3$) group to specific cytosine nucleotides in DNA to create 5-methylcytosines (5-mC). Specific types of proteins can bind 5-mC, including members of the MBD, Kaiso, and Kaiso-like protein families, which affect genome stability and normal patterns of gene expression. CpG islands, 1000-kb stretches of DNA with greater than 50% GC content and which occupy 60% of human gene promoters of constitutively expressed genes. Methylation of CpG sites within these promoters typically causes gene silencing, and hypomethylation of these same sites usually leads to gene overexpression.

Chromatin packaging, essential for DNA replication, is controlled by modifications of the histone proteins. Specific arginine and lysine residues in the front ends of histone proteins can be methylated, which results in

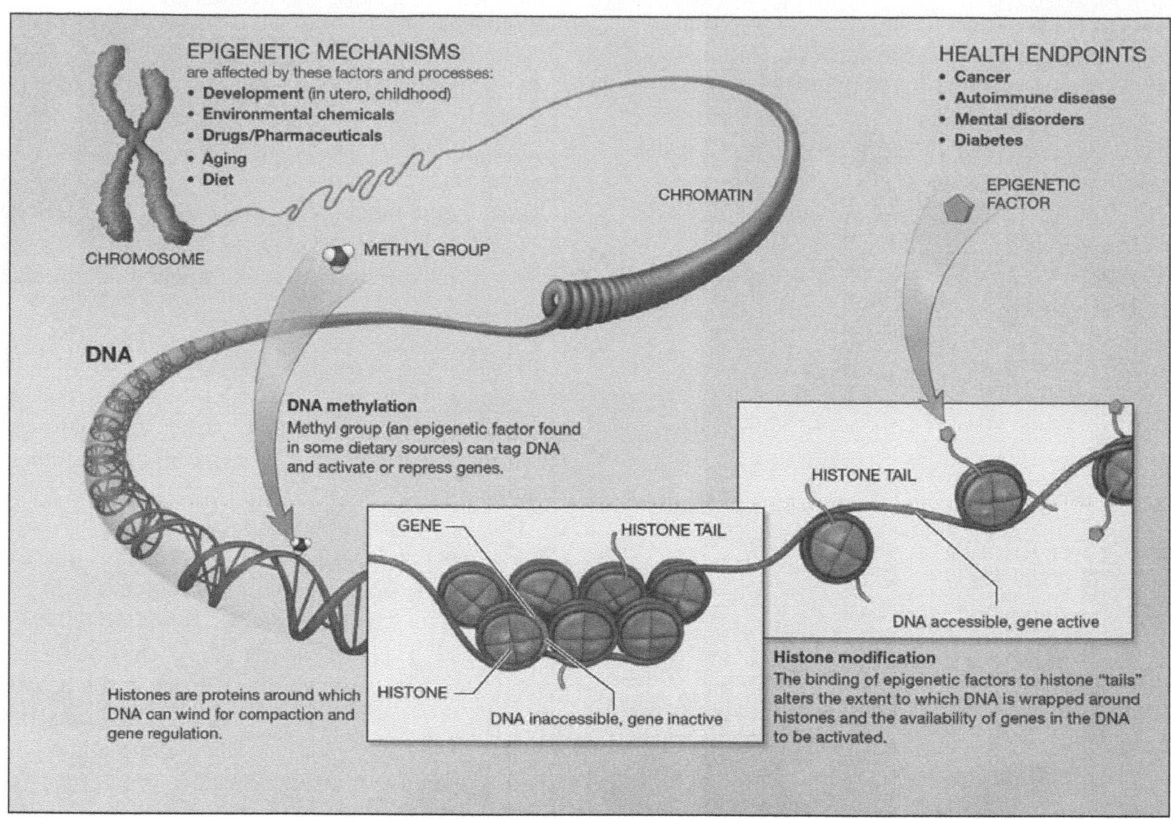

An illustration of epigenetic mechanism (Source: National Institutes of Health)

either transcriptional activation or repression downstream. Along with methylation, lysine residues on histones can also undergo acetylation which usually enhances transcription. Such epigenetic modifications of histone proteins affect their interaction with the DNA as well as with adjacent histone proteins in the chromatin structure.

Epigenetic Pathways in Cancer: A hallmark of cancer is the deregulation of gene expression and disruption of molecular networks. Changes in DNA methylation and histone modification patterns, and abnormal expression or genomic changes in those genes that encode proteins like DNA methyltransferases (DMT), methyl-CpG-binding domain (MBD) proteins, histone acetyltransferases (HATs), histone deacetylases (HDAC), histone methyltransferases (HMT) and histone demethylases (HDM) (also known as "epigenetic genes"), can cause widespread deregulation of gene expression profiles and the disruption of those signaling networks that control proliferation and cellular functions.

DNA methylation was the first epigenetic alteration identified in cancer cells and has been shown to occur very early in cancer development, which suggests that it may play a key role in cancer initiation. A cancer epigenome is marked by genome-wide hypomethylation and site-specific CpG island hypermethylation. DNA hypomethylation is known to increase genomic instability and activate proto-oncogenes, whereas site-specific hypermethylation contributes to tumorigenesis by silencing genes and transcription factors involved in DNA repair, cell cycle, cell adhesion, apoptosis, and angiogenesis. Silencing of tumor suppressor genes can lead to tumor initiation, whereas silencing of DNA repair genes leads to accumulation of genetic lesions leading to rapid progression of cancer.

Histone modification, another well-studied epigenetic mechanism, leads to gene repression during tumorigenesis. Histone modifications can occur through both acetylation and methylation pathways. HDAC-mediated histone modification results in the loss of acetylated H4-lysines. HDACs are overexpressed in various types of cancer. They work together with HATs to maintain global histone acetylation levels, which are also altered in cancer. Chromosomal translocations that involve HAT or HAT-related genes are also responsible for the altered histone acetylation patterns found in cancer. Alterations in methylation

Examples of gene and protein targets of epigenetic modifications identified in various cancers

Epigenetic Mechanism	*Genes and Proteins*	*Type of Cancer*
DNA Hypomethylation	*R-Ras, MAPSIN*	Gastric
	S-100	Colon
	MAGE	Melanoma
	IGF2	Wilm's tumor
DNA Hypermethylation	*Rb* promoter	Retinoblastoma
	BRCA1	Breast
	p16	Colorectal and SC Lung
	MLHI	Endometrial
	RUNX3	Esophageal
	GATA-4 and *GATA-5*	Colorectal and Gastric
Histone Modification	EZH2	Breast and Prostate
	G9a	Liver
	MLL2	Follicular lymphoma
	LSD1	Prostate cancer, breast cancer, neuroblastoma and bladder cancer
	FBXL10	Hematopoietic cancer

patterns of H3-lysines mediated by HMTs are also known to be associated with aberrant silencing of tumor suppressor genes in various forms of cancer. A precise balance of DNA methylation is critical for normal cell growth. There is evidence for both increased and decreased activity of enzymes controlling Lys27 methylation on H3 in cancer. To maintain the global histone methylation patterns, HMTs work in coordination with HMDs— lysine-specific demethylases—which are also implicated in cancer progression. The first HDM identified, a lysine demethylase, was LSD1, which can act both as a co-activator or repressor depending on its binding partner.

Epidemiological or human studies can identify physiological markers of cancer but they cannot identify the associated epigenetic changes. To establish the link between epigenetic mechanisms and cancer, researchers use *in vivo* models of carcinogenesis. For example, inflammation has been identified as an important initiator and promoter of lung carcinogenesis in human studies, but these studies were not able to identify the sequential molecular events that led to the cancer. Lung carcinogenic models were used to understand the specific epigenetic mechanisms involved—increases in methylation of cell cycle regulator genes *p27* and *p57* in cancer progression. Many such models exist that allow the characterization of those epigenetic mechanisms that link genetic susceptibility or environmental exposures to cancer.

Using a silica exposure-based inflammatory *in vivo* lung carcinogenesis model, researchers identified multiple epigenetic alterations; in particular, methylation of the promoters of cell cycle-control genes *p16, APC*, and *Cdh13* during tumor progression. Transgenic adenocarcinoma prostate mice were used to identify that the expression of the gene that encodes the oxidative stress-sensing enzyme *Nrf2* is suppressed by DNA methylation and chromatin silencing in prostate cancer. A mouse model of acute lymphoblastic leukemia showed that the tumor suppressor gene *Idb4* was silenced in leukemias but not in solid tumors. Using mouse models of T-cell lymphoma, researchers discovered that alterations of DNA methylation patterns silence the *PTEN* and p53 tumor suppressor genes and cause overexpression of the oncogene *MYC*.

Epigenetic Inhibitors in Cancer Therapy: Unlike genetic changes, epigenetic changes are reversible, and drugs that can reverse the process represent exciting potential therapeutic targets for cancer. Epigenetic changes can be effective indicators of diagnosis and prognosis of cancer, given that most of these changes precede pathological changes.

The primary types of epigenetic modification that have been targeted by drug discovery efforts in recent years are histone methylation and acetylation. These histone post-translational modifications catalyzed by HMTs, HDMs, HACTs, and HDACs are considered targets for pharmacological intervention. Acetylation and methylation of lysine and arginine residues are the most abundant modifications of the known histone marks and are often the target of such interventions. Current work in translational research seeks to identify small molecule inhibitors that target these enzymes, since drug discovery scientists believe that epigenetic dysregulation can be reversed by inhibitors of these enzyme targets.

As of 2014, the U.S. Food and Drug Administration has approved 4 epigenome-targeted anticancer drugs. Two are drugs that inhibit DNA methyltransferases: azacitidine and decitabine, and two are drugs that inhibit histone deacetylases: vorinostat and romidepsin. Azacitidine and decitabine have been approved for use in the myelodysplastic syndromes and low-blast count Acute Myelogenous Leukemia and have improved the survival of patients with these diseases. Vorinostat and Romidepsin are approved for treatment of cutaneous T-cell lymphomas.

The biggest clinical impact of epigenetic modifying agents thus far has been in hematological malignancies. Epigenetic therapies for solid tumors are yet to show promise in clinical trials. Newer studies presently focus on combination therapy in many cancers. Epigenetic modifications are also being used to evaluate potential biomarkers to diagnose patients with cancer and to identify patient populations likely to respond to specific anticancer therapies for personalized treatment regimens.

Continued study of the epigenetic landscape and its role in cancer along with improved insights into epigenetic therapies will enable the design of effective therapeutic regimens with low potential for adverse events.

Banalata Sen, Phd, MPH

For Further Information

Allis, C. D., Caparros, M-L., Jenuwein, T., Reinberg, D., & Lachlin M. (Eds.). (2015). *Epigenetics*. Cold Spring Harbor Laboratory, NY: Cold Spring Harbor Laboratory Press.

Kanwal, R., Gupta, K., & Gupta, S. (2014). Cancer epigenetics: An introduction. In Mukesh Verma (Ed.), *Cancer epigenetics: Risk assessment, diagnosis, treatment, and prognosis* (pp. 3-25). New York, NY: Springer.

Lund, A. H., & van Lohuizen, M. (2004). Epigenetics and Cancer. *Genes and Development,* 18:2315-2335. http://genesdev.cshlp.org/content/18/19/2315.full

Other Resources

What is Epigenetics?
http://www.whatisepigenetics.com/

Cancer Epigenetics
http://epigenie.com/epigenie-learning-center/epigenetics/cancer-epigenetics/

▶ Cell cycle control

Category: Cancer Biology
Also known as: Cell division control/regulation, cell cycle checkpoints

Definition: In eukaryotic organisms such as human beings, the cell cycle represents the series of events regulating the replication/duplication of individual cells. Since eukaryotic cells are characterized by a nucleus that segregates the chromosomal material from the cytoplasm, regulation must take into account both the proper duplication and separation of genetic material as well as cytokinesis (cell division).

Etiology: Cancers, regardless of their origins in the organism, in their simplest forms represent uncontrolled cell division. In describing the changes that occur when a normal cell transforms into a malignancy, it is important to understand the events that take place both during cell division (mitosis) as well as those events that occur when the cell is not actively dividing.

In 1879, the German cytologist Dr. Walther Flemming found that upon using dyes to observe structures in the cell, threadlike materials in the nucleus could be seen. Flemming further observed that as these cells prepared to undergo cytokinesis, the threads shortened and subsequently divided, each half moving to the sides of the cell. Flemming termed the process mitosis.

By the mid-twentieth century, cytologists had divided what they termed the cell cycle into two periods: 1) mitosis, which ended when the cell completed its division into two identical daughter cells, and 2) interphase, which encompassed any processes that the cell carried out between divisions. The length of interphase varied with the cell. While embryonic cells are capable of dividing in a matter of hours, most replicating cells divide only once every 12–24 hours; ironically, this is often true for cancer cells as well.

Mitosis (M) itself takes place in a matter of 30 to 45 minutes. The remaining portion of the cell cycle, interphase, can be subdivided into three phases. The period during which DNA replication takes place (the synthesis or S phase) lasts approximately six hours, and usually begins 6–12 hours after mitosis is completed. The interval (or gap) between mitosis and S phase is known as G_1. Following completion of DNA replication a second interval in time, a gap known as G_2, occurs prior to the beginning of mitosis. The G_2 phase lasts approximately six hours.

The entire process is strictly regulated, particularly during the G_1/S and G_2/M transition periods (or so-called "checkpoints") during which specific proteins monitor whether particular events in each phase have proceeded correctly. The precise mechanisms by which these proteins function vary, but they typically override the molecular events that move the cell from one phase to the next. Since mutations in these proteins are commonly

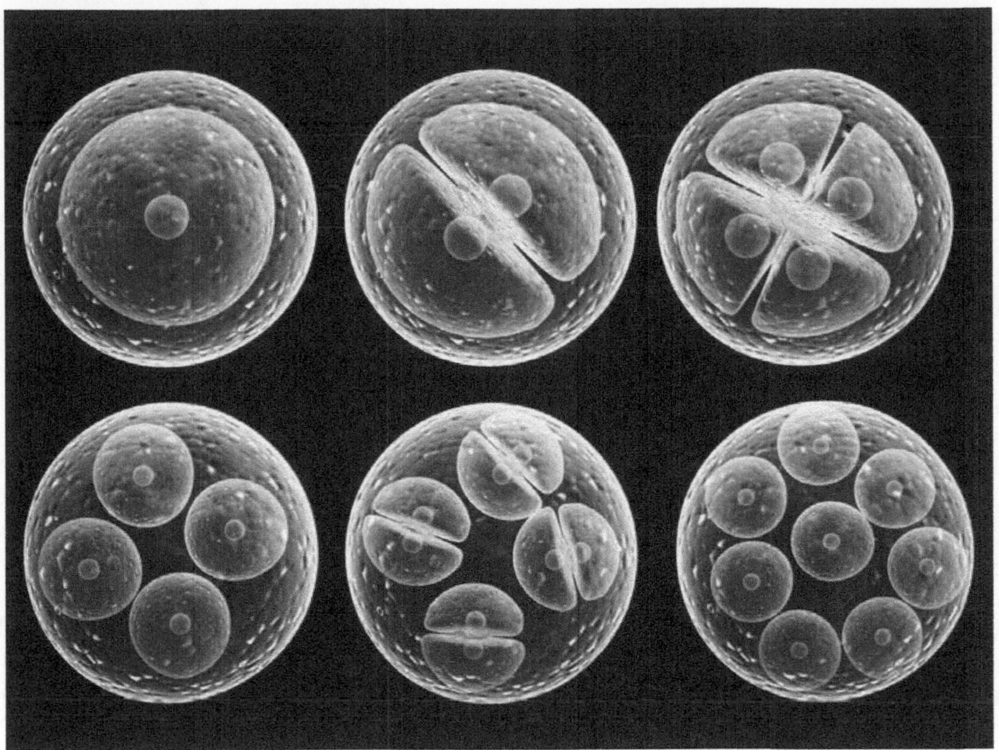

Cell division. (iStock)

associated with events that lead to the formation of cancers, the genes that encode these checkpoint molecules are known as "tumor suppressors."

Cyclins/Cyclin-dependent Kinases (CDKs): The quiescent stage following mitosis, during which the cell has not yet committed to division, is sometimes referred to as the G_0 phase. The cell will usually remain in G_0 until a triggering event, the binding of a small-molecular-weight growth factor to a specific growth factor receptor on the surface of the cell, moves the cell into G_1. At this point the cell is now committed to complete the cell cycle unless blocked by a suppressor protein. Two classes of proteins are produced sequentially, driving the cell through the remaining phases: 1) cyclin-dependent kinases (CDKs), enzymes that regulate the activity of their target substrates through phosphorylation of serine or threonine residues, and 2) cyclins, proteins that bind to a subunit on CDKs and activate their enzymatic activity. Each phase in the cell cycle is driven by the activity of the appropriate cyclin/CDK complex. The number and types of CDKs vary little during the phases of the cell cycle; regulation is maintained through the synthesis and breakdown of the specific cyclins that regulate CDK activities. Some of the substrates activated as a result of phosphorylation by CDKs are transcription factors, which are DNA-binding proteins that determine the expression of specific genes. As examples (albeit simplistic), early events in G_1 phase are regulated by the binding of D-type cyclins to CDK4 and CDK6, while the binding of cyclin E to CDK2 mediates the transition from G_1 into S phase.

CDK activity is also regulated by the removal of inhibitory phosphates by a class of enzymes known as Cdc25 (cell division cycle) phosphatases. Certain types of cancers (including prostate, breast, and ovarian cancers) overexpress cdc25B. Excessive Cdc25 activity hyperstimulates Cdks and uncontrollably drives the cells through the cell cycle. The centrality of Cdc25 to the regulation of the cell cycle and its overexpression in some cancers suggests that Cdc25 might be a suitable target for chemotherapy. Several chemical compounds are known to target the Cdc25 enzymes. Combination therapy using such compounds (in combination with microtubule-targeting compounds such as paclitaxel) has been shown to have an additive beneficial effect.

Tumor suppressors: While several families of tumor suppressors have now been identified, 2 proteins in particular appear to play the most significant roles in maintaining the checkpoints in the cell cycle: 1) the Retinoblastoma protein (RB), and 2) a protein known as p53, which has a molecular weight 53,000 daltons (a dalton is about the weight of one hydrogen atom).

The RB protein, the first tumor suppressor to be identified, was discovered in 1986 by Dr. Robert Weinberg as a result of its association with retinoblastoma, an uncommon cancer of the eye in children. Children with an inherited, mutated form of the RB gene are at greater risk not only for retinoblastoma, but for other cancers as well, including osteosarcoma (bone cancer), certain forms of muscle cancers, and cancer of the pineal gland (pinealoma).

The retinoblastoma molecule is a large 105,000 molecular weight protein, the activity of which, like many regulatory proteins in the cell, is governed by its state of phosphorylation. Movement of the cell through the G_1/S transition depends on the DNA-binding protein E2F, the function of which is to activate the expression of those genes that encode S phase-specific proteins such as DNA polymerase and cyclin E. The ability of E2F to function is determined by whether a complex is formed with the non-phosphorylated form of the RB protein; when bound to RB, the E2F transcription factor is inactive. During the G_1 phase, assuming the cell is committed to divide, the cyclin D-CDK4 enzyme begins the phosphorylation of the RB protein, resulting in its release from E2F. In a form of positive feedback, E2F transcribes the gene for another cyclin, cyclin E, which in turn (as noted previously) forms a complex with another kinase, CDK2. The cyclin E-CDK2 complex hyper-phosphorylates any remaining RB proteins bound to E2F, allowing transcription of the remaining genes necessary for movement into S phase.

In addition to mutations that might inactivate the RB molecule, certain oncogenic viruses may induce malignancy by inactivating the RB protein. Human papilloma virus (HPV), associated with cervical cancer, produces a protein known as E7 that binds and inactivates the RB protein. The adenoviruses, associated with respiratory infections in humans and malignancy in non-human animals, produce a gene product known as the E1A protein that is similar both in structure and function to the HPV E7 protein, and likewise inactivates the RB protein.

The p53 protein, which in part regulates both the G_1/S and G_2/M transitions, functions primarily in responding to cellular stresses, including damage from ultraviolet light or other forms of DNA damage. Unlike the RB protein, p53 is activated by its phosphorylation. DNA damage activates a number of kinases such as the ATM (Ataxia-telangiectasia mutated) enzyme. Mutations in the ATM gene result in ataxia-telangiectasia, a rare genetic disorder characterized by increased chromosomal breakage and a significant risk for cancer. Phosphorylated p53 inhibits movement through cell cycle transitions by activation of another protein, p21, which inactivates cyclin E-CDK2 complexes (thereby preventing the hyper-phosphorylation of the RB protein) and inhibits the cyclin D-CDK4 and cyclin A-CDK2 complexes. Mutations in the p21 gene have been associated with certain types of brain cancers, colon cancer, and leukemia. In cells with such extensive DNA damage that repair cannot take place, the p53 protein can induce apoptosis, or programmed cell death.

Regulation by CDK Inhibition: Regulation of the cell cycle, "fine tuning" so to speak, also involves a series of CDK inhibitors. One example, p21, was discussed previously. Since these inhibitors are specific for kinases, they are referred to as CDK inhibitors. A protein known as p16 has a molecular weight of 16,000 daltons and functions by forming a binding complex with CDK4 and CDK6 that prevents the phosphorylation of the RB protein, which blocks the cell from entering S phase. Because of its role in inhibiting CDK4, it is also referred to as $p16^{Ink4a}$ (Inhibitor of CDK4) in the literature. A slightly smaller protein, p15, contains amino acid sequences similar to that of p16, and has likewise been shown to inactivate both CDK4 and CDK6. Mutations in each of these genes have been observed in some tumors, including bladder cancers and melanomas. Mutations in the p16 gene have been linked to so many forms of cancers that an alternative term, multiple tumor suppressor (MTS1), is often applied to the gene that encodes p16.

Richard Adler, PhD

For Further Information

Alberts, B., Johnson, A., Lewis, J., Morgan, D., Raff, M., Roberts, K., & Walter, P. (2014). *Molecular biology of the cell* (6th ed.). New York: Garland Science.

Dynlacht, B. (1997). Regulation of transcription by proteins that control the cell cycle. *Nature,* 389(6647):149-152.

Enders, G. (2010). *Cell cycle deregulation in cancer.* New York: Springer.

Morgan, D. (2007). *The cell cycle: Principles of control.* Sunderland, MA: Sinauer Associates.

Mullan, P.B., Quinn, J. E., & Harkin, D. P. (2006). The role of BRCA1 in transcriptional regulation and cell cycle control. *Oncogene,* 25(43): 5854-5863.

Other Resources

American Cancer Society
http://www.cancer.org/cancer/cancercauses/geneticsandcancer/heredity-and-cancer

Control of the Cell Cycle
http://highered.mheducation.com/sites/0072495855/student_view0/chapter2/animation__control_of_the_cell_cycle.html

National Cancer Institute
http://www.cancer.gov/about-cancer/causes-prevention/genetics

See also: Colorectal cancer; Chromatin; DNA repair

▶ Cell death

Category: Cancer Biology
Also known as: apoptosis, autophagy, necrosis, programmed cell death, cell suicide

Definition: Cell death refers to the methods by which a body regulates the number of cells in a healthy individual. There has been much discussion in recent years about how to define cell death and what terminology to apply to these events. Two classifications of cell death, apoptosis and necrosis, are common events for cells. Malignant cells typically have mutations that protect them from apoptosis thus, allowing them to collect rapidly and to survive longer in humans. Cells experiencing stress or deficient nutrition may go through the process of autophagy, which conserves energy and promotes survival. However, in aging cells autophagy may be extensive causing vacuolization and ultimately the death of the cell.

Etiology: The cells of humans have different life spans based on their structure and function. Barring an unfortunate accident, cells usually will fall into one of three broad groups. In some cases they live for a very short time and are rapidly replaced. These are usually simple cells such as the epithelium of the skin or lining of the intestines. A second group of cells found mainly in organs such as the liver and endocrine glands may live for many months or years and when aged or injured can be replaced. The third group of cells exists for the life of the individual unless injury destroys them. They are usually very complex cells such as neurons or striated muscle cells.

In healthy cells there is a balanced regulation between cell proliferation and cell death. This balance is an important component of embryological development, structural and physiological homeostasis, the stress response and survival. Malignant cells are unique in that they do not have a limited life span because of mutations that increase the process of cell division while decreasing the rate at which cells die. They proliferate quickly and they are very slow to die even when treated with chemotherapy or radiation.

Necrosis: The least organized form of cell death is necrosis. It can occur as a result of physical or pathological cellular injury such as accidents, burns, radiation, infections, infarcts or other events that would cause energy levels to fall. The main cause of physiological events in necrosis is the decrease in energy availability. This could result from decreased nutrient supply, decreased oxygen level and/or injury to mitochondria. Once the energy levels decrease the cell is no longer able to maintain the integrity of the cell membrane and especially the membrane Na+-K+ pumps. Without fully functional membrane pumps the cell cannot maintain osmotic balance. Consequently, ions such as sodium and calcium and others can enter the cell causing the cell to swell and burst, releasing the cell contents into the surrounding environment.

When cells burst some toxic substances are released, especially dangerous enzymes from the lysosomes. This makes cells in the surrounding area vulnerable to injury or destruction. Cell rupture leads to inflammation in the area and the influx of fluid and immune cells. When the original cell underwent necrosis there was no prior signal that the cell was in danger. Therefore, the inflammatory response in the area was slow, allowing the cycle of cell damage to extend beyond the cells in the immediate area.

Apoptosis: While the process of necrosis is unstructured, the process of apoptosis is highly organized and is often referred to as programmed cell death. It involves a series of enzymatic steps that controls not only which cells are involved but also the number of cells and the elimination of cell organelles and cytoplasm. In development it is responsible for the removal of cells and for the restructuring of organs, while in adults it helps to maintain homeostasis through the removal of infected or dying cells caused by aging, mutation, or disease.

Cells receive signals for apoptosis in one of two ways, positive or negative signals. Cells need a constant input of cytokines from other cells to survive. If these are not present, the cell will undergo apoptosis. The negative signals include damage to DNA from ultraviolet light, X-rays, or chemotherapy; increased levels of free radicals, failure to fold proteins accurately during synthesis, disease or death activators that are cytokines such as tumor necrosis factor-alpha (TNFα) or FAS ligand.

Apoptosis will follow one of three possible pathways: 1) triggered by internal signals, the mitochondrial pathway; 2) triggered by external signals or 3) the release of apoptosis inducing factor. The mitochondrial pathway occurs as a result of internal damage in the cell. A protein called Bcl2, on the surface of mitochondria, serves as an apoptotic regulator. It is activated by Bax and subsequently creates pores in the outer membrane of the mitochondria. Cytochrome c, a necessary component in the mitochondrial energy production, leaks out of mitochondria and interacts with proteins to form apoptosomes.

Apoptosomes in the cytoplasm activate another protein, caspase 9 which leads to activation of several caspases in series. This caspase cascade has proteolytic activity which leads to degradation of structural proteins and chromosomal DNA. The DNA fragments are condensed in small nuclear elements that are no longer functional. By this time signals have been sent from the apoptotic cells to recruit phagocytes to the area. The phagocytes engulf and digest the remaining components of the apoptotic cell.

Apoptosis is triggered by external signals when Fas and tumor necrosis receptors are bound by death activators. Caspase 8 is activated, which in turn triggers the caspase 9 cascade. The cell undergoes the same events that occur when apoptosis is triggered through the mitochondrial pathways. In this circumstance, again the apoptotic cells are engulfed by phagocytes recruited to the area or by neighboring cells.

A third pathway for apoptosis is controlled by apoptosis- inducing factor (AIF), a mitochondrial protein. This pathway does not involve caspases. AIF is released from mitochondria and migrates to the nucleus. As it binds to DNA it fragments the DNA, which results in the formation of small, sealed membrane vesicles called "apoptotic bodies," which are shed by cells undergoing apoptosis.

Apoptosis is important to the body because when cells go through the process of apoptosis they do not release dangerous chemicals into the extracellular environment and the body does not experience inflammation. Cancerous cells undergo mutations that alter the apoptotic proteins. This allows cancer cells to continue to grow and reproduce with no limits to the number of cells that can be formed.

Autophagy: When cells are experiencing starvation or decreased energy levels or other types of stress they can restructure the cytoplasm and organelles of the cell. This process is called autophagy or self-eating. Unlike necrosis and apoptosis, it is considered a survival technique for cells and therefore, organisms. Under conditions of physiological or environmental stress the number of components of cells can be reduced thus, conserving energy to improve the chance for survival. During cancer growth there is a significant need for nutrients to keep up with the number rapidly growing and dividing cells. If the nutrient supply is reduced cancer cells rely on autophagy to maintain the cells and while the rate of autophagy increases in cancer cells these neoplastic cells also can limit autophagy in some cells of the immune system that are trying to control the malignant growth.

The process of autophagy begins when the unwanted organelles or cytoplasm is encased in a double cell membrane. This sets the biological material off from the rest of the cell. It will fuse with the normally present lysozymes and the contents will be destroyed and recycled. This will decrease the energy needs of the cells and promote cell survival.

When this process is not controlled however, it can continue to digest components of the cell; leading to the vacuolization of the cell, which if excessive, leads to the death of the cell. This may be one of the mechanisms of aging. Learning how to decrease the rate of autophagy in health cells may lead to longer lives while increasing the rate in neoplastic cells may be a way to control cancer.

Scientists have theorized that if the nutrient and energy supply of cancer cells is low and they can block autophagy, the cancers would shrink or at least not continue growing. Previous treatment to stop autophagy had been unsuccessful because the drugs being used were toxic at the levels needed to halt autophagy. Recently as more knowledge has been gathered other drugs have been tested. Currently hydroxychloroquine in combination with other therapeutic treatments is being tested in over 20 clinical trials. They are examining effectiveness in renal, breast, prostate, pancreatic, lung and brain cancers, and multiple myeloma.

Drugs to inhibit autophagy may hold promise for the future, but scientists are aware that much more needs to be understood about the process of autophagy. The large number of steps involved in the process will provide many opportunities for development of new drugs that can serve as inhibitors.

Annette O'Connor, PhD

For Further Information

Amaravadi, R.K., Lippincott, S. J., Yin, X. M., Weiss, W. A., Takebe, N., Timmer, W., DiPaola, R.S., White, E.

(2011). Principles and current strategies for targeting autophagy for cancer treatment. *Clinical Cancer Research*, 17(4): 654-666.

Elmore, S. (2007). Apoptosis: A review of programmed cell death. *Toxicologic Pathology*, 35(4): 495-516.

Mayur V. J., Paczulla, A. M., Klonisch, T., Dimgba, F. N., Rao, S. B., Roberg, K., Schweizer F, Lengerke C, Davoodpour P, Palicharla VR, Maddika S, Łos M. (2003). Interconnections between apoptotic, autophagic and necrotic pathways: Implications for cancer therapy development. *Journal of Cellular and Molecular Medicine*, 17(1): 12-29.

Other Resources

National Center for Biotechnology Information
http://www.ncbi.nlm.nih.gov

American Cancer Society
http://www.cancer.org

Amyotrophic Lateral Sclerosis Association
http://www.alsa.org

▶ Chromatin

Category: Cancer Biology
Also known as: Chromoplasm, Karyotin

Definition: Chromatin consists of a protein-DNA complex that packages DNA into a tight, compact structure that allows large amounts of DNA to fit into the nucleus of the cell.

The structure of chromatin: Cells use the molecule deoxyribonucleic acid (DNA) to store their genetic information. However, inside the nucleated cells, DNA is never naked, but forms complexes with proteins. Linear DNA molecules in nucleated cells (chromosomes) consist of a repeating unit of chromatin known as "nucleosomes." After stripping the protein shell surrounding the chromosomes, the remaining DNA-protein complexes have the appearance of beads on a string; each bead consists of a nucleosome.

Nucleosomes are made of double-stranded DNA complexed with small proteins called "histones." The core particle of each nucleosome contains 8 histone molecules, 2 each of 4 different types of histones: H2A, H2B, H3, and H4. The histone octamer forms a tiny spool around which approximately 147 bases of DNA winds around 1.6 times. Histone proteins have a very highly positively charged front part (amino-terminus) that causes them to tightly bind the negatively charged sugar-phosphate backbone of DNA. The remaining portion of histones contains the so-called "histone fold," a portion of the protein that mediates the association of histones with each other. Histone octamers form when both an H3 and H4 histone use their histone folds to bind and form an H3-H4 dimer. Two H3-H4 dimers self-assemble to form an $H3_2$-$H4_2$ tetramer. H2A and H2B histones associate in a very similar manner to form an $H2A_2$-$H2B_2$ tetramer, which self-assembles with an $H3_2$-$H4_2$ tetramer to form the histone octamer. Because the histone octamers have their histone folds ensconced inside the nucleosome core particle and their positively charged amino-termini projecting to the outside, DNA self-assembles on it to form nucleosomes.

Nucleosomes also form higher-order structures that further package the genome. In the nucleus, another histone protein, called H1, bundles nucleosomes into a coiled fiber 30 nanometers (nm) in diameter known as a 30-nm solenoid (or 30-nm fiber). The addition of purified H1 to assembled nucleosomes in the laboratory spontaneously initiates the formation of 30-nm solenoids. Attaching the 30-nm solenoids to "nuclear scaffolding proteins" assembles them into loops that form 300-nm chromatin fibers. These 300-nm chromatin fibers also associate to form a structure 700 nm in diameter (half the diameter of a metaphase chromosome).

Variations in chromatin structure: Two main forms of chromatin exist in cells. The more densely packaged form renders the DNA less accessible to gene expression but protects it from damage. This highly compacted, transcriptionally silent form of chromatin is known as heterochromatin. The more open, relaxed form of chromatin, known as euchromatin, has higher levels of gene expression.

Cells have 2 types of heterochromatin. Constitutive heterochromatin mainly comprises repeated sequences, such as those found at centromeres (where the spindle apparatus attaches during cell division) and telomeres (ends of chromosomes). Regions of the genome assembled into constitutive heterochromatin tend to exist as heterochromatin in almost every cell in the body and tend to localize to the periphery of the nucleus. Facultative heterochromatin differs from cell to cell and even the same cell can change those regions of its genome that are assembled into heterochromatin. An excellent example of facultative heterochromatin is X chromosome inactivation. Human females have 2 X chromosomes but only 1 of these chromosomes is active in each cell of their bodies. However, the copy of the X chromosome that happens to be active differs from cell to cell, since the decision to inactivate 1 copy of the X chromosome over another occurs early in development and on a cell-by-cell basis.

Histone variants: Sometimes cells earmark particular nucleosomes for specialized tasks by assembling their core nucleosome particle with variants of the core histones. For example, in the case of X chromosome inactivation, a bulky variant of H2A called macro-H2A specifically incorporates into the nucleosomes of the inactive copy of the X chromosome, but a different variant, H2A-Bbd, is exclusively present in the active copy of the X chromosome. Likewise, an H3 variant called CENPA specifically incorporates into nucleosomes at centromeric DNA. Also, DNA damage affects chromatin structure, and several different histone variants become incorporated into nucleosomes at the site where damaged DNA appears as a way to mark these areas as substrates for the DNA repair machinery.

The histone code: Cells also contain mechanisms that convert heterochromatin into euchromatin. Particular enzymes can chemically modify histones in ways that decrease their affinity for DNA. Histone acetyltransferases (HATs) attach acetyl groups (CH_3COO^-) to histones and histone deacetylases (HDACs) remove acetyl groups from histones. Histone acetylation decreases the number of positively charged amino acids in the amino-terminus of the histone, thus, neutralizing its affinity for DNA. Conversely histone deacetylation restores the affinity of histones for DNA. Therefore, HAT activity strongly correlates with gene expression whereas, HDAC activity strongly correlates with repression of gene expression.

Histones are also subject to methylation (attachment of -CH_3 groups). Histone methyltransferases (HMTs) target specific amino acids in histones (usually lysine residues). The effect of histone methylation varies depending on the particular amino acids within H3 that are methylated. For example, methylation of lysine #4 (the fourth amino acid from the beginning of H3) tends to activate gene expression as does methylation of lysine #36. However, methylation of lysine #9 and #27 strongly correlates with repression of gene expression. In particular, methylation of lysine #9 of H3 induces the binding of a protein called HP1, which may tightly compact the DNA into a very condensed chromatin structure.

The correspondence of particular histone modification with specific changes in gene expression constitutes the "histone code." If you know the precise modifications of specific histones, you can accurately predict if the genes associated with those histones will be expressed or repressed.

Epigenetics: DNA can pass genetic information from 1 generation to another through the sequences of its bases, which encode RNAs and, ultimately, proteins. However, DNA can also pass genetic information by mechanisms that have nothing to do with the sequence of that DNA molecule. The chromatin structure of DNA can determine if particular genes are expressed or repressed. These higher-order structures of DNA are also inherited and comprise the "epigenetic" means by which genetic information is passed from one generation to another.

Chromatin, epigenetics, and cancer: Aberrations of histone modification are often observed in cancer cells. Since many genes involved with the control of the cell cycle, signal transduction, programmed cell death, DNA repair, senescence, invasion/metastasis, transcription, and drug responsiveness are epigenetically regulated; epigenetic alterations can have profound consequences for the control of cell proliferation.

The epigenetic abnormalities of cancer cells also represent a potential target for new anticancer drugs. HDAC inhibitors (eg, vorinostat, romidepsin) have the ability to kill cancer cells while minimally affecting normal cells. Epizyme, a biopharmaceutical company, has designed 2 drugs that specifically target HMTs. These 2 drugs, tazemetostat and pinometostat, target the EZH2 and DOT1L HMTs, respectively, are presently being tested in phase I clinical trials. These are only a few of the exciting new drugs either being marketed or tested as treatments that attack cancer at the epigenetic level.

Michael Buratovich, PhD

For Further Information

Alberts, B., Johnson, A., Lewis, J., Morgan, D., Raff, M., Roberts, K., & Walter, P. (2014). *Molecular biology of the cell* (6th ed.). New York, NY: Garland Scientific.

Avgustinova, A., & Benitah, S. A., (2016). The epigenetics or tumour initiation: Cancer stem cells and their chromatin. *Current Opinion of Genetics and Development*, 36, 8-15.

Oberdoerffer, P., & Sinclair, D. A. (2007). The role of nuclear architecture in genomic instability and ageing. *Nature Reviews Molecular Cell Biology*, 8, 692-702.

Other Resources

Chromatin
http://www.nature.com/scitable/definition/chromatin-182

Epizyme
http://www.epizyme.com/

HIstome – the Histone Infobase
http://www.actrec.gov.in/histome/index.php

The Cell: A Molecular Approach – Chromosomes and Chromatin
http://www.ncbi.nlm.nih.gov/books/NBK9863/

See also: DNA methylation; Histone acetylation/deacetylation; Romidepsin

▶ Chromosomes and cancer

Category: Cancer Biology
Also known as: Chromosomal instability, CIN

Definition: Cancer is usually conceived of as resulting from a series of mutations in two classes of genes: oncogenes and tumor suppressors. Cancer cells, however, typically exhibit broader changes to their chromosome structure that extend well beyond the deoxyribonucleic acid (DNA) base changes that accompany most mutations. These include changes in chromosome number as well as the deletion, duplication, inversion, and translocation of chromosomal segments. Chromosomal aberrations, however, have historically been more difficult to study than mutations, and no direct evidence of their role in carcinogenesis has been produced. Scientists continue to debate whether these chromosomal changes play a causal role in cancer or are simply an artifact of the mutations that lead to cancerous states. However, some consensus has been reached that mutations and chromosomal instability probably play complementary roles in the formation of cancer and that neither acts completely independent of the other.

Etiology and symptoms of associated cancers: Most cancer cells are aneuploid. "Aneuploidy" is the term used to describe the gain or loss of a chromosome in a cell, whether it be an entire chromosome or just a portion of one. In the latter case, the gain or loss has also been described as a DNA insertion, or duplication, respectively. Unlike single mutations, aneuploidy can affect the expression of genes by the thousands as large numbers of genes have their expression effectively doubled or cut in half by the duplication or deletion, respectively, of a chromosomal segment. Such changes in a gene's "dosage" may, in turn, lead to an increased rate of cellular mutation, especially if the affected genes are involved in the repair of DNA damage. Aneuploidy and mutation can therefore be thought of as complementary processes, with one state often leading to the other.

An extreme form of aneuploidy is polyploidy, where the entire complement of chromosomes in a cell has been duplicated, so that there are more than the usual two copies of each chromosome in the cell. Many solid tumors have been shown to be made up of polyploid cells. Subtler changes in gene expression can also result from two other chromosomal aberrations that are seen to occur in cancer cells: inversion and translocation. Here, a chromosomal segment is "flipped around" in a chromosome or is transferred to a different chromosome. Although the genes on this segment are still present in the cell, they may be differentially expressed, because precisely where a gene is located on a chromosome often affects its level of activity.

Evidence that supports a causative rather than artifactual role of aneuploidy in cancer includes that aneuploid cells have been found to be associated with certain precancerous lesions and therefore could not have been caused by the formation of a cancerous state, that there are specific chromosomal translocations that are diagnostic of certain forms of cancer (these are often referred to as marker chromosomes when used in this context), and that the degree of aneuploidy in a cancer cell often correlates with the severity of the disease and can even be predictive of clinical outcomes. Aneuploidy has also been suggested to be one of the reasons cancer cells are so well adapted for continuous growth in their particular environment. By displaying a nearly limitless number of phenotypes that result from changing the dosage of many different combinations of genes, those cells that are particularly well adapted will be selected for and will propagate more cells like themselves. However, there remains no direct evidence that an aneuploid state causes the cellular changes that lead to cancer.

Another chromosomal abnormality that is associated with almost all cancer cells, but which was not evident initially using conventional cytological techniques, is the presence of very short telomeres. Telomeres are arrays of repetitive DNA that are found on the ends of linear chromosomes. These structures protect genomic DNA from the shrinkage that occurs in chromosomes every time they are replicated. DNA polymerase, the enzyme that is used to copy DNA, is unable to copy a complete linear molecule of DNA because of its use of a ribonucleic acid (RNA) "primer" to initiate its activity. Telomeres are therefore degraded each time a cell duplicates and divides, providing a distinct limit on the number of divisions any cell can undergo. Rapidly dividing cells, such as those associated with cancer, quickly reach this limit and enter a stage deemed cellular crisis. Most cells that reach this stage stop dividing, and many die, but cancerous cells overcome this limitation, called the Hayflick limit after American cell biologist Leonard Hayflick, who first described this phenomenon in 1962. To do this, most cancer cells express an enzyme called telomerase, which adds DNA repeats to the ends of the chromosomes and allows cells to continue dividing indefinitely.

Shortened telomeres have been shown to be associated with chromosomal instability. Telomeres in this shortened state often fuse with one another or to other regions of double-stranded breaks within chromosomes to avoid further degradation. The number of such break sites in cancer cells is often increased because of mutations in the DNA enzymes used to repair such damage. Chromosomes that are fused end-to-end or to another chromosomal segment that contains a centromere are then further jumbled when their DNA is pulled apart during mitosis. The centromere is a region of DNA that typically makes up the center of a chromosome and is the area to which the mitotic spindle attaches when sister chromosomes are separated from one another. The chromosomal abnormalities associated with aneuploidy can result from such cycles of fusion followed by chromosomal breakage.

History: The concept that cancer is essentially a chromosomal disease is not a new one. In 1902 Theodor Boveri, a German zoologist, proposed that changes in chromosome number were the cause of tumor formation. He used cytological techniques to view the chromosomes of a tumor cell using a microscope. This is not to say that his aneuploidy theory did not leave room to account for the contributions of changes to specific genes. As the concept of thegene began to take shape during the early twentieth century, Boveri formulated a theory of how aneuploidy caused cancer that incorporated an early notion of mutational changes. He proposed that abnormal mitoses could lead to a combination of "chromatin determinants" that, in turn, would lead to cancer.

However, when oncogenes and tumor suppressors were discovered in the 1970's and 1980's, the concept of aneuploidy as the causative factor of cancer began to fall out of favor. The notion that the identification of specific mutations in a finite number of genes would lead to a full understanding of cancer was an appealing one. As more and more cancer-causing genes were identified, the goal of understanding cancer at a molecular level seemed attainable. However, as time progressed, the mutational theory failed to explain a number of observations, including that cancer is rare in newborns, something one would not predict if newborns inherited cancer-causing genes from their parents; that certain carcinogens are known to cause cancer without causing mutations; and that a long latency period is always present before cancer develops, even after exposure to fast-acting mutagens.

The resurgence of the aneuploidy theory of cancer formation can also be linked to the development of new techniques in the 1990's, such as microarrays, which allow the expression levels of many genes to be assayed at the same time. Using microarray analysis, cancers were seen to exhibit changes in hundreds, or even thousands, of genes—many more than could be accounted for by a purely mutational model. As cancer research progresses, the role of both mutations as well as chromosomal aberrations will need to be taken into account to fully understand their contributions to carcinogenesis.

James S. Godde, Ph.D.

For Further Information

Deusberg, P., R. Li, A. Fabarius, and R. Hehlmann. "The Chromosomal Basis of Cancer." *Cellular Onocology* 27 (2005): 293-318.

Maser, R. S., and R. A. DePinho. "Connecting Chromosomes, Crisis, and Cancer." *Science* 297 (2002): 565-569. Rajagopalan, H., and C. Lengauer. "Aneuploidy and Cancer." *Nature* 432 (2004): 338-341.

Richards, R. I. "Fragile and Unstable Chromosomes in Cancer: Causes and Consequences." *Trends in Genetics* 17 (2001): 339-345.

Weaver, B. A. A., and D. W. Cleveland. "Does Aneuploidy Cause Cancer?" *Current Opinion in Cell Biology* 18 (2006): 658-667.

Other Resources

National Cancer Institute

The Center of Excellence in Chromosome Biology
http://ccr.cancer.gov/initiatives/CECB/

National Center for Biotechnology Information
Cancer Chromosomes
http://www.ncbi.nlm.nih.gov/sites/entrez?db=cancerchromosomes

See also: Cancer biology; Childhood cancers; Cytogenetics; Family history and risk assessment; Gene therapy; Genetic testing; Genetics of cancer; Hereditary cancer syndromes; Mitochondrial DNA mutations; Oncogenes; Proto-oncogenes and carcinogenesis

▶ Circulating tumor cells

Category: Cancer Biology
Also known as: circulating carcinoma cells; circulating tumor microemboli

Related conditions: breast cancer, prostate cancer, colorectal cancer

Definition: Circulating tumor cells (CTCs) are cells that have migrated from tumor masses into the bloodstream or that have been dislodged from tumors that are in contact with blood and are now present in the circulating blood (Figure 1). These cells have the properties of the tumor from which they originate and are believed to contribute to metastasis (cancer spread).

Associated cancers: Three cancers in which CTCs have been most studied are breast, prostate, and colorectal cancers. Other cancers studied include those of the lung, bladder, liver, oral cavity, kidney, stomach, and ovaries.

Testing and treatment: In the case of testing in cancer, uses of CTC analyses include: prognosis, selection of treatments, monitoring results of treatment, discovery of drug resistance in the tumor and identification of changes in the properties of tumor cells such as which proteins they express on their surfaces and if targets for anti-cancer drugs are present.

CTC testing has advantages compared to other types of tumor tests. It uses simple blood draws to obtain samples representative of a person's tumor and is more convenient and less invasive than tissue biopsy specimens. CTCs can also be obtained sequentially to monitor the current status of a tumor's characteristics in "real time," unlike biopsy specimens. CTC information has been sometimes found to be more reliable and to supplement information from imaging and measurement of soluble biomarkers. CTCs can be cultured and used for research to better understand metastasis and development of drug resistance and new anti-tumor drugs. These advantages drive the continued research into the clinical applications of CTCs.

There are some shortcomings to CTC analyses. The rarity of CTCs in blood limits their usefulness for early detection of cancers. Some preparations of CTCs are contaminated by blood cells or show poor viability. More studies must be done in order to solve such problems and enable clinical applications and regulatory approvals for medical use.

Examples of Current Providers of CTC Clinical Tests: Cell Search is an antibody/magnetic bead-based system manufactured by Janssen Diagnostics. It is FDA approved for testing in breast, prostate, and colorectal cancer. It has been validated by several independent clinical and biomedical research studies on significant numbers of samples. Just some of the companies offering this test include: Mayo Medical Laboratory Network, Cellsee, Quest Diagnostics, Cancer Treatment Centers of America, ARUP, Molecular Pathology Network, LabCorp, MLabs—University of Michigan, Roswell Park Cancer Institute, London Health Sciences Center, and Vancouver Prostate Center. Cell Search testing is covered by Medicare but private healthcare organizations vary in their coverage of the test.

Other tests are not FDA approved but are clinically used and validated. Some are able to be used for clinical purposes by the laboratories that developed them. For example, Biocept's CTC assay is certified by CLIA (Centers for Clinical Laboratory Improvements Amendments) and accredited by CAP (College of American Pathologists) and is accepted by many health insurance policies.

A large number of companies have developed methods for isolating and analyzing CTCs as listed in Table 1 although many are for research use or for studies to eventually enable their clinical use.

Clinical and Basic Research Studies of the Significance of CTCs: CTCs have been found in all types of tumors studied. In the case of breast cancer, several studies involving large numbers of patients showed that considering CTC numbers improved prognosis, predicted disease relapse and length of cancer –free time and survival. Similar findings were made in the cases of prostate and colorectal tumors. Consequently, the Cell Search technology that was used in many studies won FDA approval.

History: Circulating tumor cells were first identified 146 years ago by the Australian pathologist Thomas Asworth. Since that time, many technological changes and advances in biomedical and clinical science have enabled many findings on CTCs and their applications. Some of the relevant methods that became available include mammalian cell culture of tumor cells and monoclonal antibodies as probes for various cellular protein biomarkers of tumors. Others include multicolor immunofluorescence staining to visualize tumor cell and tissue protein localization, microfluidic devices and magnetic bead-based cell separation to isolate CTCs, automated digital microscopy to identify tumor cells in blood without prior isolation, RNA and next-generation DNA sequencing to profile gene expression and mutations in tumor cells. Computational bioinformatic technologies and the sequencing of the human genome were developed starting in the late 20th century and provide powerful analyses and personalized medicine applications to CTCs.

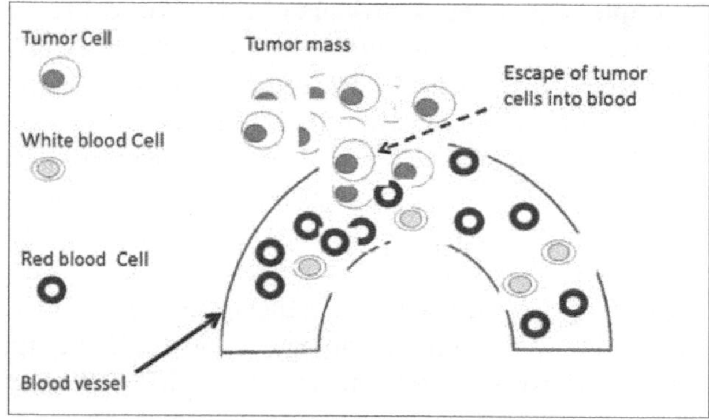

Figure 1. Circulating tumor cells. Cells escape from a tumor mass that is in contact with a blood vessel and enter the blood circulation.

In summary, CTCs appear to have great potential for use in clinical decision making to guide treatment and seem likely to find clinical use for tumors other than the currently tested breast, prostate, and colorectal ones. Research in CTCs also seems likely to provide important insight into tumor characteristics which could lead to new anti-tumor drugs, the process of metastasis, and new tumor biomarkers.

Oluseyi Adewale Vanderpuye, PhD

For Further Information

Johnson, Carolyn Y. (2014). Cancer cells may guide treatment. *Boston Globe*. https://www.bostonglobe.com/news/science/2014/07/10/rare-tumor-cells-blood-can-help-target-cancer-treatment-study-shows/OlX-6CVXbNIt51T6nu3J5QM/story.html

Table 1. Selection of Companies Developing or Applying Technologies for CTC Analysis or Isolation

COMPANY	*TYPE of TECHNOLOGY*	*APPLICATIONS*
Advanced Cell Diagnostics	Fluorescent RNA probe hybridization to target RNA	Detection of cancer relevant RNA in cells in suspension and tissue slides
Biocept	Microfluidic antibody-based CTC enrichment	Culture and characterization of lung and breast cancer cells
BioFluidica	Microfluidic antibody-based CTC capture	Isolation of viable CTC and application of other techniques
Cellsee	Microfluidic isolation of CTC automated immunohistochemistry or DNA hybridization	Counting, visualization and isolation of viable CTC for next generation DNA sequencing and PCR
Cynvenio Biosystems	Automated microfluidic isolation of CTC & Immunofluorescence staining	DNA mutation identification, 4500 mutations
CytoTrack	Immunofluorescence staining large volume sample on disc and scanner and cell picker	Imaging and counting of CTC, single cell isolation and immunofluorescence, FISH (DNA analysis) PCR
Epic Sciences	Fluorescent labeling blood cells and automated digital microscopy	Personalized medicine based on tumor cell marker analysis
Fluxion	Antibody-based magnetic bead isolation of CTCs	Next generation DNA sequencing of CTC
Janssen Diagnostics	Antibody-coated magnetic particles	Prognosis by use of CTCs for breast, prostate, and colorectal cancer
Miltenyi Biotec	Antibody-coated magnetic particles	Isolation of RNA and DNA for analysis from cells
ScreenCell	Size based CTC isolation on porous membranes	DNA and RNA analysis of isolated CTCs
SRI Biosciences	Fiber optic array scanner	Multiplex analysis- immunofluorescence, PCR, FISH, SNP analysis

Allard, W.J., Matera, J., Miller, C.J., Repollet, M., Connelly, M.C., Rao, C. ... Terstappen, L. W. M. M. (2004). Tumor cells circulate in the peripheral blood of all major carcinomas but not in healthy subjects or patients with nonmalignant diseases. *Clinical Cancer Research*, 10(20): 6897-6904.

Kolata, K. (2015, April 20). New blood test shows promise in cancer fight. *New York Times*, pp. A1. http://www.nytimes.com/2015/04/20/health/blood-test-shows-promise-as-alternative-to-cancer-biopsy.html?_r=0

Pollack, A. (2014, April 8). Sidestepping the biopsy with new tools to spot cancer. *New York Times*, pp. B1. http://www.nytimes.com/2014/04/08/business/cancer-analysis-tools-circumvent-biopsies.html?_r=0

Other Resources

Biovantra
http://www.biovantra.com/clinical-services/specialized-testing-cellsearch-ctc.php

Mayo Clinic
http://www.mayomedicallaboratories.com/articles/features/ctc/

Roswell Park Cancer Institute
https://www.roswellpark.org/pathology/laboratory-medicine/circulating-tumor-cells

WebMD
http://www.webmd.com/cancer/news/20140515/could-a-blood-test-predict-breast-cancers-return

SRI International
https://www.sri.com/blog/fastcell-testing-detects-characterizes-circulating-tumor-cells%20

See also: Breast cancer; Chemotherapy; Prostate cancer; Colorectal cancer screening

▶ Cyclin-dependent kinase inhibitor-2A (*CDKN2A*)

Category: Cancer Biology
Also known as: CDKN2, CDK4 inhibitor, multiple tumor suppressor 1 (MTS1), TP16, p16INK4a, p14ARF

Definition: Cyclin-dependent kinase inhibitor-2A (CDKN2A) is a tumor-suppressor gene located on chromosome 9p21.

The gene's role: As a tumor-suppressor gene, CDKN2A plays a major role in regulating cell division. The loss of function of a tumor-suppressor gene is a key event in the multistep process that transforms a normal cell into a cancer cell. In normal cells, these genes code proteins that play a role in regulating cell growth and proliferation. A loss of function of these genes by mutation results in uncontrolled cell growth that leads to cancer. In cancer cells, the chromosomal region where CDKN2A is located is often mutated.

The *CDKN2A* gene codes for multiple proteins; the most well studied being the p16(INK4a) and the p14(ARF) proteins. Both of these proteins function as tumor suppressors. The p16(INK4a) protein binds to two other proteins (CDK4 and CDK6) that play key roles in the process of cell growth and division. p16(INK4a) blocks the normal function of CDK4 and CDK6, and therefore, controls cell growth and division.

The p14(ARF) protein protects p53, an essential protein for regulating cell division and growth, from being degraded. By virtue of its protective role, p14(ARF) helps prevent tumor formation and functions as a tumor suppressor.

Cancer and CDKN2A: Unlike other tumor-suppressor genes that are inactivated by point mutations, inactivation of CDKN2A occurs through deletions, mutations, or promoter methylation. Mutations in the CDKN2A gene are known to occur in patients with multiple primary myelomas. Inactivation of CDKN2A has also been reported in numerous primary tumors, including bladder carcinoma, glioma, mesothelioma, gastrinomas, T-cell acute lymphoblastic leukemia, melanoma, prostate adenocarcinoma, and renal cell carcinoma. In addition, some gene alterations observed in different cancers affect the structure or function of CDKN2A. These include hypermethylation of CDKN2A in gastrinomas, germ-line mutation in CDKN2A in pancreatic cancer and melanoma, and inactivation of CDKN2A in sporadic pancreatic cancers.

An increased risk of melanoma and pancreatic cancer exists in individuals with CDKN2A mutations. Clinical observations such as detection of germ-line mutations in CDKN2A in melanoma-prone families, increased risk of pancreatic cancer among melanoma-prone families with CDKN2A mutations, and zero occurrence of pancreatic cancer in melanoma-prone families without the CDKN2A germ-line mutation suggest a link between CDKN2A mutations and occurrence of melanoma and pancreatic cancer. Families with co-occurrence of pancreatic cancer and melanoma should participate in clinical screening programs for

CDKN2A mutations. This would enable identification of high-risk family members and a more improved individual risk assessment for better outcomes for CDKN2A mutation carriers.

Banalata Bono Sen, Ph.D.

Other Resources

CDKN2A
https://ghr.nlm.nih.gov/gene/CDKN2A

Genetic Testing for CDKN2A
http://ghr.nlm.nih.gov/gene/CDKN2A/show/Genetic+Testing+Registry

See also: BRCA1 and BRCA2 genes; Hereditary cancer syndromes; MYC oncogene; TP53 protein

▶ Cytokines

Cancer Category: Cancer Biology; Chemotherapy and Other Drugs
Also known as: Lymphokines, monokines, interleukins and interferons, tumor necrosis factors, chemokines, granulocyte colony-stimulating factors

Definition: Cytokines are a class of proteins or glycoproteins produced by white blood cells in the immune system. The role of cytokines is to carry chemical messages to other immune cells when an alien cell or antigen is identified in the human body. This includes cancer cells. There are several types of cytokines, such as interleukins, lymphokines, chemokines, monokines, interferons, granulocyte colony stimulating factors, and tumor necrosis factors. They often have the same or overlapping functions.

Cancers Treated: Renal cell carcinoma, malignant melanoma, lymphoma, Kaposi's sarcoma, chronic myelogenous leukemia, and hairy cell leukemia; being studied as a treatment for breast cancer and other solid tumors

Delivery Route: Subcutaneous injection or intravenously, depending on the drug.

How these drugs work: There are three cytokines that are approved by the Food and Drug Administration to treat cancer. They are interferon-alpha, interleukin-2, and interleukin-11. Other cytokines are being studied for use in the future.

Interferon-alpha notifies the immune system when cancer cells are discovered. Interferon-alpha is produced by all the cells in the body, including those in the immune system. The immune system responds by producing cytotoxic T-cells, such as natural killer cells, and macrophages. These cells are able to interfere with the growth of cancer cells and may kill them.

Interleukin-2 cells signal the immune system when they find a cancer cell. This causes the immune system to produce B-cells, enhanced T-cells, and several subsets of T-cells. Like interferon-alpha, interleukin-2 initiates the production of natural killer cells. It also triggers the production of antibodies specific to the cancer cell antigens. These cells all concentrate on destroying the cancer cells.

Interleukin-11 has a different function than interferon-alpha and interleukin-2. It produces blood cell growth factors. Chemotherapy kills red and white blood cells, and platelets. Interleukin-11 tells the bone marrow to produce more red and white blood cells and platelets when their levels drop.

Side Effects: Common side effects are nausea, vomiting, fever, headaches, muscle pain, decreased red and white blood cells and platelets. Cytokine treatments can also induce a condition called "capillary leak syndrome" (also known as Clarkson's disease) which is characterized by episodes of plasma and other blood components leaking from blood vessels into nearby tissues. Capillary leak syndrome typically causes hypotension, increased heart rate, and peripheral edema (swelling of the extremities), but some patients can experience fluid accumulation around the heart and lungs and suffer from pulmonary edema, cardiac arrhythmias (erratic heart rates), inflammation of the heart, kidney and liver dysfunction, itching, electrolyte changes, and thrombus (blood clot) formation. Other patients may have confusion, hallucinations, depression, mania, and disorientation. A fatal side effect is sepsis (colonization of the bloodstream by microorganisms).

Janet R. Green
Updated by: Christine M. Carroll, R.N., B.S.N., M.B.A.

For Further Information

Lee, Sylvia, & Margolin, Kim. (2011). Cytokines in cancer immunotherapy. *Cancers*, 3: 3856-3893.

National Cancer Institute. (2013 June 12). Biological Therapies for Cancer. Retrieved February 7, 2016 from Http://www.cancer.gov/about-cancer/treatment/types/immunotherapy/biotheraputics-fact-sheet.

List, Thomas, Casi, Giulio, & Neri, Dario. (2014). A chemically defined trifunctional antibody-cytokine-drug conjugate with potent antitumor activity. *Molecular Cancer Therapeutics*, 13: 2641.

See also: Anthraquinones; Appetite loss; Bacillus Calmette Guérin (BCG); Beryllium and beryllium compounds; Biological therapy; Exercise and cancer; Fever; Gene therapy; Human growth factors and tumor growth; Immune response to cancer; Immunotherapy; Interferon; Interleukins; Tumor necrosis factor (TNF); Vaccines, therapeutic

▶ DNA methylation

Category: Cancer Biology
Also known as: Epigenetics

Definition: DNA methylation is a normal cellular process that turns genes off and silences them. The process of DNA demethylation turns genes back on. DNA methylation is involved with a number of bodily processes, like development of an embryo in utero, and silencing of the genes on the second X chromosome in zygotes. It also plays a role in the development of human diseases, particularly cancer. DNA methylation adds a methyl group (-CH_3) to cytosine nucleotides that are next to or across from guanine nucleotides (these are called CpG groups) and near the beginning of the start-site of transcription, ie, the synthesis of a RNA copy of the DNA gene sequence. The addition of methyl groups silences the gene by inhibiting the transcription of the gene. There are enzymes called methyltransferases that assist with the DNA methylation process.

Etiology and symptoms of related cancers: DNA methylation is common to all types of cancers. All cells possess a number of genes that are tumor suppressors. These genes are always on in normal cells, but cancer cells turn them off by DNA methylation. This is necessary to protect cancer cells from self-destructing. There are other genes that cancer cells turn on by demethylation. They include genes that enable them to invade other cells and tissues, and to repair their cells. Overall, cancer cells have predominantly non-methylated genes (hypomethylated). They have fewer methylated genes (hypermethylated).

Cancer cells develop from inherited or mutated changes in regulatory genes. There is a two-hit theory of cancer development, which states that these abnormal regulatory genes require the loss of matching normal allele of the gene, since humans have 2 copies of each chromosome and, therefore, 2 copies (alleles) of each gene. Normal alleles of these regulatory genes can be destroyed by a mutation, followed by loss of the normal allele, or, in the case of inherited mutations, by inheritance of the mutant alleles followed by loss of heterozygosity of the normal allele. So, a pair of alleles that suffers 2 losses can cause cancer. The symptoms of cancer vary by cancer location and type.

Testing and treatment: Microarray analysis is used to view the methylated parts of DNA and compare it with other DNA. The fragments of DNA are laid out on a flat surface so that they can be compared to other fragments of DNA at the same time. There are several variations in microarray analysis. These procedures include: bead arrays, short oligonucleotide arrays, long oligonucleotide arrays, and single nucleotide polymorphism arrays. The other method of analysis of DNA for methylation is called High-throughput sequencing. This process allows the methylated DNA to be sequenced without taking small pieces of DNA. High-throughput sequencing can analyze a whole piece of DNA and is quicker and less labor-intensive.

One of the ways to detect DNA methylation is the use of sodium bisulfite. It converts unmethylated cytosine to uracil. When this modified DNA molecule is amplified by means of polymerase chain reaction (PCR), the former cytosine-guanine (CG) base pairs are replaced by uracil-thymine (UT) base pairs. These molecules can be sequenced by means of the Sanger method, pyrosequencing, or mass spectrometry. Comparing the sequence of these bisulfite-treated DNA molecules with their untreated counterparts can pinpoint the precise bases that were methylated, since what is a methylated CG base pair in the untreated molecule is an UT base pair in the bisulfite-treated molecule. Methylation-sensitive restriction enzymes are a second way to look for methylation. The enzymes digest the methylated genes so that only the unmethylated genes remain. The third method to identify methylated DNA is affinity purification. The purpose of this process is to use an antibody that tightly binds to the methylated DNA, causing it to precipitate. Any of these methods of DNA methylation can be used with high-throughput sequencing.

Several enzymes that were discovered in the DNA methylation process have been exploited to treat cancer patients. Two DNA methyltransferase inhibitors, azacitidine and decitabine, have been approved by the US Food and Drug Administration (USFDA) to treat myelodysplastic syndrome. Additionally, histone deacetylase inhibitors, Vorinostat and Romidepsin, have been approved to treat Hodgkin's lymphoma, large B-cell lymphoma, and cutaneous T-cell lymphoma. While these drugs are effective, they do have limitations. Currently, there is no way to specify where in the DNA they should act. They have toxicities that could limit their use. The patient must take the medication for the rest of their life, or the cancer could reoccur. This is a significant drawback.

History: There is no formal history of DNA methylation. Research on DNA methylation appeared to begin in the late 1970s and continues to the present. In 2009, a substance called 5-hydroxymethylcytosine (5-hmC) was discovered and was found to be present in active DNA demethylation. In the past 5 years (2010 to 2015), research has turned toward finding ways to treat cancers using the DNA methylation information. Some treatments have been developed, but they can only be used to treat certain cancers.

Christine M. Carroll, RN, BSN, MBA

For Further Information

Baylin, Stephen B. (2005). Review of: DNA Methylation and Gene Silencing in Cancer. *Nature Clinical Practice Oncology*, 2, S4-S11.

Ehrlich, Melanie. (12 August 2002). Review of: DNA Methylation in Cancer: Too Much, But Also Too Little. *Oncogene*, 21(35), 5400-5413.

Kaithoju, Srikanth. (2014). Epigenetics and Cancer Therapy. *Journal of Cancer Biology and Research*, 2(3), 1052.

Phillips, Theresa, Ph.D. (2008). The Role of Methylation in Gene Expression. *Nature Education,* 1(1), 116.

Song, Chin-Xiao, and He, Chuan. (2012). Balance of DNA Methylation and Demethylation in Cancer Development. *Genome Biology*, 13: 173. http://www.genomebiology.com/2012/13/10/173

Zilberman, Daniel, and Henikoff, Steven. (2007). Genome-wide Analysis of DNA Methylation Patterns. *Development*, 3, 134, 3959-3965.

Other Resources

National Institute of Health. Genetics Home Reference

www.ghr.nlm.nih.gov/handbook/howgeneticswork/epigenome

"What is Epigenetics?" (Blog)

www.Epigenetics.com

▶ DNA repair

Category: Cancer Biology
Also known as: Genomic repair

Definition: Cells of the human body (trillions of them) are constantly being exposed to various environmental stressors (including UV light and radiation), as well as to internal errors in DNA replication. On average about one million errors occur daily in each cell. These numbers sound high, but account for less than 0.0002% of the human genome. DNA damage (especially in a critical gene) can be harmful and lead to cell or organismal death. Therefore, DNA must be repaired constantly in order to prevent these errors from dramatically affecting the cell. Fortunately, humans have multiple DNA repair processes that, collectively, eliminate more than 99.99% of mistakes that occur. These processes were the subject of the 2015 Nobel Prize in Chemistry, which was awarded to three investigators who revealed the mechanisms of DNA repair over time.

Types of DNA damage: Genetic stability requires not only a precise and accurate method for duplicating DNA, but also an extremely accurate method for proof-reading and correcting any mistakes made during the process. Most DNA damage affects the primary structure of the double helix (damage to the four chemical bases that make up DNA), and therefore most of the repair mechanisms are aimed at proofreading and correcting mistakes at this level. DNA may also be damaged at a higher level of organization, accounting for breaks either in one strand or in both strands of the DNA. Such damage is much harder to repair and often leads to cellular death.

Endogenous DNA Damage: DNA damage may result from errors in DNA replication, sometimes leading to the incorporation of the wrong base in the newly forming DNA strand. This must be corrected before cell division occurs or the incorrect base-pairing will be passed on to all future cell lines. Fortunately, DNA polymerase excises and corrects most mistakes made during replication by using its exonuclease activity.

In addition to inserting the wrong base in the DNA, bases may be altered in the cell through processes such as methylation, oxidation, or hydrolysis.

Exogenous DNA Damage: Many forms of exogenous assaults on human cells can induce DNA damage. These include UV light (both A and B), ionizing radiation (such as that found in radioactive decay), elevated temperatures, and a host of human-made chemicals (such as vinyl chloride and the tar and aromatic hydrocarbons found in cigarette smoke).

Mitochondrial DNA Damage: While most DNA resides in the nucleus (and therefore most DNA damage occurs in the 46 chromosomes of the nucleus), human cells also contain DNA in mitochondria (mtDNA). Only a small number of genes are contained in the mtDNA, but it is a very oxidative environment which increases the likelihood of DNA damage.

Repair mechanisms: In the words of Nobel Laureate (2015) Tomas Lindahl, "Life exists — so DNA must be repairable." There are, indeed, a variety of mechanisms available to our cells to reverse or repair the damage done to our DNA, whether by endogenous or exogenous means. Most require an intact (undamaged) strand of DNA that serves as the guide to repairing the other strand. The primary mechanisms for repair are direct repair, base excision repair, nucleotide excision repair, and methyl-directed mismatch repair. All rely upon a variety of enzymes present in the nucleus.

Direct repair (or direct reversal) is used predominantly with thymine dimers caused by exposure to UV light. The covalent modification causes a physical change in the backbone of the DNA strand, thus inhibiting DNA polymerase from being able to synthesize new DNA. Photolyase and other enzymes are able to split the dimer apart, thus repairing the damage and allowing replication to continue.

The process known as base excision repair removes an incorrect or damaged base by nicking the DNA backbone, removing the damaged region (a larger portion than just the incorrect base), and then resynthesizing that strand of DNA correctly. This involves enzymes known as DNA-N-glycosylases that can recognize a single damaged base and break the bond between it and the deoxyribose sugar in the DNA backbone. Nucleotide excision repair repairs DNA at the backbone damage location. For example, when UV light causes adjacent thymine bases to connect to each other (thymine dimers), DNA is removed both upstream and downstream of the dimer. Then, DNA polymerase resynthesizes that section.

The methyl-directed mismatch repair is a strand-specific method of repairing damage due to added, lost, or incorrectly positioned bases. Often this is a result of proofreading errors during DNA replication. Two or more enzymes of the Mut group are involved in the mechanism. The first recognizes the mismatch; the other alerts an endonuclease (another enzyme) that cuts the newly synthesized DNA near the error point. An exonuclease enzyme then removes the incorrect DNA. New DNA, synthesized by DNA polymerase enzyme, fills the gap.

DNA damage checkpoints in the cell cycle: When DNA is damaged, progression of the cell cycle is delayed and various checkpoints are activated. These checkpoints are natural pause buttons in the cycle, and they allow the cell time to repair the damaged DNA before continuing the process of cell division. DNA damage checkpoints are known to occur at the boundary between G_1 and S phases (prior to DNA replication in the cell), and between G_2 and M phases (prior to mitosis and separation of the chromosomes). A checkpoint also exists in the middle of the S phase (during DNA synthesis), and all checkpoints are controlled by specific mediator proteins that transmit signals to other downstream proteins.

Etiology and symptoms of associated cancers: In healthy human cells, the rate of daily DNA damage is matched by the rate of DNA repair. Periodically, however, the rate of repair lags behind the rate of damage (due to either endogenous or exogenous causes), leading to senescence, apoptosis, or cancer.

Senescence is the irreversible failure of normal cells to divide. This occurs routinely when telomeres (the ends of chromosomes) shorten to the point where DNA damage occurs. Other processes that cause DNA damage may also lead to cellular senescence, including the presence of reactive oxygen radicals. There is some evidence to suggest that a higher-than normal rate of senescence in liver cells may be associated with hepatocellular carcinoma, and that senescent cells may contribute directly to carcinogenesis.

Apoptosis is the process of programmed cell death that occurs in humans and other multicellular organisms. Apoptosis leads to the breakdown of the cellular components and (through the production of DNase enzymes) the destruction of the cellular DNA. A lack of apoptosis can signal that cancer is beginning.

Human DNA repair disorders: Poor or ineffective DNA repair pathways have now been implicated in both the onset and progression of multiple myeloma, a cancer of the blood in which there is an accumulation of malignant plasma cells. These cells produce abnormal proteins (immunoglobulins) that affect the function of the immune system, damage the kidneys, and cause cancerous tumors.

Defects in DNA nucleotide excision repair mechanisms are known to be responsible for several human disorders. These include: xeroderma pigmentosum (in which there are freckle-like spots on the skin, increased sensitivity to sunlight, increased rates of skin cancers, and premature aging); Cockayne syndrome (dwarfism, increased sensitivity to sunlight and to various chemicals, premature aging, and mental retardation); and trichothiodystrophy (hallmarks include brittle hair and nails, sensitive skin, short stature, and mental retardation). In addition, several diseases that cause premature aging (known collectively as segmental progerias, in which the young people appear elderly and suffer from various age-related diseases) are also related to poor DNA repair mechanisms. These diseases include Werner's syndrome, Bloom's syndrome, and ataxia telangiectasia. Franconi anemia (increased skin pigmentation and a predisposition to leukemia) and Li-Fraumeni syndrome (predisposition to a variety of cancers) may also be related to DNA repair mechanism failure, although the direct linkages are not as clear under these conditions.

Nearly 3 dozen mutations in DNA repair mechanisms are known to lead to an increase in cancer susceptibility. In many cases, these mutations lead to slow or error-prone repair systems and a greater probability of certain cancers. Hereditary nonpolyposis colorectal cancer (also known as Lynch syndrome) is particularly well studied and strongly associated with mutations in the mismatch repair system. Variations in the MLH1, MSH2, MSH6, and PMS2 genes may prevent proper repair of DNA replication mistakes during normal cell cycles. Mutations in the EPCAM gene (which is adjacent to the MSH2 gene) may also interrupt DNA repair mechanisms and lead to accumulated DNA mistakes. Although mutations in these genes predispose individuals to cancer, not all people who carry these mutations develop cancerous tumors.

Testing and treatment: Cancer therapies, including both chemotherapy and radiation therapy, overwhelm the ability of cells to engage in DNA repair, thus leading to cell death. Cells that are rapidly dividing, such as cancer cells, are most affected by these therapies. Of course, these therapies also affect other rapidly dividing cells (such as skin, gut, and blood cells).

Two drugs are currently used to treat multiple myeloma: Melphalan (an alkylating agent) and Bortezomib (a proteasome inhibitor). Both have direct effects on DNA repair pathways. New experimental drugs (yet to be approved for use in treating multiple myeloma) include Aplidin, Marizomib, Panobinostat, Treanda, and Zolinza.

Kerry L. Cheesman, PhD

For Further Information

Alberts, B., Johnson, A., Lewis, J., Morgan, D., Raff, M., Roberts, K., & Walter, P. (2014). *Molecular Biology of the Cell* (6th ed.). New York: Garland Science.

Clancy, S. (2008). DNA damage and repair: Mechanisms for maintaining DNA integrity. *Nature Education* 1(1):103.

Cooper, G.M., & Hausman, R.E. (2016). *The Cell: A Molecular Approach* (7th ed.). Sunderland (MA): Sinauer Associates.

Gourzones-Dmitriev, C., Kassambara, A., Sahota, S., Rème, T., Moreaux, J., Bourquard, P., … Klein, B. (2013). DNA repair pathways in human multiple myeloma: Role in oncogenesis and potential targets for treatment. *Cell Cycle* 12(17): 2760–2773.

Machado, Carlos R., & Menck, Carlos F.M. (1997). Human DNA repair diseases: From genome instability to cancer. *Brazilian Journal of Genetics*, 20(4) Retrieved February 10, 2016, from http://www.scielo.br/scielo.php?script=sci_arttext&pid=S0100-84551997000400032&lng=en&tlng=en.

University of Rochester. (2011, June 17). Protein found that improves DNA repair under stress. *ScienceDaily*. Retrieved February 10, 2016 from www.sciencedaily.com/releases/2011/06/110616142722.htm.

Other Resources

Howard Hughes Medical Institute (2003) Mismatch repair
http://www.hhmi.org/biointeractive/mismatch-repair

Josh Fischman (2015) Chemistry Nobel Prize for 2015 Goes to Discovery of DNA Repair
http://www.scientificamerican.com/article/chemistry-nobel-prize-for-2015-goes-to-discovery-of-dna-repair/

The Multiple Myeloma Research Foundation
http://www.themmrf.org/

The Nobel Prize Committee 2015
http://www.nobelprize.org/nobel_prizes/chemistry/laureates/2015/press.html

Weston, K. (2014) Country Life: Repair and Replication. In *Blue Skies and Bench Space: Adventures in Cancer Research*. Long Island, New York, Cold Spring Harbor Laboratory Press. http://blueskiesbenchspace.org/index.php?pag=4

See also: Ataxia telangiectasia; Multiple myeloma

▶ DNMT3A

Category: Cancer Biology
Also known as: DNA (cytosine-5-)-methyltransferase 3 alpha

Definition: *DNMT3A* is an enzyme that transfers a methyl group to the 5 carbon of cytosine in CpG dinucleotides to form 5-methyl cytosine (5meC). The enzyme plays a role in epigenetic modification of DNA and gene expression relative to many biological processes.

Etiology: *DNMT3A* is an enzyme that is responsible for the genome-wide *de novo* methylation of cytosine and found in virtually all tissues. Methylation of CpG-rich regions immediately upstream from genes is correlated with downregulation of gene expression. Studies in mice have indicated that the gene is essential for normal development. It has been demonstrated that aberrant *de novo* DNA methylation is common in human tumors.

Recurrent mutations in *DNMT3A* along with mutations in other genes regulating genomic methylation are common in various cancers, especially acute myeloid leukemia (AML) (also known as acute myeloblastic leukemia, acute granulocytic leukemia, and acute nonlymphocytic leukemia) and other hematological malignancies.

Studies suggest that mutations in *DNMT3A* are relevant to AML tumorigenesis. About 30% to 35% of AML patients have a heterozygous somatic mutation in *DNMT3A*. The most common mutations are missense mutations affecting amino acid 882, most commonly arginine to histidine (R882H) which significantly reduces its DNA methyltransferase activity. AML patients with a *DNMT3A* R882 mutation have poor prognosis with significantly shortened survival time. Thus, the R882H mutation is thought to be directly involved with AML by altering its methyltransferase activity which may interfere with apoptosis. Mutations in *DNMT3A* at sites other than 882 probably contribute to leukemogenesis by mechanisms that do not involve methylation.

Testing and treatment: AML is usually detected through a complete blood count. Confirmatory tests may include bone marrow aspiration and bone biopsy, cytogenetic analysis, mutation analysis, and immunophenotyping.

Treatment of most AML cases usually involves 2 chemotherapy and/or radiation treatment phases: remission induction and consolidation. Both phases use drugs and/or radiation that inhibit DNA synthesis. The consolidation phase often involves stem cell transplants.

AML can also be treated with cytosine nucleoside analogues such as azacitidine, decitabine, and zebularine which are DNA methylation inhibitors. The response rate of AML to *DNMT3A* inhibitors alone is low and unpredictable, and seems not to be related to methylation state. Response rates are better if DNA methylation inhibitors are used in combination with histone methylation and deacetylase inhibitors. Upregulation of microRNA-29b (miR-29b), which targets and inhibits *DNMT3A* mRNA translation, improves the clinical response to decitabine.

Charles L. Vigue, PhD

For Further Information

Im, A. P. (2014). DNMT3A and IDH mutations in acute myeloid leukemia and other myeloid malignancies: associations with prognosis and potential treatment strategies. *Leukemia* 28: 1774-1783.

Li, Y & Zhu, B. (2014). Acute myeloid leukemia with DNMT3A mutations. *Leukemia and Lymphoma* 55(9): 2002-2012.

Rendl, Michael. (Ed.). (2014). *Stem Cells in Development and Disease, Volume 107 (Current Topics in Developmental Biology)*. Boston: Elsevier Academic Press.

Sharma, Shikhar. (2012). *Epigenetic Inheritance of DNA Methylation Patterns: A DNMT3A and 3B Perspective*. Saarbrücken, Germany: LAP LAMBERT Academic Publishing.

Other Resources

GeneCards®—DNMT3A
http://www.genecards.org/cgi-bin/carddisp.pl?gene=DNMT3A

Online Mendelian Inheritance in Man (OMIM)—DNA Methyltransferase 3A; DNMT3A
http://www.omim.org/entry/602769

▶ Epidemiology of cancer

Category: Cancer Biology

Definition: Cancer epidemiology is the study of the distribution, determinants, and frequency of malignant disease in specific populations. Three broad objectives related to the use and importance of epidemiologic cancer research are to identify factors related to the etiology of specific cancers; to use cancer-risk data to formulate theories regarding cancer prevention and control; and to educate a diverse public regarding the prevention and control of cancer. These strategies attempt to match educational and dissemination methods to population needs with attention to cancer risk, literacy, trust of medical professionals, and palatability of information, factors known to vary widely across population subgroups.

Three types of epidemiologic research apply to the field of cancer. Descriptive epidemiology focuses on the trends and frequency of cancer in specific populations. Analytic epidemiology identifies causes and predisposing risk factors associated with the development of specific cancers. Clinical epidemiology delineates screening programs and evaluates outcomes for the range of prevention strategies implemented.

Descriptive epidemiology: In 1995 the American Cancer Society estimated 1,252,000 new cancer cases and 547,000 cancer deaths in the United States. Cancer incidence and mortality rates are higher among men than women. Furthermore, African Americans have a higher cancer mortality rate than whites, which has been a source of discussion and controversy. Some argue that inherent genetic factors account for the discrepancy, whereas others attribute the difference to an overrepresentation of poverty among African Americans and superior health care received by affluent versus impoverished groups.

The leading cancers in the United States are lung, breast, prostate, colorectal, and ovary, accounting for about 61 percent of cancer diagnoses. Americans over the age of sixty-five have a tenfold greater risk of developing cancer than do younger Americans. Despite an increase in overall cancer mortality rate between 1950 and 1990, mortality rates for all cancers combined have declined substantially for individuals under age forty-five. They have increased in people over age fifty-five, with that increase primarily related to lung cancer deaths. Many reports identify a decline in cancer mortality of about 14 percent since 1950, although these reports exclude deaths from lung cancer.

These data seem biased and problematic, as smoking is the primary etiologic factor in lung cancer diagnoses and a leading public health issue. Excluding lung cancer from cancer death statistics implies that if lifestyle issues and behaviors relate to etiology, science is not responsible or interested in research to develop effective prevention and treatment strategies. This denies the role of social, political, and economic factors in promoting increasingly prevalent maladaptive behaviors among vulnerable members of society and is an area worthy of aggressive debate and action in terms of research funding.

U.S. Cancer Statistics: 2004 Incidence and Mortality marks the sixth time that the Centers for Disease Control (CDC), the National Program of Cancer Registries (NPCR), and the National Cancer Institute's (NCI's) Surveillance, Epidemiology, and End Results (SEER) Program have combined their data sources to produce a collaborative set of federal cancer incidence statistics (newly diagnosed cases) for a single year. Mortality statistics from the CDC's National Vital Statistics System are also included and report 2003 cancer deaths both nationally and by state. The report was produced in collaboration with the North American Association of Central Cancer Registries.

Analytic epidemiology: The goal of analytic cancer epidemiology is to identify the factors that predispose individuals to a cancer diagnosis and to quantify risk. Cancer risk factors include environmental exposures, genetic susceptibility, and immunosuppressive state and may be secondary to a history of malignancy, viral infection, or medical therapy. These risk factors can account for various aspects of carcinogenesis and assume varied degrees of causal primacy.

Clinical epidemiology: Epidemiologic research plays an important role in the development of cancer-screening modalities and prevention strategies. Cancer prevention focuses on decreasing incidence by lowering risk through changes in lifestyle patterns and behavior. Primary prevention attempts to stop the development of cancer. Secondary prevention aims to improve cure rates by cancer screening and early diagnosis and treatment.

Cancer screening involves testing to detect early-stage cancer in asymptomatic individuals. Ideally, screening tests should be easy to administer, noninvasive, and inexpensive. To be beneficial, early detection should alter prognosis and improve survival.

Emerging data and discovery: New data are rapidly emerging that are changing cancer screening and prevention practices. Although these changes are quite positive, the proliferation of data can create confusion among health consumers and avenues to receive reliable information are needed.

For example, the human papillomavirus (HPV), types 16 and 18, has been causally related to cervical intraepithelial neoplasia. A history of genital warts is linked to human papillomavirus types 6 and 11 and may explain the increased risk associated with multiple sexual partners. Other sexually transmitted viruses, such as herpes simplex virus 2, may interact as etiologic factors. The vaccine Gardasil protects against four HPV types, which together cause 70 percent of cervical cancers and 90 percent of genital warts. Ideally, girls and young women should get the vaccine before they are sexually active because the vaccine is most effective in those who have not yet acquired any of the four HPV types covered by the vaccine. Girls and women who have not been infected with any of those four HPV types will get the full benefits of the vaccine; those who are sexually active may also benefit from the vaccine, although they may get less benefit from the vaccine if they may have already acquired one or more of the HPV types covered.

One would assume that the worldwide annual rate of 300,000 deaths from cervical cancer could easily be reduced by application of the vaccine—but this new technology raises questions and obstacles to care, along with offering care: First, there is no test available to tell if a woman has had any or all of these four HPV types. Second, the need to vaccinate women before they become sexually active raises ethical issues, particularly among populations that fear the vaccine will send a message condoning teenage sexual activity. Other issues revolve around who should advertise and promote the vaccine, how it should be promoted in developing nations, and whether parents who resist vaccination should be held liable for their children's sexual health. These and a host of other issues demonstrate how medical advances complicate cancer epidemiology as well as offering hope.

Sociocultural issues: A sensitive issue regarding cancer screening relates to the fact that cancer prevention and control efforts center on the development of strategies to benefit the general population rather than individual lives. As new knowledge and technologies have proliferated at unprecedented rates, many ethical questions—such as fair and equitable allocation of health resources across diverse populations, the priority of individual needs versus those of the social aggregate, and the unfair distribution of resources to privileged groups—have come under considerable scrutiny. Some of these issues have become especially poignant as genetic technologies have identified specific ethnic factors to enhance the risk for certain cancers. The incidence increases fiftyfold in whites and thirty-fold in African Americans between the ages of fifty and eighty-five. African Americans have the highest incidence of prostate cancer in the world, whereas Japanese have one of the lowest rates. Japanese who migrate to Hawaii develop a risk for prostate cancer higher than that of Japanese who remain in their home country, but only half that of American whites. African American men tend to have metastatic disease at diagnosis—indeed, 40 percent more often than whites do. The overall survival rate for African American men is 10 percent lower than that for white men, even when they are diagnosed at the same stage of disease. Endometrial carcinoma is the most common gynecologic malignancy. Its incidence is highest among white women, whereas its mortality rates are higher among African American women. For the past two decades, the incidence rates have been declining, except among African American women over fifty years old. Cultural, psychosocial, and demographic factors may discourage the use of genetic testing services among individuals who could benefit from them or, conversely, may promote use when testing has the potential to create more harm than benefit.

To develop effective cancer detection and prevention programs, therefore, it is essential to consider cultural, demographic, and psychosocial issues that may foster or hinder utilization. Consumer lead advocacy groups have taken a grassroots approach to soliciting research dollars to fund basic and clinical research programs. That fact alone may skew inquiry toward those cultural, ethnic, and socioeconomic subgroups who value and can interpret results of medical research and who have sufficient personal resources to advocate on their own behalf. Lack of interest in genetic testing has been associated with less education, minority status, lower socioeconomic status, and less performance of other health-promoting behaviors.

Culture plays a central role in determining health beliefs, attitudes, and behavior, but few health care providers realize that health is a cultural concept defined differently across cultures. Many are unaware that the health care system is culturally designed and administered largely according to mainstream values. In genetics, cultural consideration is particularly important. Although knowledge that certain diseases run in families spans all societies, beliefs about causation of familial diseases vary considerably. Cultural attitudes toward disease also differ among ethnic populations. Moreover, culture comes into play in provider-client interaction and communication, which are both key components of genetic counseling. People from cultures that expect authority figures to be directive may find nondirective genetic counseling confusing and bewildering. Between 1970 and 1990, the minority population grew at a rate about three times that of the total population. The U.S. Census Bureau projects that minorities will account for about one-third of the U.S. population by the year 2010. Given these trends, attention to ethnocultural barriers is paramount in achieving universal access to genetic services.

Although cultural competency is not a licensing requirement for health professionals, it is vital in view of the sensitive nature of the issues to be discussed and the need for privacy and confidentiality of information exchanged. The professional genetics community includes few minorities, despite demographic trends—further limiting the access of minorities to culturally sensitive and relevant genetic services. This lack of input from minority communities also limits the shaping of public policy and planning of genetic research and counseling in ways meaningful to ethnic minorities.

For individuals to benefit from genetic services, those services must be available, culturally appropriate, accessible, and affordable. Unless such issues are addressed, any attempt to broaden access to genetic services will be limited and perhaps even hazardous to a less informed population. Few primary care providers are ready to take on these new tasks. They need education in understanding not only the scientific advances in genetics but also their ethical, legal, cultural, and psychosocial implications.

Inadequate appropriations to develop the needed service infrastructure have resulted in an inadequate number of genetic specialists, primary care providers, and public health providers prepared to incorporate genetics into practice. Among primary care providers, inadequate preparation in genetics is compounded by the severe time constraints imposed on virtually all service providers and by a lack of reimbursement for cognitive services.

Most consumers also have low scientific literacy and know little about basic genetics or genetic testing. Without a degree of genetics literacy and an understanding of the limitations and risks involved including insurance and employment discrimination, psychological trauma, intrafamilial conflict, and social stigmatization, people cannot make truly informed decisions.

Chemoprevention: A relatively new approach to cancer prevention is through chemoprevention (as opposed to chemotherapy, or drug treatment, following a cancer diagnosis). Cancer chemoprevention is defined as the reversal of carcinogenesis in the premalignant phase. The observation that retinoids, acting as modulators of cell differentiation, are effective in suppressing oral carcinogenesis and, therefore, in preventing second primary tumors in squamous cell carcinoma of the head and neck has led to the evaluation of these agents as chemopreventive therapy for tumors of the upper aerodigestive tract in high-risk populations. Studies of adjuvant hormonal therapy with tamoxifen for breast cancer have shown a 50 percent reduction of contralateral disease, which led to a national tamoxifen chemoprevention trial to evaluate risk reduction for primary breast cancer in women at high risk. With the development of new molecular techniques, chemoprevention trials will be aided by the identification of markers for premalignant lesions.

Prognosis for cancer epidemiology: Decision making regarding genetic susceptibility testing, health surveillance, chemoprevention and preventative surgery are being quickly added to the realm of health care options without adequate knowledge among professionals and the public regarding the meaning and practical relevance of this information. Psychosocial, cultural, and economic factors may affect the study, dissemination, and utilization of genetic discoveries to create service barriers and widen the gap between the haves and have nots among health care consumers. Genetic information is received against a backdrop of deeply held personal beliefs. The influence of culture on health beliefs and actions is enormous, and the role that culture, ethnicity, and religion play in formulating an individual's motivation toward health-seeking behaviors must be addressed in all educational and clinical activities.

Jeannie V. Pasacreta, Ph.D., A.P.R.N.

For Further Information

Centers for Disease Control. *U.S. Cancer Statistics: 2004 Incidence and Mortality*. Washington, D.C.: Author, 2004.

Dennis, Leslie K., and Deborah Dawson. "Meta-analysis of Measures of Sexual Activity and Prostate Cancer." *Epidemiology* 13, no. 1 (January, 2002): 72-79.

Gandini, S., H. Merzenich, C. Robertson, and P. Boyle. "Meta-analysis of Studies on Breast Cancer Risk and Diet: The Role of Fruit and Vegetable Consumption and the Intake of Associated Micronutrients." *European Journal of Cancer* 36 (March, 1990).

Green, Lawrence W., and Marshall W. Kreuter. *Health Promotion Planning: An Educational and Ecological Approach*. 3d ed. Mountain View, Calif.: Mayfield, 1999.

Little, Jullian. *Epidemiology of Childhood Cancer*. IARC Scientific Publications 149. Lyon, France: International Agency for Research on Cancer, 1999.

Moolgavkar, S., et al., eds. *Quantitative Estimation and Prediction of Human Cancer Risks*. IARC Scientific Publications 131. Lyon, France: International Agency for Research on Cancer.

Other Resources

Centers for Disease Control and Prevention
National Program of Cancer Registries
http://www.cdc.gov/cancer/npcr

National Cancer Institute
Cancer Clusters
http://www.cancer.gov/cancertopics/factsheet/risk/clusters

North American Association of Central Cancer Registries
http://www.naaccr.org

See also: African Americans and cancer; Africans and cancer; Ashkenazi Jews and cancer; Asian Americans and cancer; Cancer clusters; Childhood cancers; Elderly and cancer; Ethnicity and cancer; Family history and risk assessment; Geography and cancer; Latinos/Hispanics and cancer; Native North Americans and cancer; Occupational exposures and cancer; Poverty and cancer; Singlehood and cancer; Statistics of cancer; Survival rates; Young adult cancers

▶ Estrogen Receptor Downregulator (ERD)

Category: Cancer Biology; Chemotherapy and Other Drugs

ATC code: 102BA03

Definition: Estrogen receptor downregulator (ERD) is a compound that prevents the action of estrogen by attenuation of estrogen-receptor-mediated transcription and suppression of estrogen-dependent gene expression. The only known ERD is fulvestrant (Faslodex), which is described as "pure" ER antagonist, as it lacks the agonistic effects exhibited by other estrogen receptor modulators.

Subclasses of this drug group are antiestrogens and selective estrogen receptor modulators (SERMs), the latter of which also downregulate the estrogen receptor but are selective in their antagonistic action.

Cancers treated or prevented: Breast cancer

Delivery routes: Intraperitoneal injection

How this drug works: Estrogen is the female hormone that is mainly secreted in the ovaries and acts on female organs such as the breasts and uterus. Estrogen is responsible for activating the endothelial cells of the uterus during menstrual cycles. It performs its function by binding with specific receptors, called estrogen receptors (ER), that are present in various parts of the body. This binding is critical in inducing conformational changes of the ER protein, resulting in induction of expression in associated genes, ultimately leading to proliferation of endothelial cells. In cancer patients, proliferation of cancerous cells is triggered by estrogen binding to ER. Preventing estrogen from binding to its receptor is therefore a viable pharmacological strategy in cancer research.

The estrogen receptor downregulator fulvestrant is a steroidal analog of the hormone 17β-estradiol. Fulvestrant was approved by the Food and Drug Administration (FDA) in 2002 for treating cancer. It binds to estrogen receptors and blocks downstream processes such as receptor dimerization, leading to blockade of induction of gene expression. Fulvestrant also expedites degradation of ER protein, resulting in drastic downregulation of ER levels. Estrogen cannot exert its proliferative action in the absence of ER, and thus the progression and spread of cancer can be controlled by fulvestrant treatment.

Fulvestrant is administered to postmenopausal women whose cancer has metastasized and does not respond to traditional medications, such as the classic antiestrogen tamoxifen. Fulvestrant has about a hundredfold higher affinity for ER than tamoxifen and, unlike tamoxifen, does not have any agonistic effects on ER. Tamoxifen prevents proliferation of cells in the breast but acts like estrogen and exerts agonistic effects in the uterus. Clinical trials using fulvestrant have shown decelerated cancer growth and delayed recurrence rates. Using fulvestrant in combination therapy for cancer is now considered a treatment option.

Side effects: The side effects of fulvestrant are nausea, vomiting, constipation, diarrhea, abdominal pain and hot flashes.

Geetha Yadav, Ph.D.

See also: Antiestrogens; Breast cancers; Estrogen-receptorsensitive breast cancer; Hormonal therapies; Hormone receptor tests; Hormone replacement therapy (HRT); Phytoestrogens; Progesterone receptor assay; Receptor analysis

▶ Exosomes

Category: Cancer Biology

Definition: Exosomes are the smallest known extracellular, membrane-bound vesicles released by cells. Found in almost all biological fluids, they play integral roles in cell-cell communication.

Exosome formation: Cells are delimited by a two-layered sheet of specialized lipids known as the cell or plasma membrane into which cholesterol, proteins, and other molecules are embedded. The endosomal sorting complexes required for transport (ESCRT) machinery enables cells to internalize small patches of their plasma membranes to form small, internal, membrane-bound spheres (vesicles) known as "endosomes." Endosomes can utilize the ESCRT machinery to internalize small portions of their membranes to form smaller vesicles within the original vesicle. Cells can fill these intracellular structures, known as "multivesicular bodies" or "multivesicular endosomes" (MVEs), with nucleic acids, proteins, and other molecules. Fusion of MVEs with the plasma membrane releases their internal vesicles into environment, where they are known as "extracellular vesicles" (EVs). Exosomes are the smallest identified EVs, ranging in size from 10 to100 nanometers in diameter.

Exosome function: Exosomes mediate intercellular communication. They can fuse with the plasma membranes of neighboring or distant cells, and transfer lipids, proteins, and nucleic acids (mainly RNAs) between them.

Many different cell types release exosomes, and they use them to affect the behavior of other cells or modify their surrounding microenvironment. In the immune system, antigen-presenting cells show foreign substances or "antigens" to immune cells in order to sensitize them to the antigen and stimulate them to act against it. Exosomes from antigen-presenting cells known as dendritic cells can regulate the activity of other immune cells. However, in the thymus, where developing immune cells, in particular T-cells, that attack the body's own proteins are deleted, exosomes from the cells that line the inner cavities of the thymus (thymic epithelial cells) transfer proteins to thymic dendritic cells. Thymic dendritic cells use these exosomal components to determine if a developing T-cell will attack our own proteins and cells, and should be killed. These represent but a few of the many roles of exosomes in biological systems.

Exosomes and cancer cells: Tumor cells actively release exosomes into their surroundings, and there is even a correlation between the concentration of tumor-derived exosomes in the blood of cancer patients and the aggressiveness of their cancers.

Cancer cells use exosomes to enhance the proliferation, malignancy, and invasiveness of other cancer cells, and to transfer drug resistance. For example, exosomes released by metastatic breast cancer and melanoma tumor cells can transfer their metastatic potential to nonmetastatic or poorly metastatic tumor cells, respectively. Also, exosomes from the drug-resistant cancer line MCR-7 can confer drug resistance upon drug-sensitive cells.

Alternatively cancer cells can use exosomes to signal to support cells, or tumor-associated stroma cells (TASCs), that surround tumors. TASCs include fibroblasts, inflammatory cells, and endothelial cells, which form the walls of blood vessels. Cancer cell exosomes can modify the behavior of TASCs in profound ways to aid tumor progression and metastasis. For example, several different types of cancers secrete exosomes that induce stromal endothelial cells to form new blood vessels. Since tumors require a blood supply for their ample expansion, the formation of new blood vessels (neoangiogenesis) is an integral step for tumor growth and spread.

Tumors can also deploy their exosomes to convert TASCs into tumor-enhancing cells that augment the growth, survival, and malignancy of the cancer. Exosomes from chronic myelogenous leukemia cells stimulate bone marrow stromal cells to make a small protein called interleukin-8, which promotes the survival of the cancer cells, their adhesion to stromal cells, and cancer cell migration.

Tumor-derived exosomes can also recruit nearby cells to enhance their invasiveness. Tumor cells often degrade the surrounding matrices that keep them in one place by secreting matrix-destroying enzymes. However, exosomes from gastrointestinal tumors engineer the nearby smooth muscle cells to secrete matrix-destroying enzymes, which allow the tumor cells to break free of their original location and spread to other parts of the body.

Cancer cell-derived exosomes also help cancers escape the immune response against the tumor. Exosomes from a variety of cancer cells decrease the activity of cancer-killing natural killer cells, and inhibit the maturation of the antigen-presenting dendritic cells that are required to sensitize the immune system to the cancer. Such exosomes also expand regulatory T-cell populations that staunch the immune response in general.

Testing and treatment: Several different exosomal components have been identified as potentially useful biomarkers for specific cancers. Because exosomes are released into bodily fluids and are relatively easily isolated, stored, processed, and in many cases, provide unique molecular signatures for many cancers, they represent a convenient diagnostic tool for identifying several distinct types of cancers.

Exosomes may provide a way to treat cancer patients or even vaccinate people against particular cancers. They have a unique ability to target specific tissues of the body and deliver a wide variety of specific molecules to tissues, and can even cross the blood-brain barrier and target brain tissue.

Delivering cancer-specific molecules to antigen-presenting cells by means of exosomes can prime the immune system against specific cancers and vaccinate the patients. Likewise, exosomes loaded with specific molecules can activate immune cells against already-existing cancers.

History: Bin-Tao Pan and Rose Johnstone first discovered exosomes in 1983 when they reported that immature sheep red blood cells released the receptor for transferrin (a blood iron-binding protein) in small extracellular vesicles as they matured. Johnstone called these vesicles exosomes in 1989, and regarded them as cellular waste disposal units. Then in 1996, Graça Raposo and others showed that antibody-secreting B lymphocytes secreted exosomes, and two years later, antigen-presenting dendritic cells were found to also release exosomes. Since then, exosomes have been shown to be secreted by a wide variety of cells types and mediate a wide range of biological processes.

Michael Buratovich, PhD

For Further Information

Neviani, P. & Fabbri, M. (2015). "Exosomic microRNAs in the tumor microenvironment." *Frontiers in Medicine* 2(47). doi: 10.3389/fmed.2015.00047.

Tang, Y., & Dawn, D. (2015). *Mesenchymal Stem Cell Derived Exosomes: The Potential for Translational Nanomedicine*. Salt Lake City, UT: Academic Press.

Ter-Ovanesyan, D. (2011). Exosomes: The little vesicles that could. *Boston Biotech Watch*,

Retrieved from http://bostonbiotechwatch.com/2011/04/20/exosomes-the-little-vesicles-that-could.

Wood, M. J. A. (2015). *Exosome Biology and Therapeutics*. Hoboken, New Jersey, Wiley-Blackwell.

Other Resources

ExoCarta database
http://www.exocarta.org

Exosome RNA
http://www.exosome-rna.com

▶ Genetics of cancer

Category: Cancer Biology

Definition: Genetics of cancer can be defined as the study of heredity and variation in the development of cancer.

Description: Inheritance of characters or traits occurs through basic units of heredity called genes. Each human cell consists of twenty-three pairs of chromosomes containing genes inherited from both biological parents. Twenty-two pairs are called autosomes and one pair are the sex chromosomes. Some genes come in forms (alleles) that are dominant, requiring only one copy to exert their effects, while others are recessive, requiring both autosomal copies to be in place to exert their effects. Aberrations in chromosomes on the whole or mutations in specific genes without chromosomal modifications can lead to cancer development. However, only about 5 to 10 percent of cancers are attributed to heredity. Most cancers are acquired during the course of a person's life, primarily because of changes (called mutations) that occur in normal genes. Exposure to chemicals (for example, in smoking) and radiation (emitted by various sources, including the sun) poses a high probability of inducing mutations in genes. Chromosomal aberrations such as deletion of an entire chromosome, multiplication of certain chromosomes, or translocation of certain parts of chromosomes are probable causative agents for cancer.

A normal cell gets transformed into a malignant cancer cell in a multistep process and as a consequence of a series of events leading to modifications in many of its genes. These changes primarily enable normal cells to acquire uncontrolled growth potential, resulting in the formation of tumors. Tumor development culminates in metastasis, a process in which cancerous cells travel through blood vessels and invade other organs of the body. Genetic changes suggested as hallmarks of cancer include the following:

- Self-sustained growth that is independent of availability of external growth factors
- Resistance to signals controlling cell growth and proliferation
- Methods to evade mechanisms of the programmed cell death pathway (apoptosis)
- Uncontrolled capacity to replicate
- Sustained capability to produce new blood vessels (angiogenesis) required for growth and survival of tumors and resistance to antiangiogenesis factors
- Capability to overcome stringent physiological barriers and get transported to other regions of the body and spread (metastasis)

Broadly, these properties can be encompassed within three categories of gene mutations: mutations occurring in proto-oncogenes, mutations of tumor-suppressor genes, and mutations in deoxyribonucleic acid (DNA) repair genes.

Mutations of proto-oncogenes: Proto-oncogenes are genes that are responsible and required for normal growth and development. Normal growth and development are

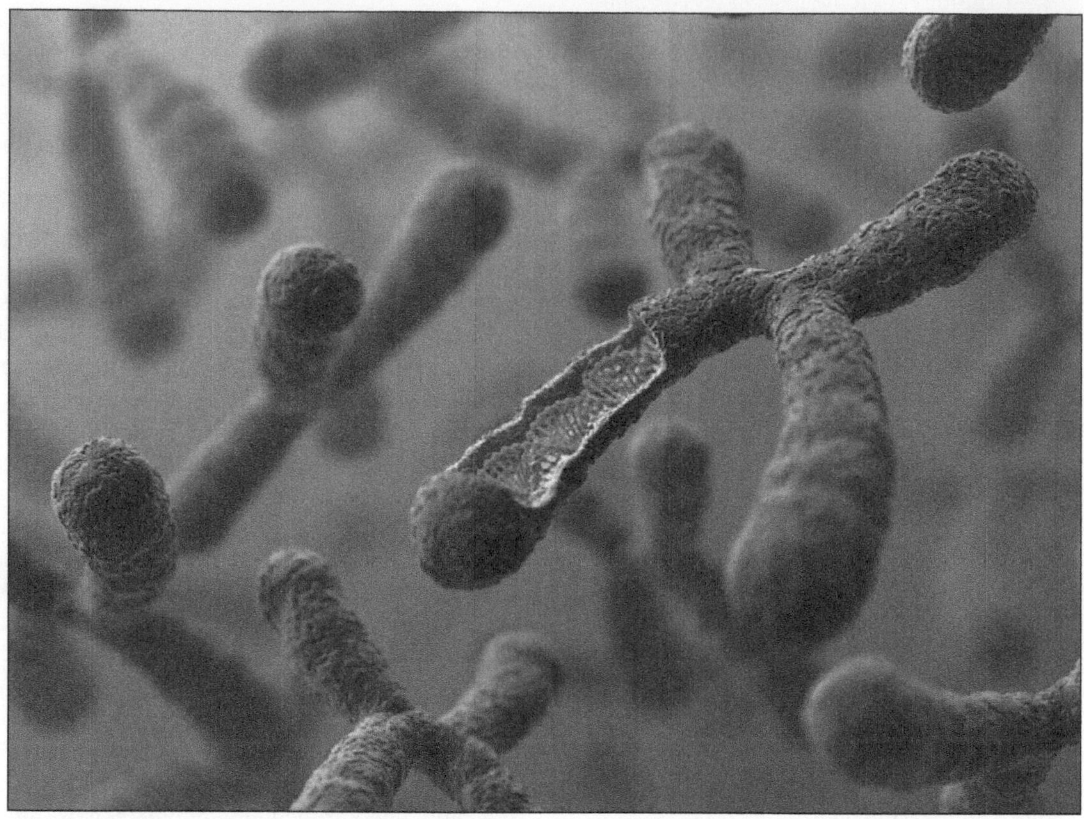

Chromosome with DNA strand. (iStock)

complex physiological processes that require activation of a number of genes. These gene activations are made possible by signal transduction mechanisms that are inherent in cells. Signal transduction is a process whereby a signal received by the cell from its external environment is processed and transduced to the internal milieu, resulting in activation of a variety of genes. Physiological processes such as cell division and proliferation are initiated by many signal transduction pathways.

Of the approximately 30,000 genes that have been mapped in the human genome, nearly 100 have been identified as proto-oncogenes. Mutated or damaged proto-oncogenes are called oncogenes. Presence of oncogenes in cells has been directly correlated with development of most types of cancers. A wide array of genes has been identified as oncogenes in humans. These genes are called gain-of-function genes, as they gain the capacity to induce tumor development as a result of mutations. They become hyperactivated in the mutated state and, consequently, initiate multitudes of cell signal transduction pathways, ultimately resulting in uncontrolled cell division and growth.

The mitogen-activated protein kinase (MAPK) pathway is one such signal transduction pathway that has been implicated in most cancers. Mutations occurring in genes involved in this signal transduction cascade impede communication within and between cells. This results in abnormal growth and ultimately tumor development. Specific examples include the RAS and BRAF gene families. About 25 percent of all cancers have recorded some kind of mutation in RAS family members. The MAPK signal transduction cascade is initiated by the activation of cell-surface receptors such as tyrosine kinase and epidermal growth factors that traverse cell membranes. Inhibitors of receptor activation are being tested as possible therapeutic agents for cancer.

Mutations of tumor-suppressor genes: Tumor-suppressor genes are a class of genes whose protein products control cell division and death. Most often, the protein products of these genes act directly on cells and usher them toward the so-called "suicidal" or apoptotic pathway. In cancer cells, such an entry into the apoptotic pathway is rendered impossible because of mutations in tumor-suppressor genes. Tumor-suppressor genes are called loss-of-function genes because mutations in these genes result in the loss of their normal tumor suppression function. It is noteworthy that these genes belong to the recessive class of genes. The significance of this is that a single copy of a normal tumor-suppressor gene is enough to exert a beneficial effect. Mutations in both copies of the genes could result from hereditary factors, environmental factors, or aging. Most tumor developments document mutations in tumor-suppressor genes.

A classic example of a tumor-suppressor gene is TP53. A majority of the cancers reported in human cells exhibit either an abundance of abnormal TP53 genes or the absence of normal TP53 genes and signaling pathways. There is also overwhelming evidence that mutant TP53 protein acquires novel oncogenic traits that provide a favorable environment for development, sustenance, and resistance of tumor cells. Replacement of the normal, wild-type TP53 gene using a retroviral TP53 expression vector is an attempted method of controlling cancer cell growth in gene therapy. In addition to the TP53 gene, its homologs TP73 and TP63 have also been identified in the induction of cancer.

Mutations in DNA-repair genes: Exposure to certain types of radiation such as ultraviolet (UV) light can induce damage in DNA. Cells have evolved normal repair mechanisms that can detect and correct such damage through specific genes called DNA-repair genes. Therefore, most mistakes usually go unnoticed. However, when mutations occur in DNA-repair genes, damaged and malfunctioning DNA accumulates in cells, interfering with normal processes and inducing tumor development. Mistakes occurring in genes such as tumor-suppressor genes, if not repaired in time, can lead to cancer formation. DNA-repair genes are recessive genes. Therefore, for visible effects to occur it is imperative to have mutations in both copies of the gene. Examples for this category of mutations are observed in the skin cancer condition xeroderma pigmentosum, as well as in some forms of colon cancer. In these colon cancers, DNA-repair genes MLH1 and MSH2, located on chromosomes 3 and 2, respectively, are mutated and damaged.

Chromosomal aberrations: Chromosomes have distinct sizes and characteristics, and accordingly, each chromosome has been designated a unique number and can be distinguished easily in modern karyotyping tests. Sometimes, for various reasons (including being fertilized by more than one sperm) cells can acquire an abnormal number of chromosomes (a condition called aneuploidy). In other cases, the number of chromosomes may not be different from the normal 46, but portions of chromosomes may be deleted, added, or translocated to a different chromosome. Some of these modifications could shuffle relevant genes, leading to cancer development. Chronic myeloid leukemia (CML) is a classic example of such a cancer. In this case, a small portion of genetic material from chromosome 22 is translocated to chromosome 9 and vice versa (a condition called reciprocal translocation). A consequence of this translocation is the transfer of a normal proto-oncogene called ABL1 from chromosome 9 to chromosome 22. Movement of ABL1 to chromosome 22 is responsible for its conversion to an oncogene and ultimately to malignancy. Other cancers resulting from a similar translocation between chromosomes 9 and 22 are acute lymphoblastic leukemia and adult acute myelogenous leukemia. Burkitt lymphoma, a B-lymphocyte malignancy most common in African children, is induced by translocation of genetic materials between chromosomes 8 and 14, resulting in activation of the oncogene MYC.

Heritability of cancer: Whether the incidence of cancer is caused by alterations of whole chromosomes or of specific genes, its inheritance is variable. In some cancers such as retinoblastoma, a childhood eye cancer, tumor development occurs only with deletions in both copies of chromosome 13. Children with deletion in one copy of the chromosome are at risk for the disease because every cell in these patients possesses this deletion. However, a second mutation, in the remaining complete copy of the chromosome, is required for disease development. Similar is the case of Wilms' tumor (a childhood kidney cancer condition) in which the abnormality in chromosome 11 is inherited in one copy, but a second mutation is necessary for tumor expression. Other kinds of cancers that have genetic predispositions include xeroderma pigmentosum, Paget disease of bone, ataxia telangiectasia, and Fanconi anemia.

There are several common examples of familial cancer syndromes that predispose subsequent generations of patients to cancers. Common examples are colon cancers, breast cancers, and prostate cancers. Colon cancers occur because of two kinds of hereditary conditions: familial adenomatous polyposis (FAP) and hereditary nonpolyposis colon cancer (HNPCC). FAP involves mutations of a tumor-suppressive gene called APC and interactions between TP53 and KRAS genes. HNPCC occurs as a result of mutations in MLH1 and MSH2 genes that are involved in DNA repair.

Approximately 80 percent of patients with familial early-onset breast and ovarian cancers exhibit mutations in a tumor-suppressor gene called BRCA1. This and another gene called BRCA2 are examples in which mutations have penetrated into the reproductive cells (germline mutations) and therefore are inherited, predisposing women to these cancers. Similarly, mutations in the gene HPC1 (hereditary prostate cancer 1), located on chromosome 1, are responsible for most familial cases of prostate cancer.

Epigenetics and cancer: Epigenetics can be defined as the study of those factors other than traditional DNA sequences that are inherited during cell division. These can be monogenic (involving a single gene) or multigenic (involving multiple genes). The prefix "epi," which is of Greek origin, means "upon," "near," "outside of," "before," or "after." Epigenetic factors affect DNA transcription, but do not involve changes in the nucleotide sequence of the genome. Therefore, epigenetic alterations may or may not be heritable. Epigenetic factors include modifications of histone proteins, such as histone deacetylation and acetylation, and histone demethylation and methylation. Histone methylation changes, for example, may decrease the activity of tumor suppressor genes and cancer regulatory genes and significantly contribute to the development of cancerous changes. Considerable attention is therefore being focused on epigenetic aspects of cancer development.

Progress and perspectives: Progress in discovering, analyzing, and profiling genetic determinants of cancer has been excellent. Advances in molecular biological techniques and the cracking of the human genome have enabled forays into various aspects of cancer. Techniques such as array comparative genomic hybridization (aCGH), which can measure DNA copy number alterations (CANs), are important contributions toward correlating genetic factors with human diseases. The advent of therapeutic strategies such as gene therapy has advanced researchers' ability to overcome various impediments posed by traditional treatment strategies. Proteins involved with epigenetic regulation of genes provide fertile ground for the development of effective cancer treatments. Current epigenetic cancer treatments include DNA methyltransferase inhibitors and histone deacetylase inhibitors, along with continued research and development regarding the modification of epigenetic factors contributing to cancer.

Previously unimaginable approaches, such as introduction of a supernumerary artificial chromosome with relevant beneficial genes to cure cancer and other diseases, have begun to be attempted. However, because of its ability to alter genes, which are the basic units of heredity and variation, gene therapy encounters multitudes of social and ethical concerns. Similarly, other benefits offered by diagnostic tools such as genetic testing should be handled with caution. Statistics show that only about 5 percent of cancers are inherited or due to heredity; therefore, being aware of and cautious about various risk factors (such as carcinogens and viruses) remains the recommended way of preventing cancer.

Geetha Yadav, Ph.D.

Updated by: Richard P. Capriccioso, M.D.

For Further Information

Albini A, & Tímár J. (2010). Genomics of metastatic progression. Clinical and Experimental Metastasis, 27(6):453. http://www.ncbi.nlm.nih.gov/pubmed/20711639

Coghlin C, & Murray GI. (2014). The role of gene regulatory networks in promoting cancer progression and metastasis. Future Oncology, 10(5): 735-48. http://www.ncbi.nlm.nih.gov/pubmed/24799055

Hanahan, D., & Weinberg, R. A. (2011). Hallmarks of cancer: The next generation. Cell, 144(5): 646–674.

McKinnell, G. R., Parchment, R. E., Perantoni, A. O. Barry Pierce, G., & Damjanov, I. (Eds.). (2006). The biological basis of cancer (2nd ed.). New York: Cambridge University Press.. http://www.cambridge.org/us/academic/subjects/life-sciences/cell-biology-and-developmental-biology/biological-basis-cancer-2nd-edition?format=AR. ISBN-13: 000-0521606330

Nguyen, D. X., & Massague, J. (2007). Genetic determinants of cancer metastasis. *Nature Reviews (Genetics)*, 8: 341-352. http://www.ncbi.nlm.nih.gov/pubmed/17440531.

Vanharanta S, & Massagué J. (2013). Origins of metastatic traits. *Cancer Cell*, 24(4):410-21. http://www.ncbi.nlm.nih.gov/pubmed/24135279

Other Resources

Cancer Genetics Web
http://www.cancerindex.org/geneweb

Centers for Disease Control and Prevention
National Office of Public Health Genomics.
http://www.cdc.gov/genomics

Genetics Home Reference
http://ghr.nlm.nih.gov

Human Genome Project Information
http://web.ornl.gov/sci/techresources/Human_Genome/index.shtml

National Cancer Institute
Cancer Genetics.
http://www.cancer.gov/cancertopics/prevention-genetics-causes/genetics

See also: APC gene testing; BRAF gene; BRCA1 and BRCA2 genes; Cancer biology; Childhood cancers; Chromosomes and cancer; Cytogenetics; DPC4 gene testing; Family history and risk assessment; Gene therapy; Genetic testing; Hereditary cancer syndromes; HRAS gene testing; Mitochondrial DNA mutations; MLH1 gene; MSH genes; MYC oncogene; Oncogenes; PMS genes; Proteomics and cancer research; Proto-oncogenes and carcinogenesis; RB1 gene; RhoGD12 gene; SCLC1 gene; TP53 protein; Tumor markers; Tumor-suppressor genes

▶ Genomics of cancer

Category: Cancer Biology
Also known as: Cancer Genetics, Genes and Cancer

Definition: Changes in genes that affect the development, progression, and treatment response of cancers.

Etiology and symptoms of associated cancers: Changes in a person's genes can affect his or her risk of developing certain cancers. These changes cause a normal cell to transform into a cancer cell, ie, one that divides and grows abnormally.

Gene changes that lead to cancer usually occur in 1of 2 types of genes: proto-oncogenes and tumor suppressor genes. Proto-oncogenes are normal genes that include growth factors, growth factor receptors, transcription factors, and proteins that control steps in the cell cycle. Mutations in proto-oncogenes change the genes into oncogenes (eg, *RAS* and *RAF* gene families) that cause the cell to divide and grow uncontrollably. Besides mutations, chromosomal translocations can cause a piece of DNA from 1 chromosome to be moved next to an oncogene on a different chromosome in such a way that the oncogene is activated. A well-known example is the *BCR-ABL* fusion gene in chronic myelogenous leukemia, whereby the *ABL* kinase gene is placed next to the *BCR* gene by translocation, causing *ABL* to be always turned on. This leads to increased cell division and cancer.

Tumor suppressor genes, such as the tumor protein 53 (*TP53*) and retinoblastoma (*RB*) genes, normally keep cell growth and division in check. Mutations in these genes remove these checks, allowing the cells to divide and grow uncontrollably. Mutations in the *TP53* gene are involved in a wide variety of cancers.

There are 2 main types of gene changes that affect cancer development: 1) so-called "germline" mutations present in the genes of the egg or sperm that are inherited from 1 generation to the next; and 2) mutations and other changes in somatic genes (any other gene besides those in egg and sperm).

Inherited cancers, which are caused by inherited gene changes, tend to manifest at a younger age than acquired cancers. Arguably the most well-known of the inherited cancer gene mutations are in the *BRCA1* and *BRCA2* genes. Inheriting one of these mutations considerably increases a woman's risk of developing breast and ovarian cancer. According to the National Cancer Institute, a woman's risk of developing breast cancer by age 70 increases from 12% to 55–65% if she has a loss-of-function mutation in the *BRCA1* gene–a 5-six-fold increase. The risk increases by 4-fold if the woman has a harmful mutation in the *BRCA2* gene. Having a harmful mutation in 1 of these genes also greatly increases a woman's risk of developing ovarian cancer by age 70: a *BRCA1* gene mutation is associated with a 30-fold increased risk, while a *BRCA2* gene mutation is associated with a 9–13–fold increased risk.

The effects of inherited cancer mutations are especially striking in Lynch syndrome, an inherited condition that predisposes individuals in a family for many cancers. These include colorectal, uterine, stomach, ovarian, small intestinal, pancreatic, urinary tract, kidney, bile duct, and brain cancers, as well as some skin cancers. Doctors will suspect Lynch syndrome if colorectal cancer has affected several members of the same family, and especially if it manifests at a younger age than in the general population. Lynch syndrome families typically have mutations in one or more of the following genes: *MLH1*, *MSH2*, *MSH6*, *PMS2*, and *EPCAM*, although mutations in *MLH1* and *MSH2* are especially common in the syndrome.

Other inherited cancers include familial adenomatous polyposis, juvenile polyposis, and von Hippel-Lindau disease.

Mutations in somatic genes make up the remainder (and majority) of cancer mutations. These mutations are not inherited from 1 generation to the next, but are acquired by cells over time. Somatic mutations may be caused by environmental factors such as cigarette smoke, radiation, and diet, or may occur spontaneously. These mutations can affect how cancer progresses in an individual and also how well the person responds to specific treatments. For example, patients with acute myeloid leukemia (AML) who have certain mutations in the *FLT3* gene are more likely to have more severe disease and a poorer prognosis compared with AML patients lacking these mutations (wild-type AML). Patients with AML who have mutations in the *NPM1* and *CEBPA* genes, on the other hand, tend to have a better prognosis than do wild-type AML patients.

Not all mutations result in cancer. Mutations that always lead to cancer are said to have complete penetrance. Most inherited mutations only cause cancer if both copies of the gene are mutated or other factors are present. These mutations are considered to have incomplete penetrance. In addition, some mutations (high-penetrance mutations) dramatically change the function of a gene to cause disease, while others (low-penetrance mutations) only slightly alter the gene function and may not cause disease in and of themselves. They may instead increase the risk for developing certain types of cancer. Another type of gene change, gene variants, may also be associated with an increased risk for cancer. These variants could involve changes as small as alterations to a single nucleotide in a gene.

The gene changes described so far are all ones that affect the gene sequence, ie, the sequence of nucleotides that make up a particular gene. Besides these changes, epigenetic changes (eg, to the methylation state of the DNA and modifications to histones around which the DNA is spooled) can also play a role in the development of cancer. Generally speaking, the DNA in a gene needs to be demethylated and the histones need to be deacetylated for the gene to be expressed. In cancer, drugs that control DNA methylation and histone acetylation are used to regulate the expression of cancer genes and stop the cancer transformation process.

Testing and treatment: Individuals who are at risk for inherited cancers can be tested for specific germline mutations by gene sequencing. Some indicators that these individuals may be at higher risk include a family history of specific cancers, having a relative with at least 2 different types of cancer, and having 2 or more relatives who developed cancer at an early age.

For example, if an individual has Lynch syndrome, his or her blood will be tested to identify the specific Lynch syndrome-associated mutations present. His or her family members would likely be tested for these mutations as well. Should a family member test positive for 1 or more of the mutations associated with Lynch syndrome, he or she would have an increased risk for developing colorectal and other cancers. Doctors may recommend genetic counseling and preventive measures. At the end of 2014, the Food and Drug Administration approved olaparib (Lynparza®), an inhibitor of the PARP enzyme, to treat breast cancer with a mutation in either the *BRCA1* or *BRCA2* gene. Olaparib appears to be especially useful in preventing ovarian cancer recurrence in women with a *BRCA* gene mutation.

Patients who have received a cancer diagnosis but do not have inherited cancers could still be tested for somatic mutations. Such mutations can be identified by analyzing the tumor material. Instead of treating all patients with the same type of cancer in the same way, treatment can be tailored or personalized according to the specific cancer mutations. Theoretically, this personalized approach should lead to more effective treatments, better outcomes, and fewer adverse effects.

For example, AML patients may be classified according to the types of somatic mutations they possess. Patients within each group could benefit from a specific type of treatment that is effective for the particular mutation. For example, *NPM1* and *CEBPA* mutations are associated with a less severe form of AML, which could respond to less intense treatment. On the other hand, certain mutations in the *FLT3* gene are associated with more severe disease and a poorer prognosis. Patients with these types of mutations would probably need more intense treatment such as stem cell transplantation. Classifying patients and tailoring treatments by class could result in AML patients with *NPM1* and *CEBPA* mutations being successfully treated with fewer side effects.

In breast cancer, some patients have mutations in the *HER2/neu* gene (which produces the HER2 protein) and are known as HER2-positive. Although HER2-positive patients have a more aggressive type of breast cancer than HER2-negative patients, they can be treated with the drugs trastuzumab (Herceptin®), lapatinib (Tykerb®), pertuzumab (Perjeta®), or Ado-trastuzumab emtansine (Kadcyla®), with relatively good outcomes. For this reason, breast cancer patients are usually tested for *HER2/neu* mutations to determine whether they would be good candidates for these drugs. Tests include those that assess the gene directly or those that evaluate the protein produced by the gene. In HER2-positive breast cancer, the mutations cause multiple copies of the gene to be made. Thus, the tests determine whether too many copies of the gene are present, or whether too much of the HER2 protein is present. If the protein (immunohistochemistry) test is used, the amount of HER2 protein must be above a certain threshold for the patient to be classified as "HER2-positive" and be slated for HER2-targeting treatments.

Instead of being used to select patients for a specific treatment, some mutations are used to exclude patients from certain treatments. For example, patients with colorectal cancer who have mutations in the *KRAS* gene do not respond well to cetuximab (Erbitux®) and panitumumab (Vectibix®). Doctors would thus, choose different treatments for such patients.

History: In the early 1980s, J. Michael Bishop and Harold Varmus discovered the first oncogene in humans, *SRC*, through their work with retroviruses. The *SRC* oncogene comes from the Rous sarcoma virus. Similarly, the other oncogenes that were subsequently discovered were also identified in retroviruses from birds and rodents. These genes included the MYC, RAS, ERBB, and PI3K oncogenes. Discovery of these oncogenes was prompted by the observation that several mutant retroviruses caused host cells to transform into abnormally shaped cells.

Another gene was initially incorrectly classified as an oncogene, but later discovered to perform the opposite function—that of a tumor suppressor. In 1979, six independent groups of researchers reported the discovery of the TP53 gene. In the 1990s, researchers defined the role of p53, the protein coded for by *TP53*. They found that, in response to DNA damage, p53 either halted the cell cycle or induced cell death to prevent errors from becoming incorporated into the genome and being propagated in future cell generations.

Inherited cancer syndromes were known as far back as 1931, when Alfred Warthin described a family with a high incidence of stomach and uterine cancers. Lynch and Krush further characterized the inherited condition, now known as Lynch syndrome, in 1971. Since then, many other inherited cancers have been reported, including the inherited breast and ovarian cancer syndrome associated with the *BRCA1* and *BRCA2* gene mutations. The *BRCA1* and *BRCA2* mutations were discovered in 1994 and 1995, respectively.

For the remainder (and large majority) of cancers, the cancer-causing mutations are not inherited but are instead present in all other cells besides the egg and sperm. Scientists originally thought that the more of these somatic cancer mutations an individual acquired, the higher the risk of developing cancer. This meant that cancer risk would always increase with age. However, some cancers such as retinoblastoma typically strike in childhood. In 1971, Alfred Knudson proposed the "two-hit" hypothesis to explain the genetic cause of such cancers. The hypothesis suggests 2 possible paths to such cancers: 1) an individual has 1 inherited cancer mutation at conception, and acquires one somatic mutation after conception; and 2) an individual acquires 2 somatic mutations after conception. This hypothesis explains the development of several cancers caused by mutations in tumor suppressor genes, which are usually recessive. In contrast, oncogenes are usually dominant. Thus, only 1 mutant oncogene is needed for cancer to occur.

Although much progress has been made in the past several decades in unraveling the role of genes in cancer, many more cancer genes remain to be discovered and the genetic basis of many cancers have yet to be characterized. Discovering the genomic pathogenesis of more cancers will result in more accurate prognoses and more specific and effective treatments.

Ing Wei Khor, PhD

For Further Information

American Cancer Society. (2014). Genes and cancer. Retrieved from http://www.cancer.org/acs/groups/cid/documents/webcontent/002550-pdf.pdf

National Cancer Institute. (2015, April 1). BRCA1 and BRCA2: Cancer risk and genetic testing. Retrieved from http://www.cancer.gov/about-cancer/causes-prevention/genetics/brca-fact-sheet

American Society of Clinical Oncology. (n.d.) Retrieved from http://www.cancer.net/cancer-types/lynch-syndrome

Moynihan, T.J. (2015, March 25). HER2-positive breast cancer: What is it? Retrieved from http://www.mayoclinic.org/breast-cancer/expert-answers/faq-20058066

Vogt, P.K. (2012). Retroviral oncogenes: a historical primer. *Nature Reviews Cancer,* 12(9), 639-648. http://www.ncbi.nlm.nih.gov/pmc/articles/PMC3428493/

Other Resources

American Cancer Society
www.cancer.org

Genetic Testing for Cancer Risk. Cancer.Net
http://www.cancer.net/navigating-cancer-care/cancer-basics/genetics/genetic-testing-cancer-risk

See also: Oncogenes

▶ Histone acetylation/ deacetylation

Category: Cancer Biology
Also known as: Epigenetic regulation of genes

Definition: Cell DNA is not characterized as a naked molecule. Rather, it is filled with proteins that fold and compact it into chromatin. The level of DNA compaction is intermediate during most of the cell cycle; not reaching its maximum level until cell division takes place. The most structural unit of chromatin is the nucleosome, in which nearly 2 turns of DNA are looped around a spool of 8 histone proteins (these 8 proteins include 2 copies of histones H2A, H2B, H3, and H4). Chromatin is a highly dynamic entity. Its chromosomal regions fold/unfold and open/close as the genetic information encoded by DNA is transcribed into RNA (or "expressed" in the cell). While particular DNA sequences can influence chromatin structure, the main contributors to chromatin dynamics are covalent chemical modifications of either the DNA or the histones.

The term "epigenetics" is used to describe changes to genetic traits that are not brought about by accompanying changes in the DNA sequence. In histones, epigenetic changes are present as post-translational modifications (PTMs) that occur after a gene's messenger RNA has been translated into the protein encoded by the gene. All histones have a three-part structure consisting of 2 "tails" of highly extended polypeptide chains that protrude from a compact core made of a histone-fold motif. Histone tails are rich in positively charged amino acids such as lysine; especially the longer tail (of the 2) that is found in front of the core (the protein's N-terminus). These lysine residues in the N-terminal tail of the histones are the main targets for PTMs.

The addition of an acetyl group ($COCH_3$) to such lysines was one of the first PTMs to be characterized in histones. Enzymatic attachment of acetyl groups serves to neutralize the positive charges found on histone tails, thereby reducing its interaction with the negatively charged DNA molecule. In the cell, PTMs are fully reversible by enzymatic activity. Histone acetylation is generally associated with open chromatin conformations, while histone deacetylation is generally associated with closed conformations. Enzymes that acetylate histones are called histone acetyl-transferases (or HATs) while those that remove the acetyl group are called histone deacetylases (or HDACs). The former have been called epigenetic "writers," while the latter have been termed epigenetic "erasers." The full set of PTMs associated with histones has been referred to as the "histone code," in contrast to the genetic code found in DNA.

Etiology and symptoms of associated cancers: Many cancer cells have been found to bypass the cell's epigenetic controls on growth and proliferation by simply erasing it via an overexpression of HDACs. Hypo-acetylated histone H4 is a common hallmark of human cancer cells and an aberrant expression of individual HDACs is associated with a long list of diseases, including breast, colon, gastric, liver, lung, ovarian, pancreatic, prostrate, and renal cancers. In addition, HDAC overexpression is usually associated with a poor prognosis in many of the cases listed above. Abnormally high HDAC activity has been associated with cell proliferation, angiogenesis (the formation of new blood vessels to feed a tumor), and metastasis, as well as a loss of cell adhesion, differentiation, and apoptosis (programmed cell death).

Testing and treatment: Compounds that act as HDAC inhibitors (HDACis) have been developed to block the epigenetic erasers employed by certain cancer cells. HDACis function to induce proliferation arrest, differentiation, and apoptosis of cancer cells; while having significantly less effects on normal cells. Due to the widespread nature of histone acetylation/deacetylation, normal cells may be more apt to cope with such an "epigenetic insult" by engaging alternate compensation mechanisms. Meanwhile, cancer cells have become over-reliant on epigenetic pathways and are unable to adapt. This adaption inability has been termed "epigenetic vulnerability."

Unfortunately, patients still experience adverse effects from HDACi treatment due to the epigenetic gene regulation disrupting normal cells. Side effects include fatigue, vomiting, and diarrhea. However, HDACis are still considered to have low toxicity overall. They are often combined with other DNA-altering agents such as topoisomerase-inhibitors or cross-linking agents like cisplatin in order to induce the synergistic effects.

History: Histone acetylation was first characterized in the mid-1960s and by the early 1970s it was linked with cancer, along with other epigenetic markers. Around this same time, butyrate was the first compound described to have activity as an HDACi. Butyrate is present in the fermentation products of dietary fiber, leading to the possibility that a high-fiber diet protects against colon cancer. Following almost 4 decades of research with HDACis, several of these compounds (vorinostat, romidepsin, and belinostat) have recently been approved by the US Food and Drug Administration for use in the treatment of various T-cell lymphomas.

James S. Godde, PhD

For Further Information

Konstantinopoulos, P. A., Karamouzis, M. V., & Papavassiliou, A. G. (2007) Focus on acetylation: The role of histone deactylase inhibitors in cancer therapy and beyond. *Expert Opinion on Investigational Drugs,* 16(5): 569-571. Short and somewhat technical review of the promise of HDACis as anticancer treatments.

Li, Z., & Zhu, W. (2014). Targeting histone deacetylases for cancer therapy: From molecular mechanisms to clinical implications. *International Journal of Biological Sciences,* 10(7): 757-770. Technical but excellent description of how basic research can lead to clinical applications.

Parbin, S., Kar, S., Shilpi, A., Sengupta, D., Deb, M., Rath, S. K., & Patra, S. K. (2013). Histone deacetylases: A saga of perturbed acetylation homeostasis in cancer. *Journal of Histochemistry & Cytochemistry,* 62(1): 11-33. Readable summary of the consequences of inhibiting HDACs in cancer cells.

Other Resources

Cancer Quest, Emory University
Histone Acetylases (HATs) and Histone Deacetylases (HDACs).
http://www.cancerquest.org/hat-hdac-introduction.html
WhatIsEpigenetics.com, an epigenetics blog

Histone Modifications
http://www.whatisepigenetics.com/histone-modifications/

▶ Histone methylation/ demethylation

Category: Cancer Biology
Also known as: Gene regulation, gene transcription repression or activation, epigenetics

Definition: Deoxyribonucleic acid (DNA) stores genetic information in all cells. Nucleated cells bundle their DNA into a compact structures called chromatin (a molecular package of DNA and protein). Histone proteins, the primary protein component of chromatin, shape and organize DNA into 3- dimensional structures. Gene expression in chromatin-packaged DNA often requires the chemical modification of histones. One such histone-specific modification includes histone methylation (the transfer of methyl groups (— CH_3) to specific amino acids in histones) and demethylation (the removal of attached methyl groups). Histone methylation and other types of histone modifications constitute an aspect of epigenetics. Epigenetics consists of anything other than DNA sequences that influences the growth, development, and adaptation of organisms. Epigenetic factors deeply influence gene transcription (the synthesis of an RNA copy of a DNA template). Consequently, epigenetic mechanisms also play profound roles in the genesis and maintenance of cancer cells, and interfering with histone methylation and demethylation can disrupt the growth and survival of tumors.

Histone methylation and demethylation can profoundly affect gene regulation. Histone protein methylation targets 2 different positively charged amino acids: lysine and arginine. These amino acids are located in the amino terminus (front part) of histones. Depending on the site of modification, methylation or demethylation of these amino acids can either deactivate or activate gene transcription. Enzymes called histone methyltransferases (HMTs) transfer methyl groups from a co-factor known as S-adenosyl methionine to specific lysine and arginine residues in histones. Enzymes that remove methyl groups from histones are known as lysine-specific histone demethylases (KDMs).

Histone methylation (an epigenetic process) has important implications for cancer diagnosis, treatment, and potential cure. Epigenetic events influence tumor progression and the development of cancerous malignancies. Gradual epigenetic changes contribute to the progressive inhibition of genes that control cell growth. This results in tumor development and, eventually, malignancy.

Histone Methylation and Demethylation: Histone methylation is one of the mechanisms cells use to regulate transcription. Healthy cells use epigenetic modifications like histone methylation and demethylation for normal cellular function during development. For example, human females have 2 X chromosomes. One of them undergoes inactivation early in development and is assembled into very a tight chromatin structure known as heterochromatin. X chromosome heterochromatin-dependent inactivation depends upon precise patterns of methylation of the histone complexes assembled on the X chromosome DNA.

Specific types of histone methylation result in distinct effects on gene expression. For example, genes wrapped around histone complexes whose H3 histone protein is methylated on the 4th or 79th lysine residue tend to show increased transcriptional activation. Alternatively, genes wrapped around histone complexes that have either the 9th or 27th lysine of the histone H3 protein or the 20th lysine of histone H4 protein usually show transcriptional repression.

Changes in histone methylation patterns can result in faulty activation or deactivation of particular genes. This disturbs the control of cell proliferation, resulting in cancerous cells. For example, certain cancers overexpress various types of KDMs. Lymphomas and adenocarcinomas overexpress KDM2; and esophageal squamous carcinomas, medulloblastomas, and breast cancers over-express KDM4. Likewise, acute myeloid leukemias consistently show loss of function mutations in the gene that encodes DNMT3A, a DNA methyltransferase.

Testing and Treatment: Since epigenetic modifications (like histone methylation) can be reversed, epigenetic cancer treatments can potentially undo the epigenetic characteristics of cancer cells and make them more like healthy cells. Cancer cells usually have hypermethylated (excessively methylated) histones and DNA. Such hypermethylation of histones decreases the expression of tumor suppressor genes, which inhibit tumor growth. Chemical agents that inhibit methyltransferases can decrease histone methylation, reactivate the expression of tumor suppressor genes, and reduce tumor growth.

Azacitidine and decitabine are medications that treat cancer by reducing histone methylation. When taken by cancer patients, these antineoplastic drugs are incorporated into DNA where they inhibit DNA methyltransferases. Additionally, because of profound interactions between DNA methyltransferases and HMTs, these drugs reorganize histone methylation patterns in cancer cells. Both drugs can reduce the development of full-blown leukemia from myelodysplastic syndrome.

A deeper understanding of how histone methylation and demethylation control gene expression will ultimately provide better treatments for disorders like cancer.

Richard P. Capriccioso, MD

For Further Information

Arrowsmith, C. H., Bountra, C., Fish, P. V., Lee, K., & Schapira, M. (2012). Epigenetic protein families: a new frontier for drug discovery. *Nature Reviews Drug Discovery,* 11(5): 384–400.

Gozani, O., & Shi, Y. (2014). Histone methylation in chromatin signaling. In J. L. Workman & A. M. Abmayr (Eds.), *Fundamentals of chromatin* (pp. 213–256). New York, NY: Springer.

Okamura, M., Inagaki, T., Tanaka, T., & Sakai, J. (2010). Role of histone methylation and demethylation in adipogenesis and obesity. *Organogenesis,* 6(1): 24–32. http://www.ncbi.nlm.nih.gov/pmc/articles/PMC2861740/

Other Resources

Histone Methylation Research Kits
https://www.epigentek.com/catalog/histone-methylation-c-23.html

New England Biolabs, Inc.
https://www.neb.com/applications/epigenetics/histone-methyltransferases

See also: Chromatin

▶ Human Chorionic Gonadotropin (HCG)

Category: Cancer Biology

Definition: The hormone human chorionic gonadotropin (HCG) is secreted by a specialized type of cell (syncytiotrophoblasts) in the developing placenta during embryonic development. HCG is composed of two subunits (alpha and beta) and is normally found in the blood and urine during a normal pregnancy. The alpha subunit of HCG is shared with the pituitary hormones: follicle-stimulating hormone (FSH), luteinizing hormone (LH), and thyroid-stimulating hormone (TSH). The beta subunit is unique to HCG and determines its functional properties. HCG is needed to maintain pregnancy until the placenta is fully developed. Detection of HCG in the urine is the basis for pregnancy detection kits.

Gestational trophoblastic disease: Gestational trophoblastic disease (GTD) includes several types of tumors, including hydatidiform mole and choriocarcinoma. These tumors develop because of an anomaly in pregnancy when placental (trophoblastic) cells grow out of control. Hydatidiform moles can progress to choriocarcinomas, which are generally aggressive and, if left untreated, tend to metastasize widely. HCG is elevated in almost all patients with trophoblastic tumors and is a very useful diagnostic marker for monitoring treatment. Gestational trophoblastic disease can be diagnosed and followed by measuring HCG hormone levels in the blood and urine. Ultrasound, computed tomography (CT), positron emission tomography (PET), or magnetic resonance imaging (MRI) scans can also be used to look for tumors. However, when scans show no evidence of tumor presence, HCG levels are often relied on to determine whether the disease may be present.

HCG as a diagnostic marker: HCG is used as a diagnostic indicator of tumor formation in gestational trophoblastic disease because of an association between elevated HCG levels and trophoblastic tumors as well as nonseminomatous testicular tumors. Trophoblast-derived tumors often secrete only the free beta-HCG subunit. Diagnostic assays that are specific for the free beta-HCG subunit are most useful for monitoring tumor development and progression. A negative result is generally less than 5 milli international units/milliliter (mIU/ml) of beta-HCG in the blood. Gestational trophoblastic disease is treatable, and HCG levels can be used to monitor the success of treatment, in that as the tumor decreases, so does the level of HCG. In some cases, elevated HCG levels may be due to factors other than gestational trophoblastic disease. Certain hormones and proteins in the blood may interfere with the blood test results; therefore, HCG tests should be performed on both the blood and the urine in the diagnosis of gestational trophoblastic disease.

Thomas L. Brown, Ph.D.

See also: Choriocarcinomas; Cryptorchidism; Germ-cell tumors; Gestational Trophoblastic Tumors (GTTs); Gynecologic cancers; Hydatidiform mole; Malignant tumors; Testicular cancer

▶ IDH1

Category: Cancer Biology
Also known as: Isocitrate dehydrogenase 1

Definition: Isocitrate dehydrogenase 1 (IHD1) is 1 of 3 metabolic isozymes that catalyzes the conversion of isocitrate to alpha ketoglutarate via oxidative decarboxylation, using the cofactor nicotinamide adenine dinucleotide phosphate (NADP+) as an electron receptor. This is an essential metabolic function common to all eukaryotic organisms. A mutant form containing the R132H amino acid substitution is common in aggressive cancers with a poor prognosis, and specific therapies targeting cells with the mutant form show promise in treating these cancers.

Etiology of Associated Cancers: IDH1 substitutions were first identified in glioblastomas, the most common and malignant form of brain tumor. The rapid development, generally poor prognosis, and resistance to traditional chemotherapy shown by these tumors led cancer biologists to focus on their underlying biological processes in the hopes of developing new therapeutic agents. IDH1 mutations have also been shown to be frequent in acute myeloid leukemia, central chondrosarcomas, Ollier disease and Maffucci syndrome, and other central nervous system tumors.

The frequency of IDH1 substitutions in tumors ranges from 10%-50%, which indicates that the mutation is not a necessary condition or primary cause of tumor formation. It is not even clear that it increases malignancy; some studies have shown a slightly better survival time in glioma patients that have the mutation, as opposed to the wild type. The mechanism whereby the mutation contributes to carcinogenesis is complex and imperfectly understood, but it may involve suppression of cellular differentiation and consequent preservation of a stem-cell like state, which promotes rapid proliferation and metastasis. The IDH1 mutation always co-occurs with other genetic abnormalities that contribute to disrupted growth regulation.

The IDH1 mutation is a gain-of-function mutation. Being a mutation in a somatic cell, it is always present on only one pair of chromosomes. One of its effects is to promote the production of hypoxia-inducible factors that favor cell survival and proliferation under conditions of low oxygen. This aids tumor growth. The gene also interferes with the maturation of collagen, which affects the integrity of the blood/brain barrier, facilitating the spread of brain and central nervous system tumors. Mutant IDH1 is also associated with DNA hypermethylation, which may be implicated in deactivation of tumor suppression genes.

Testing and Treatment: The study of this mutation and its implications for clinical practice is still in its infancy, and no treatment based on it has been approved for clinical practice, although at least one therapeutic agent has shown promise in clinical trials. In the absence of any treatment protocol that depends on the presence or absence of mutant IDH1 in a tumor, testing is of limited value. That situation is likely to change rapidly.

Initially, the presence of the mutant IDH1 gene could only be determined by labor-intensive DNA sequencing of tissues from biopsies, surgical procedures, or autopsies. A more streamlined procedure that utilizes high resolution melting analysis appeared in 2011. Unfortunately, this remains a costly procedure, performed only in specialty laboratories, and is not recommended except as an adjunct to research. It is probable, for example, that the mutation occurs in many commoner and less malignant cancers, but efforts to identify it have understandably concentrated on the most malignant and least treatable types.

The greatest potential value of identifying mutant IDH1 cells is the potential to develop therapies that target only cells carrying the mutation. Two such agents are currently being tested. One is a vaccine, which stimulates the patient's body to produce antibodies against cancerous cells. The other is a chemotherapeutic agent which inhibits metabolism, growth, and cell division. Early trials indicate that it is less toxic and has fewer side effects than older chemotherapeutic agents which target dividing cells in general, including those unaffected by cancer.

A potential drawback of this strategy is the presence of unmutated or wild-type malignant cells in most tumors. Eliminating the mutant form in this instance shrinks the tumor and produces temporary remission, but this effect is expected to be short-lived. Without more research and clinical experience it is impossible to tell whether the advantage to be gained is of sufficient duration to justify the procedure.

History: The connection between IDH1 mutations and cancer came to light in 2008 as a result of the Cancer Genome Atlas project (TCGA), which was founded in 2005. TCGA consists of collaboration between the National Cancer Institute and National Human Genome Research Institute. The goal of this research program is to generate comprehensive, multidimensional maps of the key changes in the genomes of the major types and subtypes of cancer, and those abnormal metabolic processes involved in the onset of cancer (carcinogenesis). Examining abnormalities at the molecular level— the genetic code itself, the proteins specified by that code and how those proteins contribute to abnormal cellular functioning — give cancer biologists an incredibly powerful tool for developing targeted therapies, as well as for identifying how environmental carcinogens work.

The R132H-substituted form of IDH1 was the first such tumor-specific genetic abnormality to be identified through the cancer genome atlas project, and attracted immediate interest because of its association with glioblastoma. The discovery stimulated intensive research efforts to clarify the prevalence, mechanism of action, and therapeutic potential of the discovery. As of 2015, the advantages to be gained from this specific discovery appear to be modest, but the whole field of molecular genetics holds great potential for reducing cancer mortality and morbidity in the developed world.

Martha A. Sherwood, PhD

For Further Information

Dimitrov, L., Hong, C. S., Yang, C., Zhuang, Z., & Heiss, J. D. (2015). New developments in the pathogenesis and therapeutic targeting of the IDH1 mutation in glioma. *International Journal of Medical Sciences*, 12(3): 201-213.

Ichimura K. (2012). Molecular pathogenesis of IDH mutations in gliomas. *Brain Tumor Pathology*, 29(3): 131-139.

Pelengaris, Stella, & Khan, Michael. (Eds.). (2013). *Molecular biology of cancer: A bridge from bench to bedside.* 2nd ed. Hoboken, NJ: Wiley-Blackwell.

Other Resources

The National Center for Biotechnology Information
http://www.ncbi.nlm.nih.gov

PubMed (online access to research papers on cancer biology)
http://www.ncbi.nlm.nih.gov/pubmed

Cancer genome atlas
http://cancergenome.nih.gov

▶ Immune response to cancer

Category: Cancer Biology
Also known as: T-cell or cellular immune response, B-cell or humoral immune response

Definition: The body's immune response to cancer, in which tumor cells are recognized and killed, relies on T cells (also known as the cellular immune response) and B cells (also known as the humoral immune response). T cells are a type of lymphocyte (white blood cell) that matures in the thymus gland in the neck, and B cells are lymphocytes produced in the bone marrow. To escape immune-mediated cell death, tumor cells use several strategies. However, because of the potential benefits of generating tumor-specific immunity, tumor immunotherapy is being studied as a treatment for cancer.

Tumor-associated antigens: T cells and B cells recognize specific proteins, known as antigens, expressed on tumor cells. These immune cells can then become activated and develop antigen-specific immune responses that kill cells expressing these antigens.

There are many types of tumor-associated antigens. They may be reactivated embryonic gene products that are generally not found in normal adult cells but are turned on in some types of tumors (such as the MAGE proteins expressed in melanoma, breast, esophageal, and gastric cancers). Viral gene products are another category, which includes components of the Epstein-Barr virus and the human papillomavirus present in nasopharyngeal and cervical cancers, respectively. Tumor antigens may also be mutated, overexpressed, or dysregulated self-proteins. Common mutations in self-proteins include KRAS and beta-catenin, both found in multiple tumor types. Examples of overexpressed and dysregulated self-proteins include prostate-specific antigen (expressed in prostate cancers) and HER2/neu (expressed in breast, ovarian, and colorectal cancers). By mutating or overexpressing proteins involved in cell-cycle regulation and growth control, tumors can divide more and survive longer.

Cellular immunity: For a T cell to become activated, its T-cell receptor (TCR) must recognize antigen fragments (also called peptides) that are bound to the major histocompatibility complex (MHC) expressed on antigen-presenting cells, such as dendritic cells. The interaction of the T-cell receptor and the major histocompatability complex/peptide complex is referred to as signal 1. T cells must also interact with costimulatory molecules on antigen-presenting cells, commonly referred to as signal 2. T cells can multiply and carry out their effector functions only when they receive both signals.

Two major types of T cells are classified by whether they express the CD4 or CD8 protein. T cells expressing the CD4 protein recognize peptides bound to major histocompatability complex class II. Here, extracellular proteins are taken up by antigen-presenting cells and digested into twelve to twenty amino acid fragments that associate with major histocompatability complex class II as it traffics to the cell surface. CD4+ T cells are referred to as helper T cells because they secrete proteins called cytokines that provide survival factors to other immune cells, including interleukin (IL)-2, IL-12, and interferon (IFN)-gamma.

In contrast, CD8+ T cells recognize peptides bound to major histocompatability complex class I. Here, intracellular proteins are broken down into eight to ten amino acid fragments. These fragments are transported into the endoplasmic reticulum via the transporter associated with antigen processing (TAP), loaded onto major histocompatability complex class I molecules, and exported to the cell surface. CD8+ T cells may also be activated by cross-presentation, in which extracellular antigens released from dying cells are taken up by antigen-presenting cells and associate with major histocompatability complex class I.

CD8+ T cells are referred to as killer T cells or cytotoxic T lymphocytes. CD8+ T cells release factors such as perforin and granulysin, which poke holes in the plasma membrane of a target cell and allow water to rush in, ultimately leading to cell death in a process called osmotic lysis. CD8+ T cells also secrete granzyme, which can enter target cells and activate caspases (enzymes involved in apoptosis or programmed cell death).

Humoral immunity: Whereas T cells recognize peptides bound to major histocompatability complex molecules, B cells recognize whole or unprocessed antigens on the surface of target cells.

B cells can activate T cells by serving as antigen-processing cells because they express major histocompatability complex class II. When B cells interact with CD4+ helper T cells, the T cells can activate the B cells and mature them into plasma cells. Plasma cells produce proteins called antibodies, which are specific for an antigen. Antibodies can bind to antigens on a target cell and cause cell death via the complement pathway (which causes osmotic lysis) and antibody-dependent cellular cytotoxicity (which recruits natural killer cells that, similar to CD8+ killer T cells, can secrete perforin and granzyme to induce tumor cell death). Antibodies can also bind to antigens, such as growth factor receptors, and block their activity.

Immune tolerance: There are mechanisms that control the body's ability to recognize and respond to foreign, or non-self, antigens, while not responding to self antigens. However, since most cancers develop as uncontrolled growths within the body, tumor-associated antigens may be seen as self proteins. As a result, the immune response to cancer may be limited by immune tolerance.

Central tolerance occurs in the thymus during T cell development and involves the deletion of T cells that would respond too well to self-proteins. A similar process of deletion occurs in the periphery (outside the thymus). Other mechanisms of peripheral tolerance include ignorance and anergy. Ignorance occurs when self-reactive T cells are present but not activated by the antigen because the antigen is at low concentrations or not easily accessible to the peripheral blood. T-cell anergy is a state of unresponsiveness and may occur when there is T-cell-receptor ligation (signal 1) in the absence of costimulation (signal 2).

Tumors themselves also have mechanisms to escape immune recognition. They can downregulate antigen-processing factors such as major histocompatability complex molecules, the TAP transporter, or tumor-specific antigens, which makes it harder for T cells to recognize the antigens on tumor cells. Tumors can also express proteins that provide negative costimulation, leading to reduced T-cell activity or cell death. Some tumors secrete inhibitory cytokines, such as interleukin (IL)-10 and tumor growth factor beta (TGF-β), which may inhibit antigen-presenting cells and recruit regulatory T cells. Regulatory T cells account for approximately 5 to 10 percent of CD4+ cells and are characterized by expression of the CD25 protein and the *FOXP3* transcription factor. Regulatory T cells can suppress activation of other T cells and have been found to be more prevalent in human cancer patients compared with normal donors. Therefore, mechanisms of immune tolerance and a tumor's ability to produce an immunosuppressive environment may limit the activity of the immune cells, allowing cancer to grow within the body.

Immunotherapy: Since T cells and antibodies can specifically target tumor-associated antigens, anticancer therapies that use the immune system may be more specific than traditional cancer therapies such as chemotherapy, which targets all dividing cells (both normal and cancerous). Therefore, tumor immunotherapy may be less toxic and could lead to the development of immunological memory responses.

Tumor vaccines are one type of immune-based therapy, where tumor cells (or nontumor cells engineered to express tumor antigens) are modified to boost immune responses. These cells can be genetically modified to express major histocompatability complex molecules or costimulatory molecules and would serve as the antigen-presenting cell to activate T cells. Other types of tumor vaccines use cells that secrete cytokines to recruit and activate the body's own antigen-presenting cells. Tumor vaccines are being tested in a variety of cancers including melanoma, breast cancer, and prostate cancer.

The use of antibodies represents another immune-based platform. For example, rituximab is an antibody specific for the protein CD20. CD20 is expressed on both normal and cancerous B cells, such as those in B-cell non-Hodgkin lymphoma and B-cell leukemia. Depletion of CD20-expressing B cells with rituximab rids the body of cancerous B cells and has been shown to be effective as a first-line therapy and in relapsed cancers. Similarly, HER2/ neu is overexpressed in about 30 percent of breast tumors and is associated with a more aggressive cancer. The HER2/neu-specific antibody trastuzumab has been shown to increase survival rates in metastatic breast cancer and reduce relapse rates in early breast cancers.

Tumor immunotherapy represents a different type of cancer treatment and may have benefits over traditional cancer therapies, including higher specificity and better tolerability. Although the Food and Drug Administration has approved several tumor-specific antibodies, the use of tumor vaccines remains investigational, although promising.

Elizabeth A. Manning, Ph.D.

For Further Information

Fazekas de St. Groth, B. "DCs and Peripheral T Cell Tolerance." *Seminars in Immunology* 13, no. 5 (2001): 311-322.

Janeway, C. A., ed. *Immunobiology*. 5th ed. New York: Garland, 2001.

Marincola, F. M., E. M. Jaffee, D. J. Hicklin, and S. Ferrone. "Escape of Human Solid Tumors from T-Cell Recognition: Molecular Mechanisms and Functional Significance." *Advances in Immunology* 74 (2000): 181-273.

Pardoll, D. M. "Therapeutic Vaccination for Cancer." *Clinical Immunology* 95, no. 1, pt. 2 (2000): S44-S62.

Stern, M., and R. Herrmann. "Overview of Monoclonal Antibodies in Cancer Therapy: Present and Promise." *Critical Reviews in Oncology/Hematology* 54, no. 1 (2005): 11-29.

Other Resources

Immune Central
Immune System
http://www.immunecentral.com/immune/general.cfm

Immunotherapy for Cancer
http://www.meds.com/immunotherapy/index.html

See also: Biological therapy; Cytokines; Gene therapy; HIV/AIDS-related cancers; Immunotherapy; Lymphomas; Medical oncology; Neutropenia; Radiation therapies; Vaccines, preventive; Vaccines, therapeutic

▶ Lysine Histone Demethylases (KDMs)

Category: Cancer Biology
Also known as: Lysine (K)-Specific Demethylase (LSD), Lysine-Specific Histone Demethylase, Flavin-Containing Amine Oxidase Domain-Containing Protein, Amine Oxidase (Flavin Containing) Domain.

Definition: Lysine Histone Demethylases (KDMs) are enzymes that remove epigenetic methyl groups from histone molecules and influence transcriptional activity and gene expression. Histone modification is one of the primary epigenetic marks that influences transcriptional activity and gene expression. One histone modification (involved with epigenetic changes in gene expression) is lysine methylation and demethylation, which are catalyzed by histone-lysine N-methyltransferases and lysine histone demethylases (KDMs), respectively. There are at least seven families of human lysine histone demethylases (KDM1 through KDM7). These 7 families consist of over 20 different demethylases that remove methyl groups from different substrates. The substrates of KDMs vary with regard to the specific histone protein (H1, H2A, H2B, H3, H4) they recognize, the specific lysine residue in that histone they target, and whether that residue is mono-, di- or tri-methylated. The most studied KDM is Lysine histone demethylase 1A (KDM1A), which specifically demethylates mono- and di-methylated lysine residues 4 and 9 on histone 3 and certain other polypeptides.

Biological roles: Lysine histone demethylases play roles in various biological processes, including embryogenesis, differentiation, oocyte development, spermatogenesis, chromosomal segregation, and neuronal development.

Relation to cancer: The state of lysine histone methylation strongly correlates with cancer. Therefore, mutations in *KDM* genes and/or the aberrant expression of *KDM* genes play a role in cancer, although the precise role of KDMs in the genesis of cancer is yet to be determined. Overexpression of *KDM* genes has been associated with cancers of the bladder, lung, breast, colon, and esophagus as well as lymphomas, medulloblastomas, and adenocarcinomas. Underexpression has been associated with glioblastomas and prostate cancer. Since KDMs also demethylate other polypeptides besides histones, their histone-independent activities may also be responsible for the onset of cancer. For example, KDM1A demethylates tumor suppressor p53, which reduces the ability of p53 to suppress tumor growth. KDM1A also demethylates and stabilizes DNA methyltransferase 1 (DNMT1), which results in the silencing of genes involved with tumor suppression.

Since overexpression of KDMs is associated with tumorigenesis, the inhibition of their activity is a potential target for small molecules and/or siRNA therapy. Several drugs, some of which have entered clinical trials, are in development. Two drugs presently in clinical trials are ORY-1001, an inhibitor of KDM1A, which is active against acute myelogenous leukemia (AML), and GSK2879552, an inhibitor of LDS1, which is active against AML and small cell lung cancer.

Charles L. Vigue, PhD

For Further Information

Egger, Gerda, & Paola, Arimondo. (Eds.). (2016). *Drug discovery in cancer epigenetics.* Waltham, MA: Academic Press.

Emili, Andrew & Wodak, Shoshana. (Eds.). (2014). *Systems analysis of chromatin related protein complexes in cancer.* New York: Springer Science-Business Media.

Mould, D. P., McGonagle, A. E., Wiseman, D. H., Williams, E. L., & Jordan, A. M. (2015). Reversible inhibitors of LSD1 as therapeutic agents in acute myeloid leukemia: Clinical significance and progress to date. *Medicinal Research Reviews,* 35: 586–618.

Thinnes, C. C., England, K. S., Kawamura, A., Chowdhury, R., Schofield, C. J., & Hopkinson, R. J. (2014). Targeting histone lysine demethylases — Progress, challenges, and the future. *Biochimica et Biophysica Acta - Gene Regulatory Mechanisms,* 1839(12): 1416–1432.

Other Resources

What is DNA Methylation?
http://www.news-medical.net/life-sciences/What-is-DNA-Methylation.aspx

DNA Methylation
http://www.promega.com/~/media/files/promega%20worldwide/north%20america/promega%20us/webinars%20and%20events/epigeneticwebinarsept2012.pdf?la=en

▶ Menopause and cancer

Category: Cancer Biology

Definition: A natural occurrence in a woman's body, menopause occurs when the ovaries stop releasing eggs for twelve consecutive months. Menopause is a result of a woman's body producing less estrogen and progesterone hormones, bringing on the cessation of menarche (menstruation). Menopause does not cause cancer, but as a woman ages, her risk of developing cancer increases.

Etiology and symptoms of associated cancers: The onset of menopause can act as a powerful cue for a woman to reassess her general health and lifestyle choices during midlife and beyond. The physiological changes associated with menopause can indicate a need to evaluate health risks, particularly susceptibility to cardiovascular disease, neurological problems and cancers of the breast, lung, and colon. The symptoms of menopause include hot flashes and sweats, anxiety, depression, lowered libido (sex drive), dry skin, dryness in the vagina, and osteoporosis, among others. While the average age of entering menopause is 51 years, it is normal for a woman to first experience a perimenopause stage where her period is less regular and she develops some menopausal symptoms. Perimenopause lasts 4 years on average but in some instances it can last up to 10 years.

Menopause does not cause cancer. However, menopause is directly associated with aging, and bodily processes associated with aging are correlated with some forms of cancers. For example, 95% of women diagnosed with breast cancer are over the age of 40. Not all cancers carry the same risks across the life span; for example, the chances of a diagnosis of cervical cancer levels off at middle age, while endometrial cancer risk continues to increase into late adulthood.

A significant link has been found between survivors of childhood cancer and the onset of premature menopause. A report from the Childhood Cancer Survivor Study on females who had continued ovarian function after completing cancer treatment revealed that they were 13 times more likely to experience premature menopause (meaning they had ceased menstruating prior to age 40) compared to their female siblings. One possible link between cancer and premature menopause focuses on exposure to alkylating agents used in chemotherapy. These drugs modify the bases of DNA, interfering with DNA replication and transcription and leading to mutations.

Testing and treatment: For women who seek relief from the symptoms of menopause, as well as those who want to address the prospect of osteoporosis (bone loss) due to declining levels of estrogen and progesterone, menopausal hormone therapy (MHT) can be considered. This treatment involves taking estrogen alone (usually for women who have had a hysterectomy), or estrogen plus progesterone. A study by the National Institutes of Health's Women's Health Initiative found that women taking combined hormone therapy (both estrogen and progesterone or its synthetic equivalent progestin) to manage menopausal symptoms led to a higher risk of developing breast cancer. Additionally, the breast cancers in these women were more likely to have spread to the lymph nodes by the time they were diagnosed. The number of breast cancers diagnosed increased with the length of time during which they took MHT and decreased after they stopped taking the treatment. Furthermore, there was an increased breast cancer risk for women who started MHT at the onset of menopause or shortly thereafter. The risk associated with MHT was mitigated if MHT began five years or more after menopause. This study also showed that women who were diagnosed with breast cancer prior to menopause have an increased risk of recurrent breast cancer. For this reason, MHT is not recommended for cancer survivors. Besides breast cancer, MHT is associated with an increased risk of dying from a specific form of lung cancer.

For women who wish to avoid the cancer risks associated with MHT, alternative treatments are available. As hormone depletion occurs during and after menopause, changing to a diet rich in calcium and vitamin D (or taking supplements) can help prevent osteoporosis. In addition, the Food and Drug Administration has approved several medications which have been shown to be effective in treating hot flashes (eg, venlafaxine, fluoxetine, etc.).

In terms of general health metrics, excess body weight and obesity is a contributing risk factor for postmenopausal breast cancer. Given the high incident rate of overweight women in the US, it is reasonable to consider strategies to reduce risk by addressing weight. However, some investigators have suggested that adult weight gain might be a better predictor of postmenopausal breast cancer than weight or body mass index. Research from the Iowa Women's Health Study that studied a cohort of postmenopausal women over a 15-year period made two significant discoveries: (1) women who gained weight throughout adulthood had the highest rates of postmenopausal breast cancer; (2) loss

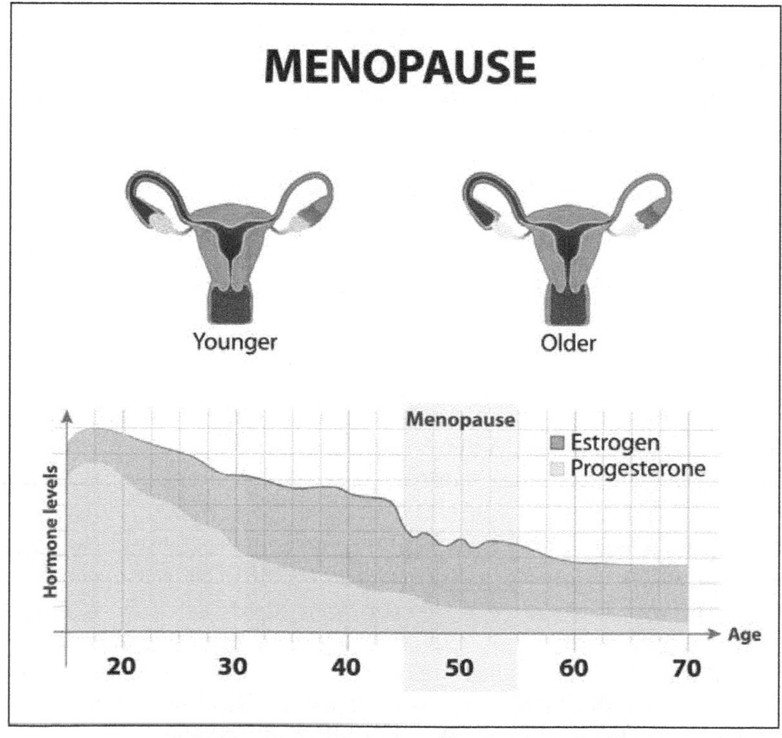

Female hormone levels during various life stages. (iStock)

of weight that occurred after adult weight gain was associated with a lower risk of postmenopausal breast cancer. These findings can serve as motivation for women to lose weight, even at midlife, as a breast cancer reduction strategy. Even a 5% weight loss has been shown to reduce breast cancer incidents.

History: Compared with previous generations, cancer incidents are increasing due to increased life expectancy. Women living in middle-to-upper-income countries have a life expectancy of 82.4 years. Although cancer is not the primary cause of death (this is reserved for cardio/circulatory diseases), in most developed countries it accounts for between 20% and 25% of female deaths. The significance of the relationship between aging processes and cancer will continue to grow.

Two landmark studies sponsored by the National Institutes of Health as part of the Women's Health Initiative began in 1991. One study examined the most common causes of death, disability, and poor quality of life in postmenopausal women. The second study investigated a subgroup of 27,000 healthy postmenopausal women between the ages of 50 and 79 years who were treated with hormone therapy (or a placebo control condition). Designed to last 15 years, the study was prematurely stopped due to the increased cancer risks associated with combined hormone therapy.

Bryan C. Auday, PhD
Maria C. Rossi

For Further Information

de Magalhães, J. P. (2013). How ageing processes influence cancer. *National Reviews Cancer*, 13(5), 357-365. doi: 10.1038/nrc3497.

Harvie, M., Howell, A., Vierkant, R. A., Kumar, N., Cerhan, J. C., Kelemen, L. E., ... Sellers, T. A. (2005). Association of gain and loss of weight before and after menopause with risk of postmenopausal breast cancer in the Iowa women's health study. *Cancer Epidemiology Biomarkers & Prevention*, 14, 656-66. doi:10.1158/1055-9965.

Nathan-Garner, L. (2013). Menopause and cancer risk: Get answers. *MD Anderson Cancer Center*. Retrieved from: http://www.mdanderson.org/patient-and-cancer-information/cancer-information/cancer-topics/prevention-and-screening/health/menopausecancer.html.

Rosenberg, S. M., & Partridge, A. H. (2013). Premature menopause in young breast cancer: Effects on quality of life and treatment interventions. *Journal of Thoracic Disease*, 5(1), 55–S61. doi: 10.3978/j.issn.2072-1439.2013.06.20.

Other Resources

National Cancer Institute
http://www.cancer.gov

American Society of Clinical Oncology
http://www.asco.org

Women's Health Initiative
https://www.nhlbi.nih.gov/whi/background.htm

See also: Breast Cancer; Ovarian Cancer; Menopause and cancer

▶ Mesenchymal stem cells and cancer

Category: Cancer Biology
Also known as: MSC, hMSC, Mesenchymal stromal cells

Related conditions: Stem Cell Transplantation, Bone Marrow Transplantation, Graft versus Host Disease

Definition: Stem cells are rare cells that are able to develop into any kind of cell in the human body. They can renew and replace themselves over and over again, creating millions of new cells. Mesenchymal Stem Cells (or MSCs) refer to non-blood adult stem cells from a variety of tissues. They were first isolated and described by Friedersen and his colleagues. MSCs can readily differentiate into osteoblasts (bone cells), chondrocytes (cartilage cells), myocytes (smooth muscle cells), and adipocytes (fat cells). The youngest type of MSCs can be found in umbilical cord tissue and cord blood, as well as tissue from developing tooth buds, amniotic tissue, and adipose tissue (body fat/connective tissue). MSCs can also be grown and expanded in laboratory settings. Although the main work of MSCs is to maintain and repair host tissue, MSCs have been found to have potential for clinical use, especially within the field of cancer. They are now the most commonly used type of stem cell in clinical and experimental trials.

MSC and Cancer: It is important to note that the use of MSCs in cancer treatment is still very controversial, as use of MSCs in cancer experimentation and trials have had mixed results. On the one hand, MSCs can migrate and incorporate into tumor tissues, creating wide-ranging effects in the tumor microenvironment. MSCs found in bone marrow have the ability to differentiate into bone, cartilage, fat, and even neural tissue. MSCs can also suppress immune reactions, and decrease time of recovery during a bone marrow or cord blood transplant. One of the biggest benefits of MSCs may be that their transformational power can play a role in treating graft versus host disease (GVHD), which can be a complication of allogeneic stem cell transplants.

Samples of clinical studies using MSCs that have been approved by United States National Institutes of Health in 2015 include:

- A study centered on finding the highest tolerable dose of MSC with beta interferon (a protein that has particular importance in terms of cell signaling) that can be given to patients with ovarian cancer
- A clinical trial centered on studying the use of MSCs and donor umbilical cord blood in treating patients with hematological malignancies such as leukemia and lymphoma
- A study focused on the safety and efficacy of human cord blood MSCs to prevent graft rejection/graft versus host disease after stem cell transplantation in children with acute leukemia
- A clinical trial using donor MSC infusions for acute and chronic graft versus host disease caused by a donor stem cell transplant
- A study focused on using MSCs for treatment of late pulmonary complications after allogeneic hematopoietic stem cell transplantation
- A clinical trial to test genetically modified MSCs to be used in the treatment of head and neck cancer

MSCs have also been used to assist in the treatment of pancreatic cancer, brain tumors, sarcomas, liver cancers, and breast cancer.

Despite the large number of clinical trials using human and genetically modified MSCs, there are still large knowledge gaps regarding the use of MSCs. For example, researchers are still trying to determine how to effectively use both freshly isolated human MSCs (hMSCs) that have not been subjected to laboratory manipulation and MSCs grown in a lab environment. Questions still remain regarding optimal time of delivery of MSCs and the number of cells needed for healing. MSC effectiveness is also dependent on tissue source and donor variability. More concerning is the paradoxical nature of MSCs themselves. They have profound anti-tumor and anti-inflammatory effects, but they also can enhance tumor growth through direct and indirect interactions with tumor cells.

Although there are many questions and issues surrounding the use of MSCs in cancer therapy, the regenerative and homing properties of MSCs make them a bright light in the field of cancer research and therapies. Usage of MSCs in treating different types of cancer will increase, and because of the increase, more specific protocols regarding the use of human and non-human MSCs will be tested and created. MSCs have been and will continue to be an important part of the future landscape of management and treatment of cancers and other immunologically based disorders.

Gina Riley, PhD

For Further Information

Wei, X., Yang, X., Han, Z., Qu, F., Shao, L., and Shi, Y. (2013). Mesenchymal stem cells: A new trend for cell therapy. *Acta Pharmacologia Sinica,* 34, 747 – 754.

Hong, I., Lee, H., & Kang, K. (2014). Mescenchymal stem cells and cancer: Friends or enemies? *Mutation Research/Fundamental and Molecular Mechanisms of Mutagenesis,* 768, 98 – 106.

Yagi, H. & Kitagawa, Y. (2013). The role of mesenchymal stem cells in cancer development. *Frontiers in Genetics.* Retrieved from http://dx.doi.org/10.3389/fgene.2013.00261. Shah, K. (2014). *Mesenchymal Stem Cells in Cancer Therapy*. Cambridge, Mass: Academic Press.

Other Resources

The University of Texas: MD Anderson Cancer Center
http://www.mdanderson.org

Columbia University Medical Center
http://newsroom.cumc.columbia.edu/blog/2015/01/15/bone-stem-cells-shown-regenerate-bones-cartilage-adult-mice

Memorial Sloan Kettering Cancer Center: Center for Stem Cell Biology
https://www.mskcc.org/research-areas/programs-centers/stem-cell-biology

Tri Institutional Stem Cell Initiative
http://www.triscistemcell.org/about_us.html

See also: Bone marrow aspiration and biopsy; Clinical trials

▶ Mitochondrial DNA mutations

Category: Cancer Biology
Also known as: Mitochondrial heteroplasmy (different mitochondrial mutations are present), homoplasmy

(only a single type of mitochondrial DNA, or deoxyribonucleic acid, sequence is present)

Related conditions: Warburg effect

Definition: Mitochondria are organelles in eukaryotic cells that produce energy (adenosine triphosphate, or ATP) by oxidative phosphorylation. Mitochondria are made from the proteins encoded by both nuclear genes and genes from the mitochondrion's own genome. The mitochondrial genome is sixteen kilobase pairs and encodes thirty-seven genes, which function in the mitochondrion. The majority of proteins in the mitochondrion are products of nuclear-encoded genes. There are multiple copies of the mitochondrial genome in each mitochondrion and multiple mitochondria in each cell. Mitochondrial DNA mutates at a high rate, and mitochondrial dysfunction is a factor in the development of cancers. Many defects in mitochondrial function are found in tumors.

The mutation process: Mitochondrial DNA (mtDNA) mutates at a rate about ten times greater than that of nuclear DNA. Likely reasons for this high mutation rate are an error-prone DNA polymerase, inefficient DNA repair enzymes, and exposure to mutagens such as oxygen radicals that are present in the mitochondrion.

Cancer cells have metabolic imbalances and a decrease in mitochondrial apoptosis (programmed, or planned, cell death). In cancer, the rapid growth of tumors is possible because of the shift in the mitochondria to glycolysis rather than the normal respiration (oxidative phosphorylation) to make ATP. Changes are observed in cancer cells, including the production of more of the rate-limiting enzymes of glycolysis and the accumulation of mutations in mitochondrial DNA. Often these mutations are in genes involved in mitochondrial respiration and ATP generation. In addition, sometimes people have mitochondrial mutations (germ-line mutations) that predispose that person to develop cancer. It is thought that most mtDNA mutations are acquired during or after the start of the cancer.

Mitochondrial DNA mutations are divided into two classes. The first class is severe mutations that inhibit oxidative phosphorylation and cause an increase in reactive oxygen species. Such mutations will promote tumor growth. The second class is milder mutations, which will allow tumors to adapt to new microenvironments as a tumor progresses and metastasizes.

Cancer cells are resistant to apoptosis because the induction of mitochondrial outer membrane permeabilization (MOMP) is inhibited. MOMP is a process that mediates apoptosis. In hematological cancers, when this process is inhibited, a neoplasm will occur. Some genes that code for proteins that function in the mitochondrion are located on nuclear chromosomes.

Associated cancers: Changes in mtDNA sequences have been found in many different types of cancers, including lung, breast, pancreatic, gastric, colorectal, thyroid, cervical, and prostate cancers. Mutations in the nuclear DNA-encoded mitochondrial genes for fumarate hydratase and succinate dehydrogenase are associated with uterine leiomyomas and paragangliomas. Studies have shown that the presence of certain mitochondrial DNA sequences (single nucleotide polymorphisms) is associated with an increase (or for other sequences, a decrease) in the risk of developing breast cancer. Germ-line mutations in mitochondrial DNA at nucleotides 10398 and 16189 are linked to breast and endometrial cancer. If the mitochondrial electron transport chain reactions are not functioning well, reactive oxygen species are made that cause oxidative stress and increase the risk of developing breast cancer. Other germ-line mtDNA mutations are associated with an increased risk of prostate cancer. Note that mutations in mtDNA show maternal inheritance because sperm mitochondria are generally eliminated from the embryo, so that mtDNA comes from the mother via the egg.

Mutations and monitoring: Somatic mutations in the displacement loop (D-loop, where the mtDNAstarts replication) occur frequently in colorectal cancers. There are hot spots in the D-loop where mtDNA mutations frequently occur. A colorectal tumor with a mutation in the D-loop is associated with a poor prognosis and resistance to fluorouracil-based adjuvant chemotherapy in Stage III colon cancers. Thus changes in mtDNA sequences are involved in the initiation and progression of cancers. Examining the mtDNA mutations in populations of cancer cells may be useful to monitor tumor progression. Analysis of these mutations may be useful for the diagnosis and treatment of the cancer. Targets for drug treatment might include glycolysis and inducing apoptosis in mitochondria.

Susan J. Karcher, Ph.D.

For Further Information

Alirol, E., and J. C. Martinou. "Mitochondria and Cancer: Is There a Morphological Connection?" *Oncogene* 25 (2006): 4706-4716. Bai, R. K., et al. "Mitochondrial Genetic Background Modifies Breast Cancer Risk." *Cancer Research* 67, no. 10 (2007): 4687-4694.

Brandon, M., P. Baldi, and D. C. Wallace. "Mitochondrial Mutations in Cancer." *Oncogene* 25, no. 34 (2005): 4647-4662.

Chatterjee, A., E. Mambo, and D. Sidransky. "Mitochondrial DNA Mutations in Human Cancer." *Oncogene* 25, no. 34 (2006): 4663-4674.

Garber, K. "Energy Boost: The Warburg Effect Returns in a New Theory of Cancer." *Journal of the National Cancer Institute* 96, no. 24 (2004): 1805-1806.

_______. "Energy Deregulation: Licensing Tumors to Grow." *Science* 312 (2006): 1158-1159.

Kroemer, G. "Mitochondria in Cancer." *Oncogene* 25 (2006): 4630-4632.

Maitral, Anirban, et al. "The Human MitoChip: A High-Throughput Sequencing Microarray for Mitochondrial Mutation Detection." *Genome Research* 14 (2004): 812-819.

Ohta, S. "Contribution of Somatic Mutations in the Mitochondrial Genome to the Development of Cancer and Tolerance Against Anticancer Drugs." *Oncogene* 25 (2006): 4768-4776.

Ruiz-Pesini, Eduardo, et al. "An Enhanced MITOMAP with a Global mtDNA Mutational Phylogeny." *Nucleic Acids Research* 35 (January 1, 2007): D823-D828.

Other Resources

MITOMAP
A Human Mitchondrial Genome Database
http://www.mitomap.org/

National Cancer Institute
Cancer Genetics
http://www.cancer.gov/cancertopics/ prevention-genetics-causes/genetics

See also: Breast cancers; Cancer biology; Cytogenetics; Genetics of cancer; Germ-cell tumors; Molecular oncology

▶ *MLH1* gene

Category: Cancer Biology
Also known as: MutL homolog 1, colon cancer nonpolyposis type 2 (E. coli); HNPCC; FCC2; HNPCC2; mutL (E. coli) homolog 1 (colon cancer, nonpolyposis type 2)

Definition: The *MLH1* gene encodes a protein that is involved in deoxyribonucleic acid (DNA) mismatch repair.

Normal cellular function: When a cell divides, it must replicate its genetic material, which is contained within the DNA. During DNA replication, errors can be made that need to be corrected. The DNA mismatch repair machinery recognizes the errors that are made and recruits other proteins to repair the errors. If errors are not corrected, mutations are made that could affect the production or function of important proteins.

Relevance to cancer: *MLH1* and *MSH2*, another gene that is part of the DNA mismatch repair machinery, are the two genes most frequently mutated in hereditary nonpolyposis colorectal cancer (HNPCC). Inheriting mutations in either *MLH1* or *MSH2* predisposes patients to developing colorectal, stomach, ovarian, and biliary duct cancers. Mutations in DNA mismatch repair genes are also present in 10 to 20 percent of sporadic (noninherited) cancers.

Defects in mismatch repair proteins are correlated with tumors that show microsatellite instability (MSI). Microsatellites are regions of the genome that contain highly repetitive DNA sequences that are more likely to generate errors during DNA replication. If the DNA mismatch repair machinery does not correct these errors, this can lead to further mutations within the genome that may promote tumor formation and progression.

Diagnostic and genetic testing: There are a number of tests that can identify people with inherited mutations in mismatch repair genes as well as characterize the levels of these proteins in tumor cells, both of which have important clinical implications. DNA sequencing tests are currently available for both *MLH1* and *MSH2*, the two mismatch repair genes that are most commonly mutated in cancer. In addition to mutations in the genes themselves, other types of chromosome modifications can alter levels at which these proteins produced by these genes are expressed within the cells. Therefore, immunohistochemical analysis of tissue samples can be used to detect how much of the mismatch repair proteins are being produced.

Clinical implications: Because mutations in *MLH1* or *MSH2* significantly increase the risk of developing cancer, patients carrying these mutations should undergo frequent screening for colon and endometrial cancer. In addition, levels of MLH1 and MSH2 protein within tumor cells can be prognostic indicators, since differential protein levels are associated with differences in cancer progression, recurrence, and treatment response. For example, one study found that cells lacking MLH1 protein were more resistant to DNA damage-inducing chemotherapy than cells that contain MLH1.

Lindsay Lewellyn, B.S.

See also: Ashkenazi Jews and cancer; Bethesda criteria; Cancer biology; Family history and risk assessment; Genetics of cancer; Hereditary cancer syndromes; *MSH* genes; Turcot syndrome

▶ *MSH* genes

Category: Cancer Biology
Also known as: MSH—MutS homolog 2, colon cancer, nonpolyposis type 1 (E. coli); HNPCC; HNPCC1; MSH3—mutS homolog 3 (E. coli); DUP; divergent upstream protein; mismatch repair protein 1; MRP1; MSH4—mutS homolog 4 (E. coli); MSH5—mutS homolog 5 (E. coli); MSH6—mutS homolog 6 (E. coli); GTBP

Definition: *MSH* genes are a class of genes that are normally involved in deoxyribonucleic acid (DNA) mismatch repair but can be mutated in many types of cancer.

Normal cellular function: DNA mismatch repair is the process whereby errors in DNA replication are recognized and repaired by proteins in the cell. If the mismatch repair machinery is defective, either by mutation of the genes encoding the proteins or by altering the expression levels of the proteins, errors are no longer repaired.

Relevance to cancer: Cells that contain defects in DNA mismatch repair show mutation rates that are one hundred to one thousand times higher than normal cells. Most mutations may not have negative effects, but if mutations are made in genes required to regulate cell growth and proliferation, this can lead to cancer. A readout of this increased mutation rate is microsatellite instability (MSI). Microsatellites are repetitive DNA sequences that are prone to replication errors, and cells that are defective in mismatch repair show variability in the length of these sequences.

One of the genes in this class, *MSH2*, is among the most frequently mutated genes in hereditary nonpolyposis colorectal cancer (HNPCC). Inheriting a mutation in this gene causes a genetic predisposition to cancer. In addition, *MSH* genes are often mutated in noninherited forms of cancer such as skin cancer and ovarian cancer. Other *MSH* genes—*MSH3* and *MSH6*—are also mutated in cancer, but at a lower frequency than *MSH2*.

Diagnostic and genetic testing: A number of tests are available to monitor the status of the mismatch repair machinery, which can provide diagnostic and prognostic information. DNA sequencing of the *MSH2* gene can be done to look for mutations that can predispose patients to cancer. Protein levels can be measured by immunohistochemical analysis of tissue samples, and tests to monitor the MSI status of tumor cells can also be performed.

Clinical implications: Because they strongly predispose people to developing cancer, patients carrying mutations in mismatch repair genes should undergo frequent colonoscopy as well as screenings for endometrial cancers. In addition, levels of mismatch repair proteins as well as MSI status can be strong predictors of tumor progression and prognosis. For example, although tumors that show high MSI tend to be aggressive, the outcome is usually favorable. Further, cells defective in mismatch repair have been shown to be less sensitive to platinum-based chemotherapy as well as methylating agents, which both work by inducing DNA damage.

Lindsay Lewellyn, B.S.

See also: Ashkenazi Jews and cancer; Cancer biology; Family history and risk assessment; Genetics of cancer; Hereditary cancer syndromes; *MLH1* gene

▶ Mutagenesis and cancer

Category: Cancer Biology

Definition: Mutagenesis refers to the process by which the genetic information of an organism undergoes a stable change, resulting in a mutation. Cancer-causing mutations are either inherited or are a result of long-term or frequent exposure to carcinogenic substances, or ionizing and/or ultraviolet radiation.

Etiology and symptoms of associated cancers: Mutations can be inherited from one or both parents. Parents can also pass on unknown genetic mutations that result from their life choices and experiences (e.g., smoking and routine consumption of charbroiled foods). Genetic mutations can only be detected by genetic testing.

There are several types of mutations. Base changes involve the substitution, insertion, or deletion of single or multiple bases in DNA. These types of mutations can involve only one base (point mutations) or more than one or even a few bases at a time. Base changes can affect regulatory sequences that control when and where genes are expressed. Mutations that disrupt or change the modes of gene expression are called “regulatory mutations.” However, not all sequences within genes are essential for either gene expression or protein coding. Mutations in such nonessential sequences will typically produce no effect and are known as "silent mutations." Mutations that occur within the protein coding region may cause the production of a mutant protein that is nonfunctional, sub-functional, or possesses new or unregulated functions. Not all base changes mutations are passed on to progeny cells because DNA repair systems can repair minor changes to DNA. Some base changes can also occur in stretches of repeated bases of DNA. The enzyme that replicates DNA (DNA polymerase) can slip when it tries to replicate stretches of repeated DNA sequences. This phenomenon is known as "replication slippage" and is responsible for the expansion or deletion of repeated stretches of repeated sequences. Expansion and reduction of arrays of repeated sequences can also occur by means of aberrant recombination.

The second type of mutation includes gross chromosomal rearrangements, which are much more complex. There are four kinds of gross chromosomal rearrangements: deletions, inversions, translocations, and duplications. Gross chromosomal rearrangements can affect a small number of bases or multiple chromosomes and thousands of base pairs. This type of mutation usually is not correctable. Deletions remove large segments of chromosomes. Inversions reverse the order of a large segment of bases within a chromosome. Translocations cause a segment of DNA from one chromosome to be switched to another chromosome. Duplications reiterate parts of a chromosome. These complex mutations can cause problems if they re-program the expression of particular genes or generate novel fusions between genes.

The third type of mutation, insertional mutations, includes viruses that randomly insert their genome into chromosomes (such as retroviruses) or transposons (mobile segments of DNA that can jump from one location in the genome to another). Insertional mutations can activate proto-oncogenes, or inactivate tumor suppressor genes. Proto-oncogenes drive cell division and inappropriate activation of proto-oncogenes predisposes cells to become tumorous. Tumor suppressor genes down-regulate cell division, and inactivation of tumor suppressor genes is a prelude to the onset of cancer.

Mutations can be spontaneous or induced. Spontaneous mutations occur randomly and are usually not due to exogenous agents. They typically result from errors made by the enzyme DNA polymerase during the DNA replication. DNA can also be damaged by substances or physical agents that can chemically attack it and alter it. Such molecules are often referred to as mutagens (since they can induce mutations). If mutagens can induce mutations in cells so efficiently that exposing cells to them predictably transforms them into cancer cells, then such mutagens are called "carcinogens." Carcinogens include such things as ultraviolet radiation, X-rays, antibiotics, viruses, and the components of cigarette smoke. DNA that has incurred mutations by any of these means is subject to the process of DNA repair. DNA repair mechanisms typically correct some mutations but these systems are also imperfect and can miss or even perpetuate some mutations. Thus, by attempting to save the cells, DNA repair systems can actually stabilize particular mutations in multiple genes.

Currently, researchers have identified mutations in specific genes that cause some types of cancer. Many are inherited, such as mutations in the BRCA1 and BRCA2 genes, which can cause breast and ovarian cancer in women. The presence of the mutant forms of these genes makes women more likely to develop cancer. A woman can inherit a harmful mutation in BRCA1 or BRCA2 from mother or father. If she carries only one copy of a harmful mutation, she will have an increased risk for breast and ovarian cancer. The only way to determine the presence of these mutant genes is to use genetic tests to detect them.

As cancer cells proliferate, their fast growth rate predisposes them to acquire new mutations that confer upon them the ability to grow faster and faster. As a result of natural selection, the fastest-growing cells will predominate in the tumor. In their quest to grow even faster and outcompete other cells, some cells will abandon mechanisms within to ensure that chromosomes are properly segregated to daughter cells. This leads to abnormal number of chromosomes, a condition known as aneuploidy. The intense competition within the tumor drives cells to acquire the ability to remodel the vasculature (angiogenesis) so that the tumor can receive nutrients from blood. Other cells acquire the ability to break through natural barriers around them and spread to other parts of the body (metastasis). Cells may also acquire resistance to chemotherapy drugs. This stepwise development of cancer is driven by mutations and the process of natural selection, which promotes the advantageous ones and discards the deleterious ones.

Tests and treatment: In order to identify mutations in chromosomes, a procedure called a DNA microassay (also known as a gene chip, DNA chip, or biochip) is used. DNA microassays utilize DNA microarray technology, which begins with glass slides that have the entire DNA from the human genome segregated into thousands of tiny dots (complex robotic apparatuses make such slides). The DNA on these slides is single-stranded. Then, a DNA sample is taken from the patient, often from a scraping from the inside of the mouth. The DNA from the patient's cells is isolated, cut into smaller pieces, and labeled with fluorescent dyes. Then the patient's labeled DNA is incubated with the genomic DNA (gDNA) sample on the slide. Because the DNA on the slide came from an individual who does not harbor such mutations, any mismatches between the patient's DNA and the DNA on the slide, will be easily detected by the degree of fluorescence on the particular spots on the slide. Such mismatches are the sites where mutations have occurred in the patient's DNA. Such microarray techniques are highly precise and sensitive, but, unfortunately, are also labor-intensive and expensive.

Spotted microarrays use smaller probes (oligonucleotides) made by means of polymerase chain reaction (PCR) or DNA synthesizing machines. Probes from cancer cells and from non-cancerous cells are hybridized to the same gDNA microarray and compared in side-by-side experiments. Differences in hybridization between these two experiments can tell scientists exactly what genetic mutations a cancer might possess. Both types of microarrays require the slides to be scanned with either lasers or radiographic imaging machines. This testing allows scientists to look for mutations in selected genes.

History: In 1865, Gregory Mendel identified genes while studying pea plants. In 1869, Johann Miescher discovered DNA in body cells while examining open wounds with a microscope. In 1927, Hermann Muller created mutations in fruit flies by using x-rays. In the 1940s, Charlotte Auerbach and J.M. Robson used mustard gas to generate mutations in fruit flies. In 1953, Watson and Crick determined the structure of DNA, as well as the substances making up the DNA. In 2000, the National Institute for Health completed the Human Genome Project which provided a map of the human genome.

Lindsay Lewellyn

Updated by: Christine M. Carroll, R.N., B.S.N., M.B.A.

For Further Information

Baaj, Y., Magdelaine, C., Ubertelli, V., Valat, C., Talini, L., Soussaline, F., … Sturtz, F. G. (2008). A highly specific microarray method for point mutation detection. *BioTechniques*, 44(1), 119–126. A paper that describes a new technique for using microarrays to detect mutations in patients with neurological diseases.

Ennis, Don G. (2001). Mutagenesis. Encyclopedia of life sciences. Retrieved on February 15, 2016 from http://www.els.net/WileyCDA/ELSarticle/refid-a0000559.html. This author describes the different types of mutations.

National Cancer Institute. (2015 April 1). BRCA1 and BRCA2: Cancer risk and genetic testing. Retrieved on February 15, 2016 from http://www.cancer.net/about-cancer/causes-prevention/genetics/brca-fact-sheet. This article discusses specifically about the BRCA1 and BRCA2 genes.

Steen, Francis F. (1998). Landmarks in the history of genetics. Retrieved on February 15, 2016 from http://www.cogweb.ucla.edu/ep/dna-history.html. This document is a listing of landmarks in genetics.

Loeb, Keith R. & Loeb, Lawrence A. (1999 September 20). Significance of multiple mutations in cancer. Retrieved on February 12, 2016 from http://www.Carcin.oxfordjournals.org/content/21/3/379.full. These authors discuss mutations in cancer in more depth.

Other Resources

American Cancer Society
WWW.Cancer.org.

See also: Antioxidants; Ashkenazi Jews and cancer; Bioflavonoids; Cancer biology; Carcinogens, known; Carcinogens, reasonably anticipated; Chromosomes and cancer; Free radicals; Gene therapy; Genetic testing; Genetics of cancer; Herbs as antioxidants; Hereditary cancer syndromes; Oncogenes; Proto-oncogenes and carcinogenesis; Tumor-suppressor genes

▶ *MYC* oncogene

Category: Cancer Biology

Also known as: *c-Myc*, v-myc myelocytomatosis viral oncogene homolog (avian)

Definition: First identified in humans based on its homology to the chicken viral oncogene (*v-myc*), *MYC* belongs to a family of *MYC* genes that codes for a transcription factor containing the basic-helix-loop-helix Leucine zipper (bHLH/LZ) domain. The MYC protein binds to the enhancer box (E-box) sequence and activates the expression of a larger number of genes. By modifying the expression of its target genes, *MYC* is able to activate numerous biological effects. It affects cell proliferation (downregulates *CDKN1A*,or *p21*), regulates cell growth (upregulates *TP53*), induces apoptosis (upregulates *BCL2*), and regulates differentiation (downregulates *C/EBPA*).

Role in cancer biology: The role of *MYC* in influencing critical aspects of the cell cycle machinery makes it a centerpiece and key to the enigma of cancer biology. In normal cells, *MYC* expression is under tight regulation, with the gene being expressed only in actively dividing cells. In contrast, genetic aberrations result in the uncontrolled expression of *MYC* in cancer cells. Aberrant expression of *MYC* plays a significant role in a wide variety of human cancers: 80 percent of breast cancers, 70 percent of colon cancers, 90 percent of gynecological cancers, 50 percent of hepatocellular carcinomas, and a variety of hematological tumors possessing abnormal *MYC* signatures. An estimated 100,000 cancer deaths per year in the United States are associated with changes in the *MYC* gene or its expression. The clinical significance of *MYC* gene alterations in human cancers is best illustrated by the amplification of *MYCN* (*N-myc*) in neuroblastoma and the translocation of *MYC* from its normal position on chromosome 8 to chromosome 14 in Burkitt lymphoma.

Inhibiting *MYC*: Experimental evidence shows that inhibiting *MYC* significantly halts tumor cell growth and proliferation; consequently *MYC* is an attractive target for cancer therapy. Another advantage of *MYC* as a therapeutic target is the fact that it is downstream of multiple converging signaling pathways that are affected by mutations in a number of genes in different cancer types. Major advances in drug development aimed at eliminating *MYC* include targeting it by antisense mitochondrial ribonucleic acid (mRNA) and deoxyribonucleic acid (DNA) oligonucleotides, triple-helix-forming oligonucleotides, ribozymes, porphyrins, and small interfering RNA (siRNA). Inhibition of *MYC* can be achieved with many of these approaches; however, for increased clinical efficacy it is probable that intervention, possibly in combination with traditional chemotherapy, will be necessary.

Banalata Sen, Ph.D.

See also: Burkitt lymphoma; Cancer biology; Free radicals; Gene therapy; Genetics of cancer; Oncogenes; Protooncogenes and carcinogenesis; Tumor markers; Tumor-suppressor genes

▶ Myeloid-derived suppressor cells

Category: Cancer Biology
Also known as: MDSCs

Definition: Myeloid-derived suppressor cells (MDSCs) are a diverse population of cells that increases in number during cancer, inflammation, and infection, and possess a remarkable ability to suppress immune responses against foreign substances.

Etiology and symptoms of associated cancers: One of the hallmarks of cancer is the ability of tumors to evade the immune system. Tumors co-opt several different types of immune cells to accomplish this (eg, regulatory T-cells, tumor-associated macrophages, type 2 NKT cells), but myeloid-derived suppressor cells (MDSCs) seem to play the most pivotal role among these immunosuppressive cells.

MDSCs descend from hematopoietic stem cells (HSCs) in the bone marrow. HSCs divide throughout our lives and constantly renew themselves. The progeny of HSCs are progenitor cells that differentiate into 1 of 2 cell lineages; the lymphoid or myeloid lineage. The lymphoid progenitor form a special group of white blood cells called lymphocytes, be they B-lymphocytes, T-lymphocytes, or natural killer (NK) cells. Myeloid progenitors (there seems to be more than 1) can form several different types of white blood cells (eg, monocytes, neutrophils, eosinophils, red blood cells, or megakaryocytes) which form platelets. The myeloid lineage also gives rise to MDSCs.

A host of tumor-derived factors (eg, interleukin-6 and granulocyte-macrophage colony-stimulating factor) activate the formation of MDSCs in bone marrow and their proliferation, expansion, and migration. MDSCs tend to be immature, and once activated, they infiltrate the spleen and liver and help form an immunosuppressive microenvironment around the tumor.

MDSCs suppress T-cell function and the cytotoxic activities of NK cells, but they must make cell contact to do so. MDSCs also produce enzymes that degrade molecules that immune cells need to mount an immune response. For example, MDSCs produce an enzyme called arginase, which degrades the amino acid arginine; an essential factor for T-cell activation. MDSCs also secrete a host of immunosuppressive molecules that can shut down immune cell activation.

In addition to suppressing the patient's immune response against the tumor, MDSCs also promote the formation of new blood vessels (angiogenesis) to feed the tumor and aid its spread (metastasis) to other tissues. MDSCs also facilitate cancer cell invasion by secreting enzymes that degrade basement membranes and other barriers. Abundant evidence in laboratory animals has also established that MDSCs play a critical role in cancer cell drug resistance and that liquidation or inactivation of MDSCs can sensitize the tumor to anticancer drugs.

Testing and treatment: The number of circulating MDSCs correlates quite well with the stage of the cancer and the capacity of the tumor to metastasize. The San Diego-based biotechnology company Seramatrix Corporation has developed a blood test to measure the levels of MDSCs in cancer patients. Such a test might be an excellent diagnostic indicator of a patient's prognosis.

Because of the centrality of MDSCs to tumor immune evasion, inhibiting MDSC function can make tumors vulnerable to the patient's immune system. While this approach remains experimental for now, some drugs show some promise. Some examples include: 1) sunitinib, which reduces MDSC proliferation in cancer patients; 2) MDSC-specific peptides fused to antibodies (peptibodies), which can delete MDSCs from circulation without affecting levels of other immune cells; 3) cyclooxygenase-2 inhibitors (eg, celecoxib), which suppress activation of MDSCs; 4) phosphodiesterase-5 inhibitors (ie, sildenafil, tadalafil, and vardenafil), which down-regulate MDSC functions and restore the activities of T-cells; and 5) vitamin A derivatives, which force MDSC differentiation and essentially delete them from circulation.

History: MDSCs were first isolated and characterized in tumor-bearing mice or human cancer patients. Transplanting tumors into laboratory mice causes a marked increase in the number of MDSCs in the body of the animal. Further work has shown that MDSC numbers also increase during infectious or inflammatory diseases.

Michael Buratovich, PhD

For Further Information

Diaz-Montero, C. M., Finke, J., & Montero, A. J. (2014). Myeloid-derived suppressor cells in cancer: Therapeutic, predictive, and prognostic implications. *Seminars in Oncology*, 41(2), 174-184.

Gabrilovich, D. I., & Nagaraj, S. (2009). Myeloid-derived suppressor cells as regulators of the immune system. *Nature Reviews Immunology*, 9(3), 162-174.

Katoh, H., & Watanabe, M. (2015). Myeloid-derived suppressor cells and therapeutic strategies in cancer. *Mediators of Inflammation*, doi:10.1155/2015/159269.

Other Resources

R & D Systems–Myeloid-derived Suppressor Cells (MDSC)
https://www.rndsystems.com/research-area/myeloid–derived-suppressor-cells–mdsc

Serametrix–MDSC-based blood test for predicting response to cancer therapy commercialized by Serametrix
http://www.serametrix.com/Press-Releases/mdsc-blood-test.html

▶ NK cells

Category: Cancer Biology
Also known as: Natural Killer cells

Definition: Natural Killer Cells (NK cells) are lymphocytes that normally circulate throughout the bodies of humans and other vertebrates. They have the ability to recognize cells that are foreign to the body which includes aged, injured, virally infected and cancerous cells and destroy them quickly and efficiently.

Etiology: In the blood of humans about 1 in 1000 cells is a white blood cell. These cells are further subdivided and about 30% to 40% are classified as lymphocytes. The major lymphocytes in blood include T-lymphocytes, B-lymphocytes, and the NK cells. The NK cells represent about 10% of circulating lymphocytes.

The NK cells are a part of the innate immune system. They do not need to have previously encountered their targets to be effective. Unlike T and B lymphocytes, they are not uniquely assigned to attack or create antibodies against only one type of antigen. Because they are always in circulation and nonspecific, they can respond to a threat more quickly than T or B lymphocytes. They are capable of identifying and destroying any cells that are damaged, infected by viruses, or cancerous. The NK cells are widely distributed in the body and are produced primarily in the bone marrow in response to interleukins, IL-2, IL-12, IL-15, and IL-18.

Human cells have identifying characteristics on their cell surface which are unique in every human being. These cell surface markers are the genetically determined major histocompatibility complex (MHC). Because of the large number of genes involved in determining which markers appear on an individual's cells, it is highly unlikely that any 2 individuals will have the same MHC markers with the exception of identical twins who would inherit the same MHC genes. The NK cells recognize any cell that does not have the same major histocompatibility complex that they do.

All cells with the same MHC markers are considered "self" while any cells lacking the same MHC are considered non-self-cells. Non-self-cells are attacked by NK cells in an effort to prevent them from injuring the normal healthy cells of the body. The NK cells can be activated when the individual is suffering from a viral infection or has a tumor. When a cell is invaded by a virus, typically the virus will destroy the markers on the cell. Similarly, when a cell is transformed into a malignant cell, it will no longer express the MHCs that normally would appear on its surface. Once these cells without markers are recognized, they will be targeted by the NK cells for destruction.

In a normal, healthy cell, the MHC markers will block the attachment of NK cells to its surface receptors. Once there are no longer any "self" markers on the surface of infected or malignant cells, the NK cells are able to directly attach to receptors on the modified cell's surface. The attached NK cells release two lysosomal chemicals into the target cell: perforin and granzymes. Perforin is a protein that produces pores in cell membranes of the target cell. Once the pores are created, proteases, called granzymes, are released into the cell. Granzyme signals the initiation of a process called programed cell death or apoptosis. Under such controlled circumstances, the dying cell goes through several biochemical steps that destroys its internal components but does not release potentially toxic substances into the surrounding environment, thus preventing injury to the surrounding tissues. In the early stages of a neoplasm, this action may be adequate to prevent the development of a cancer, limit the extent of the cancer, and/or prevent metastasis.

Testing and treatment: Since NK cells can recognize and destroy precancerous and cancerous cells, scientists have been devising ways to use NK cells as a tool to treat cancer quickly and effectively. In some hematologic cancers such as acute myeloid leukemia and chronic lymphocytic leukemia, NK cell-based treatments have produced good results, but in other cancers they have been less successful. There are several reasons that immunotherapies that utilize NK cells have taken some time to become successful:

1) Some cancerous cells have mechanisms that protect them from NK cells. In some cases they produce chemicals that block recognition of the cancerous cell or block receptor binding at the cell surface, which prevents the NK cells from attaching to the cell surface and releasing perforin and granzymes.

2) The number of NK cells varies in individuals under different biological conditions. Scientists have tried to stimulate the production of NK cells in vivo by using cytokines, in particular interleukins and interferon, but the amount required can have serious side effects. They have also isolated NK cells and grown them in culture for a return to the body. Only recently have they been able to grow adequate quantities to fight cancer. This technique holds great promise as a way to treat patients quickly and effectively.

3) Obtaining NK cells from an external source such as umbilical cord blood or cultured NK cell lines is another technique presently under investigation. Now that laboratories can grow large numbers of NK cells in culture, it is possible to use exogenous NK cells to treat a wide variety of cancers.

4) In some studies NK cells have been genetically modified. Some cells have been modified to produce interleukins that will stimulate their own production. When returned to the patient, these genetically-modified NK cells would stimulate the production of other NK cells that can fight the cancer. Genetically modified NK cells that produce cytokines that destroy the receptor blocking agents produced by the neoplastic cells have also been made.

Most of the techniques described here are expected to be administered following chemotherapy. There are many clinical studies underway to test these techniques, and researchers believe that they will be successful either on their own or in combination with other therapies. They hold promise for the future as more information on the growth and genetic modification of NK cells becomes available.

Annette O'Connor, PhD

For Further Information

Topham, N. J., & Hewitt, E. W. (2009). Natural Killer Cell Cytotoxicity: How Do They Pull the Trigger? *Immunology,* 128(1): 7-15.

Mandal, A. & Viswanathan, C., (2015) Natural Killer Cells: In Health and Disease. *Hematology Oncology and Stem Cell Therapy,* 8(2): 47-55.

Moussa, P., Marton, J., Vidal, S. M. & Fodil-Cornu, N. (2012) Genetic dissection of NK cell responses. *Frontiers in Immunology*, 3(425): Retrieved at http://dx.doi.org/10.3389/fimmu.2012.00425.

Other Resources

American Cancer Society

HOPE Foundation Gift Helps Study "Natural Killers" That Can Heal http://www.cancer.org/research/dr-michael-verneris

MD Anderson Cancer Center
Natural Killer Cell Therapy May Augment Treatment of Hematological Cancers
http://www.mdanderson.org/publications/oncolog/previous-issues/2015-february/natural-killer-cell-therapy-may-augment-treatment-of-hematological-cancers.html

▶ Oncogenes

Category: Cancer Biology; Carcinogens and Suspected Carcinogens
Also known as: Proto-oncogenes

Related cancers: Leukemias, lymphomas, most sarcomas (of bone and muscle), carcinomas (of epithelial origin)

Exposure routes: Inherited as genetic information

Where found: Proto-oncogenes are genes found within the chromosomes of all eukaryotic (nucleated) cells and organisms.

At risk: Proto-oncogenes are universal among all eukaryotic cells and organisms, which include humans and all animals. Congenital mutations in some of these genes are associated with a significantly increased risk for certain cancers.

Definition: Oncogenes are variations of cellular proto-oncogenes that normally function in the regulation of cell division. Mutations in these genes may result in the cell becoming cancerous. The term "proto-oncogene" refers to the normal cell copy of the gene, while the term "oncogene" refers to a mutated, or activated, form of the same gene that results in disruption of cell regulation.

Most oncogenes have a three-letter name based on their initial identification or the type of cancer with which they were first found to be associated. For example, the src gene was first identified in the Rous sarcoma virus. The ras oncogene was first identified as a gene in rat sarcomas.

Etiology and symptoms of associated cancers: More than one hundred proto-oncogenes have now been recognized in cells. Most are involved in regulating movement through the cell cycle (regulation of chromosome replication followed by cell division). The cell cycle is characterized as having four phases: G1, which regulates events leading to deoxyribonucleic acid (DNA) replication; S, in which cell chromosomes replicate; G2, which regulates events leading to cell division; and mitosis, the period in which the chromosomes separate and the cell divides. Each phase is regulated by specific enzymes, signals, and other molecules, as well as suppressors that prevent movement through the phase. Many of the regulatory proteins involved in these events are encoded by proto-oncogenes. Not all proto-oncogenes are expressed in every cell, and the type of cancer that potentially develops is related to the particular oncogene that has undergone a mutation.

Proto-oncogenes are subdivided into four categories, each of which represents a particular set of steps that regulate the cell cycle: growth factors, growth factor receptors, signal mechanisms, and tumor suppressors/regulators of apoptosis (cell death).

Growth factors are small proteins that bind specific cell surface receptors and set in motion events that will result in cell division. Overproduction of growth factors may result in repeated cell division, setting the stage for development of cancer. For example, the PDGFB (commonly known as sis) oncogene, originally isolated from the simian sarcoma virus, encodes one of the protein chains that make up the platelet-derived growth factor. PDGFB is secreted by platelets and binds receptors on certain fibroblast cells. Overproduction of PDGFB may induce uncontrolled cell division, resulting in a sarcoma.

Growth factor receptors are cell surface proteins that bind specific growth factors. Each cell type expresses a particular form or forms of receptors, and the ability of

Selected Oncogenes and Tumor-Suppressor Genes and Their Related Cancers

Gene	*Associated Cancers*
APC	Colorectal cancer
BCL2	B-cell lymphoma
BRC-ABL1	Chronic myelogenous leukemia
BRCA1, BRCA2	Breast, ovarian
EWSR1 (EWS)	Ewing sarcoma
HER2/neu (ERBB2)	Breast, ovarian
MLH1, MSH2	Colorectal
MYC (c-myc)	Burkitt lymphoma, others
MYCN (N-myc)	Neuroblastoma
RB1	Retinoblastoma, others
TP53 (p53)	Brain, skin, lung, head and neck

Source: American Cancer Society

any growth factor to stimulate a cell depends on expression of these surface molecules. Some of these receptor proteins are actually enzymes that, when activated, begin a series of signals within the cell, resulting in cell division. Certain mutations in the genes that encode these receptors may, in effect, cause a "short circuit" in regulation, resulting in loss of control and continuous movement of the cell through the cell cycle.

One example of such a receptor mutation is that of the HER2/neu proteinHER2/neu (also known as ERBB2) receptor protein expressed on certain breast cells. The HER2/neu protein is similar in its amino acid sequence to the human epidermal growth factor receptor molecule and is an example of a transmembrane enzyme that begins the signal transmission in the cell. A mutation in the HER2/neu proto-oncogene converts it into the HER2/neu oncogene (named for the neuroblastoma in which it was first identified). Overexpression of the HER2/neu protein is associated with the aggressive nature of certain forms of breast cancer. The basis for the chemotherapeutic action of Herceptin is its ability to inhibit the activity of the HER2/neu protein.

Signal mechanisms represent a series or cascade of enzymatic reactions that move the cell through the cell cycle and regulate cell division. Regulation generally involves phosphorylation by kinases at either tyrosine or serine residues on the substrate. Mutations in the signaling pathway arguably represent the most common forms of genetic mutation which result in cell transformation. The reason is the critical role played by these proteins in regulation of cell activity. Intermediates in this pathway are primarily kinase enzymes that activate DNA-binding proteins (DBPs), inducing gene expression. Examples include the src (tyrosine) kinase and Jun kinase. Other oncogenes in this category include transcription factors such as the *myc* gene, which also regulates cell replication. Translocation of the *myc* gene is associated with Burkitt Lymphoma.

The RAS supergene family and the greater than one hundred proteins its members encode are examples of such inducers. RAS proteins are also called G proteins, reflecting their utilization of guanosine triphosphate (GTP) for their activity. Mutations in these genes may result in a continuous activating signal within the cell and uncontrolled cell division. Certain forms of colon and bladder cancers are the result of such mutations, and some forms of mutations are associated with mutations in the DNA-binding protein substrates for these RAS proteins. RAS gene mutations have been observed in nearly one-third of all cancers.

Tumor-suppressor genes/regulators of apoptosis control steps at the end of the cell cycle. The proto-oncogenes that regulate apoptosis can either promote or inhibit cell death. The BCL2 gene family produces proteins that are pro-apoptosis and anti-apoptosis (the BCL2 gene itself inhibits apoptosis, and its overexpression has been implicated in cancers such as lymphoma). Proto-oncogenes and tumor suppressors provide the cell with the means not only to block division if chromosome replication is incomplete or if a mutation has occurred that could cause the cell to become cancerous, but also to actually cause the cell to die. Tumor suppressors promote apoptosis and therefore are usually deactivated in cancers.

The first of the tumor suppressors to be discovered was the retinoblastoma RB1 protein, isolated in the 1980's. The RB1 protein regulates the steps that allow DNA replication to begin in the cell. The p53 protein, named for its size, detects mutations that have occurred in DNA and induces repair of the DNA site or, if the mutation is too extensive, induces steps that culminate in the death of the cell.

As is true for other genes that regulate cell division, mutations in the genes associated with tumor suppression are associated with certain forms of cancer. For example, mutations in the RB1 gene may predispose the person for retinoblastoma. Mutations in the p53 gene have been found in nearly 50 percent of all forms of cancer. The ability of oncogenic viruses such as hepatitis B, the etiological agent for hepatocarcinoma, or the human papillomavirus, the agent for cervical carcinoma, to initiate cancer is related to their abilities to inactivate tumor suppressors. Mutations at these sites may be caused as a result of infection by certain viruses or by exposure to carcinogens, most of which are also mutagens, chemicals that induce DNA mutations. In some cases, the mutation is congenital, the individual having been born with that specific mutation. Childhood retinoblastoma, for example, results from congenital mutations in the RB1 gene.

In some cases, it is not "simply" a point mutation in a proto-oncogene that leads to a cancer. Certain forms of the disease are known to result from chromosomal breaks and translocations, the movement of pieces of chromosomes from one site to another in the cell chromatin. One example is the aforementioned myc oncogene in Burkitt Lymphoma. The DNA in patients suffering from chronic myelogenous leukemia was also found to possess a specific type of translocation. What became known as the Philadelphia chromosome is characterized by translocation of the ABL1 oncogene, on chromosome 9, into the region of the BCR oncogene on chromosome 22. The combined gene product disrupts the normal signaling mechanism in these cells, resulting in uncontrolled cell division. Inhibition of this activity is the basis of action for at least one type of antileukemic drug, imatinib mesylate (Gleevec), lending further support to this mutation as being the actual cause of chronic myelogenous leukemia.

Cancer, however, generally is not the result of any individual mutation. The molecules previously described regulate cell division, The difference between a benign growth and a true malignancy is the result of accumulated mutations over time. For example, a malignancy would require not only a mutation in the signal pathway but also, at a minimum, additional mutations in tumor-suppressor genes or in steps that inhibit cell death.

History: The evidence for existence of oncogenes dates to the early history of retroviruses, viruses with genomes of ribonucleic acid (RNA), which are copied into DNA following infection and which were found to be etiological agents for some forms of cancer. In the late nineteenth century, leukemia in animals was demonstrated to be transmissible using extracts from cells. However, leukemia was not considered to be a true cancer at the time. It was only when Peyton Rous demonstrated in 1911 that solid tumors in chickens sarcomas could be transmitted using cell-free extracts that scientists began to believe cancer, at least in animals, was associated with infectious agents. Eventually what became known as the Rous sarcoma virus (RSV) was isolated and identified with this disease in chickens.

As an increasing number of such tumor viruses, in which RNA was shown to be the genetic material, were isolated by the 1950's, the question that followed was how these viruses could change, or transform, cells from normal to cancerous. In 1958 Howard M. Temin and Harry Rubin demonstrated that single virus particles could transform chicken cells. Further work by Temin indicated that it was possible to disrupt viral replication and transformation by adding inhibitors acting at the level of DNA. Temin proposed that such viruses act using a DNA intermediate and that they encode an enzyme that copies RNA into DNA, allowing what has become viral DNA to integrate into the cell chromosome. By the late 1960's Temin and David Baltimore independently discovered an enzyme, popularly known as reverse transcriptase, that carries out this function. Viruses that encode the enzyme have become known as retroviruses and include the RNA tumor viruses. Temin and Baltimore were each awarded the Nobel Prize in Physiology or Medicine in 1975.

The seemingly simplistic genetic structure of the RNA tumor viruses lent itself to determining which viral genes are associated with cancers. The discovery of a temperature-sensitive mutation in one of these genes led to the identification of the src gene from the Rous sarcoma virus, the first such oncogene to be discovered.

The src gene was shown to be required for transformation by the Rous sarcoma virus. However, strains of the virus that lacked the gene were found to replicate normally, suggesting the src gene was superfluous for the virus and may even have originated as genetic material extraneous to the virus. In 1976 J. Michael Bishop and Harold Varmus provided the answer. Creating DNA probes from transformation defective mutants of the Rous sarcoma virus, they found that normal avian cells contained cellular homologs of the viral SRC gene that is, a cellular proto-oncogene. The proto-oncogene product of the gene was subsequently shown to be an enzyme critical in the signaling pathway that regulates cell division.

Through the 1980's, an increasing number of cellular proto-oncogenes were identified, and evidence for their association with cancers was increasingly demonstrated. When carcinogens were used to transform cells growing in laboratory cultures, mutations were found in proto-oncogenes carried by these cells. Indeed, the only difference found between proto-oncogenes in normal cells and oncogenes expressed in cancer cells was often a mutation at a single site. For example, the RAS oncogene found in cases of bladder cancer differed from its counterpart in a normal cell at only one amino acid position.

Transformation and tumor development require more than "simply" a mutation in a regulatory protein. The cell cycle includes a number of checkpoints, each monitored by forms of tumor suppressors. The most common of these suppressors include the aforementioned RB and p53 proteins, and mutations in their respective genes are associated with a number of cancers. Since the year 2000, over a dozen additional proteins have been found to regulate cell cycle checkpoints. It has become clear that a series of progressive mutations must take place, most of which are associated with growth regulation, for cancer to progress.

Richard Adler, Ph.D.

For Further Information

Bignold, Leon. *Principles of Tumors.* San Diego, CA: Academic Press, 2015.

Bishop, J. Michael. How to Win the Nobel Prize. Cambridge, Mass.: Harvard University Press, 2003.

Lynn, Jorde, et al. *Medical Genetics,* 5th ed. Philadelphia, PA: Elsevier, 2015.

Pelengaris, Stella, and Michael Khan. The Molecular Biology of Cancer. Malden, Mass.: Blackwell, 2006.

Vogelstein, Bert, and Kenneth Kinzler. The Genetic Basis of Human Cancer. New York: McGraw-Hill, 2002.

Other Resources

American Cancer Society
Oncogenes and Tumor Suppressor Genes.
http://www.cancer.org/docroot/ETO/content/ETO_1_4x_oncogenes_and_tumor_suppressor_genes.asp

CancerQuest
Important Oncogenes.
http://www.cancerquest.org/index.cfm?page=181

See also: Angiogenesis; Ataxia Telangiectasia (AT); Biological therapy; BRAF gene; Breast cancer in pregnant women; Breast cancers; Cancer biology; Carcinomas; Chromosomes and cancer; Craniosynostosis; Cytogenetics; Endocrine cancers; Free radicals; Gene therapy; Genetics of cancer; Giant Cell Tumors (GCTs); Hemangiosarcomas; HER2/neu protein; HIV/AIDS-related cancers; HRAS gene testing; Hypercalcemia; Mesothelioma; Mitochondrial DNA mutations; Monoclonal antibodies; Multiple endocrine neoplasia; Mutagenesis and cancer; MYC oncogene; Myelofibrosis; Neuroendocrine tumors; Oncogenic viruses; Parathyroid cancer; Proto-oncogenes and carcinogenesis; RhoGD12 gene; SCLC1 gene; Tumor-suppressor genes; Viral oncology; Virus-related cancers

▶ Personalized medicine/whole genome sequencing

Category: Cancer Biology
Also known as: Precision Medicine

Definition: Personalized medicine is a medical strategy that focuses on the unique characteristics of the individual patient. This strategy differs from the more traditional "broad strokes" approach of treating diseases based on what has statistically proven effective for the majority of the population. The personalized medicine approach takes the unique genetic makeup of the patient into account in order to find the treatment(s) that will be most effective and cause the least harmful side effects. This is usually accomplished by exploring the patient's genetics and family medical history as well as testing and analyzing the tumor to come up with a personalized treatment plan. While this approach can be used for nearly all aspects of healthcare, currently one of the main focuses of personalized medicine has been on the treatment and prevention of cancer.

Whole genome sequencing is the process of analyzing and identifying the approximately 3 billion nucleotides that compose the human genome, usually from a small DNA sample. Nucleotides are sugar-phosphate-nitrogenous base compounds that serve as the structural units of DNA. While most genetic testing focuses on a few genes (mostly common problem genes), whole genome sequencing allows physicians and researchers to see the big picture. This allows them to better identify which drugs and/or treatments will be most ideal based on the patient's unique genetic makeup.

History and uses: The benefits of personalizing treatments to the individual patient have been known in the medical community since the 1960s. However, the term "personalized medicine" did not appear in journal articles until 1999. It only recently has started to become a feasible reality for the broader population due to advances and inventions of new technologies. Many innovations in the realms of science, technology, and an increased understanding of human genetics have come together to make this more precise and personalized approach to medicine possible. Several major discoveries have specifically paved the way for this approach, and are thus, worth discussing here.

The Human Genome Project (HGP), an international research project that decoded and mapped all of the genes of the human genome, paved the way for genetic testing to become more accurate and accessible. The successful completion of the first human genome in 2003 (accomplished as part of the HGP) was a great victory for science and personalized medicine, as it aided the scientific understanding of human genetics. Also, this discovery significantly furthered the medical community's understanding of how genetic variables play an important role in prescribing the most ideal treatments for individual patients while minimizing adverse side effects. The HGP discovered that 99.1% of the human genome is identical, regardless of genetic factors, and 0.9% is variable.

Additionally, 2 technological and innovative extensions have been developed from HGP: single nucleotide polymorphism (SNP, ie, single base pair variations in a DNA sequence) genotyping and the invention of the microarray biochip. SNP genotyping is the process of measuring and analyzing genetic variations of SNPs that are common in the population. This information helps the medical community gauge the general public's susceptibility to certain diseases and to fine-tune treatment approaches to be more effective and precise and to minimize side effects. The microarray biochip is a technology that has the capability to store and analyze the whole human genome within a single biochip. Doctors and researchers trained in genome analysis use this tool to further the development of new drugs and treatments. These drugs and treatments can then be used for people of specific genetic constitutions as well as for the general public.

Uses and cost of whole genome sequencing: Whole genome sequencing (WGS) can be used to diagnose diseases, identify genetic mutations, help physicians come up with personalized treatment plans, and expose uncommon genetic issues that are often overlooked by the more limited types of normal genetic testing. The first entire human genome that was sequenced as part of the HGP in 2003 cost $2.7 billion and took over a decade to complete. However, the DNA sequencing technology has become much more efficient and effective. Today, WGS can be done for approximately $10,000 and typically takes less than a week. As sequencing technology continues to advance, the process may eventually become even more affordable, convenient, and accessible to the general public.

Ethical concerns of WGS: Despite the potential benefits of WGS, the ability to identify and analyze a person's entire genome does present some ethical issues. Because genome sequencing is a relatively new technology, the security measures and policies designed to protect the privacy of the patient are still in the early stages. This is especially worth noting because of the very large volume of information that can be gleaned from the results of whole genome sequencing. This information used by the wrong hands could cause major problems for the medical and scientific communities as well as the broader population. Also, results from WGS can reveal potential ailments that the patient does not want to know about.

Disadvantages of WGS: Because WGS is still quite new, much in the field remains unknown or not fully understood. Scientists and physicians still do not fully understand the role and function of the majority of genes in the human genome. WGS technology has come a long way but still has a ways to go before the human genome is even close to being fully understood. While some physicians are trained in interpreting this type of data, the majority of physicians are not.

Benjamin Noah Riley

For Further Information

Pucheril, D. & Sharma, S. (2011). The history and future of personalized medicine. *Managed Care Magazine*. Retrieved from: http://www.managedcaremag.com/content/history-and-future-personalized-medicine.

Mendes, E. (2015). Personalized medicine: Redefining cancer and its treatment. Retrieved from: http://www.cancer.org/research/acsresearchupdates/more/personalized-medicine-redefining-cancer-and-its-treatment.

Stein, R. (September, 2012). Scientists see upside and downside of sequencing their own genes. Retrieved from: http://www.npr.org/sections/health-shots/2012/09/19/160955379/scientists-see-upside-and-downside-of-sequencing-their-own-genes.

Other Resources

Whole Genome Sequencing
http://knowgenetics.org/whole-genome-sequencing/
PMC. http://www.personalizedmedicinecoalition.org/

What Is Personalized Medicine?
http://genomemag.com/what-is-personalized-medicine/#.VoAzi5g5cUU
A High-Resolution View of the Entire Genome
http://www.illumina.com/techniques/sequencing/dna-sequencing/whole-genome-sequencing.html

Personalized Medicine In Oncology
http://www.personalizedmedonc.com/

See also: Gene therapy; Genomics of cancer

▶ Placental Alkaline Phosphatase (PALP)

Category: Cancer Biology

Definition: Placental alkaline phosphatase (PALP) is one of the four isoenzymes of alkaline phosphatase, a group of enzymes that hydrolyze organic phosphate esters. Alkaline phosphatase isoenzymes associated with the liver, bone, and intestine are normally present in serum. When the serum alkaline phosphatase level is above established reference ranges, determining which fraction is elevated may be helpful in pinpointing the source of disease.

PALP is normally produced by the syncytiotrophoblast of the placenta. This unique cell layer is in direct contact with maternal blood during pregnancy and is considered the source of rising PALP levels in maternal plasma during gestation, with the highest levels occurring right before delivery.

PALP-like isoenzymes are similar to PALP but different enough in their biochemical and physical properties to be considered separate proteins. Several PALP-like isoenzymes have been identified, characterized, and named: Regan, Nagao, and Kasahara. Some authors refer to the PALP-like isoenzymes as germ-cell alkaline phosphatases.

Related cancers: When pregnancy is not a condition of consideration, elevated levels of PALP have been associated with cancers of the testis, ovary, colorectal tract, and lung. In the 1970's and 1980's, researchers investigated the relationship between malignant changes in many tissues with the serum concentration of several fetal-type proteins. They pursued PALP along with alpha-fetoprotein (AFP) and carcinoembryonic antigen (CEA) as tumor markers. Of these, PALP and the PALP-like isoenzymes have yet to be demonstrated as useful markers for screening or monitoring cancer and related conditions.

Ongoing research: Cancer researchers continue to explore a role for PALP as a tumor marker. Antibodies to detect and differentiate PALP and the related PALP-like isoenzymes are being designed and tested. Some of the antibodies are used in immunohistochemistry protocols, requiring a biopsy of the organ where the suspicious tumor is located. These tissue biopsy studies can confirm the presence of PALP and PALP-like isoenzymes, which further choracterizing the tumor and leading to a more specific diagnosis and targeted therapy.

Other researchers are designing antibodies that target PALP and PALP-like isoenzymes in an individual's plasma and thus can serve as noninvasive markers for cancer. To date elevated concentrations of PALP and PALP-like enzymes have been found to be no better than cancer antigen 125 (CA 125) and AFP in monitoring ovarian cancer. However, there is some evidence that PALP and PALP-like isoenzymes may become useful indicators of cancer recurrence in survivors.

Jane Adrian, M.P.H., Ed.M., M.T. (ASCP)

See also: Alkaline Phosphatase Test (ALP); Cancer biology; Immunocytochemistry and immunohistochemistry; Paget disease of bone; Pregnancy and cancer; Staging of cancer; Tumor markers

▶ *PMS* genes

Category: Cancer Biology

Also known as: PMS1 postmeiotic segregation increased 1 (*Saccharomyces cerevisiae*); postmeiotic segregation increased (*S. cerevisiae*) 1; PMS2 postmeiotic segregation increased 2 (*S. cerevisiae*); postmeiotic segregation increased (*S. cerevisiae*) 2

Definition: *PMS* genes, *PMS1* and *PMS2*, encode proteins that are part of the cellular mismatch repair machinery that corrects errors made during deoxyribonucleic acid (DNA) replication. Defects in mismatch repair proteins are seen in hereditary nonpolyposis colorectal cancer, or HNPCC.

Normal cellular function: Each time a cell divides, it must faithfully replicate its genetic material contained within the DNA. Due to the inherent properties of the replication machinery, a number of mutations are made each time the genome is replicated. These mutations are rarely permanent, though, because of the action of a set of proteins that recognize and repair DNA damage. One type of repair mechanism is called the mismatch repair pathway.

Role in cancer: Individuals who inherit a mutation in one of the mismatch repair genes are strongly predisposed to developing certain types of cancer, including colorectal, ovarian, and endometrial. *MLH1* and *MSH2* are the most commonly mutated genes in this pathway, but *PMS1* and *PMS2* are also mutated in some cases of hereditary nonpolyposis colorectal cancer. Cells that have defects in mismatch repair proteins have a mutator phenotype; that is, because the machinery that normally corrects errors is compromised, the frequency of mutations is significantly higher than in normal cells. These cells are more likely to accumulate mutations within genes that are critical for limiting cell growth and proliferation and inducing cell death when damage has been done to the DNA, which are characteristics of cancer cells.

Clinical implications: Because inheriting a mutation in one of the DNA mismatch repair genes greatly predisposes an individual to developing cancer, it is important to identify at-risk individuals so that they can be frequently screened for tumors. People with a strong family history of early-onset colorectal cancer are urged to undergo genetic testing to identify mutations in the mismatch repair genes. Once a tumor has formed, the levels of mismatch repair proteins can provide insight into the patient's prognosis and cancer progression. In addition, knowing the levels of mismatch repair proteins within tumor cells can have implications for the method of treatment that is prescribed. Although the effects vary based on tumor type, there have been data showing that the state of the mismatch repair machinery can affect the efficacy of certain types of chemotherapeutic agents. For example, patients with ovarian cancer resulting from defective mismatch repair show higher levels of cancer recurrence following treatment with cisplatin.

Lindsay Lewellyn, B.S.

See also: Endometrial cancer; Family history and risk assessment; Genetic testing; Genetics of cancer; Hereditary cancer syndromes; Ovarian cancers; Turcot syndrome

▶ Proteasome

Category: Cancer Biology

Also known as: Proteosome (alternate spelling), protein degradation pathway

Definition: The proteasome is a "machine" found in the cell whose job it is to degrade/destroy proteins and return small strings of amino acids from the protein to the cell for reuse (think of the disposal unit on a kitchen sink). The proteasome itself is made from proteins, and the principal target of proteasomes is endogenous proteins (proteins synthesized in the cell). This includes proteins that were incorrectly folded and those that were coded incorrectly by either translation errors or faulty genes (various DNA mutations). It also includes proteins whose work has been completed, such as those that control the cell cycle (eg, cyclins needing to be destroyed in order to prepare for the subsequent cycle) and proteins involved in transcriptional control that need to be cleared at regular intervals. Excess enzymes within the cell are also destroyed through the proteasome. Finally, proteasomes are involved in the destruction of proteins coded by viruses and other intracellular parasites. An average human cell contains about 30,000 proteasomes, which are constantly built, repaired, and recycled.

The core protein (or core particle) of the proteasome consists of two copies of each of 14 different proteins. These are assembled into rings and stacked 4-high, each consisting of 7 proteins. The result is a barrel-shaped assembly with openings at each end. The site of active enzymatic work is on the inside. Regulatory peptides, stationed at either end of the barrel, act as a lock and allow entry to the barrel only when proteins have been tagged properly. Each regulatory peptide consists of 19 different proteins (none the same as the 14 proteins of the core particle).

The process of protein destruction in the cell begins with a protein molecule known as ubiquitin. This small protein (76 amino acids) is tasked with identifying and binding to the terminal amino group of lysine residues within proteins. As soon as one ubiquitin tags a protein, other molecules of ubiquitin bind to the first, thus forming a chain (poly-ubiquitylated proteins). This process is mediated by a cascade of enzymes (E1, E2, and E3) that activate, conjugate, and transfer multiple ubiquitin molecules to proteins targeted for destruction. This ubiquitin chain is then recognized by a special ubiquitin-recognizing sequence of the regulatory peptide, allowing the complex to bind to the proteasome and unfold. This process of protein unfolding requires ATP (active process), and is produced by 6 of the regulatory peptides that are ATPases.

Denatured (unfolded) proteins are then moved into the central cavity of the barrel where the active sites for destruction are located. Proteins are broken apart into small peptides of about 8 amino acids each before exiting the opposite end of the proteasome. These small peptides are usually further broken down into individual amino acids by peptidases in the cytoplasm, thus returning to the cellular amino acid pool to be reutilized in the construction of needed proteins. As this occurs, the ubiquitin molecules are released from the regulatory proteins and reused in the cell.

A secondary side of proteasomes is their role in the human immune system. Cytotoxic T cells (one group of lymphocytes found in humans) detect other cells of the body that express, on their surface, foreign or mutated protein molecules. They then remove/destroy these cells. Recognition of these cells depends entirely on the binding of these "antigenic" proteins by MHC (major histocompatibility complex) class I molecules. The proteasome is responsible for generation of appropriately-sized peptide fragments from viruses or tumors that may then be presented to the MHC class I molecules in the endoplasmic reticulum (via specific transporter molecules) and subsequently moved to the surface of the cell.

Etiology and symptoms of associated cancers: The ubiquitin-proteasome pathway, as has been shown, is important in regulating many pathways in the cell that are important for cell growth and survival. This is true also for tumor cells, and since the rate of protein synthesis and degradation in cancer cells is higher than normal, any errors or blockage of the pathway may lead to cell death.

Defects in the pathway are associated with a number of diseases, including Spinocerebellar ataxia type 1 and multiple myeloma. Spinocerebellar ataxia type 1 is a neurological disorder in which patients experience declining balance and coordination that eventually leaves them unable to walk or even talk. It is caused by a buildup in nervous system cells of a mutated protein (ataxin-1) that is unable to be unfolded for entry into the proteasome. As a result, it accumulates in the cell and eventually kills it. As more and more cells die, symptoms of the disease increase.

Multiple myeloma is a cancer of the blood in which there is a clonal proliferation of neoplastic plasma cells in the bone marrow. These cells produce abnormal proteins (immunoglobulins) that affect the function of the immune system, damage the kidneys, and may cause cancerous tumors. The growth of myeloma cells relies on the proteasome-dependent degradation IκB-alpha (a protein involved in regulation of transcription). In non-malignant cells, the proteasome carefully regulates IκB-alpha.

Testing and treatment: Drugs that elicit proteasome-inhibiting action (proteasome inhibitors) provide a mechanism for blocking cancer cell growth.

Bortezomib (Velcade) was approved in 2003 for use in treating multiple myeloma. Bortezomib blocks the proteolytic action of the proteasome. As a result, the degradation of IκB-alpha (a protein involved in regulation of transcription) ceases, and IκB-alpha induces the degradation of the transcription factor NF-κB. This prevents the transcription of dozens of genes required for proliferation and adhesion of myeloma cells, effectively stopping the progression of the disease. In addition, the failure to degrade cyclins in a timely manner inhibits the cell cycle and therefore, the mitotic activity of the myeloma cells.

Several new proteasome inhibitors have been introduced in recent years, including carfilzomib, marizomib, and MLN9708. Trials of these "second-generation" proteasome inhibitors have demonstrated positive results for patients with multiple myelomas.

History: The 2004 Nobel Prize in Chemistry was awarded to 3 biochemists (Aaron Ciechanover, Avram Hershko, and Irwin Rose) "for the discovery of ubiquitin-mediated protein degradation."

Kerry L. Cheesman, PhD

For Further Information

Adams, J. (2003). The proteasome: structure, function, and role in the cell. *Cancer Treatment Reviews*, 29(suppl 1): 3–9.

Crawford, L., Walker, B., & Levine, A. (2011). Proteasome inhibitors in cancer therapy. *Journal of Cell Communication and Signaling*, 5(2): 101–110.

Devoy, A., Soane, T., Welchman, R., & Mayer, R.J. (2005). The ubiquitin-proteasome system and cancer. *Essays in Biochemistry*, 41: 187–203.

Goldberg, A.L., Elledge, S.J. & Harper, J.W. (2001). The cellular chamber of doom. *Scientific American*, 284(1): 56–61.

Moreau, P., Richardson, P.G., Cavo, M., Orlowski, R.Z., San Miguel, J.F., Palumbo, A., & Harousseau, J.L. (2012). Proteasome inhibitors in multiple myeloma: 10 years later. *Blood*, 120: 947–959.

Other Resources

HHMI Biointeractive — a 3-D animation
http://www.hhmi.org/biointeractive/proteasome

The Nobel Prize Committee 2004
http://www.nobelprize.org/nobel_prizes/chemistry/laureates/2004/press.html

See also: Bortezomib (Velcade); Cell cycle control

▶ Proteomics and cancer research

Category: Cancer Biology

Definition: The term "proteome" was coined in 1994 to describe the study of all the protein forms expressed within an organism, tissue, or group of cells as a function of time, age, state, and external factors. Many technological advances have led to the emergence of the discipline termed proteomics, which is now widely employed in the cancer field.

Background: Many scientists are using the rapidly emerging technologies of proteomics in an effort to identify new cancer biomarkers, specific protein species in the body that are helpful for disease prediction or treatment, and to understand the underlying mechanisms associated with cancer onset and progression. These technologies are also being applied to drug development and the identification of patients who might benefit from targeted therapies. Proteomics integrates some key fundamental technologies such as high-throughput protein separation and profiling, mass spectrometry, large databases, and bioinformatics tools to analyze and extract information from these databases.

Scientific rationale: After the human genome was sequenced, it consisted of fewer genes than scientists had expected—approximately 30,000, about twice as many genes as a worm or fly. This raised the question of how human complexity can be explained by a genome with such a relatively small number of genes. Scientists realized that such complexity is achieved in part by the economical use of genes. The effective number of distinct protein species present in a cell is greatly increased through a wide variety of ways in which proteins can be modified after being synthesized, collectively called posttranslational modifications. These modifications range from the addition of biochemical functional groups such as phosphate groups (resulting in phosphorylation) and carbohydrate groups (resulting in glycosylation), the addition of other proteins or peptides, chemical changes to the amino acids of the protein, and structural changes to the protein such as formation of disulfide bridges or proteolytic cleavage of the protein.

Besides their ability to undergo modifications, another characteristic of proteins is their dynamic state. They have the ability to constantly move around and bind to other proteins or cellular components. Proteins are able to respond quickly to a changing cellular environment, and they play an important role in the elaborate communication pathways within and between cells. A cell's complement of proteins in their specific posttranslationally modified forms is increasingly being recognized as playing an important role in many cellular processes and states, including cancer.

Scientists believe that cancer develops through a multistep process involving the accumulation of genetic alterations that lead to altered gene expression patterns, protein structures, and functions. Because the transformation of a normal cell to a cancerous one involves changes in the proteins present in the cell, the aim of proteomics in cancer research is to monitor these changes and use the information to provide valuable information that may aid diagnosis, prognosis, and monitoring response to therapy.

One goal of proteomics in cancer research is to define the expression patterns of proteins that are expressed at different levels in cells in different physiological states, such as cancer cells compared with noncancerous cells, or late-stage cancer cells compared with early-stage cancer cells. Another goal is the identification of tumor markers, proteins that are associated with particular types of cancer. Ideally, such markers would be sensitive, selective, and measurable by a noninvasive procedure (such as by analysis of blood or urine). In addition, the emergence of proteomics offers the promise of helping to elucidate the complex molecular events involved in cancer, as well as those that control clinically important tumor behaviors such as metastases, invasion, and resistance to therapy. Biomarkers may also be used to help devise optimal therapeutic treatment plans for different patient subsets and to monitor the effect of treatment.

Technologies: Proteomics consists of sample preparation, protein separation, and protein identification. Since the late 1990's, mass spectrometry has increasingly become the method of choice for analyses of complex protein samples. Mass spectrometry is a technique that generates electrically charged fragments from the proteins present in the mixture and measures particular properties of those fragments. The end product is a spectrum or chart with a series of peaks. The size of the peaks and the distance between them provide a "fingerprint" of the sample. Mass spectrometry offers the ability to measure, rapidly and inexpensively, thousands of proteins in a few drops of blood. The entire process, from collection of a few drops of blood to analyzing the "fingerprint," can take less than one minute. Hundreds of samples can be analyzed sequentially and very small amounts of protein can be detected.

The spectrum obtained from mass spectrometry experiments is difficult to analyze manually, but computers are being used to analyze such patterns and distinguish small differences in patterns between patients. Bioinformatics tools are the computer-based algorithms that are used to convert raw proteomics data into a useful form that can be analyzed, compared, interpreted, and stored in large databases.

Of particular interest in the field of proteomics research are high-throughput technologies that are capable of simultaneous and rapid analysis of multiple samples. One example is microarray technology, an automated technique for the simultaneous analysis of thousands of different samples affixed to a thumbnail-sized "chip" of glass or silicon.

Examples of tumor markers: The tumor marker prostate-specific antigen (PSA) is indispensable in the management of prostate cancer. Patients at high risk for primary liver cancer are screened by the tumor marker alphafetoprotein, in combination with ultrasonography, a regimen that has been shown to result in earlier detection and therefore more effective treatment and longer survival for patients with this type of cancer. Available screening tests for ovarian cancer include the biomarker cancer antigen 125 (CA125), which has also proved to be a useful marker for monitoring response to chemotherapy. A rapid fall in the CA 125 level during chemotherapy predicts a favorable prognosis. In another example for ovarian cancer, a blood test for the levels of four proteins (leptin, prolactic, osteopontin, and insulin-like growth factor II) has been shown to discriminate with high accuracy between patients with early ovarian cancer and those who were disease free.

Challenges: The identification of large numbers of proteins from complex biological samples is a continuing challenge in this field. Techniques to address this challenge are evolving quickly. The biological variability among patient samples and the large concentration range over which proteins can be present also present challenges to deducing diagnostic patterns that are unique to specific types of cancer. The fast pace of technological innovation in this area should result in the identification of new biomarkers for different cancers and their use to improve diagnosis and treatment.

Standardization of proteomics techniques is needed to allow for the reproducibility required for medical applications. Alarge knowledge base is needed to allow for the accurate interpretation of proteomics data. Large databases, such as the publicly available Protein Atlas, are being assembled. Frozen tissue banks will be useful to preserve tissue samples for future analysis and comparison of samples taken at different times.

The main bottlenecks for proteomics research are the rapid accumulation of data and the lack of suitable computational tools for analysis. Data are being collected at a faster pace than researchers can validate, interpret, and integrate with other known data. Software tools are needed in all areas of data analysis, including data collection, searching, evaluation, archiving, and retrieval.

Prospects: With the ongoing rapid technological developments in this field, the prospects for identification of new highly sensitive and specific biomarkers for different cancers and their use for making significant contributions to the understanding, diagnosis, and treatment of cancer patients seems very hopeful.

Jill Ferguson, Ph.D.

For Further Information

Brusic, V., O. Marina, C. J. Wu, and E. L. Reinherz. "Proteome Informatics for Cancer Research: From Molecules to Clinic." *Proteomics* 7 (2007): 976-991.

Cho, W. C. S. "Contribution of Oncoproteomics to Cancer Biomarker Discovery." *Molecular Cancer* 6 (2007): 25-37.

Liang, S.-L., and D. W. Chan. "Enzymes and Related Proteins as Cancer Biomarkers: A Proteomic Approach." *Clinica Chimica Acta* 381 (2007): 93-97.

Pastwa, E., S. B. Somiari, M. Czyz, and R. I. Somiari. "Proteomics in Human Cancer Research." *Proteomics—Clinical Application* 1 (2007): 4-17.

Reid, J. D., C. E. Parker, and C. H. Borchers. "Protein Arrays for Biomarker Discovery." *Current Opinion in Molecular Therapeutics* 9 (2006): 216-221.

Wu, W., W. Hu, and J. J. Kavanagh. "Proteomics in Cancer Research." *International Journal of Gynecological Cancer* 12 (2002): 409-423.

Other Resources

The Human Genome/Wellcome Trust
Proteomics and Cancer
http://genome.wellcome.ac.uk/doc_WTD020926.html

National Cancer Institute
Clinical Proteomic Technologies for Cancer
http://proteomics.cancer.gov

See also: Alpha-Fetoprotein (AFP) levels; American Association for Cancer Research (AACR); CA125 test; Cancer biology; Chemotherapy; Pathology; Prostate-Specific Antigen (PSA) test; Screening for cancer; Tumor markers

▶ Proto-oncogenes and carcinogenesis

Category: Cancer Biology
Also known as: Precursors of oncogenes

Definition: Proto-oncogenes are cellular genes that may be transformed into oncogenes (cancer-causing genes). Proto-oncogenes provide signals that promote the division and specialization of normal cells or regulate programmed cell death (apoptosis). Changes in their genetic sequence or their expression level due to chromosomal translocation, point mutation, or amplification can trigger a sequence of events leading to the neoplastic transformation (abnormal growth) of a cell and subsequently to tumor formation.

Particularly at risk are persons carrying chromosomal translocations or molecular rearrangements in their genome and persons infected with distinct viruses: Epstein-Barr virus (EBV) in Burkitt lymphoma, sinonasal lymphoma, and lymphomas in immunocompromized patients; human T-cell lymphotropic virus type 1 (HTLV-1) in adult T-cell lymphoma/leukemia; and human herpesvirus 8 (HHV-8) in body-cavity-based lymphomas in patients infected with the human immunodeficiency virus (HIV).

Etiology and symptoms of associated cancers: B-cell lymphomas are caused by malignant B-cell lymphocytes. Through a chromosomal translocation, the *BCL2* protooncogene may become rearranged, resulting in overexpression of its protein product. The protein product blocks apoptosis, thereby enabling continued growth of the malignant B cells.

T-cell lymphomas show a high frequency of a characteristic chromosomal translocation, resulting in the combination of the *NPM1/ALK* genes and a fused oncogenic protein product.

Nephroblastoma (Wilms' tumor) is the most common malignant tumor of the kidney in children. Mutations of the *WT1* proto-oncogene are found in approximately 20 percent of Wilms' tumors, half of which additionally carry mutations in *CTNNB1*, a proto-oncogene encoding betacatenin.

Plasmacytomas frequently show chromosomal translocations resulting in dysregulation of oncogenes followed by proliferation of a plasma cell clone. Genomic instability leads to further mutations and translocations.

The oncogene *CCND1* product cyclin D1 is overexpressed in 45 to 50 percent of primary ductal mammary carcinomas, in part because of amplification of the region of the genome where the proto-oncogene is located. Other oncogenes that play roles in mammary carcinomas are *HER2/neu* (*ERBB2*), *MYC* (*c-myc*), and *WNT1*.

History: Oncogenes were first discovered in certain retroviruses and were later identified as cancer-causing agents in many animals. In 1976 it was demonstrated by J. Michael Bishop and Harold Varmus that cancer-causing genes (oncogenes) carried by certain viruses are derived from normal genes (proto-oncogenes) present in the cells of their host. Further research showed that such genes can cause cancer even without viral involvement. By 2008 scientists had identified more than one hundred oncogenes in animals.

Nicola E. Wittekindt, Dr.Sc. (ETH Zürich)

See also: Burkitt lymphoma; Cancer biology; Carcinogens, known; Carcinogens, reasonably anticipated; Carcinomas; Endocrine cancers; Epstein-Barr Virus; Free radicals; Gene therapy; Genetics of cancer; Giant Cell Tumors (GCTs); HIV/AIDS-related cancers; *HRAS* gene testing; Leukemias; Lymphomas; Mesothelioma; Mitochondrial DNA mutations; Molecular oncology; *MYC* oncogene; Nephroblastomas; Oncogenes; Oncogenic viruses; Viral oncology; Virus-related cancers; Wilms' tumor

▶ *RB1* gene

Category: Cancer Biology
Also known as: Retinoblastoma 1 (including osteosarcoma), OSRC

Definition: The *RB1* gene (a tumor-suppressor gene), which is 180 kilobase pairs with 27 exons, can become inactivated and cause retinoblastoma, a rare childhood cancer of the retina, occurring from in utero to about five years of age.

Gene location and function: The retinoblastoma gene, *RB1*, is on chromosome 13q14.2. This ubiquitously expressed gene codes for a 110 KDa tumor suppressor (pRB), which regulates cell division. The retinoblastoma protein regulates the progression of cells through the cell cycle and the exiting of differentiating cells from the cell cycle. This protein controls cell cycle by sequestering transcription factors and by deacetylating histones, involved in gene silencing. To lose the tumor-suppressor ability, both copies of the *RB1* gene must be mutated. Individuals with an inherited form of retinoblastoma have a germ-line mutation of one *RB1* gene. During development, the second copy of the *RB1* gene is mutated; control of the cell cycle is lost, and tumors develop. These tumors may be in both eyes. Other individuals have sporadic retinoblastoma in which mutations occur in the same somatic cell to inactivate both copies of the *RB1* gene. Sporadic retinoblastoma is often in only one eye.

***RB1* gene inactivation:** Causes of *RB1* gene inactivation include chromosome rearrangements of the 13q14 region; nucleotide changes, loss of heterozygosity (loss of the normal copy); and CpG hypermethylation in the *RB1* promoter region (which silences the gene).

Molecular screening: Methods to screen for *RB1* gene mutations include multiplex polymerase chain reaction (PCR) sequencing of the gene, a protein truncation test, and methylation analysis. The usual clinical screening for retinoblasoma requires examination of the eyes under anesthesia. Molecular screening could eliminate anesthesia-related risks and reduce the financial and psychological costs of clinical screening. Individuals without germ-line *RB1* mutations will not need the clinical screening. Fetuses that have highly penetrant germ-line mutations could be delivered early and treated sooner to save their vision. People with inherited forms of retinoblastoma (have one defective *RB1* gene) have an increased risk of developing other cancers, such as those of the bladder, pineal gland, bone, and skin.

Incidence: Retinoblastoma accounts for 3 percent of cancers in children under the age of fifteen. The frequency of retinoblastoma is about 1 in 20,000. About 60 percent of those with retinoblastoma have *RB1* mutations only in the tumor and not in other cells. Some 40 percent of retinoblastoma cases are hereditary. Of hereditary cases, 90 percent are due to new mutations occurring near the time of conception; 10 percent are due to a mutation inherited from a parent.

Susan J. Karcher, Ph.D.
Updated by: Richard Adler

See also: Cancer biology; Childhood cancers; Fibrosarcomas, soft-tissue; Oncogenes; Pineoblastomas; Retinoblastomas; Simian virus 40; Tumor-suppressor genes

▶ Regulatory T-cells

Category: Cancer Biology
Also known as: Tregs, suppressor T-cells

Definition: A type of lymphocyte having the ability to down-regulate or suppress the cell-mediated immune response. Yolk-sac or bone marrow derived stem cells travel to the thymus or to lymph nodes where the lymphocytic cells mature and acquire surface receptor proteins. The differentiation of Tregs in the thymus results from interactions with self-antigens. Tregs differentiating in the lymph nodes appear to do so in response to non-self-antigens such as allergens, foods, and the host microbes. The mature T (for thymus)-lymphocytes, or T cells, are categorized on the basis of the surface protein receptors and those bearing a CD4 receptor have the ability to control the cell-mediated immune response. The CD4 T cells that increase the immune response are called helper cells and those that decrease the response are called regulatory T cells. In the thymus developing lymphocytes with a high level of receptor proteins matching self-antigens are killed and those with no or very few matches with self-antigens develop into CD4 helper cells. The intermediate level of self-antigen matching lymphocytes are able to avoid destruction and form the pool of cells that develop into Tregs.

Etiology and symptoms of associated cancers: Tregs fulfill a critical role in maintaining a balanced immune system in health and disease. Early in carcinogenesis prolonged inflammation is an important driver of malignant mutations and Tregs may help prevent the development of cancer by suppressing the local inflammation. Additionally, infiltration of $FOXP3^+$ Tregs into tumors may decrease inflammatory stimuli and help limit carcinogenesis. An increase in the number of Tregs in lymphomas, head and neck cancers, and colorectal cancers has been associated with better outcomes, presumably due to the suppression of inflammation associated with these neoplasms, which reside in a highly microbial environment.

However, Tregs play a dual role in the development of cancer, and while the down regulation of inflammation limits the growth of some cancers, most cancers associated with an expansion of Tregs have a poorer prognosis. Tregs can suppress anti-tumor immunity. Cancer cells display a variety of antigens on their surfaces, some of which are self-antigens while others are unique to the cancer cells. It has been shown that the immune response to cancer is in part an immune response to self-antigens and is a type of autoimmunity. This is not surprising in that these unique cancer antigens are modified or aberrantly expressed self-antigens. Tregs have a role in protecting normal cells displaying self-antigens from damage or destruction by the immune system. This same beneficial protective mechanism can also protect cancer cells displaying self-antigens along with tumor-associated antigens from immunological targeting and subsequent destruction. Increased numbers of Tregs in cancers of the breast, lung (non-small cell), liver, kidney, pancreas, stomach, ovary, and cervix are associated with a poor prognosis. Furthermore, it has been shown that both tumor-infiltrating macrophages and tumor cells themselves can attract Tregs to the site of the tumor.

Testing and treatment: The concept of cancer immunosurveillance is generally accepted and the model of immuno-editing with 3 stages (elimination, equilibrium, and escape) demonstrates the dual role of the immune system. An intact immune system may find, attack, and eliminate new neoplasms, but may also interact with cancers to produce variants that are less immunogenic and thus able to suppress or evade the immune system. Tumor-associated antigens are modified variants of self-antigens and there is now evidence that Tregs suppress lymphocytic activity against tumors. Strategies have been devised to facilitate immune system effectiveness in eliminating tumors by reducing the number of Tregs. Monoclonal antibodies against $CD25^+$ lymphocytes in combination with a peptide vaccine have been reported to enhance anti-tumor immune responsiveness in metastatic breast cancer patients. Similar studies have also shown immunological enhancement in T cell lymphoma and renal cell carcinoma patients. However, these study treatments have failed to slow progression or improve mortality in non-small cell lung cancer, metastatic melanoma, or renal cell carcinoma patients.

There are numerous variables to consider with therapies depleting Tregs. First, Treg depletion is relatively short-lived as repopulation can occur in 48 days thus, providing a small, but potentially useful, window of therapeutic opportunity. Second, monoclonal antibody targeting CD25 is not specific for Tregs as approximately 25% of human T cells bear this antigen. Therefore, lymphocytes other than Tregs, which may be necessary for an optimum immune response to a tumor, may be depleted. Third, it has been shown that depletion of Tregs may lead to the undesirable adverse effect of autoimmunity.

In order to craft more effective strategies for treating cancer by immune enhancement, a better understanding of Treg function overall and in the microenvironment of the tumor will be needed. The balance between immune surveillance and autoimmunity is delicate and a carefully targeted approach based on a thorough understanding of the molecular mechanisms involved will be necessary to achieve success.

History: The concept of cancer immunosurveillance was first proposed in the early 1950s, but suppressors cells were not identified until 1971. Unfortunately, no specific surface markers could be found to identify and isolate these suppressor T cells thus, hampering further research until 1995 when a subset of CD4 T cells with high levels of interleukin-2 receptor alpha-chain (CD25) was identified. These cells had high levels of suppressor activity and were called regulatory T cells. It was subsequently found that all CD4 cells were capable of being unregulated to express CD25 thereby limiting the usefulness of this as a specific marker for Tregs. Recent research has revolved around the discovery of another more specific marker called forkhead/winged-helix transcription factor box P3 (FOXP3). Researchers now concentrate their efforts on $CD4^{+}CD25^{+}FoxP3^{+}$ T cells. A FOXP3 is a transcription factor located on the X chromosome and appears to be the key to the suppressor function of Tregs by controlling a number of other genes.

H. Bradford Hawley, MD

For Further Information

Corthay, A. (2010). How do Regulatory T Cells Work?" *Scandinavian Journal of Immunology*, 70(4): 759-767.

Josefowicz, S. Z., Lu, L-F., & Rudensky, A. Y. (2012). Regulatory T cells: Mechanisms of differentiation and function. *Annual Review of Immunology*, 30: 531-564.

Nishikawa, H., & Sakaguchi, S. (2014). Regulatory T cells in cancer immunotherapy. *Current Opinions in Immunology*, 27: 1-7.

Oleinika, K., Nibbs, R. J., Graham, G. J., & Fraser, A. R. (2013). Suppression, subversion and escape:The role of regulatory T cells in cancer progression. *Clinical and Experimental Immunology*, 171(1): 36-45.

Whiteside, T. L. (2012). What are regulatory T cells (Treg) regulating in cancer and why? *Seminars in Cancer Biology*, 22(4): 327-334.

Other Resources

National Cancer Institute (NCI)
www.nih.gov

National Cancer Center for Biotechnology Information
www.ncbi.nlm.nih.gov

▶ *RhoGDI2* gene

Category: Cancer Biology
Also known as: Guanine nucleotide binding protein, Guanine nucleotide dissociation inhibitor, tumor-suppressor gene

Definition: RhoGDI2 is an oncogene, the product of which suppresses the metastatic potential of several types of tumors, including those of the bladder, lung, prostate, ovarian, breast, and colon. The RhoGDI2 gene at one time was thought to "merely" regulate hematopoietic (blood cell) production, but was subsequently found to be expressed in other normal (non-cancerous) cells as well as in cancers. The method of regulation of expression of the gene is unknown. Tumors that have undergone metastasis appear to downregulate the gene, while increased expression is correlated with reduced levels of metastasis.

Significance: Mortality associated with cancer can be the result of two separate but interrelated processes: growth of the primary tumor and metastasis of the growth to distal sites, potentially any organ in the body, which may result in damage to that organ. Removal of the primary tumor by surgery may eliminate one growth, but if metastasis has taken place, the tumor may recur at other sites, potentially proving fatal. Elimination of metastatic growth sites has been addressed using chemotherapy, a method of treatment that may have significant side effects.

The discovery of the RhoGD12 suppressor gene potentially opens another method to limit metastasis. The gene product has been found to suppress metastasis associated with some, but not all cancers, apparently by interfering with the function of endothelin-1, a member of a protein family involved in cell signaling and cell dissemination from primary tumors. Endothelin-1 was found to be overexpressed in several forms of cancers, particularly ovarian cancers, and appears to play an important role in the development of these forms of cancers.

While the expression of RhoGDI2 is reduced in certain forms of cancer, particularly cancer of the bladder, levels are increased in ovarian cancer, some forms of colon cancer and stomach cancer. Whether this is the result of variations in cell type remains uncertain.

Recent studies have also suggested a possible role for the RhoGDI2 gene product in the induction of apoptosis – programmed cell death – in certain cells. The N-terminal portion of the protein has been shown to activate the cell caspase system, leading to cell death; reduced expression of the gene may provide a means for certain types of tumor cells to survive, through prevention of apoptosis. While it is intriguing to project a means of inhibiting metastasis through increasing the level of RhoGDI2 expression, increased expression seen in colon or stomach cancers has suggested a conflicting role for the gene.

History: In 2002 cancer researchers attempted to correlate the likelihood of metastasis of various types of neoplasms with the expression of specific genes. Using a technique known as microarray analysis, a method to measure expression of large numbers of genes in a cell, it was discovered that the level of expression of one specific gene, now called RhoGDI2, correlated with lack of metastasis in bladder cancers. That is, the greater the level of expression, the less likely metastasis would take place.

Richard Adler, Ph.D.

For Further Information

Golen, Kenneth van. *The Rho GTPases in Cancer.* New York: Springer, 2010.

Griner, Erin and Dan Theodorescu. "The faces and friends of RhoGDI2." *Cancer and Metastasis Review* (December 2012) 31(3): 519-528.

Tannock, Ian, et al. *The Basic Science of Oncology.* 5th ed. New York: McGraw-Hill, 2013.

See also: Bladder cancer; Breast cancers; Cancer biology; Chemotherapy; Colorectal cancer; Lung cancers; Metastasis; Oncogenes; Oncogenic viruses; Ovarian cancers; Prostate cancer; Proto-oncogenes and carcinogenesis; Tumor-suppressor genes

▶ *SCLC1* gene

Category: Cancer Biology
Also known as: Small-cell carcinoma of lung, small-cell lung cancer (SCLC)

Definition: The *SCLC1* gene is located on a region on the short arm of chromosome 3 that is frequently deleted in neoplastic lung cells associated with small-cell carcinomas, cells of epithelial origin.

Significance: Approximately 110,000 cases of small-cell carcinomas of the lung are diagnosed annually, accounting for some 60 percent of all forms of lung cancer diagnosed yearly. Small-cell carcinomas of the lung are most commonly associated with people exposed to airborne carcinogens, particularly those associated with cigarette smoke. This form of lung cancer is particularly aggressive and has undergone metastasis at the time of diagnosis. SCLC cells frequently express a number of unusual neuroendocrine markers, including dopa-decarboxylase (DDC), and evidence suggests that these cells originate from a form of neuroendocrine cells that differentiate into epithelial cells in the lung.

Cancer cells in general arise from mutations that disrupt normal regulation of cell divisions, frequently at the level of internal cell signaling. Expression of neuroendocrine markers in SCLC neoplasms appears to affect the *RHOA* (*ras* homolog) family of genes in particular, the products of which are part of the signaling mechanism to stimulate cell division. Other oncogenes also appear to be altered in cell lines originating from SCLC neoplasms.

Regulation of oncogenes in a cell in part involves the production of tumor suppressors, proteins that either regulate oncogene expression or serve as stop signals to prevent the cell from undergoing replication. The region of the short arm on chromosome 3 that is deleted, 3p14-23, and specifically the *SCLC1* gene, appears to encode one or more tumor suppressors.

Deletions of this region of chromosome 3, the region which encodes the *SCLC1* gene, appears to take place during the early stages of formation of the neoplasm. Whether the deletion is required for development of this form of cancer is unknown, but this specific mutation seems to occur in nearly all cases of SCLC that have been analyzed. The mechanism of the deletion is also unknown.

History: The presence of this particular deletion in small-cell carcinomas of the lung was first noted in 1982. Scientists had established a number of lung-cancer cell lines in the laboratory, the purpose of which was to study characteristics unique to each group; twelve lines originated as SCLC cases. All were observed to have the same deletion on chromosome 3, while cells from other lines did not.

Richard Adler, Ph.D.

See also: Bronchial adenomas; Bronchoalveolar lung cancer; Cancer biology; Cigarettes and cigars; Lambert-Eaton syndrome (LEMS); Lung cancers

▶ Telomerase

Category: Cancer Biology
Also known as: telomere terminal transferase, telomerase reverse transcriptase, TERT

Definition: Telomerase is a naturally occurring enzyme. It is present in higher concentrations in rapidly growing cells, such as stem cells, developing cells, and tumor cells. Telomerase activity participates in the uncontrolled cell growth and proliferation characteristic of cancer cells.

Etiology and symptoms of associated cancers: Telomerase is not specific for any single type of cancer. Rather, a broad range of human cancer types express telomerase in high concentrations.

In the majority of adult human stem cells telomerase levels are either low or absent. However, telomerase levels increase in cells undergoing rapid expansion. Rapidly expanding cells include committed hematopoietic progenitor cells (that form blood cells), activated lymphocytes (a type of white blood cell), keratinocytes (skin cells), and even within tissues with a low cell turnover (such as the brain).

Mutations in telomerase core components, TERT and TERC, have been found in patients who with aplastic anemia and dyskeratosis congenital. Both diseases are characterized by bone marrow failure and/or skin abnormalities, which result from defects in maintaining the hematopoietic stem cell compartment in bone marrow.

Testing and treatment: Cancer cells contain much higher concentrations of telomerase than normal cells. Therefore, inhibiting the action of telomerase should limit the typically uncontrolled growth of cancer cells. Telomerase inhibition is a key area of focus in cancer research, and telomerase inhibitors are currently being tested in clinical trials.

History: The enzyme telomerase was discovered in 1984. In 2009, the Nobel Prize in Physiology or Medicine was awarded to 3 scientists, Elizabeth H. Blackburn, Carol W. Greider, and Jack W. Szostak for the discovery of telomerase. Most cells are only capable of dividing a limited number of times before they reach senescence (growth arrest) and stop proliferating. Cancer cells, however, can continue to divide indefinitely without becoming senescent. Each time a cell divides, a small amount of DNA is lost from the ends of chromosomes. Chromosome ends are also known as "telomeres" and are important for maintaining genome stability. As a result of losing DNA from chromosome ends, each time a cell divides, telomeres shorten. Once telomeres become critically short, cells can no longer replicate DNA without compromising essential genetic material. At this point, normal cells enter senescence and stop growing. Therefore, each cell generally has a finite number of times that it can divide.

Cancer cells have about 10 to 20 times more telomerase than normal cells do. The higher levels of telomerase in cancer cells may be one mechanism through which cancer cells avoid senescence and continue proliferation. Telomerase functions in maintaining cell viability by adding specific DNA sequences to telomeres to maintain the ends of chromosomes. The activity of telomerase prevents telomeres from becoming too short and also promotes continued cell growth and tumor progression.

Catherine J. Walsh, Ph.D.

For Further Information

Greider, Carol W., & Blackburn, Elizabeth H. (2009). Telomeres, telomerase and cancer. *Scientific American*. Retrieved from http://www.scientificamerican.com/article/telomeres-telomerase-and/

Skloot, R. (Winter 2001). The marvels of telomerase. *Hopkins Medical News*. Retrieved from http://m.hopkinsmedicine.org/hmn/W01/top.html

Armanios M., & Greider, C.W. (2005). Telomerase and cancer stem cells. *Cold Spring Harbor Symposia on Quantitative Biology*, 70: 205-208.

Other Resources

Facts About Telomeres and Telomerase. Shay/Wright Lab.
www.utsouthwestern.edu/labs/shay-wright/research/facts-about-telomeres-telomerase.html

iBiology - Blackburn, Elizabeth - Telomeres and Telomerase: Their Implications in Human Health and Disease. Retrieved from http://www.ibiology.org/bioseminars/genetics-gene-regulation.html

Telomerase
www.geron.com/telomerase
Meštrović, T., 2015. Telomeres and Cancer. Retrieved from www.news-medical.net/health/Telomeres-andCancer.aspx

See also: Chromosomes and cancer

▶ T-lymphocytes

Category: Cancer Biology

Also known as: T-cells

Definition: T-lymphocytes are white blood cells of the adaptive immune system that help fight disease. There are several subgroups of T-lymphocytes with different immune system functions: cytotoxic T-lymphocytes (CTLs), helper T-lymphocytes, memory T-lymphocytes, regulatory T-lymphocytes, and tumor-infiltrating T-lymphocytes (TILs). TILs can be manipulated in the laboratory for use in cancer treatment.

Function: Some background on the immune system is helpful in understanding how T-lymphocytes function and the role they play in fighting cancer. The immune system is a complex of tissues, cells, and chemicals produced by these cells that spread throughout the body. Its function is to rid the body of foreign microbes and damaged or abnormal body cells (such as cancer cells). The major organs of the immune system are the bone marrow, lymph nodes, thymus, and spleen. Immune system cells and a clear fluid called lymph move throughout the body in a series of channels called lymphatic vessels that are separate from the blood-based circulatory system.

The immune system has 2 divisions, the innate immune system and the adaptive immune system. The innate system consists of white blood cells (leukocytes) that respond rapidly to a wide range of microbes but that cannot confer immunity against disease. While a cell in the innate system can attack many different kinds of microbes, each cell of the adaptive system recognizes and attacks only one type of microbe or damaged cell. T-lymphocytes and B-lymphocytes (see B-Lymphocyte entry) are the major cells of the adaptive immune system. Adaptive system cells respond more slowly when first encountering a microbe but have the ability to "remember" exposure to that microbe in a way that creates long-lasting immunity to a particular disease.

All cells have marker molecules on their surface that act as a "uniform" that identifies them as "self cells" or "non-self cells." Self markers do not cause an immune response in a healthy person. Non-self marker molecules, also called antigens, stimulate an immune system reaction. As a distinctive feature of the adaptive immune system, every T-lymphocyte or B-lymphocyte develops a unique receptor on its surface that will interact only with one highly specific non-self antigen.

Development: T-lymphocytes originate in bone marrow from hematopoietic stem cells, which are cells that have the potential to differentiate into many different kinds of blood cells. Immature T-lymphocytes leave the bone marrow and travel to the thymus, an organ behind the breastbone. Here they undergo a complicated maturation process that results in 2 major types of T-lymphocytes. One type has the CD8 protein on its surface and is called a $CD8^+$ cell. The other carries the CD4 protein and is called a $CD4^+$ cell. In addition to these proteins, every one of these cells has a different T-cell-specific antigen receptor on its surface. T-lymphocytes that develop antigen receptors that bind to marker molecules on healthy tissue cells are killed before they leave the thymus so as not to harm the body.

At this point, the T-lymphocytes in the thymus need to be activated. Dendritic cells, part of the innate immune system, constantly circulate through the body. When a dendritic cell finds a foreign microbe or an abnormal cell, it engulfs or "eats" the cell and takes some of the engulfed cell's proteins and moves them to their own surfaces. This process is called "antigen presentation." The dendritic cell then moves to the thymus to find a T-lymphocyte whose receptor matches the foreign antigen. When a dendritic cell finds a match with a CD8+ T-cell, it presents the antigen to the CD8+ cell and activates it. The CD8+ cell undergoes clonal expansion, dividing rapidly to produce a large number of identical cells.

Most activated CD8+ cells become CTLs. CTLs leave the thymus and move through the body looking for microbes or abnormal cells that match their receptors. When a CTL finds a match, it attaches to the cell and releases a chemical that causes the cell to burst. CTLs play a particularly important role in fighting viral infections.

A few CD8+ cells become memory T-lymphocytes instead of CTLs. Memory cells remain in the body for many years and are the basis for long-term immunity.

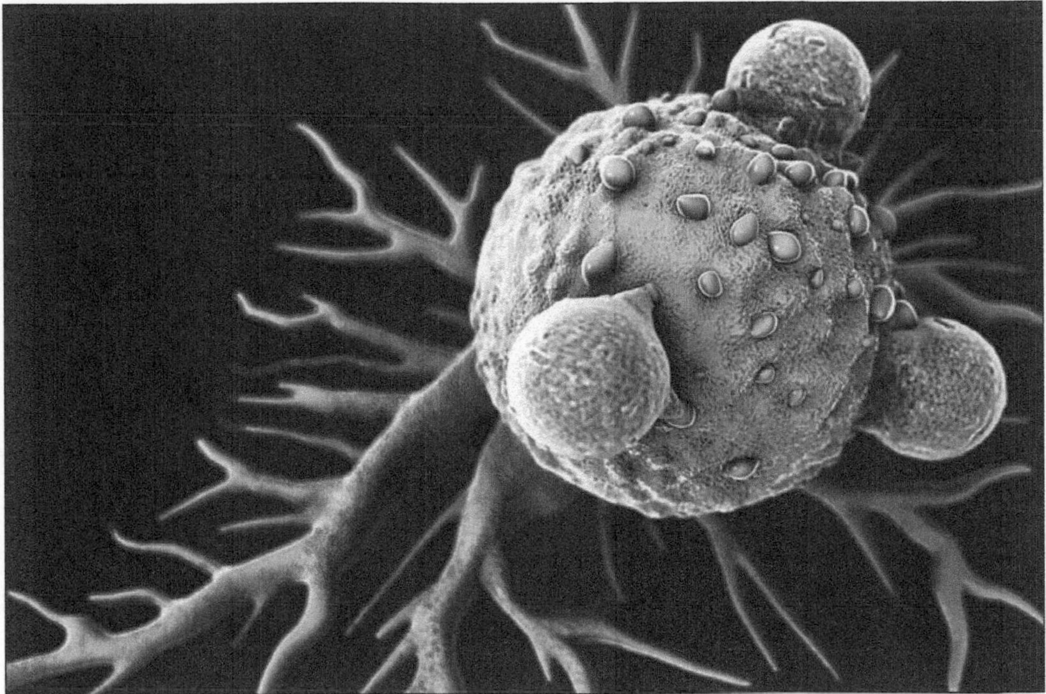

T-Lymphocytes and cancer cell. (iStock)

If the same microbe invades the body again, memory T-lymphocytes and memory B-lymphocytes respond quickly to control the invader before the individual becomes sick.

When a dendritic cell presents an antigen to a CD4+ T-lymphocyte whose receptor matches its foreign surface protein, the CD4+ cell is activated and becomes either a helper T-lymphocyte or a regulatory T-lymphocyte. There are at least 3 subgroups of helper T-lymphocytes: Th1, Th2, and Th17. Helper cells cannot kill other cells directly. Instead, they secrete chemicals that coordinate the immune system response. One subset of helper cells, Th2, secretes a chemical that stimulates B-lymphocytes to produce antibodies against foreign or abnormal cells. Another, Th1, helps CTLs become more effective killers. In addition, some T-helper cells become memory T-lymphocytes.

Some CD4+cells become regulatory T-lymphocytes instead of helper cells. Regulatory T-lymphocytes (refer to *Regulatory T-lymphocytes* entry) monitor the activity of other T-lymphocytes, help prevent immune response against normal body cells, and wind down the immune response once a microbe has been eliminated.

Both CD4+ and CD8+ cells can become tumor-infiltrating T-lymphocytes (TILs). Researchers are still learning about TILs and how they can be used to fight cancer.

Treatment: The body is exposed to thousands of different microbes each day, and a healthy immune system effectively eliminates most of them before an individual becomes sick. The immune system, however, has challenges in eliminating cancer cells. Cancer cells start out as normal body cells with all the surface proteins that identify them as self cells. At some point, these normal cells transform into cancer cells, but they often continue to have enough the surface proteins that originally marked them as self cells to escape detection by dendritic cells and T-lymphocytes. If the immune system does respond to transformed cells, the response may not be effective since the growth of cancer cells is not limited the way it is in healthy cells. In addition, some cancer cells make chemicals that turn off or disrupt the functioning of immune system cells.

As of 2015, the US Food and Drug Administration has approved only 1 T-lymphocyte cancer treatment vaccine. Unlike preventative vaccines, treatment vaccines are given after a person already has cancer. The drug, called Sipuleucel-T, is used to treat advanced prostate cancer. Scientists take cells from the patient's immune system and expose them in the laboratory to chemicals that turn them into dendritic cells with a special molecule artificially attached to stimulate a strong immune response against prostate cancer cells. The drug does not cure the cancer, but can prolong life.

Another approach to treating cancer uses TILs and manipulates them in the laboratory to fight certain cancers. The process is called adoptive cell therapy (ACT), and it was first used to successfully treat metastatic melanoma. A piece of the patient's melanoma tumor that contains TILs is removed. In the laboratory the tumor is separated into tiny pieces that are grown in culture with interleukin 2 (IL-2), a chemical that stimulates T-cell growth. In a few weeks, the T-lymphocytes destroy the tumor leaving a culture of billions of TIL cells—many more than the body could make— that are re-introduced into the patient. Since these cells are clones of self TILs, the immune system does not reject them, and they are able to infiltrate and successfully attack metastic melanoma tumors.

Originally, ACT worked only with melanoma tumors, but researchers are working on perfecting ways to use a harmless virus to genetically engineer the patient's own TIL cells to make them more effective against difficult to treat cancers such as acute lymphoblastic leukemia. The cells are taken from the patient, manipulated and cloned in the laboratory, and then re-introduced into the patient. This process is called chimeric antigen receptor (CAR) T-cell therapy (see separate entry). Although results are promising, problems still exist because some genetically engineered cells appear to be short-lived once they are re-introduced into the patient. As of 2015, treatment with TILs and CAR T-cell therapy was being tested in clinical trials against many different kinds of cancer. A searchable list of current clinical trials can be found at http://www.clinicaltrials.gov.

Tish Davidson, AM

For Further Information

Kershaw, Michael H., Westwood, J. A., Slaney, C. Y., & Darcy, P. K. (2014). Clinical Application of Genetically Modified T Cells in Cancer Therapy. *Clinical and Translational Immunology,* 3: e16. Retrieve at http://www.nature.com/cti/journal/v3/n5/full/cti20147a.html

Man, Yang-gao, Stojadinovic, A., Mason, J., Avital, I., Bilchik, A., Bruecher, B., ... Jewett, A. (2013). Tumor-infiltrating immune cells promoting tumor invasion and metastasis: existing theories. *Journal of Cancer,* 4(1): 84-95

Pardoll, Drew. (2012). T cells take aim at cancer. *Proceedings of the National Academy of Sciences,* 99(25): 15840-15842.Retrieve at http://www.pnas.org/content/99/25/15840.full

Other Resources

American Cancer Society
What's New in Cancer Immunotherapy Research? Retrieve at
http://www.cancer.org/treatment/treatmentsandsideeffects/treatmenttypes/immunotherapy/immunotherapy-whats-new-immuno-res

Cancer Research United Kingdom
The Immune System and Cancer. Retrieve at
http://www.cancerresearchuk.org/about-cancer/what-is-cancer/body-systems-and-cancer/the-immune-system-and-cancer

National Cancer Institute
Immunotherapy: Using the Immune System to Treat Cancer. Retrieve at
http://www.cancer.gov/research/areas/treatment/immunotherapy-using-immune-system

See also: B-lymphocytes

▶ TP53 protein

Category: Cancer Biology
Also known as: Tumor protein P53, P53, cellular tumor antigen P53, tumor suppressor P53, phosphoprotein P53, antigen NY-CO-13, guardian of the genome

Definition: Proteins TP53 The TP53 protein is the product of the *TP53* tumor-suppressor gene. As the molecular weight appears to be 53 kilodltons (kDa) when electrophoresed in a sodium dodecyl sulfate (SDS) polyacrylamide gel, it is referred to as TP53. The actual molecular weight is 43.7 kDa. The TP53 protein functions as a transcription factor that controls the expression of many target genes. The *TP53* gene is often referred to as the "guardian of the genome" because of its many anticancer functions. It also seems to be important in the process of sun tanning.

Biological function: The *TP53* tumor-suppressor gene is located on chromosome 17 at 17p13.1 and is essential for cell function. The TP53 protein's anticancer activity is exhibited by one of several mechanisms, many of which have not been clearly elucidated: activating mechanisms that repair DNA, arresting the cell cycle and preventing it from entering the DNA synthesis phase and passing damaged DNA on to daughter cells until damaged DNA can be repaired, initiating senescence and/or apoptosis to prevent damaged DNA from being replicated and distributed to its daughter cells, inhibiting angiogenesis, and promoting genome stability.

TP53 has many downstream targets affecting many pathways. One well-characterized pathway involves the *CDKN1A* (Cyclin-Dependent Kinase Inhibitor 1A) (also known as CIP1, WAF1, and *p21*) gene. Normally, TP53 is sequestered in the nucleus by the protein HDM2. When bound to HDM2, TP53 is inactive and targeted for breakdown, keeping its cellular concentration low. If the cell detects damage to its DNA, oxidative stress, or membrane damage, TP53 becomes phosphorylated on its N-terminus by enzymes called kinases. These kinases include DNA-PK, CHK1, CHK2, ATM, ATR, CAK, and members of the MAPK (mitogen-activated protein kinase) family. When phosphorylated, TP53 dissociates from HDM2, becomes more stable, increases in concentration, changes its conformation, and becomes an active transcription factor that stimulates transcription of several genes including the *CDKN1A* gene. The CDKN1A protein binds to and inactivates polypeptides that are required for the cell to enter the DNA synthesis phase of the cell cycle. Thus the cell is prevented from replicating damaged DNA that could cause cancer and passing it on to its daughter cells.

The TP53 protein can also activate genes that stimulate senescence and/or apoptosis of cells with damaged DNA, activate genes necessary for the repair of damaged DNA, and stimulate genes involved with the tanning reaction to protect cells from damaging ultraviolet (UV) light. By these and other mechanisms, TP53 prevents cell growth and even causes cell death to suppress the formation of cancer **cells**.

Structure of the protein: Active TP53 protein is a tetramer consisting of four identical polypeptides of 393 amino acids each. Many of the amino acid residues can be assigned to distinct functional domains. The 39 amino acid residues at the N-terminus are involved with HDM2 binding and activation of transcription of the *CDKN1A* gene. Residues 80 to 94 are responsible for TP53's apoptosis activity, while amino acid residues 101 to 306 are responsible for TP53's DNA-binding activity, an activity essential to its role as a transcription activator. The ability of TP53 monomers to polymerize into tetramers depends on amino acid residues 307 to 355. The C-terminus amino acids (356 to 393) are responsible for TP53's localization in the nucleus and nonspecific binding to damaged DNA.

Cancer involvement: Mutations, usually simple amino acid replacement (missense) mutations, and deletions in the *TP53* gene that alter the function of its product can severely limit its tumor-suppressor activity. People who inherit one defective *TP53* gene are highly predisposed to developing Li-Fraumeni syndrome, which is characterized by cancer in a variety of tissues. More than 50 percent of all human cancers involve the *TP53* gene, including 60 percent of head and neck cancers, 50 percent of ovarian and lung cancers, 45 percent of colon cancers, 35 percent of stomach cancers, 30 percent of bladder cancers, and 20 to 40 percent of breast cancers.

Of the mutations in TP53 that result in cancer, 90 percent affect the DNA-binding domain (amino acids 101 to 306). These mutations result in the inability of TP53 to bind to the *CDKN1A* gene and stimulate its expression.

Mutations in the *TP53* gene affecting amino acid residues 307 to 355 are in the domain that allows TP53 to form tetramers with other TP53 molecules, a function necessary for its activity. TP53 molecules with one of these mutations form dimers with normal TP53 molecules, preventing their activity. Thus, these mutations are referred to as dominant loss-of-function mutations.

Charles L. Vigue, Ph.D.

For Further Information

Armstrong, Sue. (2014). P53: The gene that cracked the cancer code. New York: Bloomsbury Sigma.

Hainaut, Pierre, & Wiman, Klas G. (1999). Twenty-five years of p53 research. New York: Springer.

Mukhopadhyay, Tapas, Maxwell, Steven A., & Roth, Jack A. (1995). p53 suppressor gene. New York: Springer, 1995.

Zambetti, Gerald, (Ed.). (2005). Protein reviews: The p53 tumor suppressor pathway and cancer. New York: Springer.

Other Resources

Cornell University

Tumor Suppressor Genes: Guardians of Our Cells.
http://envirocancer.cornell.edu/FactSheet/Genetics/fs6.TSgenes.cfm

HUGO Gene Nomenclature Committee

Symbol Report: TP53.
http://www.genenames.org/data/hgnc_data.php?hgnc_id=11998

International Agency for Research on Cancer
IARC TP53 Mutation Database.
http://p53.iarc.fr/
p53 Knowledgebase.
http://p53.bii.a-star.edu.sg/index.php

The p53 Web Site
http://p53.free.fr

TP53 Mutations and Cancer
http://p53.fr/

Genetics Home Reference
http://ghr.nlm.nih.gov/gene/TP53

Online Mendelian Inheritance in Man
http://www.omim.org/entry/191170

See also: Adenoid Cystic Carcinoma (ACC); Ataxia Telangiectasia (AT); Bowen disease; BRAF gene; Breast cancer in pregnant women; Cancer biology; Cytogenetics; Dilation and Curettage (D&C); Drug resistance and multidrug resistance (MDR); Endocrine cancers; Endometrial cancer; Fallopian tube cancer; Family history and risk assessment; Fibrosarcomas, soft-tissue; Free radicals; Gene therapy; Genetics of cancer; Giant Cell Tumors (GCTs); Gynecologic cancers; Li-Fraumeni Syndrome (LFS); Liver cancers; Mutagenesis and cancer; MYC oncogene; Nasal cavity and paranasal sinus cancers; Neuroectodermal tumors; Oncogenes; Sarcomas, soft-tissue; Simian virus 40; Spermatocytomas; Thymus cancer; Tumor-suppressor genes; Virus-related cancers; Vulvar cancer

▶ Tumor biomarkers

Category: Cancer Biology
Also known as: biological markers, molecular biomarkers, genetic testing

Definition: Biomarker, a biological molecule located in blood, body fluids, or tissues, is a sign of normal or abnormal processes such as cancer. Biomarkers consist of substances, including proteins, nucleic acids, antibodies, peptides, and other biological constituents. In cancer, biomarkers include changes in the genes or abnormal byproducts of gene metabolism.

Use in cancer medicine: Biomarkers are used in cancer medicine for several reasons. First, the measurement of biomarkers may establish a patient's risk of developing a malignancy and motivate them to initiate lifestyle changes to prevent cancer. For instance women with strong family histories of ovarian cancer may be carriers of BRCA1, a specific cellular mutation indicative of an increased risk of breast or ovarian cancer. Once discovered the patient may employ preventative options including increased screening, prophylactic drug therapy, or surgery to decrease risk of developing malignancy.

Second, biomarkers can distinguish between two or more conditions that share similar signs or symptoms. In this way, biomarkers can help physicians determine if a questionable illness is actually cancer, infection, inflammation, or another benign process.

Third, biomarkers may help identify the tissue of origin in cancer and determine prognosis or likelihood of disease recurrence in patients diagnosed with cancer. This helps physicians prescribe drugs to target specific cancers.

Most healthcare professionals use biomarkers cautiously as multiple factors can lead to erroneous diagnosis based solely on their presence or absence. Although biomarkers are widely used in oncology, most clinicians use biomarkers as only one factor in determining a patient's risk, disease presence, and treatment modality of cancer.

Associated Cancers: No one biomarker can detect all types of cancer. However, some biomarkers are frequently linked with specific types of malignancy (see table). The presence or absence of biomarkers raises a clinician's suspicion that cancer may be present.

Testing: There are 3 types of biomarker tests on material derived from blood, body fluids, or tissues: chromosome, gene, and biochemical tests. Each test provides the physician with specific information when evaluating cancers.

Chromosome tests can detect gross chromosomal changes such as the loss (deletions), expansion (duplications), or rearrangement (inversions or translocations) of chromosomal material. Bone marrow cytogenetics chromosome tests require evaluation of a small bone marrow sample obtained through puncturing the iliac crest (hip) or sternum (breastbone) with a special needle.

Gene testing identifies additional gene copies (duplicated or amplified genes), missing genes (deleted genes), or incorrectly placed genes (translocated genes). Gene tests can assess for altered nucleotide bases within DNA.

In some cancers, proteins produced by genes are atypical. These abnormal proteins can promote cancer growth. Oncologists search for abnormal proteins with biochemical tests that may indicate the presence of cancer. Other

Biomarkers frequently used in oncology

Biomarker	*Most Notable Cancer Types*	*Use in Oncology*
ALK gene (Anaplastic Lymphoma Kinase)	• Non-small cell lung cancer • Anaplastic large cell lymphoma	Aids in determining treatment and prognosis.
Alpha-fetoprotein (AFP)	• Liver cancer • Germ Cell tumor (tumor that begins in the cells that give rise to sperm or eggs)	Aids in the diagnosing liver cancer and following treatment response. Used to assess stage, diagnosis, and reaction to therapy of germ cell tumors.
Beta-2-microglobulin (B2M)	• Multiple myeloma • Chronic lymphocytic leukemia • Various types of lymphoma	Used to ascertain prognosis and monitor response to treatment.
BRCA1 and BRCA2 gene mutations (Breast Cancer suscepti-bility gene)	• Breast cancer • Ovarian cancer	Determines appropriate treatment with a particular type of therapy.
BCR-ABL fusion gene (Philadelphia chromo-some)	• Chronic myeloid leukemia • Acute lymphoblastic leukemia • Acute myelogenous leukemia	Aids in the diagnosis, predicts response to therapies, and monitors disease progression.
BRAF V600 mutations	• Cutaneous melanoma • Colorectal cancer	Helps to determine which patients are likely to benefit from treatment with certain therapies.
Calcitonin	• Thyroid cancer	Assists in the diagnosis. Checks if treatment is effective. Assesses for recurrence of cancer.
Carcino-embryonic antigen (CEA)	• Colorectal cancer	Monitors progress of cancer treatments. Determined if cancer has returned.
EGFR (epidermal growth factor receptor) gene mutation	• Non-small cell lung cancer	Helps determine the treatment and prognosis of cancer.
Estrogen receptor(ER)/ progesterone receptor (PR)	• Breast cancer	Helps determine whether treatment with hormone therapy is appropriate.
ER2 (human epidermal growth factor receptor) gene amplification or protein overexpression	• Breast cancer • Gastric cancer	Aids in determining that certain therapies will be effective.
KRAS gene mutation	• Colorectal cancer • Non-small cell lung cancer	Determines whether treatment with a particular type of therapy is appropriate.
Lactate dehydrogenase	• Lymphoma • Leukemia • Melanoma • Neuroblastoma	Assesses stage, prognosis, and response to therapy.
Programmed death ligand 1 (PD-L1)	• Non-small cell lung cancer	Aids in deciding which treatment with a particular type of therapy is correct.
Prostate-specific antigen (PSA)	• Prostate cancer	Aids in diagnosis and assesses response to treatment and recurrence of disease.

biochemical tests such as blood chemistry tests detect the possible effects of cancer.

History: The use of biomarkers in health science dates to the early 1970s when Harvard Medical School Professor Herbert Needleman published his groundbreaking work on lead toxicity in children. Needleman linked lead biomarkers to cognitive decline. However, the term biomarker did not appear in the scientific literature until the early 1980s when researchers Perera and Weinstein proposed the term to link human environmental exposures with illness, creating a new approach to the study of cancer.

In 1987, The National Research Council published its seminal paper describing biomarker groupings that are still used today in healthcare. The paper officially proposed that biomarkers could be used in medicine to delineate events in the healthcare continuum.

Robert W. Koch, DNSc, RN

For Further Information

Ransohoff, D. F. (2003). Developing molecular biomarkers for cancer. *Science*, 299(5613): 1679-1680.

Saporito, B. (2013, May 20). Blood work. *Time Magazine*, 181(19). http://content.time.com/time/magazine/0,9263,7601130520,00.html

Schmidt, C.W. (2006). Signs of the times: Biomarkers in perspective. *Environmental Health Perspectives,* 114(12): A700-A705. http://www.jstor.org/stable/4119581

Other Resources

National Cancer Institute
http://www.cancer.gov

National Comprehensive Cancer Network
http://www.nccn.org

OncoLink
http://www.oncolink.org

See also: Oncology

▶ Tumor Necrosis Factor (TNF)

Category: Cancer Biology; Chemotherapy and Other Drugs

Also known as: Tumor necrosis factor-alpha (TNF), tumor necrosis factor-beta (TNF-β, or lymphotoxin); the colloidal gold-bound form of TNF is also called Aurimmune

Definition: TNF is a protein belonging to the class of cytokines (immunoregulatory proteins) that is made by the body's white blood cells in response to an infection, or antigen. It can also be synthesized in the laboratory. Because it causes necrosis (cell death), it is being investigated as a possible immunotherapeutic drug to induce death of some types of tumor cells.

Cancers treated: Breast, ovarian, colon, kidney, and liver cancers, as well as melanomas.

Delivery routes: Tumor necrosis factor is generally delivered as an injection in a vein or muscle. Injection may also be under the skin. A colloidal form of TNF bound to small particles of gold has also been tested for improved specificity for cancer tissue, reducing the ability of the drug to bind normal tissue and possibly permitting systemic delivery.

How this drug works: The term TNF actually refers to a family of trimeric proteins produced by certain types of white blood cells that can attack blood vessels in tumors, thereby destroying certain types of cancer cells. The most common forms are TNF; and TNF-β. TNF is the form used for cancer therapy. Its existence was discovered fortuitously in the early twentieth century. On rare occasions, but frequently enough to come to the attention of physicians, cancers would occasionally spontaneously regress. In 1893, William Coley observed such regression when some patients were injected with killed gram-negative bacteria. Coley's toxin, as the preparation was called, was used as frequently as the 1960s in addressing cancers, at which time it was supplanted by better methods of treatment.

The response to TNF is dose-dependent and can result either in inflammation, augmenting the immune response, or in binding to a cell surface, inducing the destruction of that cell. The induction of apoptosis, or "cell suicide," appears to be the primary mechanism by which TNF may cause tumor regression. Depending upon the state of the particular cell, either tumor cells or the cells of the blood vessels that feed those tumors may express receptors on their respective surfaces for the drug. The binding of TNF to these receptors sets in motion a series of intracellular signals that culminates in the death of the cell.

Testing has also been carried out using a human recombinant form of TNF (rTNF), as well as treatments utilizing a combination of chemotherapies in conjunction with TNF.

Side effects: Like other forms of chemotherapy, TNF has the potential to interact with other medications. Specific side effects of TNF may include a mild fever, chills or sweating, fatigue, and vomiting. Since most cells in the body have surface receptors to which TNF may bind, the drug is potentially toxic if given systemically. TNF may adversely affect muscles. It can reduce smooth muscle tone and even disturb cardiac contraction, potentially resulting in shock. The ability of TNF to reduce the anticoagulant properties of capillaries may also result in formation of blood clots within small capillaries (likely a reason for its anti-tumor properties as well).

Richard Adler, Ph.D.

For Further Information

Abbas, Abul & Lichtman, Andrew. (2015). *Cellular and molecular immunology* (8th ed.). Philadelphia, PA: Elsevier/Saunders.

Dembic, Zlatko. (2015). *The cytokines of the immune system.* Waltham, MA: Elsevier.

Moticka, Edward. (2016). *A historical perspective on evidence-based immunology.* Waltham, MA: Elsevier.

Murphy, Kenneth. (2011). *Janeway's immunobiology* (8th ed.). New York: Garland Science, 2011.

See also: Biological therapy; Cancer biology; Chemotherapy; Crohn disease; Cytokines; Gene therapy; Histiocytosis X; Hyperthermic perfusion; Immune response to cancer; Immunotherapy; Liver cancers

▶ Tumor-suppressor genes

Category: Cancer Biology

Definition: Tumor-suppressor genes are found in normal cells, and encode proteins that control cell division, repair damage to deoxyribonucleic acid (DNA), and control cell death. Mutated tumor-suppressor genes lose their regulatory function, which leads to uncontrolled cell growth, a hallmark of cancer.

What they do: The protein products of tumor-suppressor genes regulate cell division and growth by participating in many different biochemical pathways. When these pathways are disrupted due to loss-of-function mutations in the tumor suppressor genes, normal cell growth is disrupted and normal cells can become cancerous. The proteins encoded by tumor-suppressor genes can inhibit cell division if proper conditions for growth are not met (e.g., DNA damage, a lack of growth factors, or a malfunction of the cell's division machinery). Scientists have identified about fifty tumor-suppressor genes.

Types of tumor-suppressor genes: There are several types of tumor-suppressor genes. Some, like the first tumor suppressor gene to be identified, the retinoblastoma (RB) gene, control cell division and growth. A second type repair errors in DNA. The process of DNA replication leads to occasional mistakes, and cells have a set of proteins (e.g., BRCA1 and BRCA2) that repair these mistakes. A third type induces cells to undergo programmed cell death (apoptosis) if their DNA is damaged beyond repair or if the process of cell division malfunctions. This protects the organism from the effects of runaway cell replication. The TP53 (also known as p53) gene is an example of such a tumor-suppressor gene.

Because the presence of tumor-suppressor genes contributes to normal cell division and function, both copies of a tumor-suppressor gene must be inactivated to result in a maximum increased risk of cancer development. An increased risk of developing a specific type of cancer in some families is often the result of the presence of one defective copy of a tumor-suppressor gene. Although there is a low likelihood that the good copy of the tumor-suppressor gene will be mutated in any given cell, there is a much higher likelihood that the necessary second mutation will occur somewhere in the vast number of cells in a human body. Many of the identified tumor-suppressor genes have been shown to be implicated in familial cancers. Inheritance of a defective copy of one of these genes carries a greatly increased risk of developing one or more specific types of cancer, often types that are otherwise rare. In some cases, mutant copies of these genes are linked to susceptibility to multiple cancer types, as is the case with the retinoblastoma (RB1) gene. The two most important tumor-suppressor genes code for the TP53 protein and the retinoblastoma protein (RB1 or pRB).

TP53 gene: The TP53 gene has been found to be involved in numerous cellular processes and is considered to be one of the most important cancer-related genes. The TP53 protein belongs to a class of proteins containing covalently bound phosphate groups, called phosphoproteins. It is located in the nucleus of the cell and interacts directly with the cell's DNA to function as a transcription factor by binding to a specific DNA sequence in the control regions of the genes it controls. The number of bound phosphate groups modulates the activity of TP53. Normal TP53 function results in a global transcriptional response that can negatively regulate cell division, or induce apoptosis. TP53 function is activated in response to various kinds of cell stress that increase the cell's need for DNA repair and surveillance of the cell's physiological status, including irradiation, lack of oxygen, oncogene activation, and DNA damage.

The TP53 gene is the single most frequently inactivated gene in human cancers. More than 90 percent of small-cell lung cancers and more than 50 percent of breast and colon cancers have been shown to be associated with mutant forms of TP53.

Retinoblastoma (RB1) gene: The RB1 gene encodes another phosphoprotein located in the nucleus of the cell. The RB1 protein acts as a negative regulator of cell division by binding to other transcription factors to alter their function. The action of these other transcription factors in turn regulates the level of expression of a number of other genes. The number of phosphate groups bound to the RB1 protein controls its ability to bind to other transcription factors and varies in a regular controlled manner during a normal cell cycle. The RB1 protein is responsible for a major "checkpoint," or regulatory step, in the cell cycle, in which cells must make a decision whether to undergo another round of cell division. Normal RB1 protein function results in a coordinated progression of the cell through the division process. Loss of the RB1 protein leads to unregulated and increased cell division, characteristic of cancer cells. The RB1 gene is mutated in many types of cancer, including retinoblastoma (a cancer of the eye from which the gene got its name), as well as bone, lung, breast, and bladder cancers.

Another tumor suppressor gene that many are familiar with is the BRAC family of genes (which includes BRAC1 and BRAC2). Inherited mutations in BRAC1 and BRAC2 are commonly associated with increased risk of breast and ovarian cancer. Mutations in BRAC1 and BRAC2 genes account for 20-25% of all hereditary breast cancers, and 5-10% of all breast cancers. Mutations in these genes also account for 15% of all ovarian cancers. The United States Preventive Services Task Force recommends that women who have a family history of breast and gynecologic cancers, consider genetic testing for mutations in BRAC1 and BRAC2.

Jill Ferguson, Ph.D.
Updated by: Banalata Bono Sen

For Further Information

Hanahan, D., & Weinberg, R. A. (2000). The hallmarks of cancer. *Cell*, 100, 57-70.

Sherr, C. J. (2004). Principles of tumor suppression. *Cell*, 116, 235-246.Strano, S., Dell Orso, S., Di Agostino, S., Fontemaggi, G., Sacchi, A., & Blandino, G. (2007). Mutant p53: An oncogenic transcription factor. *Oncogene*, 26, 2212-2219.

Weinberg, R. A. (2007). *The biology of cancer*. New York: Garland Science.

Vogelstein, B., Sur, S. & Prives, C. (2010). p53: The most frequently altered gene in human cancers. *Nature Education,* 3(9): 6,

Other Resources

BRAC1 and BRAC2
Cancer Risk and Genetic Testing
http://www.cancer.gov/about-cancer/causes-prevention/genetics/brca-fact-sheet#q6

American Cancer Society
Genes and Cancer
http://www.cancer.org/acs/groups/cid/documents/webcontent/002550-pdf.pdf

Emory University
CancerQuest: Important Tumor Suppressors.
http://www.cancerquest.org/index.cfm?page=52

Tumor Suppressor Genes
http://users.rcn.com/jkimball.ma.ultranet/BiologyPages/T/TumorSuppressorGenes.html

Vanderbilt University
Tumor Suppressor gene database
http://bioinfo.mc.vanderbilt.edu/TSGene/

Proto-Oncogenes and Tumor-Suppressor Genes Molecular Biology, 4th Edition
http://www.ncbi.nlm.nih.gov/books/NBK21662/#_A7100_

See also: APC gene testing; BRCA1 and BRCA2 genes; Cancer biology; Cowden syndrome; Endocrine cancers; Gene therapy; Genetic testing; Genetics of cancer; Mutagenesis and cancer; Oncogenes; Oncogenic viruses; RB1 gene; RhoGD12 gene; TP53 protein

▶ Acrylamides

Category: Carcinogens and Suspected Carcinogens
RoC status: Reasonably anticipated human carcinogen since 1991
Also known as: 2-propenamide, propenamide, acrylic amide, vinyl amide, ethylene carboxamide

Related cancers: Although an acrylamide-cancer connection in humans has not been established with certainty, the level of suspicion is high because under laboratory conditions in rats and mice, the following cancers have been associated with acrylamide: adrenal pheochromocytomas and mesotheliomas in the testes; adenomas in the pituitary and mammary glands; adenocarcinomas of the clitoris, uterus, and thyroid gland; squamous cell carcinoma of the skin; and adenomas of the lung.

Definition: Acrylamide is a compound of carbon, hydrogen, nitrogen, and oxygen resulting in the chemical formula, C_3H_5NO. This white, odorless, and crystalline compound is soluble in water, ethanol, ether, and chloroform, accounting for not only its many industrial uses but also its potential for uncomplicated entry into the human body. Many of its industrial and agricultural uses require the conversion of acrylamide to the polymer polyacrylamide.

Exposure routes: Experimentally in rats and mice, cancer-inducing exposure routes include administration in the drinking water, intraperitoneal injection, and topical application. In humans, during everyday activity and work, acrylamide gains entrance through unbroken skin, mucous membranes, lungs, and the gastrointestinal tract. The primary occupational exposure routes are skin contact and through the inhalation of dust and vapor.

Where found: Acrylamides are used in the treatment of wastewater, drinking water, and sewage; in the production of paper, plastics, and dyes; and in the manufacture of permanent press fabrics, adhesives, and food packaging. It is also fundamental to ore processing. Acrylamide finds its way into a number of everyday products such as building materials, contact lenses, textiles, soap, food, and gelatin capsules. Acrylamides have also established a place on people's dining tables: It is found in fried and baked goods, coffee, olives, and prune juice. Smoking is also a major acrylamide producer.

Some acrylamide contaminates drinking water because of its use in water treatment facilities, but curiously, the amount of acrylamide in a large order of fast-food french fries is more than three hundred times what the U.S. Environmental Protection Agency allows in a single glass of water. This pervasiveness of acrylamide prompted Dale Hattis, a risk analysis expert at Clark University, to speculate that "acrylamide causes several thousand cancers per year in Americans."

Additionally, polyacrylamide, the polymer of acrylamide, finds widespread global use in pesticides and in soil treatment formulations. This has resulted in notable residues of polyacrylamide in the most widely consumed vegetables such as potatoes and grains. There is little government oversight or measurement of polyacrylamide in foods.

At risk: Because of its almost ubiquitous presence at the dinner table and its known neurotoxic and carcinogenic potential, acrylamide poses a health risk to humans. Microwaving, baking, and frying will produce acrylamide, and as the food continues to cook, ever larger amounts of acrylamide are produced. As the risk potential for acrylamides in foods becomes more publicized, some steps are under way to modify food production methods, such as using vacuum frying at lower temperatures. Raw or boiled foods pose little risk for acrylamides.

Workers engaged in oil drilling, paper and pulp manufacture, general construction, plastics manufacture, mining, food processing, textile and cosmetics processing, and agricultural industries are at increased risk of acrylamide exposure.

Etiology and symptoms of associated cancers: Although research has not firmly established the acrylamide-cancer connection in humans, there is no question that acrylamide is a serious neurotoxin. Depending on dosage levels, exposure can cause damage to the male reproductive glands, skin, and eyes. Additionally, it may result in urinary incontinence, numbness, weakening in the legs and hands, and irritation of the mucous membranes.

The National Institute for Occupational Health and Safety (NIOSH) lists the common acrylamide exposure symptoms in an industrial setting: irritation of the eyes and skin, ataxia, numbness of the limbs, paresthesia, muscle weakness, absent deep tendon reflex, hand sweating, lassitude (weakness, exhaustion), drowsiness, and reproductive effects. The institute further cautions that acrylamide is a potential occupational carcinogen.

History: Production of acrylamide in the United States exceeds one million pounds per year. It was not until 2002 that Swedish scientists found high levels of acrylamide in certain fried and baked starchy foods. In the same year, the Center for Science in the Public Interest in the United

States reported finding high levels of acrylamide in popular brands of snack chips, french fries, taco shells, and breakfast cereals. Government action concerning these findings has been very slow, but in 2005 the California attorney general filed a lawsuit requiring a warning label for french fries and potato chips.

Although NIOSH considers the compound dangerous to life and health, the Food and Drug Administration allows acrylamide to be used for packaging, in plastics that are in contact with food, and in treating food to maximum levels ranging up to 0.20 percent.

Although research has firmly established the cancer-acrylamide connection in rats and mice, the findings are still mixed in human studies. Some experts claim the very pervasiveness of acrylamide in the Western diet confuses the results.

Richard S. Spira, D.V.M.

For Further Information

Brown, L., M. M. Rhead, K. C. C. Bancroft, and N. Allen. "Model Studies of the Degradation of Acrylamide Monomer." *Water Research* 14, no. 7 (1980): 775-778.

Rice, Jerry M. "The Carcinogenicity of Acrylamide." *Mutation Research/Genetic Toxicology and Environmental Mutagenesis* 580, nos. 1/2 (2005): 3-20.

Smith, E., S. Prues, and F. Ochme. "Environmental Degradation of Polyacrylamides: Effect of Artificial Environmental Conditions." *Ecotoxicology and Environmental Safety* 35 (1996): 121-135.

Tareke, E., et al. "Analysis of Acrylamide, a Carcinogen Formed in Heated Foodstuffs." *Journal of Agriculture and Food Chemistry* 50, no. 17 (2002): 4998-5006.

U.S. Department of Health and Human Services, Public Health Service, National Toxicology Program. *Eleventh Report on Carcinogens*. Research Triangle Park, N.C.: Author, 2005.

Weiss, G. "Acrylamide in Food: Uncharted Territory." *Science* 27 (2002): 297.

Other Resources

National Institute for Occupational Safety and Health
http://www.cdc.gov/niosh

National Library of Medicine
Toxicology Data Network
http://toxnet.nlm.nih.gov

U.S. Food and Drug Administration
Draft Action Plan for Acrylamide in Food
http://www.cfsan.fda.gov/~dms/acrypla3.html

See also: Adenocarcinomas; Endocrine cancers; Testicular cancer; Vulvar cancer

▶ Aflatoxins

Category: Carcinogens and Suspected Carcinogens
RoC status: Known human carcinogen since 1980
Also known as: Aflatoxin B^1, aflatoxin B^2, aflatoxin G^1, aflatoxin G^2, aflatoxin M^1

Related cancers: Liver cancer, primary liver cell cancer, hepatocellular carcinoma, lung cancer

Definition: Aflatoxins are naturally occurring toxic metabolites produced by certain fungi that grow on some agricultural products. At least thirteen different aflatoxins are produced in nature, with the four major aflatoxins called aflatoxin B^1, B^2, G^1, and G^2. Aflatoxin B^1 is typically the most predominant as well as the most toxic. Aflatoxin M^1 is found primarily in milk.

Exposure routes: Ingestion and inhalation

Where found: Numerous agricultural commodities, including corn and other grains, peanuts, tree nuts, and cottonseed meal. Milk, eggs, and meat products can be contaminated if animals consume aflatoxin-contaminated feed.

At risk: Those living in countries where agricultural products that readily support the growth of aflatoxin-producing fungi are a dietary staple. Farmers and other agricultural workers are at risk for occupational exposure through inhalation of dust generated during handling of contaminated crops and feeds.

Etiology and symptoms of associated cancers: Aflatoxin-producing fungi can grow on a wide range of agricultural products. Corn and groundnuts are major sources of human exposure because of greater susceptibility to contamination and widespread consumption. Worldwide, corn is probably of greatest concern because it is grown in climates that readily support the growth of fungi and is a dietary staple in many countries. Aflatoxin-producing fungi often grow on crops in the field before harvest, particularly if the crops have experienced drought stress. After harvest, contamination can occur during storage. The growth of aflatoxin-producing fungi and subsequent production of aflatoxins are influenced by weather conditions such as temperature and humidity. As a result, aflatoxin contamination varies with geographic location, agricultural and agronomic practices, and the susceptibility of crops to fungal growth.

Exposure to aflatoxins occurs primarily by consuming contaminated food. Aflatoxin consumption is commonplace in developing countries where food supplies are limited and regulations of aflatoxin levels are not enforced or nonexistent. In developed countries, food supplies are generally more abundant and diverse, and aflatoxin levels are monitored to limit toxin ingestion. Although the sale of heavily contaminated food supplies is not permitted in developed countries, chronic exposure to low levels of aflatoxins may still be a concern.

The most common aflatoxin-producing fungi are *Aspergillus flavus* and *Aspergillus parasiticus*. Although many aflatoxins are produced by these fungi, aflatoxin B^1 is the most prevalent and the most toxic. Aflatoxin B^1 is also the most potent naturally occurring carcinogen. Aflatoxins are both toxic and carcinogenic, with exposure to high levels resulting in toxic effects referred to as aflatoxicosis and chronic exposure to low levels potentially resulting in cancer. Susceptibility to aflatoxin-related diseases is influenced by many factors, including age, exposure level, duration of exposure, health, nutritional status, and exposure to other agents, such as the hepatitis B virus (HBV).

The liver is the primary target organ of aflatoxin exposure, although other organs can also be affected. Metabolic activation by liver enzymes is required for the carcinogenic effects of aflatoxin B^1. In the liver, aflatoxin B^1 is metabolized to a highly reactive form that readily binds deoxyribonucleic acid (DNA) and proteins and can lead to liver damage and subsequent formation of tumors in the liver. Exposure to aflatoxins in the diet has been shown to be one of the major etiological factors in the development of primary hepatocellular carcinoma in some countries, such as China and many African countries. Concurrent infection with HBV and exposure to aflatoxins results in significantly greater liver damage than either infection or exposure alone, a synergy that is likely produced because HBV interferes with the liver's ability to detoxify aflatoxins. Although aflatoxin is most well known as an agent that promotes liver cancer, inhalation of contaminated grain dust has been associated with an increased incidence of lung cancer.

Liver cancer is not associated with any symptoms in the early stages. As the cancer progresses, symptoms may include pain in the upper abdomen on the right side, which may also extend to the back and shoulder. Other symptoms include a swollen or bloated abdomen, weight loss, loss of appetite, feeling of fullness, weakness, fatigue, nausea and vomiting, yellowish skin and eyes, dark urine, and fever.

History: Aflatoxins have been recognized as a significant contaminant since the 1960's, when more than 100,000 young turkeys on poultry farms in England died from what was termed turkey X disease. The mortalities were traced to consumption of mold-contaminated peanut meal. In 1961 the toxin-producing fungus, *A. flavus*, was identified and the toxin given the name aflatoxin. The International Agency for Research on Cancer (IARC) first recognized aflatoxins as carcinogenic in 1976. In 1987 naturally occurring mixtures of aflatoxins and AFB_1 were classified as Group I carcinogens.

Aflatoxins are considered unavoidable contaminants of food and feed, even when good manufacturing practices have been followed. Although absolute safety can never be achieved, many countries have attempted to limit exposure to aflatoxins by imposing regulatory limits on commodities intended for consumption. The Food and Drug Administration has established specific guidelines that regulate this toxin to very low concentrations in human food and animal feed.

Catherine J. Walsh, Ph.D.

For Further Information

Bennet, J. W., and M. Klich. "Mycotoxins." *Clinical Microbiology Reviews* 16, no. 3 (2003): 497-516.

Eaton, D. L., and J. D. Groopman. *The Toxicology of Aflatoxins*. New York: Academic Press, 1994.

Goldblatt, L., ed. *Aflatoxin: Scientific Background, Control, and Implications*. New York: Academic Press, 1969.

U.S. Department of Health and Human Services, Public Health Service, National Toxicology Program. *Eleventh Report on Carcinogens*. Research Triangle Park, N.C.: Author, 2005.

Other Resources

Centers for Disease Control and Prevention
http://www.cdc.gov

National Cancer Institute
http://www.cancer.gov

National Toxicology Program
http://ntp.niehs.nih.gov

U.S. Food and Drug Administration
Center for Food Safety and Nutrition
http://www.cfsan.fda.gov

See also: Free radicals; Hepatomegaly; Infectious cancers; Liver cancers; Risks for cancer

▶ Agent Orange

Category: Carcinogens and Suspected Carcinogens
Also known as: Super Orange

Related cancers: Soft-tissue sarcoma, non-Hodgkin lymphoma, Hodgkin disease, chronic lymphocytic leukemia (CLL), acute myelogenous leukemia (AML)

Definition: Agent Orange was a chemical mixture used in the United States to control weeds and in Vietnam during the Vietnam War to remove forest cover. So named because of the orange stripes painted on its storage drums, Agent Orange is a blend of two herbicides: 2,4-dichlorophenoxyacetic acid (2,4-D) and 2,4,5-trichlorophenoxyacetic acid (2,4,5-T). Although 2,4,5-T is not highly poisonous, the manufacturing process generates a toxic by-product called TCDD, or 2,3,7,8-tetrachlorodibenzo-*p*-dioxin. This dioxin, classified as a human carcinogen, tainted Agent Orange formulations.

Exposure routes: Inhalation, ingestion, skin contact, ocular absorption

Where found: Herbicide mixtures formerly used for agricultural, forestry, and military purposes

At risk: Combatants and civilians exposed to Agent Orange during the Vietnam War and their children, workers occupationally exposed to the chemical, and populations exposed through domestic herbicide spraying

Etiology and symptoms of associated cancers: Because epidemiologic data on Vietnam veterans is limited, the health effects of Agent Orange have been studied indirectly in certain populations highly exposed to dioxin or dioxin-tainted herbicides. These studies provide sufficient evidence linking Agent Orange to chloracne, an acnelike skin disorder, and to certain cancers, induced when TCDD activates a protein receptor in target cells. The soft-tissue sarcomas develop from fat, muscle, or deep body tissues and usually appear as a lump. Hodgkin disease (highly curable) and non-Hodgkin lymphoma originate in lymphatic tissue and result in painless swelling of lymph nodes under the skin. Chronic lymphocytic leukemia, which develops from white blood cells, is often asymptomatic, but later is marked by enlarged lymph nodes. Paternal exposure to Agent Orange has been associated with acute myelogenous leukemia in children. This fast-growing cancer of the bone marrow produces abnormal white blood cells and results in fatigue, shortness of breath, and increased susceptibility to infection. Only limited evidence links Agent Orange to respiratory cancer, prostate cancer, and multiple myeloma.

History: Phenoxy herbicides, including the 2,4,5-T component of Agent Orange, were developed in the 1940's and widely used in agriculture and forestry. Starting in 1960 during the Vietnam War, the United States military sprayed Agent Orange onto lands in Vietnam and Laos. It suspended this activity in 1970, after a study in laboratory animals linked 2,4,5-T to birth defects. Since the 1980's, various groups of Vietnam veterans have filed lawsuits against the makers of Agent Orange. The United States has permanently banned all uses of 2,4,5-T and, consequently, Agent Orange.

Anna Binda, Ph.D.

See also: Dioxins; Multiple myeloma; Mycosis fungoides; Organochlorines (OCs); Pesticides and the food chain

▶ Air pollution

Category: Carcinogens and Suspected Carcinogens
RoC status: Asbestos, known human carcinogen since 1980; diesel exhaust particulate, reasonably anticipated human carcinogen since 2000. Other air pollutants that are known human carcinogens include benzene, 1,3-butadiene, radon, and tobacco smoke; those that are reasonably anticipated human carcinogens include formaldehyde and polycyclic aromatic hydrocarbons. Air pollutants such as ozone, oxides of nitrogen, and sulfur oxides are not listed in the Report on Carcinogens (RoC); however, epidemiologic studies (studies on populations) provide some evidence of their association with lung cancer. Of the many components of particulate matter (PM), only diesel exhaust particulate has been the subject of studies that led to its current classification.
Also known as: Criteria air pollutants, toxic air pollutants

Related cancers: Lung cancer, pleural and peritoneal mesotheliomas, gastrointestinal cancers, laryngeal cancer, cancers of the lymphatic and blood-forming systems (1,3-butadiene).

Definition: Air pollution is the presence of contaminants, many of which are carcinogens, in the air. Outdoors, pollution is largely a consequence of the combustion of fossil fuels for transport, power generation, and other human activities. Indoors, pollution is also generated by burning solid fuels, but the air may also contain asbestos, radon gas, environmental tobacco smoke, formaldehyde, and volatile organic compounds. In 2013, the International Agency for Research on Cancer (IARC) first classified outdoor air pollution overall as a carcinogen.

Exposure routes: Inhalation

At risk: Populations exposed to smog and particulate matter in air pollution, including inner-city residents; people living near electric-power-generating plants, factories, and refining plants; occupationally exposed railroad workers and synthetic rubber industry workers; people cooking indoors with solid fuels. The most recent data from the Global Burden of Disease Project indicates that in 2010, 3.2 million deaths worldwide resulted from air pollution, including 223,000 from lung cancer.

Etiology and symptoms of associated cancers: The World Health Organization describes air as containing a complex mixture of pollutants. These include primary emissions such as diesel soot particles, oxides of nitrogen produced during combustion processes, the products of atmospheric transformation such as ozone, and the sulfate particles formed by burning sulfur-containing fuels. Some carcinogens associated with air pollution do not affect DNA directly, but lead to cancer by other means. For instance, they may cause cells to divide at a more rapid rate than normal and increase the chances that DNA changes will occur. Moreover, air pollutant carcinogens may have different levels of cancer-causing potential. Some may cause cancer only after prolonged, high levels of exposure. For some individuals the risk of developing cancer depends on many factors such as the length and intensity of the exposure, and the person's genetic makeup.

Although air pollution is a minor contributor to lung cancer compared with tobacco smoke, it can affect entire populations, and components of the pollutant mix might interact with other carcinogens, possibly enhancing their effects.

In 2009, Krewski and researchers conducted an extended follow-up of a 1995 epidemiological study and found that there continues to be consistent evidence suggesting that ambient air pollution, chiefly as a result of the incomplete combustion of fossil fuels, is responsible for increased rates of lung cancer.

The major outdoor air pollutants linked to lung cancer are particulate matter, sulfur oxides, ozone, oxides of nitrogen, and volatile organic compounds. Particulate matter is the term for a mixture of solid particles and liquid droplets found in the air that come from soot, smoke, and diesel exhaust.

In 2012 Attfield, and researchers published a cohort mortality study of 12315 workers exposed to diesel exhaust at eight US non-metal mining facilities. The study's findings provided evidence that exposure to diesel exhaust increases risk of mortality from lung cancer and have important public health implications.

The particles of most concern are those smaller than 10 micrometers in diameter. Once inhaled, the smaller particles can travel to the deepest regions of the lungs, where chemicals (such as those adsorbed to diesel exhaust particulate) can be released. Some of these chemicals cause deoxyribonucleic acid (DNA) mutations that can lead to cancer.

Many studies have demonstrated that exposure to indoor air pollutants has adverse effects on health. More than three billion people worldwide depend on solid fuels, including biomass fuels and coal, for their cooking and energy needs. Combustion of these materials indoors produces high levels of smoke that contains many pollutants, and according to the World Health Organization, there is consistent evidence of lung cancer in adults exposed to coal-generated pollutants. Inhaling asbestos fibers released from damaged or crumbled insulating materials or other products containing this material can lead to mesothelioma and several other cancers. Other common indoor air pollutants include formaldehyde, environmental tobacco smoke, radon gas, and polycyclic aromatic hydrocarbons (a class of volatile organic compounds).

History: Many of the components of air pollution are recognized as known or reasonably anticipated carcinogens, such as asbestos, benzene, 1,3-butadiene, radon, tobacco smoke, diesel exhaust particulate, formaldehyde, and polycyclic aromatic hydrocarbons. Other components have scientific research supporting their link to human cancer.

The Clean Air Act as amended in 1990 requires the U.S. Environmental Protection Agency to set national ambient air quality standards for ozone, oxides of nitrogen, particulate matter, and sulfur oxides. The agency is mandated to work with state and local governments to reduce the release of other air pollutants classified as toxic air pollutants. From 1970 to 2014, emissions of the six common pollutants alone dropped an average of 69 percent while gross domestic product grew by 238 percent. This progress reflects efforts by state, local and tribal governments, the EPA, private sector companies, environmental groups, and others. Air pollution Pollution, air

Bernard Jacobson, Ph.D.

Updated by: Jeffrey Larson PT, ATC

For Further Information

Attfield, M. D., Schleiff, P. L., Lubin, J. H., Blair, A., Stewart, P. A., Vermeulen, R., ... Silverman, D. T. (2012). The diesel exhaust in miners study: A cohort mortality study with emphasis on lung cancer. *JNCI Journal of the National Cancer Institute*, *104*(11), 869–883. http://doi.org/10.1093/jnci/djs035

Brunekreef, B., Beelen, R., Hoek, G., Schouten, L., Bausch-Goldbohm, S., Fischer, P., ... van den Brandt, P. (2009). Effects of long-term exposure to traffic-related air pollution on respiratory and cardiovascular mortality in the Netherlands: the NLCS-AIR study. *Research Report (Health Effects Institute)*, 139: 5–71.

EPA; Progress Cleaning the Air and Improving People's Health (2015). http://www.epa.gov/clean-air-act-overview/progress-cleaning-air-and-improving-peoples-health#pollution

Beeson, W. L., Abbey, D. E., & Knutsen S. F. (1998). Long-term concentrations of ambient air pollutants and incident lung cancer in California adults. *Environmental Health Perspectives*, 106: 813-822.

Pope, C.A. III, Majid, E., & Dockery, D. W. (2009). Fine particle air pollution and life expectancy in the United States, *New England Journal of Medicine*, 360: 376-386.

Krzyzanowski, M., Kunnadibbert, B., & Schneider, J. (Eds.). (2005). Health effects of transport-related air pollution. Geneva, Switzerland: World Health Organization.

McGranahan, G., & Murray, F. (2003). Air pollution and health in developing Countries. London: Earthscan.

Pluschke, P. (Ed.). (204). Indoor air pollution. New York: Springer.

Ramachandran, G. (2005). Occupational exposure assessment for air contaminants. New York: CRC Press.

U.S. Department of Health and Human Services, Public Health Service, National Toxicology Program. (2005). *Eleventh report on carcinogens*. Research Triangle Park, N.C.: Author.

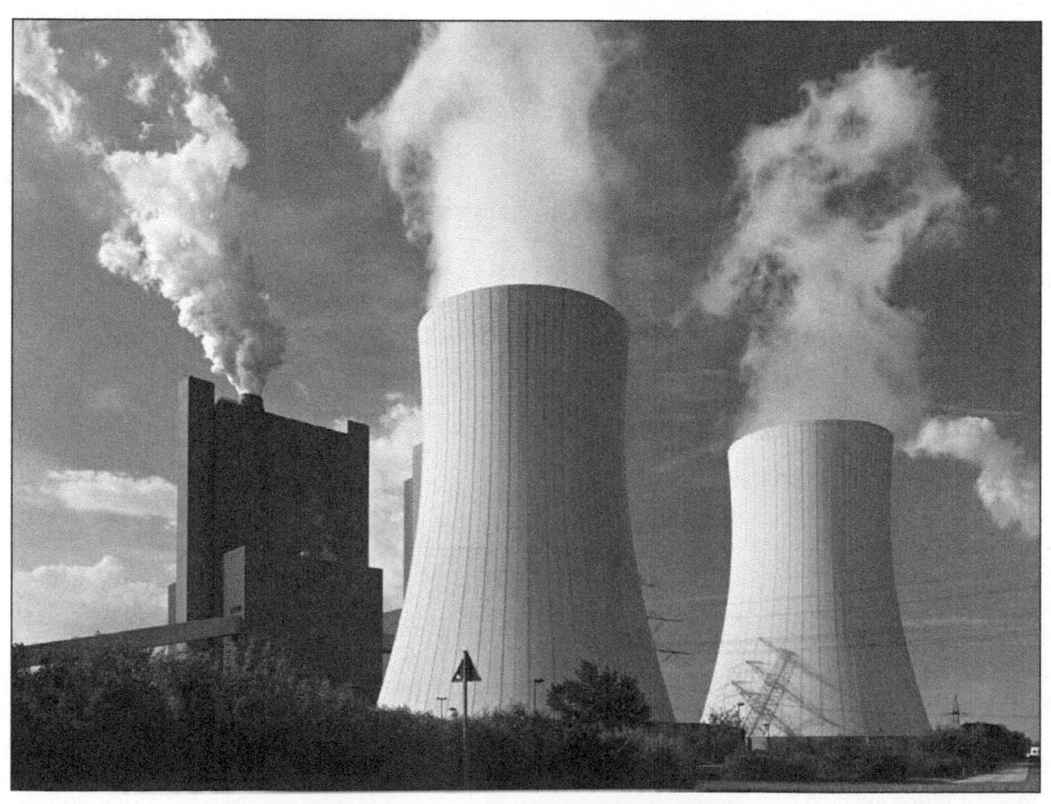

Air pollution from a coal power plant. (iStock)

Other Resources

U.S. Environmental Protection Agency.
Pollutants/Toxics: Air Pollutants.
http://www.epa.gov/ebtpages/pollairpollutants.html
World Health Organization. Air Pollution.
http://www.who.int/topics/air_pollution/en/
American Cancer Association
250 Williams Street NW
Atlanta, Georgia, 30303

See also: Arsenic compounds; Bronchoalveolar lung cancer; 1,3-Butadiene; Cigarettes and cigars; Coke oven emissions; Dioxins; Lung cancers; Occupational exposures and cancer; Polycyclic aromatic hydrocarbons; Radon; Smoking cessation; Tobacco-related cancers; Wood dust

▶ Alcohol, alcoholism, and cancer

Category: Carcinogens and Suspected Carcinogens

Definition: Alcohol is a chemical that is generated during fermentation of sugar. Ethyl alcohol is the specific chemical that is generally referred to as alcohol. Alcohol is the most commonly used intoxicating agent around the world. Alcoholism (also called alcohol-dependence syndrome) is a phenomenon of continuous intake of alcohol, with a compulsive need to consume it. Alcohol has been linked to several cancers but a direct causal relationship between the two has not been established.

Alcohol as carcinogen: Intake of alcohol is considered a risk factor for developing various kinds of cancers, and therefore, alcohol has been classified as a carcinogen. Ethyl alcohol, the form in which alcohol is commonly consumed, undergoes an array of metabolic changes when ingested. The main enzymes that are involved in metabolism of alcohol are alcohol dehydrogenase and aldehyde dehydrogenase. A small amount (approximately 10 percent) is metabolized by microsomal cytochrome P4502E1 (CYP2E1). Alcohol dehydrogenase converts about 80 percent of ethanol to acetaldehyde. Acetaldehyde is a mutagen and a carcinogen and is considered a risk factor in many cancers of the upper gastrointestinal tract.

Acetaldehyde is implicated in a variety of processes such as inflammation of the tracheal epithelium, delaying of cell cycle progression, induction of apoptosis, chromosomal damages and aberrations, and sister chromatid exchanges. Much of the carcinogenic effect of alcohol is attributed to this single metabolite. Direct association between the concentration of acetaldehyde in saliva and development of cancer has been reported. Acetaldehyde covalently bonds with deoxyribonucleic acid (DNA) and forms structures called DNA-adducts. The most common DNA-acetaldehyde adduct is N^2-ethyl-dG, which is not mutagenic. Acetaldehyde also induces the formation of the mutagenic DNA adduct called Cr-PdG (alpha-methyl-gamma-hydroxy-1, N2-propano-2′-deoxyguanosine). Polyamines are one of the basic molecules essential for cells and are implicated in cell growth and differentiation, nucleic acid synthesis, and protection against oxidative damage. Polyamines facilitate acetaldehyde-induced formation of Cr-PdG adducts. Cr-PdG adducts are highly mutagenic and interfere with DNA replication and repair, inducing cancer formation. Polyamines also react with acetaldehyde and form crotonaldehyde, which is highly carcinogenic.

Response to alcohol is individualistic and differs among people and races. This is because of polymorphisms in the genes for the enzymes alcohol dehydrogenase (ADH) and aldehyde dehydrogenase (ALDH). Presence of the *ALDH2*1/2* allele significantly increases the risk of upper aerodigestive tract cancer. In addition to these enzymes, oral bacteria also generate acetaldehyde. High amounts of acetaldehyde are detected in saliva after alcohol consumption. Saliva is directly in contact with the upper aerodigestive tract, and this contact is considered a possible mechanism for its carcinogenic effects.

Alcohol and breast cancer: Alcohol is one of the most ancient intoxicants known to humankind. Consuming one or two drinks a day is not just common but is also a social custom in many cultures. However, research suggests that even one or two drinks a day could put women at a greater risk for developing breast cancer. A study conducted at the National Cancer Institute tested postmenopausal women for differences in hormone levels after alcohol consumption (15 or 30 grams of alcohol per day) for eight weeks. Results showed a significant elevation of estrone sulfate (an estrogen metabolite) and the hormone DHEAS (dehydroepiandrosterone sulfate). DHEAS is secreted by the adrenal glands, and increased levels of DHEAS indicate induction of a process called adrenal steroidogenesis, reflecting stimulation of the hypothalamic-pituitary-adrenal axis in the brain as a response to alcohol consumption.

How Much Is Too Much?

The risk for cancers of the mouth, esophagus, pharynx, larynx, and liver in men and women and breast cancer in women increases after about two drinks per day for men and one per day for women. One drink is defined as 12 ounces of beer, 5 ounces of wine, or 1.5 ounces of 80- proof liquor. The risk for liver cancer goes up significantly after five or more drinks per day.

Source: National Cancer Institute

Alcohol and liver cancers: Excessive consumption of alcohol leads to alcohol liver disease. One type of alcohol liver disease is called alcoholic cirrhosis of the liver, a condition in which normal liver tissue is completely destroyed. Cirrhosis of the liver is considered the primary risk factor for development of hepatocellular carcinoma (liver cancer). Even though alcohol does not seem to cause liver cancer directly, there is a strong association between alcohol and liver cancer.

Alcohol and other cancers: Drinking two or more drinks per day increases the risk of oral and upper gastrointestinal tract (GI) cancers in both men and women. Alcohol-related cancers include those of the mouth, esophagus, and larynx. Drinking alcohol together with smoking increases the risk of developing cancer more than drinking alone. Alcohol is addictive, and alcoholism leads to enhanced tolerance levels, loss of control, cravings for alcohol, and an inability to stop drinking even when people wish to stop or need to stop for their health. Evidence shows that the nutritional status of the body is also negatively affected by alcohol.

Perspectives and progress: According to World Health Organization statistics, alcohol is responsible for about 1.8 million deaths a year, and alcohol-related cancer is the most common cause of these deaths. Some 3.6 percent of all cancer-related deaths are caused by chronic alcohol consumption. Education to make people aware of the link between alcohol consumption and cancer should aid in prevention of such cancers.

Geetha Yadav, Ph.D.

For Further Information

Cho, Chi Hin, and Vishnudutt Purohit, eds. *Alcohol, Tobacco, and Cancer*. New York: Karger, 2006.

Dorgan, J. F., et al. "Serum Hormones and the Alcohol-Breast Cancer Association in Postmenopausal Women." *Journal of the National Cancer Institute* 93 (2001): 710-715.

Seitz, H. K., B. Maurer, and F. Stickel. "Alcohol Consumption and Cancer of the Gastrointestinal Tract." *Digestive Diseases* 23 (2005): 297-303.

Seitz, H. K., and F. Stickel. "Molecular Mechanisms of Alcohol-Mediated Carcinogenesis." *Nature Reviews* 7 (2007): 599-612.

Yirmiya, Raz, and Anna N. Taylor, eds. *Alcohol, Immunity, and Cancer*. Boca Raton, Fla.: CRC Press, 1993.

Other Resources

American Cancer Society

Alcohol and Cancer

http://www.cancer.org/docroot/PRO/content/PRO_1_1x_Alcohol.pdf.asp?sitearea=PRO

National Cancer Institute

Alcohol Consumption

http://progressreport.cancer.gov/doc_detail .asp?pid=1&did=2007&chid=71&coid=706&mid=

See also: Esophageal cancer; Gastrinomas; Gastrointestinal cancers; Hepatomegaly; Laryngeal cancer; Liver cancers; Pancreatic cancers; Pancreatitis

▶ 4-Aminobiphenyl

Category: Carcinogens and Suspected Carcinogens
RoC status: Known human carcinogen since 1980
Also known as: 4-Biphenylamine, p-aminobiphenyl, para-aminobiphenyl, p-aminodiphenyl

Related cancers: Bladder cancer, liver cancer

Definition: 4-Aminobiphenyl, an aromatic amine, occurs as a colorless to yellowish brown crystalline solid that turns purple in air and has an floral odor.

Exposure routes: When heated, 4-aminobiphenyl emits toxic fumes. For the general public, exposure to 4-aminobiphenyl comes from inhalation of tobacco smoke. Occupational exposure occurs from inhalation by laboratory personnel who are doing research with 4-aminobiphenyl. When most of the 4-aminobiphenyl was disposed of by injection into underground wells in the late 1980's, small amounts of it were released into the air, subjecting some individuals to possible contamination.

Where found: 4-Aminobiphenyl is a by product of tobacco smoke and is found as a contaminant in diphenylamine.

Its use is confined to laboratory research, although it may still be found in some dyes, particularly in cosmetics and drugs that contain yellow dye number 1 and in rubber compounds that were manufactured before the mid-1950's.

At risk: Scientists and laboratory technicians who work where 4-aminobiphenyl is used in research as a chemical antioxidant have a high risk for 4-aminobiphenyl contamination. Because 4-aminobiphenyl is generated in tobacco smoke, people who smoke are at high risk for contamination. The general public is at risk for contamination from secondhand tobacco smoke.

Etiology and symptoms of associated cancers: Inhalation of 4-aminobiphenyl can produce headaches, lethargy, urinary burning, and blood in the urine (hematuria). When metabolized, it can be activated by liver enzymes to form adducts with blood serum proteins, particularly hemoglobin and albumin. Hemoglobin adducts are associated with an increased risk for liver cancer. In some cases, 4-aminobiphenyl can undergo additional metabolism to form reactive compounds that are transported to the bladder, where they bind to deoxyribonucleic acid (DNA) molecules. In laboratory tests on cultured human cells, 4-aminobiphenyl caused genetic damage that included cell transformation and inhibition of DNA repair. 4-aminobiphenyl can cross the human placenta and has been detected in fetal blood.

History: 4-Aminobiphenyl was commercially produced in the United States from the early 1930's until the mid-1950's. It was used in the detection of sulfates, in the production of azo dyes and yellow-dye stuffs, and as an antioxidant in the production of rubber. There are still a few companies in the United States that manufacture 4-aminobiphenyl for use in laboratory research.

Alvin K. Benson, Ph.D.

See also: Bladder cancer; Cigarettes and cigars; Diethanolamine (DEA); Liver cancers; Tobacco-related cancers

▶ Arsenic compounds

Category: Carcinogens and Suspected Carcinogens
RoC status: Known human carcinogen since 1980
Also known as: Arsenic pentoxide, arsenic trioxide, arsenic acid

Related cancers: Lung cancer, bladder cancer, liver cancer, kidney cancer, prostate cancer, colon cancer, certain types of skin cancer

Definition: Arsenic occurs in small concentrations in earth and minerals. Leaching effects of water and wind erosion continuously release trace amounts, which can be transported over long distances via windblown dust, surface water, and groundwater flow.

Inorganic arsenic compounds are naturally occurring combinations of arsenic and oxygen, sulfur, or chlorine. These and the complex minerals they are associated with are generally water soluble and occur as white, odorless solids. They typically have high melting and boiling points and can be extremely toxic, even fatal, if inhaled or ingested in large quantities.

Exposure routes: Arsenic compounds in the form of dust and fumes can be absorbed through dermal layers of the skin or can be inhaled and absorbed in respiratory passageways. Arsenic can be ingested orally as a contaminant in food or water.

Where found: Arsenic is a naturally occurring material in soil and water and also in various ores, especially copper and lead. Therefore, arsenic compounds are found throughout the environment. Arsenic naturally combines with other naturally occurring elements including sulfur, oxygen, and chlorine to create relatively stable inorganic arsenic compounds. Often the most concentrated environmental forms of arsenic are released into the atmosphere via volcanoes and mineral and ore erosion. Because arsenic compounds cannot be destroyed, a fairly constant level of toxic inorganic compounds of arsenic always exists in the environment, either in soil, water, or as airborne particulate matter. Because most arsenic compounds are soluble in water, airborne arsenic may be transported great distances before being removed via precipitation to return to soil and water.

At risk: Compounds of inorganic arsenic are used in the manufacture of semiconductors and as a wood preservative. They are also used in making special glass. People involved in these industries are especially at risk because of direct occupational exposure. Because many arsenic compounds occur in ores, people who work in metal smelters are often exposed to higher levels of arsenic. Similarly, carpenters and contractors and others may be exposed to the fumes of burning wood treated with an arsenic preservative or inhale sawdust from treated wood. The most common arsenic poisoning incidents occur among workers involved in the production of arsine, an extremely toxic gas produced by combining arsenic and hydrogen. Finally, people who live in areas with high levels of arsenic in rock or in water are at greater risk.

Etiology and symptoms of associated cancers: Studies conducted on humans testing positive for high levels of inorganic arsenic compounds show significant correlations with various cancers, including skin, liver, lung, and bladder cancer. Studies show an especially strong positive correlation between an increase in toxicity levels of arsenic in air, soil, and water and an increase in nonmelanoma skin cancer. Internal cancers, including liver, kidney, and bladder cancer, probably result from exposure to arsenic via ingestion of food and liquid contaminated with high levels of inorganic arsenic and its compounds. As plants fairly readily absorb inorganic arsenic and its compounds, plants in habitats with high levels of arsenic will be contaminated with higher than normal amounts of this highly toxic mineral. Digestion of plant food in the gastrointestinal tract increases exposure to and absorption of certain arsenic compounds, which then are carried to the liver, kidney, aorta, and skin before they are transferred to the bladder for excretion. Note that this list of exposed organs equates to the more common types of arsenic-induced cancers.

The two most common types of nonmelanoma skin cancers associated with toxic arsenic levels are basal cell carcinoma and squamous cell carcinoma. Basal cell carcinoma begins in the lowest layer of the epidermis, called the basal cell layer. It is highly unusual for a basal cell cancer to spread to lymph nodes or to distant parts of the body. However, if a basal cell cancer is left untreated, it can grow into nearby areas and invade the bone or other tissues beneath the skin. Squamous cell carcinomas tend to be more aggressive than basal cell cancers. They are more likely to invade fatty tissues just beneath the skin, and slightly more likely to spread to lymph nodes or distant parts of the body, although this is still uncommon. Symptoms include changes in skin texture, size, or color, and the area may become sore or ooze.

Very high levels of arsenic exposure and absorption via all routes may lead to a decrease in blood cell production, lymphatic cancer, brain damage, and, in women, infertility and miscarriages.

History: In industry, inorganic arsenic compounds were used as pesticides as early as the middle of the nineteenth century. Within the next century, however, use of such compounds was curbed because of noticeable environmental effects. The most common use for inorganic arsenic since the 1980's is in wood preservation. Pressure-treated wood is made by immersing wood in chromated copper arsenate (CCA) or applying it to the wood under pressure. The arsenic component helps protect the treated wood from weather damage, insects, and decay. CCA is no longer used for residential projects but is used for industrial building. Although the United States has not produced arsenic since 1985, it is still the world's leading arsenic consumer. This puts people at risk in nontraditional ways. For example, people with decks and other housing structures constructed with preserved wood are automatically at increased risk of arsenic exposure, as are farmers who used arsenic-containing pesticides.

In medicine, diseases such as syphilis and psoriasis, leukemia, and asthma were commonly treated with inorganic arsenic solutions until the 1970's. Even in the twenty-first century, it is still used as an antiparasitic agent in veterinary medicine, especially in many countries outside the United States. Continued use of arsenic in all its forms has actually increased environmental levels in soil, water, and air—a trend that is likely to continue with increased industrial demands for this highly valuable but also highly toxic mineral.

Dwight G. Smith, Ph.D.

For Further Information

Battacharyua, Prosun, et al., eds. *Biogeochemical Interactions, Health Effects, and Remediation.* Vol. 9 in *Arsenic in Soil and Groundwater Environment.* Cambridge, Mass.: Elsevier, 2007.

Frost, Floyd J. *Cancer Risks Associated with Elevated Levels of Drinking Water Arsenic Exposure.* Washington, D.C.: AWWA Research Foundation and U.S. Environmental Protection Agency, 2004.

Naidu, R., et al., eds. *Managing Arsenic in the Environment: From Soil to Human Health.* Enfield, N.H.: CSIRO and Science, 2006.

U.S. Department of Health and Human Services, Public Health Service, National Toxicology Program. *Eleventh Report on Carcinogens.* Research Triangle Park, N.C.: Author, 2005.

Other Resources

National Library of Medicine

Environmental Health and Toxicology: Enviro-Health Links—Arsenic and Human Health

http://sis.nlm.nih.gov/enviro/arsenicandhumanhealth.html

See also: Basal cell carcinomas; Bowen disease; Chewing tobacco; Cigarettes and cigars; Coke oven emissions; Fibrosarcomas, soft-tissue; Free radicals; Hemangiosarcomas; Hepatomegaly; Liver cancers; Lung cancers; Melanomas; Nickel compounds and metallic nickel;

Occupational exposures and cancer; Pesticides and the food chain; Soots; Squamous cell carcinomas

▶ Asbestos

Category: Carcinogens and Suspected Carcinogens
RoC status: Known human carcinogen since 1980
Also known as: Chrysotile, actinolite, amosite, anthophyllite, crocidolite, tremolite

Related cancers: Pleural and peritoneal mesothelioma, gastrointestinal cancers, laryngeal cancer, possibly kidney and other cancers

Definition: Asbestos refers to six naturally occurring fibrous silicate minerals: the serpentine mineral chrysotile and the amphibole minerals actinolite, amosite, anthophyllite, crocidolite, and tremolite. The fire-resistant properties of these minerals have been known since antiquity. Their fibers are released into the environment from both natural and human sources and are found in indoor and outdoor air, soil, drinking water, food, and even some medicines. Although there are a variety of forms of asbestos, some more associated with cancer than others, all forms of asbestos share a common characteristic: Because asbestos consists of silica crystals, the fibers are inherently irritating to human tissue.

Exposure routes: Inhalation and ingestion

Where found: Materials for roofing, thermal and electrical insulation, cement pipe and sheets, flooring, gaskets, friction materials, coatings, plastics, textiles, paper, and other products

At risk: Workers in asbestos mining and milling, shipyards, building demolition, insulation, brake repair, and asbestos abatement, and their families

Etiology and symptoms of associated cancers: Several asbestos-related conditions are nonmalignant, including asbestos warts (callus-like growths that form when asbestos fibers become embedded in the skin), asbestosis, pleural plaques, pleural thickening, and pleural effusions (the collection of fluid around the lung a few years after asbestos exposure). Inhaled or ingested asbestos fibers lead to the two most serious asbestos-related disorders: the noncancerous asbestosis, in which scarred and increasingly stiff lung tissue progressively reduces breathing capacity, and the cancer known as malignant mesothelioma. These diseases may take years or decades to develop, although there have been cases of adolescents developing mesothelioma within only a few months of initial asbestos exposure.

Malignant mesothelioma takes two main forms: pleural mesothelioma, in which tumors form on the outer lining of the lungs, and peritoneal mesothelioma, in which tumors form on the peritoneum, the sac containing the abdominal organs. Both have a high mortality rate because mesothelioma is rarely detected in its early stages; the average age of diagnosis is sixty. Symptoms—chest pain, cough, weight loss, and shortness of breath—are often attributed to more common diseases such as asthma. As the cancer spreads, lung capacity is diminished, and the patient eventually succumbs to the inability to take in sufficient oxygen, if not to the failure of other organs after the cancer metastasizes.

Asbestos exposure has also been associated with cancers of the stomach, liver, and other organs. Researchers have observed digestive-tract cancers in workers exposed to crocidolite, amosite, and chrysotile, although study results are inconsistent. An excess of laryngeal cancer has been reported in shipyard workers, chrysotile miners, insulation workers, and others exposed to asbestos. People living near asbestos factories or mines or living with asbestos workers have also developed mesothelioma;

Asbestosis: Most Frequently Recorded Occupations on Death Certificate

Occupation	*Number of Deaths*	*Percent*
Plumbers, pipefitters, and steamfitters	238	8.3
Managers and administrators	129	4.5
Electricians	125	4.4
Carpenters	120	4.2
Insulation workers	108	3.8
Laborers, except construction	95	3.3
Supervisors, production occupations	85	3.0
Welders and cutters	78	2.7
Janitors and cleaners	74	2.6
Truck drivers	66	2.3
All other occupations	1,639	57.3
Occupation not reported	102	3.6
Total	2,859	100.0

Source: Multiple cause of death data from the National Center for Health Statistics
Note: U.S. residents age fifteen and over, selected states and years, 1990-1999.

however, there is no clear association between cancer risk and exposure to asbestos in drinking water. Smokers who are also exposed to asbestos are at a synergistically (rather than additively) greater risk of developing lung cancer.

History: In the 1930's, researchers established that asbestos presented especially high risks of causing lung diseases in miners, shipyard workers, and others who either manufactured or worked with materials incorporating asbestos, such as insulation. It soon became evident that exposure to minute amounts of asbestos could lead to asbestos-related disorders. Miners' spouses developed mesothelioma after being exposed to asbestos through doing laundry, for example, while children became victims through exposure to their parents' work clothes in the home.

In the United States, asbestos was one of the first hazardous air pollutants regulated by the Clean Air Act of 1970. The first lawsuits resulting from occupational exposures began in the late 1960's and increased in 1973 when the Fifth Circuit Court of Appeals applied strict liability in *Borel v. Fibreboard Paper Prods. Corp.* (493 F.2d 1076). In 1976, Congress passed the Toxic Substances Control Act, which imposed regulations regarding asbestos, including a requirement that asbestos abatement occur in schools. The International Labour Organization's Asbestos Convention of 1986 mandated that national laws should "prescribe the measures to be taken for the prevention and control of, and protection of workers against, health hazards due to occupational exposure to asbestos."

The widespread use of asbestos fibers in multiple applications means that exposure remains a concern in the twenty-first century. Although asbestos is no longer as widely used in industry, which has reduced exposure in the workplace, people still risk asbestos exposure when engaging in home improvement projects as they rip out old flooring or replace ceiling tiles.

Christina J. Moose, M.A.

For Further Information

Bartrip, Peter. *Beyond the Factory Gates: Asbestos and Health in Twentieth Century America*. New York: Continuum, 2006.

Bowker, Michael. *Fatal Deception: The Untold Story of Asbestos—Why It Is Still Legal and Still Killing Us*. Emmaus, Pa.: Rodale, 2003.

Harris, L. V., and I. A. Kahwa. "Asbestos: Old Foe in Twenty-First Century Developing Countries." *Science of the Total Environment* 307, nos. 1-3 (2003): 1-9.

Institute of Medicine of the National Academies. Board on Population Health and Public Health Practices. Committee on Asbestos: Selected Health Effects. *Asbestosis: Selected Cancers*. Washington, D.C.: National Academies Press, 2006.

Pass, Harvey I. *One Hundred Questions and Answers About Mesothelioma*. Sudbury, Mass.: Jones & Bartlett, 2004.

U.S. Department of Health and Human Services, Public Health Service, National Toxicology Program. *Eleventh Report on Carcinogens*. Research Triangle Park, N.C.: Author, 2005.

Other Resources

'Lectric Law Library
A History of Asbestos Use and Asbestos Litigation
http://www.lectlaw.com/files/med40.htm

National Toxicology Program
http://ntp.niehs.nih.gov

See also: Air pollution; Bronchoalveolar lung cancer; Cancer clusters; Carcinomatosis; Epidermoid cancers of mucous membranes; Free radicals; Head and neck cancers; Kidney cancer; Laryngeal cancer; Lung cancers; Mesothelioma; Occupational exposures and cancer; Risks for cancer; Sarcomas, soft-tissue; Statistics of cancer; Throat cancer; Urinary system cancers

▶ Azathioprine

Category: Carcinogens and Suspected Carcinogens
RoC status: Known human carcinogen since 1985
Also known as: Azasan, Imuran

Related cancers: Non-Hodgkin lymphoma, cancers of the skin and liver

Definition: Azathioprine is a drug prescribed for transplant patients and those whose immune systems attack their own tissues, but long-term usage causes cancer.

Exposure routes: Ingestion, intravenous injection, and inhalation

Where found: The drug is found in hospitals, used for transplant and autoimmune disease patients, and in manufacturing plants that make and package the drug.

At risk: Patients who take azathioprine and workers who manufacture it.

Etiology and symptoms of associated cancers: In the liver, azathioprine is converted to 6-mercaptopurine, which inhibits deoxyribonucleic acid (DNA) synthesis. This suppresses the immune system but can also cause a dangerous decrease in the number of white blood cells (leukopenia) and platelets (thrombocytopenia), increased risk of infection and bleeding, gastrointestinal disturbances, and liver damage. The substance 6-mercaptopurine also inserts between adjacent nucleotide bases in DNA molecules and causes mutations that lead to various types of cancer.

Azathioprine increases the risk of developing squamous cell carcinoma, a type of skin cancer that appears as persistent wartlike growths, scaly patches, or open sores that crust over and bleed; non-Hodgkin lymphoma, a blood-based cancer of white blood cells called T cells, the most common symptoms of which are painless swelling of the neck, or underarm lymph nodes, unexplained fever, loss of weight and appetite, itchy skin with reddened patches, and constant fatigue; and cancer of the bile ducts or hepatobiliary carcinomas, whose symptoms include jaundice, itching, stomach pain, weight loss, and fever.

History: The pioneer of liver transplantation, Sir Roy Yorke Calne, first used azathioprine to prevent organ rejection in liver transplant patients. Azathioprine was the standard antirejection drug in the 1970's for organ transplants and was later enlisted to treat patients who suffer from diseases that result when the immune system attacks the patient's own body (autoimmune diseases).

Several epidemiological studies have shown that transplant patients who took azathioprine were at a high risk for different types of tumors. Other patients who took azathioprine but were not transplant patients, including those with rheumatoid arthritis, systemic lupus, inflammatory bowel disease, and certain skin and renal diseases, have also shown higher incidences of such malignancies, but not as high as those observed in transplant patients, since the dosages to treat autoimmune diseases are lower than those used for transplant patients. Mycophenolate mofetil, which is not as carcinogenic, is gradually replacing azathioprine as the antirejection drug of choice.

Michael A. Buratovich, Ph.D.

See also: Crohn's disease; Myasthenia gravis; Pancolitis

▶ Bacteria as causes of cancer

Category: Carcinogens and Suspected Carcinogens
Also known as: Helicobacter pylori, Salmonella typhi, Streptococcus bovis, Chlamydophila (previously Chlamydia) pneumoniae

Related cancers: Gastrointestinal cancers, lung cancer

Definition: Although no bacterium has been shown to be absolutely responsible for causing cancer, very strong evidence implicates two types of bacteria in the process of cancer formation, and less convincing evidence implicates others. Each of these types of bacteria has been shown to cause a persistent (chronic) infection in which the organisms are in contact with the tissue over a long period of time. During that time, genes for cell division and other cell maintenance functions, the same ones that are damaged by other known chemical and physical carcinogens, are damaged by the metabolic and toxic products produced by these bacteria. Equally important are immune system defenses and additional genetic and environmental factors that make only certain individuals susceptible to these organisms. The two types of bacteria are Helicobacter (associated with gastric cancer) and Salmonella typhi (gallbladder cancer). Additional bacteria probably associated with different cancers include Streptococcus bovis (colorectal cancer), Chlamydophilia pneumoniae (lung cancer), strains of Escherichia coli (colorectal cancer associated with Crohn disease and ulcerative colitis), and different types of oral streptococci (oral cancers).

Exposure routes: Ingestion and inhalation

Where found: Infected and uninfected persons carrying certain bacteria; contaminated water, air, and surfaces

At risk: Genetically susceptible individuals specific to each type of bacteria

Etiology and symptoms of associated cancers: Cancer caused by H. pylori is characterized by tumors in the protective layer of mucus in the stomach, including the immune tissue. Continued high incidence of stomach cancer in areas of Asia suggests that a diet high in salted, smoked, and pickled foods is a contributory factor. Transmission of H. pylori is thought to be by the fecal-oral route.

The second strongest case for bacterial causation of cancer involves S. typhi and its role in causing cancer of the gallbladder. It has been known since the famous case of Typhoid Mary that survivors (or carriers without symptoms) of typhoid fever carry S. typhi for at least a year and can transmit the pathogen in their feces. The organism resides in the gallbladder during that entire time, thus fulfilling one of the conditions necessary to cause cancer (long exposure). Cancer formation in the gallbladder is frequently associated with gallstone formation (solid deposits of cholesterol or calcium salts).

Symptoms that may indicate a diseased gallbladder include chronic indigestion, upper abdominal pain, nausea and vomiting, and fever. All of these symptoms may also be associated with additional gastrointestinal problems, so they are not definitive for gallbladder problems, including gallbladder cancer. Associated risk factors include cholelithiasis (especially untreated symptomatic chronic gallstones), obesity, reproductive factors, environmental exposure to toxic chemicals, congenital malformation of bile ducts, and chronic infections affecting the gallbladder. The most significant risk factor for those cancers associated with S. typhi appears to be chronic infection of the gallbladder. Data show that patients with chronic infections with this organism are eight times more likely to have cancer of the gallbladder than those who had acute infections in which the organisms were cleared from their body. Genetic susceptibility of American Indians and Mexican Americans, especially women (in all populations), to gallbladder cancer suggest that these groups are predisposed to develop it primarily or secondarily due to an increased incidence of cholesterol gallstones. A secondary pathway of cancer development revolves around congenital malformation of the bile duct, and is seen primarily in people from Japan, Korea, and possibly China.

History: The first indication that a relationship existed between bacteria and cancer occurred in 1951, when researchers found that patients frequently had both infective endocarditis (infection of the heart) and colonic carcinoma. It took until 1974 to identify S. bovis as the bacterium associated with the colonic cancer and bacteremia (bacteria in blood). It is known today that S. bovis is a natural inhabitant of the human gastrointestinal tract and causes both endocarditis and bacteremia. Patients having colon carcinoma frequently also harbor S. bovis, and these cancerous lesions may develop years after having endocarditis or bacteremia.

Further research has focused on the bacteria naturally found in the gastrointestinal tract and their ability to metabolize nutrients into carcinogens. Experiments done using gastrointestinal flora from rats determined that metabolic products are mutagenic (cause mistakes in deoxyribonucleic acid, or DNA). The fact that germ-free rats did not develop tumors as frequently as normal animals was also significant in defining the relationship between diet and gastrointestinal flora.

Data from later experiments have suggested that the presence of microorganisms as a causative agent for cancer formation may be more complicated than first thought. Conflicting reports suggest that the presence of H. pylori is both detrimental and beneficial in the development of esophageal cancer. The ability to use the presence of microorganisms as an indication that cancer may also be present (in situations in which the cancer is not easily diagnosed at an early stage) is being examined. This is the case with oral tumors and specific oral bacteria. Therefore, the precise relationship between microorganisms and different types of cancer is still unclear and remains to be determined.

Steven A. Kuhl, Ph.D.

For Further Information

Hope, Mari, et al. "Sporadic Colorectal Cancer: Role of the Commensal Microbiota." *FEMS Microbiology Letters* 244 (2005): 1-7.

Lax, Alistair, and Warren Thomas. "How Bacteria Could Cause Cancer: One Step at a Time." *Trends in Microbiology* 10 (2002): 293-299.

Mager, Dixie. "Bacteria and Cancer: Cause, Coincidence, or Cure? A Review." *Journal of Translational Medicine* 4 (2006): 14.

Other Resources

Centers for Disease Control and Prevention
Helicobacter pylori
http://www.cdc.gov/ncidod/aip/research/hp.html

National Cancer Institute
H. pylori and Cancer: Fact Sheet
http://www.cancer.gov/cancertopics/factsheet/HPylori

See also: Achlorhydria; Alcohol, alcoholism, and cancer; Diverticulosis and diverticulitis; Esophagitis; Ethnicity and cancer; *Helicobacter pylori*; Infectious cancers; Mucosa-Associated Lymphoid Tissue (MALT) lymphomas; Poverty and cancer; Prostatitis; Risks for cancer; Stomach cancers; Virus-related cancers

▶ Benzene

Category: Carcinogens and Suspected Carcinogens
RoC status: Known human carcinogen since 1980
Also known as: Benzol, phenyl hydride, 1,3,5-cyclohexatriene

Related cancers: Cancers of the blood and blood-forming organs, including acute myelogenous, monocytic, erythroblastic and lymphocytic leukemias, lymphomas, and Zymbal gland carcinomas

Definition: Benzene (chemical formula C_6H_6) is a clear, colorless to light yellow, volatile and flammable liquid that has an aromatic odor. It is slightly soluble in water, is sensitive to heat, and mixes easily with alcohol, ether, chloroform, acetone, carbon tetrachloride, carbon disulfide, oils, and glacial acetic acid. It forms a solid below 42 degrees Fahrenheit.

In the United States, the Safe Drinking Water Act (1976) has legal control over benzene levels in drinking water, which cannot exceed 5 parts per billion (ppb). Exposure at 19,000-20,000 parts per million for five to ten minutes is fatal.

Exposure routes: Inhalation, skin contact, and oral ingestion are the most toxic and dangerous routes.

Where found: Benzene is an industrial chemical that is widely used as a solvent and used in inks, rubber, lacquers, paint removers, gas additives, glue backing for carpeting, high solvent paints, some furniture wax, automobile exhaust, tobacco smoke, secondhand smoke, taxidermy, firefighting, metal preparation and pouring, petroleum refining, industrial cleaning, drinking water, and closed processes to synthesize organic chemicals. It is also used to make dyes and insecticides and in the processing of numerous chemicals.

At risk: Children and pregnant woman are at higher risk. However, anyone exposed to benzene is at risk. For example, the presence of benzene in gasoline makes exposure to it a risk for anyone filling an automobile gas tank.

Etiology and symptoms of associated cancers: It is not clear how benzene causes damage to the blood-forming organs, which then leads to leukemias and lymphomas. Interaction between breakdown products (metabolites) is being studied as a likely cause. Exposure to as little as 1 part per million lowers white cell counts.

Symptoms of leukemias and lymphomas include fever, night sweats, fatigue, bleeding and easy bruising, bone pain, frequent infections, swollen lymph nodes, and weight loss.

History: Benzene is a natural component of crude oil. In 1825 Michael Faraday performed distillation experiments and extracted a gas from the oil. The gas burned, and he named it "bicarburet of hydrogen." The chemical structure of benzene remained elusive until 1865, when Friedrich August Kekulé von Stradonitz hypothesized a hexagonal structure.

Benzene was derived from the distillation of coal by A. W. Hoffman in 1846. The uses of and demand for benzene increased along with oil exploration as its usefulness in many industrial applications became apparent.

Linus Pauling, the Nobel Prize-winning physicist, was one of many scientists to attempt to elucidate the unique hybrid structure of benzene that was confirmed in 1931.

The main use of benzene prior to World War I was in gasoline blending, as it increased octane. It was used extensively in industry in World War II, and almost all organic-chemistry-related industry involves petroleum (benzene-containing) products.

Janet R. Green, M.S.P.H.

See also: Acute Lymphocytic Leukemia (ALL); Acute Myelocytic Leukemia (AML); Air pollution; Aleukemia; Aplastic anemia; Bioflavonoids; Blood cancers; 1,3-Butadiene; Carcinogens, known; Carcinogens, reasonably anticipated; Chlorambucil; Cigarettes and cigars; Coal tars and coal tar pitches; Coke oven emissions; Dioxins; Free radicals; Leukemias; Myelodysplastic syndromes; Myelofibrosis; Organochlorines (OCs); Phenolics; Urinary system cancers

▶ Benzidine and dyes metabolized to benzidine

Category: Carcinogens and Suspected Carcinogens
RoC status: Benzidine, known human carcinogen since 1980; dyes metabolized to benzidine, known human carcinogens since 2000
Also known as: Direct Blue 6, Direct Black 38, Direct Brown 95

Related cancers: Bladder cancer, and less frequently cancer of the stomach, liver, kidney, central nervous system, and pancreas

Definition: Benzidine is an organic compound used to make dyes. It is usually found in the form of a powder that is white, reddish gray, or grayish yellow.

Exposure routes: Benzidine can enter into the human body in many ways. If air containing molecules of benzidine is inhaled, the benzidine can enter into a person's system. Benzidine can also be ingested, either directly or in contaminated drinking water. It is also possible for benzidine to enter the human body through the skin if direct contact is made with benzidine or a benzidine-based dye.

Where found: For many years, benzidine was used in the production of dyes and dyeing compounds. It was also used occasionally in some clinical and laboratory settings, for example, in blood detection. Dyes that metabolize to benzidine were used in many different dyeing applications. Benzidine was used especially often to dye paper products, textiles, and leather goods. Plants manufacturing dyes were likely to contain large quantities of benzidine or dyes that metabolize to benzidine, as were plants that produced goods using such dyes. Beginning in the late 1970's use of these dyes was phased out.

Because of long usage, there remains the possibility of benzidine contamination in areas around plants and factories that once used benzidine or related dyes. Benzidine that is released into or makes its way into rivers or streams generally settles quickly on the bottom of the riverbed or streambed. Benzidine that was released into the environment through accidental contamination or as a waste product that ends up in the soil bonds strongly to particles found in the soil. It is not likely to seep into the groundwater and contaminate drinking water sources because of these strong bonds. Because its use in dyeing was phased out, benzidine and related dyes are used in only very small quantities in mostly research and laboratory settings in the United States.

At risk: People who worked in industries that manufactured dyes or regularly used dyes in the production of other goods before the late 1970's were at risk of exposure to high levels of benzidine and dyes that metabolize to benzidine. According to the Occupational Health and Safety Administration, in 1979 there were sixty-three separate occupations in which workers were at risk for benzidine exposure. Also at risk are people living near factories or plants that manufactured or used benzidine or benzidine-based dyes, especially if by-products of the plant were released into the air or water. Some residual benzidine may continue to exist at such locations. Benzidine and related dyes have also been identified as existing at many hazardous waste disposal sites and people who live near such areas may be at risk of exposure.

Etiology and symptoms of associated cancers: Benzidine and related dyes have been shown to cause cancer in laboratory animals. Studies of humans who have a history of working with benzidine or related dyes have also shown that prolonged benzidine exposure is a significant risk factor for developing bladder cancer. Scientists do not clearly understand all the complex mechanisms involved in how benzidine causes cancer, but benzidine is believed to interfere with normal cellular processes.

Bladder cancer is the cancer most commonly associated with benzidine exposure. The first signs and symptoms of bladder cancer are usually changes in bladder function or habits. This may include a person's often feeling the urge to urinate without actually being able to do so. Needing to urinate much more frequently than usual is also a possible symptom of bladder cancer, as is blood in the urine.

History: Benzidine has a long history as an important industrial dye. It was first made in 1845. Its first use as a dye was in 1884, when a dye named Congo Red was created for the first time. Benzidine and related dyes were extremely useful in dyeing because of the way they adhere to cotton and cotton products. In the 1920's some physicians and researchers began to suspect a relationship between exposure to benzidine and the development of bladder cancer. It was not until 1976, however, that major commercial production of benzidine and benzidine-based dyes ceased in the United States. There are no major manufacturers of benzidine for the purposes of dyeing or of benzidine-based dyes in the United States; however, there are still some small manufacturers of benzidine because it has some research and laboratory applications. It is considered a possible occupational carcinogen by the Occupational Safety and Health Administration. Personal protection is required for work with benzidine and related products, and it is necessary to take precautions to ensure that no benzidine is released into the environment. Benzidine is also considered a hazardous substance that requires special labeling and precautions when it is transported.

Robert Bockstiegel, B.S.

For Further Information

Bozzone, Donna M. *Causes of Cancer*. New York: Chelsea House, 2007.

Pohanish, Richard P. *Sittig's Handbook of Toxic and Hazardous Chemicals and Carcinogens*. 5th ed. Norwich, N.Y.: William Andrew, 2008.

U.S. Department of Health and Human Services, Public Health Service, National Toxicology Program. *Eleventh Report on Carcinogens*. Research Triangle Park, N.C.: Author, 2005.

Williams, Nerys R. *Atlas of Occupational Health and Disease*. New York: Oxford University Press, 2004.

Other Resources

International Agency for Research on Cancer
http://www.iarc.fr/index.html

Occupational Safety and Health Administration
http://www.osha.gov

See also: Carcinogens, known; Carcinogens, reasonably anticipated; Immunocytochemistry and immunohistochemistry

▶ Beryllium and beryllium compounds

Category: Carcinogens and Suspected Carcinogens
RoC status: Known human carcinogen since 2002
Also known as: Glucinium. Glucinium is a rarely used term, but it is noteworthy because, although the name describes beryllium's tempting, sugary flavor, it does not warn of its poisonous nature, and those working with the alkaline earth metal should be cautioned.

Related cancers: Lung cancer

Definition: Beryllium is an alkaline earth metal found in ore deposits and in some precious stones. It was discovered in 1798 in emeralds and beryl and isolated in 1828. The metal did not see large-scale industrial use until the late 1950's. In the twenty-first century, however, because of its high melting point, great elasticity, exceptional thermal conductivity, high permeability to X rays, and resistance to oxidation, beryllium finds uses across a wide range of products.

Exposure routes: Inhalation of beryllium compounds that are found in dust and fumes combined with prolonged exposure elevate the risk of pulmonary disease and lung cancer. Beryllium can also enter the body through food and drinking water, but these routes seem less harmful because of its poor absorption. However, contact through abraded skin may result in local irritation, ulceration, or granulomatous growths.

Where found: Beryllium has found uses across a variety of industries due to its properties as a light, high-strength metal combined with great elasticity and high melting point. A brief list includes uses in X-ray diagnostics; as a lightweight structural material required by the aerospace and missile industries; and as an alloying agent found in applications requiring high strength and first-rate electrical conductivity. Additionally, beryllium and its compounds find use in nonsparking tools, telecommunication devices, electrical contacts, nuclear reactors, ceramics, microwave equipment, communication satellites, space vehicles, aircraft, semiconductors, electrical insulators, everyday items such as golf clubs and bicycle frames, and many other applications requiring a hardening agent found in alloys such as beryllium copper.

At risk: Workers experiencing chronic exposure to beryllium compounds are most at risk. This would include beryllium miners (the United States is the world's largest producer); workers involved with beryllium alloys, ceramics, nuclear reactors, phosphorus manufacture, electronic equipment, and missiles; and garment workers exposed to beryllium dust. According to Environmental Protection Agency (EPA) estimates, work facilities in the United States release approximately 1 million pounds of beryllium and beryllium compounds into the environment annually, but the risk to the general population remains poorly understood. What is understood is that lung cancer risk rises with exposure time and beryllium dust concentration.

Etiology and symptoms of associated cancers: The nonmalignant disease associated with beryllium and its compounds is called berylliosis. When exposed to high levels of beryllium, the immediate response is characterized by inflammation of the nose, larynx, trachea, bronchioles, and lungs. This is the acute form of beryllium disease and requires air levels of the metal on the order of 100 micrograms/cubic meter (mcg/m^3) or more. Normally, ambient air levels are thousands of times less. As the exposure becomes more chronic, and typically from contact at much lower levels just exceeding 0.02 mcg/m^3 over ten or more years, berylliosis takes the form of a granulomatous disease of the lungs and possibly other organs. Granulomas are nodular inflammatory lesions packed with immune cells (macrophages). Both the acute and chronic forms of berylliosis are usually not fatal.

The beryllium lymphocyte proliferation test (BeLPT) is an effective blood test that measures beryllium sensitization. Although most people with beryllium sensitization will eventually develop berylliosis, further testing must be done to establish the individual's disease status. This is an important diagnostic tool because chronic berylliosis is not only a serious illness but also a significant pathway to malignancy.

The progression to chronic berylliosis follows a continuing, overzealous, and ultimately destructive immune response that leads to lung scarring and loss of respiratory capacity. This cascade of events is triggered by chemical messengers called cytokines, which repeatedly call in more immune cells than the lungs can process. This overzealous immune response leads to severe lung damage. The terrible number of deaths from the 1918 flu epidemic was a result of just such a cytokine storm and not from the destructive properties of the virus itself.

The progression to lung cancer is not completely understood, and there is some debate over just how lung cancer arises from berylliosis, but most experts accept that chronic berylliosis is a strong marker for events leading to malignancy.

History: Cancer arising from beryllium or its compounds depends on length and level of exposure. In general these exposure risks have been significantly reduced since the 1950's, when workers might have been exposed to hundreds of times the levels found in twenty-first century working conditions. In 1991 researchers confirmed the carcinogenicity of beryllium and its compounds, and in 2002 the Department of Health and Human Services officially recognized beryllium as a carcinogen. The Occupational Safety and Health Administration (OSHA) sets permissible peak exposure limits for beryllium at 0.025 mcg/m^3; however, independent occupational health organizations are urging the reduction of these limits even further. To confuse the issue, there is even some minor debate on just how well previous data support the connection between cancer risk and beryllium exposure.

What is known is that certain factors may affect the progression of chronic beryllium disease (CBD). These factors include the individual's work environment, the duration and intensity of exposure, and the particle size and solubility of the beryllium dust. Also the individual's genetic makeup, lifestyle habits, and general health are contributing issues.

Richard S. Spira, D.V.M.

For Further Information

American Conference of Governmental Industrial Hygienists. *1999 TLVs and BEIs: Threshold Limit Values for Chemical Substances and Physical Agents—Biological Exposure Indices*. Cincinnati, Ohio: Author, 1999.

American Industrial Hygiene Association. *The AIHA 1998 Emergency Response Planning Guidelines and Workplace Environmental Exposure Level Guides Handbook*. Fairfax, Va.: Author, 1998.

Kelleher, P. C., et al. "Beryllium Particulate Exposure and Disease Relations in a Beryllium Machining Plant." *Journal of Occupational and Environmental Medicine* 43 (2001): 238-249.

U.S. Department of Health and Human Services, Public Health Service, National Toxicology Program. *Eleventh Report on Carcinogens*. Research Triangle Park, N.C.: Author, 2005.

U.S. Environmental Protection Agency. *Integrated Risk Information System (IRIS) on Beryllium*. Washington, D.C.: National Center for Environmental Assessment, Office of Research and Development, 1999.

_______. *Toxicological Review of Beryllium and Compounds*. Washington, D.C.: Author, 1998.

U.S. Occupational Safety and Health Administration. *Occupational Safety and Health Standards, Toxic and Hazardous Substances*. Code of Federal Regulations 29 CFR 1910.1000. Washington, D.C.: Author, 1998.

Other Resources

Agency for Toxic Substances and Disease Registry
ToxFAQS for Beryllium
http://www.atsdr.cdc.gov/tfacts4.html

U.S. Environmental Protection Agency
CICAD Report on Beryllium and Beryllium Compounds
http://www.inchem.org/documents/cicads/cicads/cicad32.htm

See also: Carcinogens, known; Cytokines; Lung cancers

▶ Birth control pills and cancer

Category: Carcinogens and Suspected Carcinogens
RoC status: Most birth control pills contain two active ingredients, a form of estrogen and a form of progesterone. Collectively, estrogens have been classified as a known human carcinogen since 1985. Progesterone has been listed as a reasonably anticipated human carcinogen since 1985.
Also known as: Oral contraceptives

Related cancers: Carcinogens, suspected breast cancer, cervical cancer

Definition: A birth control pill is a tablet containing a synthetic estrogen, such as ethinyl estradiol; a synthetic progesterone, such as norethindrone; or both. These compounds mimic the action of naturally occurring sex hormones and are administered to alter the function of tissues that respond to these hormones. For example, a moderate, consistent dose of estrogen will prevent the typical spike in estrogen that occurs naturally during the middle of the menstrual cycle. This in turn prevents the ovary from releasing an egg.

Estrogen and progesterone have different effects on reproductive tissues that, in combination, are highly effective in preventing pregnancy. Although the majority of birth control pills contain a dose of each hormone, mini-pills that contain only progesterone are also available. Although contraception is the most common reason for using birth control pills, the pill is also commonly prescribed for other purposes, such as bothersome menstrual symptoms and acne.

Exposure routes: Birth control pills are tablets that are ingested orally. Several alternative delivery systems, such as transdermal patches, vaginal ring, and contraceptive injection contain similar active ingredients that are taken into the body through other routes.

Where found: Birth control pills are manufactured by drug makers and prescribed by health providers. The World Health Organization estimates that approximately 9 percent of all women of reproductive age worldwide use birth control pills.

At risk: At highest risk are women of reproductive age, particularly in developed countries where the pill is more widely available and pill use is more prevalent. A small minority of pill users are women who take the pills to manage menstrual symptoms, acne, or premenstrual syndrome (PMS).

Etiology and symptoms of associated cancers: Some breast cancers, though not all, involve the abnormal growth and proliferation of cells that are responsive to estrogen or progesterone. Studies in mice and rats indicate that exposure to either synthetic estrogen alone or synthetic progesterone alone caused malignant tumors to develop in mammary tissue. Likewise, combinations of synthetic estrogen and progesterone appear to cause development of both benign and malignant mammary tumors in animals. In humans, research suggests that breast cancer risk is slightly increased with birth control pill use, and that the risk increases with a longer duration of use. Birth control pills containing a higher dose of estrogen and/or progesterone may increase breast cancer risk more than low-dose pills. Triphasic pills, in which the hormone dose changes three times over the course of a month, were particularly associated with increased breast cancer risk in the Nurses' Health Study. Recent pill use is associated with greater breast cancer risk. After long-term cessation of pill use, the risk of breast cancer appears to decrease to a level comparable to that of women who never used the pill.

The risk of cervical cancer may also slightly increase with birth control pill use, and particularly with long-term use. Research to date has yet to fully explain the relationship between cervical cancer and birth control pills, yet it may be related to infection with human papillomavirus (HPV), which causes most cervical cancer cases. Researchers theorize that birth control pills may increase susceptibility to HPV infection, and with it cervical cancer risk.

Conversely, the use of birth control pills appears to reduce the risk of some types of cancer, including colorectal, ovarian, and endometrial cancers. Evidence suggests that birth control pill use reduces a woman's risk of developing ovarian cancer, possibly due to fewer cycles of ovulation over her life span. Birth control pill use also appears to decrease the risk of cancer of the endometrium (the uterine lining), with protective effects lingering for many years after the woman stops taking contraceptives.

History: The first birth control pill became available in the United States in 1960, and birth control pills were widely adopted in the decades that followed. Early concern about the safety of birth control pills linked the high doses of estrogen in birth control pills with an increased risk of serious cardiovascular events, including heart attack and stroke. Over time, drug manufacturers lowered the dosages of estrogen in birth control pills.

By the 1980's researchers had observed associations between birth control pill use and cancer risk. However, studies were inconsistent in confirming this relationship, and a number of large population-based studies were undertaken to clarify the effect of pill use on cancer risk. After review of multiple such studies, the International Agency for Research on Cancer, a division of the World Health Organization, classified combined estrogen-progesterone birth control pills as carcinogenic to humans.

Andrea Bradford, M.A.
Updated by: Stephanie Watson

For Further Information

Beaber, E.F., Buist, D.S.M., Barlow, W.E., Malone, K. E., Reed, S. D., & Li, C. I. (2014). Recent oral contraceptive use by formulation and breast cancer risk among women 20 to 49 years of age. *Cancer Research*, 74: 4078-4089.

Center for Young Women's Health. (2014). Medical uses of the birth control pill. Retrieved from http://youngwomenshealth.org/2011/10/18/medical-uses-of-the-birth-control-pill/.

Cerhan, James R. (2006). Oral contraceptive use and breast cancer risk: Current status. *Mayo Clinic Proceedings,* 81(10): 1287-1289.

Gierisch, J.M., Coeytaux, R.R., Urrutia, R.P., Havrilesky, L. J., Moorman, P. G., Lowery, W. J., ... Myers, E. R. (2013). Oral contraceptive use and risk of breast, cervical, colorectal, and endometrial cancers: A systematic review. *Cancer Epidemiology, Biomarkers & Prevention*, 22: 1931-1943.

National Cancer Institute. (2012). Oral Contraceptives and Cancer Risk. Retrieved from http://www.cancer.gov/about-cancer/causes-prevention/risk/hormones/oral-contraceptives-fact-sheet.

United Nations. (2015). Trends in Contraceptive Use Worldwide 2015. Retrieved from http://www.un.org/en/development/desa/population/publications/pdf/family/trendsContraceptiveUse2015Report.pdf.

Zonderman, Jon, & Shader, Laurel. (2006). *Birth control pills*. New York: Chelsea House.

Other Resources

Mayo Clinic.

Birth Control Pill Frequently Asked Questions: Benefits, Risks, and Choices.
http://www.mayoclinic.com/health/birth-control-pill/WO00098

National Cancer Institute.

Oral Contraceptives and Cancer Risk.
http4://www.cancer.gov/cancertopics/factsheet/Risk/oral-contraceptives

See also: Antiestrogens; Cervical cancer; Endocrine cancers; Endometrial cancer; Endometrial hyperplasia; Estrogen-receptor-sensitive breast cancer; Fertility drugs and cancer; Fibrocystic breast changes; Gestational Trophoblastic Tumors (GTTs); Hormonal therapies; Hormone receptor tests; Hormone Replacement Therapy (HRT); Ovarian cancers; Ovarian cysts; Progesterone receptor assay; Receptor analysis; Screening for cancer; Vasectomy and cancer

▶ Bis(chloromethyl) ether and technical-grade chloromethyl methyl ether

Category: Carcinogens and Suspected Carcinogens
RoC status: Known human carcinogen since 1980
Also known as: BCME, chloro(chloromethoxy) methane dichloromethyl ether, CMME, dimethylchloroether, methyl chloromethyl ether

Related cancer: Lung cancer

Definition: Bis (chloromethyl) ether (BCME) and technical-grade chloromethyl methyl ether (CMME) are chemicals known as chloroalkyl ethers. Both are clear, flammable liquids with strong, unpleasant odors.

Exposure routes: After BCME and CMME are released into the air, humans can be exposed by inhalation, dermal contact, and oral exposure via contaminated water. Potential exposure by inhalation can occur to workers who are involved in the production of BCME and CMME.

Where found: BCME and CMME are found at production sites where they have been released into the air and at landfill sites where they have been transferred for disposal. Both are found in chemical plants where they are manufactured and in research laboratories where they are used to make other chemicals. They can also be found in plants where they have been used to make several types of polymers, resins, plastics, and textiles. Small quantities of BCME can be formed as an impurity during the production of CMME. CMME can be converted to BCME through hydrolysis.

At risk: The greatest risk for contamination from BCME and CMME is to chemical plant workers, laboratory workers, ion-exchange resin makers, and polymer producers. The general public experiences some risk from both chemicals around sites where they are produced or where they are discarded, such as landfills and surface impoundments.

Etiology and symptoms of associated cancers: Individuals exposed to BCME and CMME show significant increases in the incidence of lung carcinomas, mostly of the oat-cell type, which is generally not associated with smoking tobacco. The number of lung carcinomas is much higher in people exposed to just BCME, as compared with individuals who are exposed to both BCME and CMME. When exposed to BCME or CMME, individuals have shown a slight increase of incidence of chromosomal aberrations in peripheral lymphocytes. Both chemicals can induce unscheduled synthesis of deoxyribonucleic acid (DNA) in human fibroblasts in vitro.

History: Although BCME and CMME were previously manufactured in the United States, use of both chemicals in the United States has dropped significantly since 1976. Since 1982, only CMME is produced in the United States. In the past, BCME was used to treat vulcanized rubber to increase adhesion and in the production of flame-retardant fabrics. CMME is used as an alkylating agent and solvent in manufacturing polymers, ion-exchange resins, and water repellants.

Alvin K. Benson, Ph.D.

See also: Carcinogens, known; Carcinogens, reasonably anticipated; Occupational exposures and cancer

▶ Bisphenol A (BPA)

Category: Carcinogens and Suspected Carcinogens
Also known as: 4, 4´-(1-Methylethylidene)bisphenol; 2, 2-bis (4-hydroxyphenyl) propane

Related cancers: Prostate and breast cancer

Definition: Bisphenol A (BPA) is an organic compound belonging to the aromatic class known as phenols. It is the main monomer used for the manufacture of polycarbonate plastics, which are essentially long chains of individual BPA molecules linked together. All the BPA monomers do not react to form the polymer, as a result of which small amounts of the unpolymerized free units leach into the contents of the plastic containers.

Exposure routes: Exposure to BPA is mainly through direct contact or by ingesting food or drink that has been in contact with plastic material containing bisphenol A. BPA is known to leach into the contents of polycarbonate containers under certain conditions. It is also released from epoxy resins that are used in dental sealants, food container linings, polyvinyl chloride (PVC) pipes, and flooring materials. As plastics are used ubiquitously in modern society, bisphenol A has many plausible exposure routes for humans.

Where found: Bisphenol A is a high-production-volume chemical used as the main building block for the manufacture of many polymers such as polycarbonates and epoxy resins. Polycarbonates are widely used for making food and drink containers, baby bottles, milk containers, and water pipes, and epoxy resins are used in the linings of metal food containers and in dental sealants.

At risk: Infants, children, and adults

Etiology and symptoms of associated cancers: The safety data on bisphenol A are controversial. A hazard assessment study by the National Toxicology Program is ongoing. The final peer-reviewed assessment results will be used as a basis for federal regulation of the compound. If the assessment indicates concern about carcinogenicity and other health risks associated with BPA exposure, appropriate measures will be formulated to protect public health and safety.

BPA is a known hormone disrupter, and many studies have confirmed this effect. Most research data on the adverse effects of BPA exposure have been collected in rodent studies. Low-level chronic exposure to BPA has been reported to cause endocrine disruption even at levels of 2.3 micrograms per kilogram (mcg/kg) per day, leading to aberrant growth of mammary tissue in mice, which is a precursor to breast cancer. Additionally it has been reported that prenatal exposure to low levels of BPA causes breast cancer in adult rats.

Research reports indicate that BPA at low levels causes adverse effects on the development of the prostate in fetal mice. Studies also suggest that exposure to BPA in the womb alters gene behavior in such a way as to lead to development of prostate cancer in adult rats. A small study involving Japanese women found that the serum levels of BPA were three times higher in women with a recurrent history of miscarriages, providing indirect evidence for BPA as an endocrine-disrupting chemical.

History: Bisphenol A was first synthesized in 1891. In the 1930's it was demonstrated that BPA mimicked the action of estrogens in rats. Around that time, diethylstilbestrol, a more potent estrogen, was discovered, relegating BPA to the background in terms of pharmacological use. In the 1950's polymer chemists discovered that BPA could be polymerized readily to make plastics such as polycarbonate. BPA thus became a large-volume chemical used in the plastics industry. It is also used as an inert ingredient in antioxidants, pesticides, and flame retardants. Additionally it is used in materials for making reinforced pipes, water-main filters, floorings, and enamels. Its ubiquitous use creates various exposure routes for humans.

BPA has been measured in river water, reservoirs, streams, and estuaries. There is ongoing debate about the safety limit for this compound. In the 1980's the Environmental Protection Agency (EPA) set a reference dose of up to 50 mcg/kg per day in the United States and considers intake below this dose to be safe for health. However, based on research in the late 1990's and early 2000's, scientists are of the consensus that exposure to BPA well below the EPA guideline induces adverse effects in rodents in the fetal stage, and these effects are precursors to breast cancer and prostate cancer in adulthood. The cause for concern is that the low levels inducing carcinogenicity in the rodent experiments are within the range of daily human exposure to BPA. European and American regulatory agencies have maintained that exposure to BPA from polycarbonates and epoxy resins does not pose a health risk. Bisphenol A is one of two hundred compounds selected by the Canadian regulatory agency for further safety assessment studies. The U.S. Food and Drug Administration is aware of the need for an objective assessment of the experimental data on the health risks of BPA exposure. The assessment, which will form the basis for regulation of bisphenol A by federal toxicology agencies, will affect the health of millions of people.

Lalitha Krishnan, Ph.D.

For Further Information

Haighton, L. A., et al. "An Evaluation of the Possible Carcinogenicity of Bisphenol A to Humans." *Regulatory Toxicology and Pharmacology* 35 (2002): 238-254.

Mittelstaedt, Martin. "'Inherently Toxic' Chemical Faces Its Future." *Globe and Mail*, April 7, 2007.

Stowell, Cheri L., et al. "A Role for Sulfation-Desulfation in the Uptake of Bisphenol A into Breast Tumor Cells." *Chemistry and Biology* 13, no. 8 (2006): 891-897.

U.S. Department of Health and Human Services, Public Health Service, National Toxicology Program. *Eleventh Report on Carcinogens*. Research Triangle Park, N.C.: Author, 2005.

Vom Saal, Frederick S., et al. "Chapel Hill Bisphenol A Expert Panel Consensus Statement: Integration of Mechanisms, Effects in Animals and Potential to Impact Human Health at Current Levels of Exposure." *Reproductive Toxicology* 24, no. 2 (2007): 131-138.

Wetherill, Y. B., et al. "Bisphenol A Facilitates Bypass of Androgen Ablation Therapy in Prostate Cancer." *Molecular Cancer Therapeutics* 5 (2006): 3181-3190.

Other Resources

American Cancer Society

Federal Report Looks at Risks from Plastics Chemical
http://www.cancer.org/docroot/NWS/content/NWS_1_1x_Federal_Report_Looks_at_Risks_from_Plastics_Chemical.asp

Breast Cancer Fund

Bisphenol A
http://www.breastcancerfund.org/site/pp.asp?c=kwKXLdPaE&b=2638145

National Toxicology Program

Bisphenol A
http://ntp.niehs.nih.gov/index.cfm?objectid=BC9825E3-123F-7908-7BF465F9E25681B0

Toxicology and Chemical Substances/European Chemical Bureau

http://ecb.jrc.it

See also: Acrylamides; Bis(chloromethyl) ether and technical-grade chloromethyl methyl ether; Cadmium and cadmium compounds; Carcinogens, known; Carcinogens, reasonably anticipated; Chromium hexavalent compounds; Di(2-ethylhexyl) phthalate (DEHP); Organochlorines (OCs); Pesticides and the food chain; Plasticizers; Vinyl chloride

▶ 1,3-Butadiene

Category: Carcinogens and Suspected Carcinogens
RoC status: Known human carcinogen since 2000
Also known as: Vinylethylene, bivinyl, buta-1,3-diene, α,γ-butadiene

Related cancers: Leukemia, lymphosarcoma, reticulosarcoma, hematopoietic cancers

Definition: 1,3-Butadiene is a hydrocarbon molecule made up of four atoms of carbon and six atoms of hydrogen. The first and last pairs of carbon atoms are held together by two chemical bonds or four electrons. The two and three carbons share a single pair of electrons. This atomic arrangement makes 1,3-butadiene highly flammable and extremely reactive.

Exposure routes: Inhalation, ingestion, dermal contact, exhaust from motor vehicles and cigarette smoke

Where found: Industries involved in the synthesis of rubber-like materials, resins, and polymers

At risk: Workers who deal with synthetic rubber, organic chemicals, and resins

Etiology and symptoms of associated cancers: In all species studied, including humans, 1,3-butadiene has been shown to be oxidized to rings that involve two of the carbon atoms and one atom of oxygen. Such epoxides are chemically similar to the known carcinogen ethylene oxide. Tumor production in both rodents and humans involves reaction with deoxyribonucleic acid (DNA), producing genetic alterations in tumor-suppressor genes.

History: The shortage of natural rubber in World War II caused an intense search for synthetic latex. It was determined that 1,3-butadiene reacts readily with other similar hydrocarbons to produce a wide variety of polymeric substances. An example is copolymerization with styrene, a molecule involving the carcinogen benzene. Uncertainty in early studies of 1,3-butadiene carcinogenicity resulted when conditions also involved benzene. More than 75 percent of 2 million metric tons of 1,3-butadiene produced in a typical year are consumed by the rubber industry; the compound is also involved in nylon synthesis.

Studies of workers in synthetic rubber plants beginning in 1943 gave conflicting evidence concerning the carcinogenicity of 1,3-butadiene. Later animal studies with rats and mice exhibited a strong pattern of incremental risk for a variety of cancers. More carefully controlled studies of production workers in the early 1990's documented 1,3-butadiene's carcinogenic nature.

Extensive federal regulation of 1,3-butadiene exists. The U.S. Department of Transportation (DOT) lists the chemical as hazardous and requires special marking, labeling, and transporting precautions. The U.S. Environmental Protection Agency (EPA), acting under the Clean Air Act (1970), lists 1,3-butadiene as one of thirty-three hazardous air pollutants that present the greatest threat to public health and requires that as little as ten pounds of the substance must be reported. The Occupational Safety and Health Administration (OSHA) has set the permissible exposure limit at one part per million.

K. Thomas Finley, Ph.D.

See also: Air pollution; Carcinogens, known; Carcinogens, reasonably anticipated

▶ 1,4-Butanediol dimethanesulfonate

Category: Carcinogens and Suspected Carcinogens; Chemotherapy and Other Drugs
RoC status: Known human carcinogen since 1985
Also known as: Myleran, busulfan

Related cancers: In patients receiving busulfan for chronic myeloid leukemia (CML), cytological anomalies and cancers were observed at a variety of sites, including breast cancer, female genital cancers, and leukemia. Cancer patients given busulfan for bronchial cancer developed leukemia that was not dose related.

Definition: Busulfan is a sulfonurea alkylating agent that contains reactive alkyl groups that readily combine with other molecules via cross-linking of deoxyribonucleic acid (DNA) strands in the nuclei of rapidly dividing cells, thereby destroying them. A prescription drug employed in chemotherapy of leukemias, especially CML, busulfan does not selectively harm cancer cells but kills normal cells as well, and it is considered to be mitogenic, carcinogenic, and leukemogenic. Locally it may cause blistering of the skin and damage to the eyes and respiratory tract. Systemic toxic effects include nausea and vomiting, reduction in both leukocytes and erythrocytes, and hemorrhage.

Exposure routes: Intravenous (IV), oral/ingestion of tablets

Where found: People may be exposed via chemotherapy (oral or IV) for treatment of various types of leukemia, especially CML, and before bone marrow transplants (used to treat CML), in combination with cyclophosphamide used as a conditioning regimen.

At risk: There is a potential for occupational exposure in employees who formulate and package busulfan tablets, and for health care professionals who administer IV busulfan to patients.

Etiology and symptoms of associated cancers: Busulfan may cause cellular dysplasias and cytologic abnormalities. Busulfan, which is both leukemogenic and carcinogenic, has been shown to cause cancer of the breast and female reproductive organs as well as leukemias in humans, though evidence is limited in animal studies. Related symptoms and signs vary by cancer. For leukemia, they include weakness, fever, bleeding gums, petechiae, swollen glands, and enlarged spleen or liver; for breast cancer, a new lump or mass in the breast; and, for endometrial cancer, postmenopausal, or irregular vaginal bleeding.

History: Introduced in 1950, busulfan raised the median survival time for CML to approximately 3.5 to 4.5 years. However, because busulfan proved more efficient at destroying normal stem cells than CML cells, it has been largely supplanted by more specific and less toxic agents. Malignant tumors and acute leukemias have been reported in patients who were treated with busulfan; the World Health Organization (WHO) found a cause-and-effect relationship between busulfan and secondary malignancies. The International Agency for Research on Cancer found four cases of acute leukemia among 243 patients treated with busulfan as adjuvant chemotherapy following surgical removal of bronchogenic carcinoma, suggesting that busulfan is leukemogenic.

Cynthia Racer, M.A., M.P.H.

See also: Carcinogens, known; Carcinogens, reasonably anticipated; Chronic Myeloid Leukemia (CML)

▶ Cadmium and cadmium compounds

Category: Carcinogens and Suspected Carcinogens
RoC status: Known human carcinogen since 2000
Also known as: Cadmium chloride, cadmium sulfate, cadmium nitrate, cadmium oxide, cadmium sulfide, cadmium carbonate, greenockite, capsebon, cadmopur yellow

Definition: Cadmium is a natural metal, usually occurring in combination with other elements rather than in its pure state. It is most frequently found in zinc deposits as cadmium sulfide. Commercial use of cadmium began at the end of the nineteenth century and became widespread by the middle of the twentieth century. The noncorrosive properties of cadmium led to its use in batteries, electroplating, and coating of other metals, such as steel. Workers are at risk for occupational exposure to cadmium through inhalation, but cadmium also may be released into the environment through these industrial processes. Additionally, cadmium is released into the environment from other sources, including forest fires, volcanos, weathering of rocks, and combustion of fossil fuels such as coal. Both industrial and natural releases of cadmium into the atmosphere put the general public at risk for exposure through contaminated water, air, and soil. Plants can absorb cadmium from contaminated soil, so the major exposure to cadmium in the general public is through the food supply. Tobacco plants are among those that absorb cadmium, so tobacco smoking is another source of exposure in the general public.

Related cancers: Lung cancer, possibly prostate and kidney cancer

Exposure routes: Inhalation and ingestion

Where found: Food (particularly grain cereal products, potatoes, and other vegetables), cigarette smoke, zinc and lead ores, electroplating and -coating, alloys, pigments (paint, glass, ceramics, porcelain, textiles, plastics, paper, and fireworks), stabilizers in plastics, nickel-cadmium batteries, smoke detectors, radiation detectors, and various electronics and laboratory equipment

At risk: Workers who refine and smelt zinc and lead ores, workers in industries using thermal processes (iron production or welding cadmium-coated steel), and tobacco smokers

Etiology and symptoms of associated cancers: Cadmium exposure can be acute or chronic. Acute toxicity through ingestion of cadmium may cause only short-term illness, but acute toxicity through inhalation can lead to severe damage to the lungs and even death. Chronic exposure to cadmium can cause damage to the lungs, kidneys, and sometimes bones. Studies have shown that inhalation of cadmium in the workplace is associated with lung cancer. Laboratory studies using cultured cells have shown that cadmium damages the dexoyribonucleic acid (DNA) of the cells and affects the cells' ability to repair DNA damage. These factors are likely to be the mechanism through which cadmium contributes to the formation of cancer in humans.

Lung cancer can affect one lung or both. Lung cancer detection often occurs when the disease has progressed to late stages because symptoms may take years to appear. When symptoms do appear, they often are mistaken for other less serious conditions. Common signs and symptoms of lung cancer are persistent cough (not related to smoking); persistent pain in the chest, shoulder, or back; coughing up mucus or blood; recurrent respiratory infections; shortness of breath; fatigue; unexplained weight loss; and loss of appetite. Many of these symptoms may be attributed initially to other causes before lung cancer is eventually diagnosed. Lung cancer is the only cancer that has been confirmed to be associated with cadmium exposure.

Studies from the 1960's and later have had conflicting results regarding a connection between cadmium and prostate cancer. A number of studies have shown increases in the occurrence of prostate cancer in workers exposed to cadmium in nickel-cadmium battery plants and other industrial sites, but conflicting studies have indicated no increases or increases that were too small to be statistically significant. Cadmium has also been implicated in kidney cancer, with early studies showing a correlation between exposure and increases in kidney cancer. However, further studies have not confirmed this association.

History: Industrial use of cadmium became widespread in the middle of the twentieth century, and the toxic effects due to occupational exposure began to be recognized by the early 1950's. Studies that examined workers who had been exposed to high levels of cadmium were used to examine the toxic effects, and by the 1960's researchers were investigating cadmium's potential carcinogenicity. Experimental animal studies also were conducted to research the toxicity and carcinogenicity of cadmium. Regarding the role cadmium played in the development of lung cancer, initial studies were inconclusive or conflicting. Confounding factors, such as workers who were also tobacco smokers or were exposed to additional heavy metals, contributed to the confusing results. Because of its toxic effects, many federal, state, and local agencies, including the Environmental Protection Agency (EPA), began to regulate cadmium in a variety of ways, including stipulation of allowable amounts in air and water. In 1992 the Occupational Safety and Health Administration (OSHA) ruled on permissible exposure limits (PELs) for workers exposed to airborne cadmium in the workplace. By 2000 sufficient studies reported that cadmium contributed to the development of lung cancer for it to be designated as a known human carcinogen by the U.S Department of Health and Human Services.

Michelle L. Herdman, Ph.D.

For Further Information

Klaassen, Curtis D., ed. *Casarett and Doull's Toxicology: The Basic Science of Poisons*. New York: McGraw-Hill, 2001.

Silvera, S. A. N., and T. E. Rohan. "Trace Elements and Cancer Risk: A Review of the Epidemiologic Evidence." *Cancer Causes Control* 18 (2007): 7-27.

U.S. Department of Health and Human Services, Public Health Service, National Toxicology Program. *Eleventh Report on Carcinogens*. Research Triangle Park, N.C.: Author, 2005.

Waisberg, M., P. Joseph, B. Hale, and D. Beyersmann. "Molecular and Cellular Mechanisms of Cadmium Carcinogenesis." *Toxicology* 192 (2003): 95-117.

Other Resources

Agency for Toxic Substances and Disease Registry
http://www.atsdr.cdc.gov

U.S. Department of Labor
Occupational Safety and Health Administration
http://www.osha.gov

U.S Environmental Protection Agency
http://www.epa.gov

See also: Chewing tobacco; Coke oven emissions; Free radicals; Kidney cancer; Nickel compounds and metallic nickel; Soots; Urinary system cancers

▶ Caffeine

Category: Lifestyle and Prevention; Carcinogens and Suspected Carcinogens
ATC code: N06BC01
Also known as: Trimethylxanthine, coffeine, theine, mateine, guaranine, methyltheobromine

Definition: Sometimes considered the most widely used drug in the world, caffeine is an alkaloid stimulant found naturally in coffee, tea, cocoa, and many carbonated drinks. Caffeine is a secondary metabolite substance that plants manufacture as a pesticide against insects and other invertebrates. Humans use the naturally bitter caffeine as a stimulant. Coffee, tea, and cocoa have become extraordinarily popular in most cultures of the world. In the United States, for example, it is estimated that 80 percent of adults drink either coffee or tea and over 70 percent of adults and children consume soft drinks that contain caffeine. Different studies support different arguments that caffeine has a positive or negative correlation with cancer.

Related cancers: Skin cancer, breast cancer, colon cancer, rectal cancer, bladder cancer, kidney cancer, ovarian cancer, pancreatic cancer

Delivery routes: Caffeine is most often ingested as a stimulant in coffee, tea, cocoa, chocolate, soft drinks, and "energy drinks." Caffeine tablets are also taken orally as a stimulant. Caffeine is also an ingredient in certain nonprescription drugs designed to address colds, flu, headache, and pain, as well as preparations that function as stimulants to allow users to stay awake.

How this drug works: Caffeine acts as a stimulant because it inhibits neurotransmitters that normally act as depressants. Specifically, caffeine occupies the neuron's receptor sites for adenosine, which is a neuron inhibitor. Instead of being blocked and inhibited, the neuron remains active, thereby increasing neuron activity.

Despite numerous studies, the relationships between caffeine intake and cancer risk remain inconclusive at best and contradictory at worst. Some studies show an inverse relationship between caffeine intake and cancer risk, while other studies suggest that caffeine increases the risk of certain cancers.

Links between caffeine and cancer risk are based on the suggestion that caffeine and some of its metabolites can cause changes in cell reproduction that might enhance growth and proliferation, thereby increasing the growth and spread of cancerous cells that develop.

Alternatively, other studies have suggested that caffeine and a related molecule called theophylline can block production of an enzyme that is crucial for cell growth, thereby inhibiting tumor proliferation. Studies at Rutgers University demonstrated that hairless mice treated with caffeine showed much greater resistance to skin tumors than untreated mice, but the experiment has yet to be conducted on human volunteers.

Possibly the greatest concern is about a possible relationship between caffeine consumption and breast cancer incidence, with some studies suggesting that a combination of caffeine and methylxanthines showed positive correlation to breast cancer and other diseases of the mammary glands. For example, caffeine and methylxanthines (also found in coffee and tea) are associated with increased severity of fibrocystic breast disease, which may lead to the development of breast cancer, but this finding is contradicted by other studies, leading the American Cancer Institute to announce that there is no evidence between breast cancer and caffeine intake at any level.

Although numerous studies have suggested a causal relationship between coffee intake and pancreatic cancer, none so far has provided conclusive support.

The relationship between caffeine and cancer is complex and remains unproven; both the International Agency for Research on Cancer and the American Cancer Society have concluded that there is no evidence that caffeine is carcinogenic. This verdict is echoed by the World Health Organization (WHO) and the Food and Drug Administration (FDA).

Side effects: In the short term caffeine increases attention span and simultaneously decreases the feeling of tiredness and weariness. Caffeine intake in children may cause hyperactive behavior. Caffeine can offset some of the effects of alcohol, but performance and coordination remain unaffected. Caffeine also increases plasma levels of fatty acids, cortisol, and epinephrine.

Negative effects of excessive caffeine consumption vary with age, diet, and exercise levels. Generally, higher caffeine intake may elevate blood levels of sugars and fats, increase blood pressure, irritate the lining of the stomach, and cause heartburn, irregular heartbeat, irritability, nervousness, anxiety, depression, insomnia, and the disruption of sleeping habits.

Excessive caffeine intake has also been linked to stroke and heart attack. The relationship between caffeine intake and heart problems is of great concern. Recent studies by the Adventist Health Study group reported finding a 50 percent increase in risk of serious heart disease, including heart palpitations and cardiac arrhythmias, both of which can lead to heart attacks. Other studies, however, have failed to demonstrate any relationship between coronary heart disease, stroke, and caffeine intake.

Some researchers have also suggested a relationship between caffeine doses and the severity and duration of premenopausal syndrome (PMS) in females among heavy consumers of coffee, tea, and other fluids containing caffeine.

Other studies have linked higher-than-normal caffeine consumption with lowered rates of conception, birth defects, retarded fetal growth, reduced birth weight, spontaneous abortion, premature delivery, and stillbirth. There is some evidence that caffeine intake by males prior to mating may result in significant fetal growth retardation, but this too remains problematic and awaits further study. While none of these claims is absolute, women are advised not to consume caffeine while pregnant or planning on becoming pregnant, since blood levels of caffeine can be transferred through the placenta and can be metabolized by a developing fetus.

Finally, high caffeine intake reduces the absorption of dietary iron by 40 to 60 percent and reduces calcium intake while simultaneously increasing the rate of calcium loss, all of which may lead to serious calcium imbalance in blood and body fluid levels.

Dwight G. Smith, Ph.D.

For Further Information

Gilbert, S. G. *A Small Dose of Toxicology: The Health Effects of Common Chemicals.* Boca Raton, Fla.: CRC Press, 2004.

Porta, M., et al. "Coffee Drinking: The Rationale for Treating It as a Potential Effect Modifier of Carcinogenic Exposures." *European Journal of Epidemiology* 18, no. 4 (2003): 289-298.

Rowley, R., M. Zorch, and D. B. Leeper. "Effect of Caffeine on Radiation-Induced Mitotic Delay: Delayed Expression of G2 Arrest." *Radiation Research* 97, no. 1 (January, 1984): 178-185.

Waldren, C. A., and I. Rasko. "Caffeine Enhancement of X-Ray Killing in Cultured Human and Rodent Cells." *Radiation Research* 73, no. 1 (January, 1978): 95-110.

See also: Benign Prostatic Hyperplasia (BPH); Clinical Breast Exam (CBE); Diarrhea; Esophagitis; Fatigue; Fibrocystic breast changes; Gastric polyps; Gastrointestinal complications of cancer treatment; Green tea; Hot flashes; Nutrition and cancer prevention; Side effects

▶ Carcinogens, known

Category: Carcinogens and Suspected Carcinogens

Definition: A carcinogen is any agent that causes cancer. A "known" human carcinogen is a chemical compound or an exposure identified by the National Toxicology Program of the U.S. Department of Health and Human

Services as displaying "sufficient evidence of carcinogenicity in humans [to indicate] a causal relationship between exposure to the agent, substance, or mixture and human cancer."

Cancer causing agents: Exposure to certain chemicals (such as arsenic) or environmental insults (like UV radiation) can cause cells in an organ of the body to grow uncontrollably. As early as a century ago, scientists knew of malignant growths produced by exposure to particular chemicals. The National Toxicology Program (NTP) produces a biennial Report on Carcinogens (RoC). The RoC is a scientific document that lists carcinogenic agents, substances, or exposure conditions that pose a cancer hazard in humans. It includes exposure scenarios, potential of exposure, and exposure limitations of these agents; as well as federal regulations to limit such exposures.

Definitive data on carcinogenicity is difficult to obtain, because often multiple exposures to the substance and a long induction period are needed before a tumor appears. Genetics, lifestyle, and ethnic factors are also important in the development of certain tumors. The National Toxicology Program employs a variety of approaches but considers two-year studies in rodents to be its primary method of determining what substances are carcinogenic.

International Agency for Research on Cancer Known Human Carcinogens

- Acetaldehyde (from consuming alcoholic beverages)
- Acheson process, occupational exposure associated with
- Acid mists, strong inorganic
- Aflatoxins
- Alcoholic beverages
- Aluminum production
- 4-Aminobiphenyl
- Areca nut
- Aristolochic acid (and plants containing it)
- Arsenic and inorganic arsenic compounds
- Asbestos (all forms) and mineral substances (such as talc or vermiculite) that contain asbestos
- Auramine production
- Azathioprine
- Benzene
- Benzidine and dyes metabolized to benzidine
- Benzo[a]pyrene
- Beryllium and beryllium compounds
- Betel quid, with or without tobacco
- Bis(chloromethyl)ether and chloromethyl methyl ether (technical-grade)
- Busulfan
- 1,3-Butadiene
- Cadmium and cadmium compounds
- Chlorambucil
- Chlornaphazine
- Chromium (VI) compounds
- *Clonorchis sinensis* (infection with), also known as the Chinese liver fluke
- Coal, indoor emissions from household combustion
- Coal gasification
- Coal-tar distillation
- Coal-tar pitch
- Coke production
- Cyclophosphamide
- Cyclosporine
- 1,2-Dichloropropane
- Diethylstilbestrol
- Engine exhaust, diesel
- Epstein-Barr virus (infection with)
- Erionite
- Estrogen postmenopausal therapy
- Estrogen-progestogen postmenopausal therapy (combined)
- Estrogen-progestogen oral contraceptives (combined) (Note: There is also convincing evidence in humans that these agents confer a protective effect against cancer in the endometrium and ovary)
- Ethanol in alcoholic beverages
- Ethylene oxide
- Etoposide
- Etoposide in combination with cisplatin and bleomycin
- Fission products, including strontium-90
- Fluoro-edenite fibrous amphibole
- Formaldehyde
- Haematite mining (underground)
- *Helicobacter pylori* (infection with)
- Hepatitis B virus (chronic infection with)
- Hepatitis C virus (chronic infection with)
- Human immunodeficiency virus type 1 (HIV-1) (infection with)
- Human papilloma virus (HPV) types 16, 18, 31, 33, 35, 39, 45, 51, 52, 56, 58, 59 (infection with) (Note: The HPV types that have been classified as carcinogenic to humans can differ by an order of magnitude in risk for cervical cancer)
- Human T-cell lymphotropic virus type I (HTLV-1) (infection with)
- Ionizing radiation (all types)
- Iron and steel founding (workplace exposure)
- Isopropyl alcohol manufacture using strong acids

Development of cancer: The process of carcinogenesis can be broken down into three stages: initiation, promotion, and progression. Initiation is a result of irreversible alterations by means of mutations and/or deletions in important targets including oncogenes and tumor-suppressor genes. Promotion is a reversible phase which involves expression of these target genes. The final irreversible phase of progression involves uncontrolled malignant growth.

Many carcinogenic agents are known to cause mutations. The formation of bonds between a strand of DNA and a carcinogen produces mutations that might be replicated before they can be repaired. Such an error might be passed along to future generations. Most such mutations do not affect the cell, but if a protein associated with growth is involved, it might create the potential for future rapid cell growth.

In cancer development, the promotion stage's process of proceeding is still unclear, but the nature of promoting substances provides clues. The effect of these substances is reversible; with their withdrawal, the tumor disappears. They are, however, not able to produce the cancer on their own.

During the progression stage, another genetic change results in a selective growth advantage for the mutant cell. There are several ways in which such an event might take place: additional exposures to the original carcinogen, spontaneous mutation from replication enzymes, or changes in the genes caused by initiating

International Agency for Research on Cancer Known Human Carcinogens *(continued)*

- Kaposi sarcoma herpesvirus (KSHV), also known as human herpesvirus 8 (HHV-8) (infection with)
- Leather dust
- Lindane
- Magenta production
- Melphalan
- Methoxsalen (8-methoxypsoralen) plus ultraviolet A radiation, also known as PUVA
- 4,4'-Methylenebis(chloroaniline) (MOCA)
- Mineral oils, untreated or mildly treated
- MOPP and other combined chemotherapy including alkylating agents
- 2-Naphthylamine
- Neutron radiation
- Nickel compounds
- N'-Nitrosonornicotine (NNN) and 4-(N-Nitrosomethylamino)-1-(3-pyridyl)-1-butanone (NNK)
- *Opisthorchis viverrini* (infection with), also known as the Southeast Asian liver fluke
- Outdoor air pollution (and the particulate matter in it)
- Painter (workplace exposure as a)
- 3,4,5,3',4'-Pentachlorobiphenyl (PCB-126)
- 2,3,4,7,8-Pentachlorodibenzofuran
- Phenacetin (and mixtures containing it)
- Phosphorus-32, as phosphate
- Plutonium
- Polychlorinated biphenyls (PCBs), dioxin-like, with a Toxicity Equivalency Factor according to WHO (PCBs 77, 81, 105, 114, 118, 123, 126, 156, 157, 167, 169, 189)
- Processed meat (consumption of)
- Radioiodines, including iodine-131
- Radionuclides, alpha-particle-emitting, internally deposited (Note: Specific radionuclides for which there is sufficient evidence for carcinogenicity to humans are also listed individually as Group 1 agents)
- Radionuclides, beta-particle-emitting, internally deposited (Note: Specific radionuclides for which there is sufficient evidence for carcinogenicity to humans are also listed individually as Group 1 agents)
- Radium-224 and its decay products
- Radium-226 and its decay products
- Radium-228 and its decay products
- Radon-222 and its decay products
- Rubber manufacturing industry
- Salted fish (Chinese-style)
- *Schistosoma haematobium* (infection with)
- Semustine (methyl-CCNU)
- Shale oils
- Silica dust, crystalline, in the form of quartz or cristobalite
- Solar radiation
- Soot (as found in workplace exposure of chimney sweeps)
- Sulfur mustard
- Tamoxifen (Note: There is also conclusive evidence that tamoxifen reduces the risk of contralateral breast cancer in breast cancer patients)
- 2,3,7,8-Tetrachlorodibenzo-para-dioxin
- Thiotepa
- Thorium-232 and its decay products
- Tobacco, smokeless
- Tobacco smoke, secondhand
- Tobacco smoking
- ortho-Toluidine
- Treosulfan
- Trichloroethylene
- Ultraviolet (UV) radiation, including UVA, UVB, and UVC rays
- Ultraviolet-emitting tanning devices
- Vinyl chloride
- Wood dust
- X- and Gamma-radiation

mutations. The result is an irreversible change that offers a distinct growth advantage for the affected cells. Evidence from rodent studies indicates that genetics is an important factor in these late-stage changes as well as in the early development of the cancer. Experiments reveal protein synthesis, amplification of gene creation, and further DNA reactions at this stage in the tumor cell.

Testing for carcinogens: The "long-term rodent bioassay" is the gold standard test to determine whether a substance is a carcinogen. Given the concerns for animal welfare and concerns that animal carcinogenicity data lack human specificity, alternative testing protocols are being developed. These non-animal methods include cell-based assays and computational prediction models. However, these newer methods are not considered sufficient to replace all animal testing at this time.

The realization that intermediate products from detoxification may be the cause of the initiation phase of cancer development has led to the development of tests involving bacteria and enzymes. These procedures greatly reduced cost (one-thousandth as much as mice) and time (two days compared with at least a year). It has become possible to test all new compounds for mutations and to conduct animal tests only on those showing positive results. The National Toxicology Program is actively using all these approaches.

Achieving a balance: Although carcinogenic chemicals are of concern, it is important to put their actual risk to human health in perspective. Extensive studies conducted by the National Toxicology Program and the International Agency for Research in Cancer (IARC) show that only one-third of suspected chemicals are actually carcinogenic. Approximately 96 percent of human cancer results from naturally occurring carcinogens.

Intense study of such carcinogenic compounds shows that 95 percent involve only three types of chemicals:

- Alkylating agents: Transfer small fragments (CH_3) to DNA
- Arylkylating agents: Transfer aromatic rings (C_6H_5) to DNA
- Arylhydroxylamines: Transfer amines, containing NH_2, to DNA.

A common aspect of these materials is their ability to produce structures that have a deficiency of electrons. Such structures react rapidly with the electron-rich oxygen, sulfur, and nitrogen atoms of nucleic acids.

K. Thomas Finley, Ph.D.
Updated by: Banalata Bono Sen

For Further Information

Mechanisms of Carcinogenesis. International Agency for Cancer Research, 2008 https://www.iarc.fr/en/publications/pdfs-online/wcr/2008/wcr_2008_5.pdf

Perantoni, Alan O. (1998). Carcinogenesis. In R. G. McKinnell, R. E. Parchment, A. O. Perantoni, G. B. Pierce, & I. Damjanov (Eds.), The biological basis of cancer (2nd ed.), (pp. 80-125). New York: Cambridge University Press.

Ruddon, Raymond W. (2007). Cancer Biology (4th ed.). New York: Oxford University Press.

Tomatis, Lorenzo, & Huff, James. (2002). Evolution of research in cancer etiology. In William B. Coleman & Gregory T. Tsongalis (Eds.), The molecular basis of human cancer. Totowa, N.J.: Humana Press.

NTP (National Toxicology Program). 2014. *Report on Carcinogens, Thirteenth Edition.* Research Triangle Park, NC: U.S. Department of Health and Human Services, Public Health Service. http://ntp.niehs.nih.gov/pubhealth/roc/roc13/

Yuspa, Stuart H., & Shields, Peter G. (2001). Etiology of cancer: Chemical factors. In Vincent T. DeVita, Jr., Theodore S. Lawrence, & Steven A. Rosenberg (Eds.), Cancer: Principles and practice of oncology (6th ed.), (pp 152-160). Philadelphia: Lippincott Williams & Wilkins. https://oncouasd.files.wordpress.com/2014/09/cancer-principles-and-practice-of-oncology-6e.pdf

Other Resources

American Cancer Society.
Known and Probable Carcinogens.
http://www.cancer.org/cancer/cancercauses/other-carcinogens/generalinformationaboutcarcinogens/known-and-probable-human-carcinogens

International Agency for Research on Cancer.
http://www.iarc.fr

National Toxicology Program.
http://ntp.niehs.nih.gov/

See also: Acrylamides; Aflatoxins; Agent Orange; Air pollution; Alcohol, alcoholism, and cancer; 4-Aminobiphenyl; Arsenic compounds; Asbestos; Azathioprine; Bacteria as causes of cancer; Benzene; Benzidine and dyes metabolized to benzidine; Beryllium and beryllium compounds; Birth control pills and cancer; Bis(chloromethyl) ether and technical-grade chloromethyl methyl ether; Bisphenol A (BPA); 1,3-Butadiene; 1,4-Butanediol dimethanesulfonate; Cadmium and cadmium compounds;

Caffeine; Carcinogens, reasonably anticipated; Cell phones; Chewing tobacco; Chlorambucil; 1-(2-Chloroethyl)-3-(4-methylcyclohexyl)-1-nitrosourea (MeCCNU); Chromium hexavalent compounds; Cigarettes and cigars; Coal tars and coal tar pitches; Coke oven emissions; Cyclophosphamide; Cyclosporin A; Di(2-ethylhexyl) phthalate (DEHP); Diethanolamine (DEA); Diethylstilbestrol (DES); Dioxins; Electromagnetic radiation; Epstein-Barr Virus; Erionite; Ethylene oxide; Fertility drugs and cancer; Formaldehyde; Free radicals; Hair dye; Helicobacter pylori infection; Hepatitis B virus (HBV); Hepatitis C virus (HCV); HER2/neu protein; Herpes simplex virus; Herpes zoster virus; HIV/AIDS-related cancers; Hormone replacement therapy (HRT); Human growth factors and tumor growth; Human papillomavirus (HPV); Human T-cell leukemia virus (HTLV); Ionizing radiation; Melphalan; Mineral oils; Mustard gas; 2-Naphthylamine; Nickel compounds and metallic nickel; Oncogenes; Oncogenic viruses; Organochlorines (OCs); Pesticides and the food chain; Phenacetin; Plasticizers; Polycyclic aromatic hydrocarbons; Radon; Report on Carcinogens (RoC); Silica, crystalline; Simian virus 40; Sunlamps; Thiotepa; Ultraviolet radiation and related exposures; Vinyl chloride; Wood dust

▶ Carcinogens, reasonably anticipated

Category: Carcinogens and Suspected Carcinogens

Definition: Chemical compounds similar chemically to those that have shown carcinogenicity are labeled "reasonably anticipated carcinogens" by the National Toxicology Program of the U.S. Department of Health and Human Services.

Describing cancer: Cancer has been studied intensely for a long time, yet its causes remain elusive and uncertain. There is much evidence that when certain chemical compounds are introduced to the human body, the probability of a tumor forming is increased. Scientists have used several methods to gather evidence about the carcinogenicity of a chemical before allowing general use.

A central difficulty with methods of studying cancer is that a specific chemical, introduced by a particular route, does not always produce a tumor. Therefore carcinogenicity is defined in terms of the increased risk of producing a tumor. Because the primary interest of such studies is tumors produced in human beings, there is a species problem. It is very difficult to show that susceptibility to increased rates of tumor production in test animals predicts a similar outcome in humans. The National Toxicology Program (NTP) uses animal testing in its basic studies. Research conducted with bacteria also shows great promise.

Such complications have resulted in the creation of a rather limited list of carcinogenic chemicals. It pays to take a conservative position in the field of public health, so there is a much longer list of suspected carcinogens.

The National Toxicology Program issues a biennial *Report on Carcinogens* (RoC) in which compounds may be labeled "reasonably anticipated carcinogens" if they meet the following criteria:

- There are limited studies in humans.
- Sufficient animal studies exist.
- A structural relationship to a known carcinogen exists.

Carcinogens and suspected carcinogens: Reports concerning chemicals linked to cancer make the public suspicious of all chemicals. Studies have shown that only one-fourth to one-third of suspected molecules are actually cancer causing. More than 95 percent of carcinogenic chemicals belong to three general types of compounds. Chemists who work with organic compounds have always appreciated this relationship. A powerful tool in managing such compounds has been the structure-activity relationship. A given set of atoms, arranged in a particular pattern, will often lead to very similar chemical behavior.

The chief cancer-causing molecules predominantly display one of the following chemical structural types: polycyclic aromatic hydrocarbons, aromatic amines, or alkylating agents.

Polycyclic aromatic hydrocarbons: As their name suggests, polycylic aromatic hydrocarbons are composed only of atoms of the elements carbon and hydrogen, and the carbon atoms are linked together in a ring or cycle. The simplest chemical in this class is the known carcinogen benzene, which has a single ring of six carbon atoms. Molecules of four or more benzene rings that are fused together by sharing two carbon atoms are quite common.

Aromatic amines: As with the hydrocarbons, aromatic amines generally have the six-carbon atom ring, but they also have a nitrogen atom attached to that ring. The most common example is 2-naphthylamine. This compound has two benzene rings attached to each other and an ammonia-like nitrogen atom containing two hydrogen atoms attached to the second carbon atom.

Alkylating agents: Although the first two categories of carcinogenic compounds are characterized by their structure, alkylating agents share a common chemical function. An alkyl group is a fragment of a molecule that is of high energy and therefore reacts rapidly. One of the most common is the methyl group composed of a single carbon atom and three hydrogen atoms. A methylating agent would be a molecule that can transfer such a reactive fragment during a chemical reaction. There are many compounds that can perform this function, but one of the most active subgroups is that of the nitrosamines, for example, *N*-nitrosodimethylamine. Like the aromatic amines, there is a nitrogen atom, but in place of the two hydrogen atoms, there are two methyl groups. The aromatic ring is replaced by a second nitrogen atom connected to an oxygen atom.

A summary of suspected carcinogens: Some common examples of probable carcinogens would include:

Reasonably Anticipated Human Carcinogens

- Acetaldehyde
- 2-Acetylaminofluorene
- Acrylamide
- Acrylonitrile
- Adriamycin (doxorubicin hydrochloride)
- 2-Aminoanthraquinone
- *o*-Aminoazotoluene
- 1-Amino-2,4-dibromoanthraquinone
- 1-Amino-2-methylanthraquinone
- 2-Amino-3,4-dimethylimidazo [4,5-*f*]quinoline (MeIQ)
- 2-Amino-3,8-dimethylimidazo [4,5-*f*]quinolaxine (MeIQx)
- 2-Amino-3-methylimidazo [4,5-*f*]quinoline (IQ)
- 2-Amino-1-methyl6-phenylimidazo[4,5-*b*]pyridine (PhIP)
- Amitrole
- *o*-Anisidine hydrochloride
- Azacitidine
- Benzotrichloride
- Bromodichloromethane
- 2,2-bis(Bromomethyl)-1,3-propanediol (technical grade)
- Butylated hydroxyanisole (BHA)
- Carbon tetrachloride
- Ceramic fibers (respirable size)
- Chloramphenicol
- Chlorendic acid
- Chlorinated paraffins (C_{12}, 60 percent chlorine)
- 1-(2-Chloroethyl)-3-cyclohexyl-1-nitrosourea
- bis(Chloroethyl) nitrosourea
- Chloroform
- 3-Chloro-2-methylpropene
- 4-Chloro-*o*-phenylenediamine
- Chloroprene
- *p*-Chloro-*o*-toluidine and p-Chloro-*o*-toluidine hydrochloride
- Chlorozotocin
- C.I. basic red 9 monohydrochloride
- Cisplatin
- Cobalt sulfate
- *p*-Cresidine
- Cupferron
- Dacarbazine
- Danthron (1,8-dihydroxyanthraquinone)
- 2,4-Diaminoanisole sulfate
- 2,4-Diaminotoluene
- Diazoaminobenzene
- 1,2-Dibromo-3-chloropropane
- 1,2-Dibromoethane (ethylene dibromide)
- 2,3-Dibromo-1-propanol
- tris(2,3-Dibromopropyl) phosphate
- 1,4-Dichlorobenzene
- 3,3´-Dichlorobenzidine and
- 3,3´-dichlorobenzidine dihydrochloride
- Dichlorodiphenyltrichloroethane (DDT)
- 1,2-Dichloroethane (ethylene dichloride)
- Dichloromethane (methylene chloride)
- 1,3-Dichloropropene (technical grade)
- Diepoxybutane
- Diesel exhaust particulates
- Diethyl sulfate
- Diglycidyl resorcinol ether
- 3,3´-Dimethoxybenzidine and dyes metabolized to 3,3´-dimethoxybenzidine
- 4-Dimethylaminoazobenzene
- 3,3´-Dimethylbenzidine and dyes metabolized to 3,3´-dimethylbenzidine
- Dimethylcarbamoyl chloride
- 1,1-Dimethylhydrazine
- Dimethyl sulfate
- Dimethylvinyl chloride
- 1,4-Dioxane
- Disperse blue 1
- Epichlorohydrin
- Ethylene thiourea
- di(2-Ethylhexyl) phthalate
- Ethyl methanesulfonate
- Formaldehyde (gas)
- Furan
- Glass wool (respirable size)
- Glycidol
- Heterocyclic amines
- Hexachlorobenzene
- Hexachloroethane
- Hexamethylphosphoramide
- Hydrazine and hydrazine sulfate
- Hydrazobenzene
- Iron dextran complex
- Isoprene
- Kepone (chlordecone)
- Lead and lead compounds
- Lindane and other hexachlorocyclohexane isomers
- 2-Methylaziridine (propylenimine)
- 4,4´-Methylenebis(2-chloroaniline)
- 4,4´-Methylenebis (*N,N*-dimethyl) benzenamine
- 4,4´-Methylenedianiline and its dihydrochloride salt
- Methyleugenol
- Methyl methanesulfonate
- *N*-Methyl-*N*´-nitro-*N*-nitrosoguanidine

Reasonably Anticipated Human Carcinogens *(continued)*

- Metronidazole
- Michler's ketone (4,4′-(dimethylamino)benzophenone)
- Mirex
- Naphthalene
- Nitrilotriacetic acid
- *o*-Nitroanisole
- Nitroarenes (1,6-dinitropyrene; 1,8-dinitropyrene; 6-nitrochrysene; 1-nitropyrene; 4-nitropyrene)
- Nitrobenzene
- Nitrofen (2,4-dichlorophenyl-*p*-nitrophenyl ether)
- Nitrogen mustard hydrochloride
- Nitromethane
- 2-Nitropropane
- *N*-Nitrosodi-*n*-butylamine
- *N*-Nitrosodiethanolamine
- *N*-Nitrosodiethylamine
- *N*-Nitrosodimethylamine
- *N*-Nitrosodi-*n*-propylamine
- *N*-Nitroso-*N*-ethylurea
- 4-(*N*-Nitrosomethylamino)-1-(3-pyridyl)-1-butanone
- *N*-Nitroso-*N*-methylurea
- *N*-Nitrosomethylvinylamine
- *N*-Nitrosomorpholine
- *N*-Nitrosonornicotine
- *N*-Nitrosopiperidine
- *N*-Nitrosopyrrolidine
- *N*-Nitrososarcosine
- Norethisterone
- Ochratoxin A
- 4,4′-Oxydianiline
- Oxymetholone
- Phenazopyridine hydrochloride
- Phenolphthalein
- Phenoxybenzamine hydrochloride
- Phenytoin
- Polybrominated biphenyls (PBBs)
- Polychlorinated biphenyls (PCBs)
- Polycyclic Aromatic Hydrocarbons
- Benz[*a*]anthracene
- Benzo[*b*]fluoranthene
- Benzo[*j*]fluoranthene
- Benzo[*k*]fluoranthene
- Benzo[*a*]pyrene
- Dibenz[*a,h*]acridine
- Dibenz[*a,j*]acridine
- Dibenz[*a,h*]anthracene
- *7H*-Dibenzo[*c,g*]carbazole
- Dibenzo[*a,e*]pyrene
- Dibenzo[*a,h*]pyrene
- Dibenzo[*a,i*]pyrene
- Dibenzo[*a,l*]pyrene
- Indeno[1,2,3-*cd*]pyrene
- 5-Methylchrysene
- Procarbazine hydrochloride
- Progesterone
- 1,3-Propane sultone
- β-Propiolactone
- Propylene oxide
- Propylthiouracil
- Reserpine
- Safrole
- Selenium sulfide
- Streptozotocin
- Styrene-7,8-oxide
- Sulfallate
- Tetrachloroethylene (perchloroethylene)
- Tetrafluoroethylene
- Tetranitromethane
- Thioacetamide
- 4,4′-Thiodianiline
- Thiourea
- Toluene diisocyanate
- *o*-Toluidine and *o*-toluidine hydrochloride
- Toxaphene
- Trichloroethylene
- 2,4,6-Trichlorophenol
- 1,2,3-Trichloropropane
- Urethane
- Vinyl bromide
- 4-Vinyl-1-cyclohexene diepoxide
- Vinyl fluoride

Source: U.S. Department of Health and Human Services, Public Health Service, National Toxicology Program. *Report on Carcinogens.* 11th ed. (Research Triangle Park, N.C.: Author, 2005)

- Dimethyl sulfate, which, like *N*-nitrosodimethylamine, has two methyl groups available to be transferred. The new compound has a sulfur atom and four oxygen atoms in place of the nitrogen and oxygen atoms of the carcinogen.
- Benzo[*a*]pyrene has five benzene rings, all sharing two or more carbon atoms.
- 2-Toluidine resembles 2-naphthylamine but has the second benzene ring replaced by a single methyl group.

Bear in mind that while these compounds are suspected of being carcinogenic and proper safeguards are needed when they are used, there are many examples showing that compounds with similar structure have very different, or no, carcinogenic properties.

K. Thomas Finley, Ph.D.
Updated by: Banalata Bono Sen

For Further Information

Perantoni, Alan O. "Carcinogenesis." In *The Biological Basis of Cancer*, edited by Robert G. McKinnell et al. New York: Cambridge University Press, 1998.

Ruddon, Raymond W. "Causes of Cancer." In *Cancer Biology*. 4th ed. New York: Oxford University Press, 2007.

Tomatis, Lorenzo, and James Huff. "Evolution of Research in Cancer Etiology." In *The Molecular Basis of* Human Cancer, edited by William B. Coleman and Gregory T. Tsongalis. Totowa, N.J.: Humana Press, 2002.

U.S. Department of Health and Human Services, Public Health Service, National Toxicology Program. *Eleventh Report on Carcinogens*. Research Triangle Park, N.C.: Author, 2005.

Yuspa, Stuart H., and Peter G. Shields. "Etiology of Cancer: Chemical Factors." In *Cancer: Principles and Practice of Oncology*, edited by Vincent T. DeVita, Jr., et al. 6th ed. Philadelphia: Lippincott Williams & Wilkins, 2001.

Other Resources

American Cancer Society
Known and Probable Carcinogens
http://www.cancer.org/docroot/PED/content/PED_1_3x_Known_and_Probable_Carcinogens.asp

International Agency for Research on Cancer
http://www.iarc.fr

National Toxicology Program
http://ntp-server.niehs.nih.gov

See also: Acrylamides; Aflatoxins; Agent Orange; Air pollution; Alcohol, alcoholism, and cancer; 4-Aminobiphenyl; Arsenic compounds; Asbestos; Azathioprine; Bacteria as causes of cancer; Benzene; Benzidine and dyes metabolized to benzidine; Beryllium and beryllium compounds; Birth control pills and cancer; Bis(chloromethyl) ether and technical-grade chloromethyl methyl ether; Bisphenol A (BPA); 1,3-Butadiene; 1,4-Butanediol dimethanesulfonate; Cadmium and cadmium compounds; Caffeine; Carcinogens, known; Cell phones; Chewing tobacco; Chlorambucil; 1-(2-Chloroethyl)-3-(4-methylcyclohexyl)-1-nitrosourea (MeCCNU); Chromium hexavalent compounds; Cigarettes and cigars; Coal tars and coal tar pitches; Coke oven emissions; Cyclophosphamide; Cyclosporin A; Di(2-ethylhexyl) phthalate (DEHP); Diethanolamine (DEA); Diethylstilbestrol (DES); Dioxins; Electromagnetic radiation; Epstein-Barr Virus; Erionite; Ethylene oxide; Fertility drugs and cancer; Formaldehyde; Free radicals; Hair dye; *Helicobacter pylori*; Hepatitis B virus (HBV); Hepatitis C virus (HCV); HER2/neu protein; Herpes simplex virus; Herpes zoster virus; HIV/AIDS-related cancers; Hormone replacement therapy (HRT); Human growth factors and tumor growth; Human papillomavirus (HPV); Human T-cell leukemia virus (HTLV); Ionizing radiation; Melphalan; Mineral oils; Mustard gas; 2-Naphthylamine; Nickel compounds and metallic nickel; Oncogenes; Oncogenic viruses; Organochlorines (OCs); Pesticides and the food chain; Phenacetin; Plasticizers; Polycyclic aromatic hydrocarbons; Radon; *Report on Carcinogens* (RoC); Silica, crystalline; Simian virus 40; Soots; Sunlamps; Thiotepa; Ultraviolet radiation and related exposures; Vinyl chloride; Wood dust

▶ Cell phones

Category: Carcinogens and Suspected Carcinogens
Also known as: Cellular phones

Related cancers: Gliomas, astrocytomas

Definition: Cell phones are handheld electronic communication devices that send and receive wireless electromagnetic signals. Their ubiquitous use and proximity to the brain during use has prompted concerns over their long-term impact on human health, including their potential association with cancers.

Exposure routes: Radiation that is strong enough to penetrate human tissue

Where found: Electronic devices such as mobile or cellular phones, microwave ovens, and computer monitors that emit radiofrequency radiation

At risk: Possibly people who are exposed to high levels of electromagnetic radiation, such as electric railway workers and those exposed to lower levels of radiation over many years

Etiology and symptoms of associated cancers: Of the dozens of epidemiological studies published since the 1990's on the harmful effects of cell phones, only a few have indicated a possible relationship between cell phone usage and cancer. The overwhelming scientific evidence supports the conclusion that cellular phones do not pose a health risk for the more than one billion users worldwide. The electromagnetic frequency range of cell phones is from about 850 to 1900 megahertz. Regulatory bodies in the United States do not recognize radiofrequency radiation emitted from a cell phone as a carcinogen.

At high enough levels, radiofrequency energy can damage biological tissue through the application of heat. This energy is essentially what gets produced in a microwave oven when it cooks food. Since mobile or cellular phones emit very low levels of radiofrequency radiation, it had always been assumed that these small electronic devices do not pose a health risk. However, some scientists have argued that long-term exposure to even low intensities of radiation could promote the development and growth of tumors as well as contribute to other kinds of health problems. Because cell phones are placed right against the head, in close proximity to the radiofrequency waves being sent and received, researchers wondered if they would cause damage. Brain tumors, originating from different types of cells, have received the most attention, particularly tumors that have developed on the same side of the head that the individual most often uses when talking on the phone.

Of the 47,000 new cases of brain tumors diagnosed each year in the United States alone, only a small number of cases can be understood in terms of what has caused the cancer to develop. Unfortunately, little is known about potential mechanisms that might cause brain cancers to develop in general. In terms of cell phone radiation as a possible cause of cancer, no hypothesis has been offered that adequately explains how low levels of radiofrequency energy emitted from cell phones could alter biological tissue or bring harm to the user.

History: The incidence of brain tumors began rising in the 1990's, and this increase cannot be fully explained by the improved diagnostic methods used to detect these tumors. One way to study possible external factors that might be responsible for the increase in tumors is to conduct an epidemiological study. Epidemiological studies look at the frequency of a health problem—such as cancer—in different groups of people. For example, those who have been diagnosed with a brain tumor are compared with a group who share similar characteristics except they do not have a brain tumor. Scientists can then explore how these two groups might differ in terms of frequency, duration, and exposure intensity of radiofrequency radiation from cellular phone usage. One weakness of this type of study is that it is not particularly well suited to determine cause-and-effect relationships.

In 2002, Lennart Hardell from University Hospital, Orebro, Sweden, and his colleagues found an increase in malignant brain tumors associated with the use of analog, digital, and cordless phones. He also found that risks for astrocytomas increased over time and that risk of glioma went up for periods greater than ten years. There did not appear to be an increased risk for meningioma over a long period of time. In another study, Hardell came to the conclusion that there is no association between cell phones and salivary gland tumors. Although Hardell and colleagues have published data that support claims that cellular phone use is associated with brain cancer, dozens of other studies have found results to the contrary.

Several studies conducted after 2002 have included much larger numbers of people. Increasing the number of participants can strengthen the research by making it easier for scientists to generalize the results to the overall population. In one of the largest studies on the use of cell phones and risk for cancer ever conducted, more than 420,000 Danish citizens were followed for up to twenty-one years. The researchers found no evidence for risk of tumor development from the use of cell phones either in short-term use or in those who had been using cell phones for more than ten years.

Overall, the vast majority of research supports the conclusion that cellular phones do not pose a threat for cancer development. No relationship has been reliably found when variables such as the number of years used, the cumulative hours of phone use, or the number of calls has been taken into consideration.

Bryan C. Auday, Ph.D.

For Further Information

Connelly, Jennifer M., and Mark Malkin. "Environmental Risk Factors for Brain Tumors." *Current Neurology and Neuroscience Reports* 7 (2007): 208-214.

Hardell, L., M. Hansson, and M. Carlberg. "Case-Control Study on the Use of Cellular and Cordless Phones and the Risk for Malignant Brain Tumours." *International Journal in Radiation Biology* 78 (2002): 931-936.

Schuz, J., et al. "Cellular Telephone Use and Cancer Risk: Update of a Nationwide Danish Cohort." *Journal of the National Cancer Institute* 98 (2006): 1707-1713.

Other Resources

International Commission for Electromagnetic Safety
Benevento Resolution
http://www.icems.eu/benevento_resolution.htm

National Cancer Institute
Cellular Telephone Use and Cancer: Questions and Answers
http://www.cancer.gov/cancertopics/factsheet/Risk/cellphones

See also: Electromagnetic radiation; Ultraviolet radiation and related exposures

▶ Chewing tobacco

Category: Lifestyle and Prevention; Carcinogens and Suspected Carcinogens
RoC status: Known human carcinogen since 2000
Also known as: Smokeless tobacco, chew, snuff, dip, plug tobacco

Related cancers: Oral cancers and cancers of the esophagus, larynx, pharynx, stomach, and bladder

Definition: Also called smokeless tobacco, these tobacco and tobacco-based products that are not smoked but chewed or otherwise used in the mouth, such as chew, snuff (both oral and inhaled), dip, and plug tobacco, cause or are associated with certain cancers and other disorders of the mouth.

Exposure routes: Oral by chewing, sucking, and ingestion

Where found: Sold in the form of snuff, chewing tobacco, and plug tobacco

At risk: Users of smokeless tobacco

Many individuals use tobacco by smoking it in the form of cigarettes or cigars, and in pipes. Other individuals use tobacco by simply chewing it. Some do not even chew it, but use it by keeping it inside their mouth, such as in a cheek or between the teeth and lower lip, and absorb it by sucking on it. The tobacco products release their chemicals, like nicotine, and these are absorbed into the body. Relative to cigarettes, three to four times as much nicotine is absorbed into the body per dose with smokeless tobacco. Additionally, because having these substances in the mouth will generate saliva, individuals who use them may frequently be spitting out the saliva and part of these products or their juices in the process of using them. Such products include chew, snuff, and dip.

Chew is a form of shredded tobacco leaves. Snuff is processed tobacco that is fine-grained and smaller particles, similar to prepared spices or tea; it may even be powdery. It is so fine in some cases that users may inhale or sniff it, rather than use it orally. Dip is another term for snuff and refers to how individuals will use the material. For instance, they may dip their finger into a packet or pinch it to get the dose required to place in the mouth. Plug tobacco is similar to chew, but instead of having loose leaves, the tobacco is compressed into a hard plug that is placed in the mouth between the cheek and gums for use. All serve the same function—to dispense nicotine to the user—and all are classified under the general term of chewing tobaccos.

Etiology and symptoms of associated cancers: Many individuals wrongly believe that because they are not smoking tobacco, they are skirting the normal cancer risks posed by tobacco in cigarettes. However, this is not true. In fact, chewing tobacco also carries health and cancer risks. Smokeless tobacco contains at least twenty-eight known carcinogens. These cancer-causing agents form in the tobacco while it is growing, being processed, and being aged for use. They include substances such as acetylaldehyde, arsenic, benzopyrene, cadmium, formaldehyde, hydrazine, and nitrosamines. Nitrosamines are some of the most dangerous carcinogens in smokeless tobacco.

Oral cancers are commonly associated with such tobacco use and are somewhat of a function of the direct or close contact of the substance with parts of the mouth, such as the bones, cheeks, floor of the mouth, gums, roof of the mouth, and tongue. Further, users sometimes swallow juices from these products, causing them to travel elsewhere into the body. As a result, smokeless tobacco use is associated with cancers of the esophagus, larynx, pharynx, stomach, and bladder. Often problems will show up first as sores in the mouth that will not heal, difficulty swallowing or chewing, ear pain, voice changes, or sore throats that seem to persist. Another sign might be lesions or areas of discoloration, such as white patches or red sores on the gums, tongue, or cheeks. Exposed tooth roots may also begin to have problems.

History: Reports on health problems related to smokeless tobacco use date back to the eighteenth century. Use of these products is worldwide. Approximately 90 percent of individuals with mouth cancers are tobacco users. In the United States, approximately 3 percent of adults, 8 percent of high school students, and 3 percent of middle school students are smokeless tobacco users. Many high school and middle school students learn about smokeless tobacco through its use by members of professional sports teams, such as baseball players and hockey players. Recent prevention efforts have focused on sports players who have endured problems related to oral cancers telling their stories and warning students about the risks to dissuade them from starting this habit. Relative to women, men are about two to ten times as likely to use smokeless tobacco, depending on the age group examined. In the United States, 9 percent of smokeless tobacco users are American Indians and Alaska natives, relative to 4 percent of whites, 2 percent of African Americans, 1 percent of Hispanics, and 0.6 percent of Asian Americans. Oral cancers usually occur in individuals aged forty to sixty; however, they may occur at any age. Tobacco use combined with alcohol use can dramatically increase the risk of cancers related to smokeless tobacco. Oral cancers account for only 2 to 4 percent of cancers diagnosed in the United States annually, but they have one of the lowest survival rates.

Nancy A. Piotrowski, Ph.D.

For Further Information

Bellinir, Karen, ed. *Tobacco Information for Teens: Health Tips About the Hazards of Using Cigarettes,*

Smokeless Tobacco, and Other Nicotine Products. Detroit: Omnigraphics, 2007.

Icon Health. *Smokeless Tobacco: A Medical Dictionary, Bibliography, and Annotated Research Guide to Internet References*. San Diego, Calif.: Author, 2004.

MacKay, Judith, and Michael P. Eriksen. *The Tobacco Atlas*. Geneva: World Health Organization, 2002.

Snell, Clete. *Peddling Poison: The Tobacco Industry and Kids*. Westport, Conn.: Praeger, 2005.

Winter, John C. *Tobacco Use by Native North Americans: Sacred Smoke, Silent Killer*. Norman: University of Oklahoma Press, 2000.

See also: Head and neck cancers; Oral and oropharyngeal cancers; Throat cancer; Tobacco-related cancers

▶ Chlorambucil

Category: Chemotherapy and Other Drugs; Carcinogens and Suspected Carcinogens
RoC status: Known human carcinogen since 1981
Also known as: Leukeran, chloraminophene, Ambochlorin, Ecloril, Linfolysin

Related cancers: Acute myeloid leukemia (AML), acute nonlymphocytic leukemia (ANLL)

Exposure routes: Inhalation, ingestion, dermal contact

Where found: Chemically synthesized; provided as treatment to people with cancer or autoimmune disorders as sugar-coated 2-milligram tablets

At risk: Patients receiving chlorambucil for treatment of cancer or autoimmune disorder; occupational exposure via skin contact or dust inhalation during pharmaceutical processing

Definition: Chlorambucil is an alkylating agent of the nitrogen mustard class. As with other agents in this class, chlorambucil undergoes chemical activation to the aziridinium ion, which reacts with deoxyribonucleic acid (DNA) to form a covalent bond. This alkylation damages DNA and leaves it more prone to breakage. When taken up by rapidly dividing cells (such as cancer cells), damaged DNA is unable to repair itself quickly, leading to cell death.

Etiology and symptoms of associated cancers: Acute myeloid (or nonlymphocytic) leukemia is a malignancy of blood in which myeloid precursor cells do not mature. These immature cells proliferate rapidly without normal maturation into granulocytes and monocytes. Early signs and symptoms are similar to those of influenza and include fever, weakness, fatigue, loss of appetite, and pain in the bones and joints. Infections, delayed healing of minor cuts, and unusual bruising or bleeding may occur.

AML may occur at any age but typically occurs at about age sixty-five. Prognosis varies by age. Overall, 65 to 85 percent of patients achieve complete remission, with 20 to 40 percent achieving five-year survival. Children and adults older than the age of sixty are less likely to achieve complete remission.

Alkylating agents such as chlorambucil increase the risk of acute myeloid leukemia, as does exposure to radiation and chemicals, such as benzene.

History: Chlorambucil has been used in chemotherapy since the 1960's, often for long durations. Although it is considered to be the least toxic nitrogen mustard derivative in use, sufficient evidence for carcinogenicity in animals and humans exists. Anecdotal evidence of carcinogenicity has been reported by the International Agency for Research on Cancer (IARC) since the early 1980's. In most case reports, patients were also receiving radiotherapy or other potential carcinogens. A randomized trial inpolycythemia vera patients showed a thirteenfold increase in the incidence of AML in patients receiving chlorambucil. Risk of development of acute leukemia increased with dose and length of treatment.

Karen M. Nagel, Ph.D.

See also: Antineoplastics in chemotherapy; Myelodysplastic syndromes; Waldenström Macroglobulinemia (WM)

▶ 1-(2-Chloroethyl)-3-(4-methylcyclohexyl)-1-nitrosourea (MeCCNU)

Category: Carcinogens and Suspected Carcinogens
RoC status: Known human carcinogen since 1991
Also known as: Semustine

Related cancers: Leukemia, preleukemia

Definition: MeCCNU is used to treat various cancers, including some of the brain. A nitrosourea alkylating agent, MeCCNU contains alkyl groups that mainly react with the deoxyribonucleic acid (DNA) in the cell nuclei via a process called interstrand cross-linking. Local side effects of MeCCNU may include blistering of the skin as well as damage to the eyes and respiratory tract. Systemic toxic effects include nausea and vomiting, reduction in both leukocytes and erythrocytes, hemorrhagic tendencies, and nephrotoxicity. Busulfan and cyclophosphamide are among other alkylating agents used in cancer chemotherapy.

Exposure routes: Oral (ingestion of capsules)

Where found: 1-(2-Chloroethyl)-3-(4-methylcyclohexyl)-1-nitrosourea (MeCCNU) is an investigational drug. Patients may be exposed via oral adjuvant chemotherapy for various cancers, including those of the brain, lung, and digestive system.

At risk: The National Institute for Occupational Safety and Health (NIOSH) conducted a survey from 1981 to 1983 and determined that approximately 229 workers were potentially exposed to MeCCNU.

Etiology and symptoms of associated cancers: Though the exact mechanisms are unclear, it is believed that the most significant actions of alkylating agents are those that disturb cell growth, mitosis, and differentiation of rapidly dividing cells, providing the rationale for use in cancer therapy. However, because alkylating agents such as MeCCNU do not selectively kill cancer cells, they have a toxic effect on normal cells and are considered carcinogenic, mitogenic, and leukemogenic. Symptoms of leukemia may include weakness, fever, bleeding gums, petechiae (small red spots on the skin), lymphadenopathy (swollen glands), splenomegaly (enlarged spleen), and hepatomegaly (enlarged liver).

History: Introduced in 1963 because of their lipophilicity and, therefore, ability to cross the blood-brain barrier, nitrosourea alkylating agents such as MeCCNU were designed to treat brain and meningeal cancer. However, based on scientific data, MeCCNU has been shown to be carcinogenic in humans. In 1983 researcher J. D. Boice and colleagues found a twelvefold relative risk of leukemic disorders in 2,067 patients given adjuvant treatment with MeCCNU compared with those given other therapies. In 1987 the International Agency for Research on Cancer (IARC) demonstrated a significant dose-related response to MeCCNU with an adjusted relative risk of approximately fortyfold for patients who received the highest dose of MeCCNU. Also in 1987 the IARC concluded that there was evidence that MeCCNU was carcinogenic in experimental animals. In 1977 researcher J. H. Weisburger had found an increased incidence of tumors and leukemias in animals injected with MeCCNU.

Cynthia Racer, M.A., M.P.H.

See also: Alkylating agents in chemotherapy; Chemotherapy

▶ Chromium hexavalent compounds

Category: Carcinogens and Suspected Carcinogens
RoC status: Known human carcinogen since 1980
Also known as: Hexavalent chromium, chromium 6, chromium (Vl), Cr (Vl)

Related cancers: Lung cancer, and less commonly, cancer of the nose and nasal sinus cavities

Definition: The term "hexavalent" describes how highly oxidized chromium becomes in a chemical compound and means that chromium has combined with six oxygen atoms. It is this fully oxygenated form that is associated with chromium's greatest industrial use and most serious health concerns.

Exposure routes: Primarily inhalation and to a lesser extent skin contact and water intake

Where found: Chromate dyes of plastics, inks, and photographic processing compounds; anticorrosive agent in paints, electroplated metal, and welded stainless steel; and also in leather-tanning products, textile dyes, and wood preservatives

At risk: Workers in daily contact with hexavalent chromium. There is also concern among people living near contaminated wastewater, people who breathe air polluted with chromium hexavalent compounds, and those who have skin contact with products containing these compounds. Hexavalent chromium became part of the American lexicon following the film *Erin Brockovich* (2000), a cautionary tale about a cancer cluster seemingly associated with industrial contamination of the local drinking water. In a 2001 report, the Environmental Protection Agency estimated that more than two thousand work sites released 7 million tons of chromium compounds into the environment. The health risk from this discharge is unknown.

Etiology and symptoms of associated cancers: The respiratory tract is the most common site for hexavalent chromium damage. This damage may lead to septal ulceration and perforation, bronchitis, asthma, pneumonia, decreased lung function, and cancers of the nose, sinuses, and lung. Even short-term exposure may manifest in fits of coughing, wheezing, and shortness of breath. Although the respiratory tract is the primary area of concern, injury to the kidneys, liver, teeth, eardrums, eyes, and skin is possible. Although genetic damage following hexavalent chromium exposure is clear, research has not yet described the exact cellular mechanism that results in cancer.

History: Shortly after chromium, "the red mineral," was found in Siberia toward the end of the eighteenth century, it became useful as a paint pigment and leather-tanning product. Although some of its health risks soon became apparent, it was not until 1980 that the U.S. government officially acknowledged its role as a carcinogen. In the twenty-first century, businesses using hexavalent chromium must establish the exposure rates of their workers. The Occupational Safety and Health Administration (OSHA) has mandated strict monitoring and eight-hour exposure limits to hexavalent chromium dust or fumes in targeted job sites.

Richard S. Spira, D.V.M.

See also: Cancer clusters; Cigarettes and cigars; Lung cancers; Nasal cavity and paranasal sinus cancers

▶ Cigarettes and cigars

Category: Carcinogens and Suspected Carcinogens
RoC status: Known human carcinogen since 2000
Also known as: Smoking tobacco

Definition: Cigarettes and cigars are made from dried tobacco leaves, to which manufacturers add hundreds of substances to enhance flavor and other properties. The primary difference between cigars and cigarettes is that cigars are wrapped in leaf tobacco or other substances that contain tobacco, whereas cigarettes are wrapped in paper or other substances that do not contain tobacco. Also, cigars typically do not have filters. According to the American Cancer Society, a single large cigar can contain as much tobacco as an entire pack of cigarettes.

Tobacco and tobacco smoke contain more than 4,000 chemicals, of which as many as 250 are known to be toxic or carcinogenic. The composition of smoke varies depending on the product, tobacco blend, chemical additives, and other factors. Some of the toxic compounds found in tobacco smoke include ammonia, tar, cyanide, carbon monoxide, and the carcinogens benzene, aromatic amines, arsenic, and chromium. Sidestream (second-hand) smoke contains many of the same carcinogens as mainstream smoke, sometimes in higher concentrations. Because cigars contain more tobacco than cigarettes and usually burn longer, they give off more sidestream smoke with higher concentrations of carcinogens.

Related cancers: Cancers of the lung, oral cavity, larynx, pharynx, esophagus, bladder, stomach

Exposure routes: Inhalation is the primary route of exposure to the carcinogens found in cigarettes and cigars. Smoking tobacco produces mainstream smoke that is inhaled by the smoker. Secondhand exposure via sidestream smoke (also called secondhand smoke, passive smoke, or environmental tobacco smoke) can also occur. Cigarettes are the primary source of tobacco smoke exposure; cigars are less common. Direct exposure through the mouth, gums, and swallowed saliva can also occur during smoking.

Where found: Legally sold in the form of cigarettes and cigars

At risk: All users of smoking tobacco are at risk of developing cancer. As of 2007, approximately 21 percent of adults in the United States (45.3 million people) were smokers. In 2006, about 371 billion cigarettes were consumed. The use of tobacco products varies with gender, age, and racial and ethnic background. More men smoke (23.9 percent) than women (18.0 percent). Smoking is much more common among adults ages eighteen to forty-four (48.5 percent) and forty-five to sixty-four (21.9 percent) than among those over age sixty-five (8.6 percent). In addition, of high school students, 23 percent smoke cigarettes and 14 percent smoke cigars. Overall smoking rates are highest among American Indians and Alaska natives (32 percent), whites (21.9 percent), and blacks (21.5 percent).

Each year, approximately 438,000 people in the United States die prematurely from smoking or sidestream smoke exposure; another 8.6 million suffer from smoking-related illnesses. Cancer was among the first diseases causally linked to smoking, and cigarette smoking is the primary cause of cancer mortality in the United States (responsible for at least 30 percent of all cancer deaths). It is the leading risk factor for lung cancer and causes approximately 90 percent of lung cancer deaths in men and almost 80 percent in women. Smoking light cigarettes or those with less tar does not substantially reduce lung cancer risk.

Inhalation of sidestream smoke also increases cancer risk. More than 126 million nonsmoking Americans, including children, are regularly exposed to secondhand smoke, and more than 3,000 nonsmoking Americans die of lung cancer each year, primarily because of exposure to sidestream smoke.

Cigar smoking is a popular habit in the United States. Rates more than doubled in the 1990's, and approximately 5.1 billion cigars were consumed in 2005. Cigar smoking is most common among men ages thirty-five to sixty-four who have higher incomes and educational backgrounds. Most new cigar users are teenagers and younger males (ages eighteen to twenty-four). In addition, in 2004, about 18 percent of students (grades six to twelve) smoked at least one cigar in the past thirty days.

Etiology and symptoms of associated cancers: Toxic ingredients in cigarette smoke travel throughout the body, causing damage in several different ways. Some carcinogens in tobacco smoke produce substances called epoxides when they undergo oxidation (burning). These epoxides bind to and damage the deoxyribonucleic acid (DNA) in cells, causing them to grow abnormally or divide quickly and uncontrollably, resulting in tumor development. Although nicotine is not considered carcinogenic, it can inhibit cell death, thereby promoting tumor development. Symptoms vary with the type of cancer.

History: Based on the findings of hundreds of scientific articles, the U.S. Surgeon General first reported a causal association between cigarette smoking and cancer in 1964. The health risks associated with sidestream smoke were first published by the Surgeon General in 1972.

Cigarettes are subject to several state and federal regulations. The 1964 Surgeon General's report led to laws requiring warning labels on tobacco products; however, those laws were only applied to cigars much later. Television advertising of cigarettes has been prohibited since 1971 and has since been expanded to include advertising on radio and other electronic media; these regulations do extend to cigar advertising. Cigarettes and cigars are also subject to taxes, which vary from state to state. In addition, it is currently illegal to sell tobacco products to minors, and in many states it is illegal for a minor to possess any form of tobacco. Many states also prohibit smoking in restaurants and in some public places.

Jaime Stockslager Buss, M.S.P.H., ELS

For Further Information

Brandt, A. M. *The Cigarette Century: The Rise, Fall, and Deadly Persistence of the Product That Defined America*. New York: Basic Books, 2007.

Lapointe, Martin M., ed. *Adolescent Smoking and Health Research*. New York: Nova Biomedical Books, 2008.

U.S. Department of Health and Human Services. *The Health Consequences of Involuntary Exposure to Tobacco Smoke: A Report of the Surgeon General*. Washington, D.C.: Author, 2006.

U.S. Department of Health and Human Services, Public Health Service, National Toxicology Program. *Eleventh Report on Carcinogens*. Research Triangle Park, N.C.: Author, 2005.

Wesley, Merideth K., and Ingrid A. Sternbach, eds. *Smoking and Women's Health*. New York: Nova Science, 2008.

Other Resources

American Cancer Society
Tobacco and Cancer
http://www.cancer.org/docroot/PED/PED_10.asp

American Lung Association
What Is the Connection Between Tobacco Use and Lung Disease?
http://www.lungusa.org/site/c.dvLUK9O0E/b.4061173/apps/s/content.asp?ct=5328919

Centers for Disease Control and Prevention
Smoking and Tobacco Use
http://www.cdc.gov/tobacco

See also: Chewing tobacco; Lung cancers; Oral and oropharyngeal cancers; Smoking cessation; Tobacco-related cancers

▶ Coal tars and coal tar pitches

Category: Carcinogens and Suspected Carcinogens
RoC status: Known human carcinogen since 1980
Also known as: Coal tar pitch volatiles (CTPVs)

Related cancers: Skin cancer, scrotal cancer, lung cancer, bladder cancer, kidney cancer, leukemia, digestive tract cancers including the esophagus, as well as cancers of the oral cavity and larynx

Definition: Coal tar is a product of bituminous coal distillation and is composed mainly of aromatic hydrocarbons.

Coal tar pitch is the residue produced by the distillation or heat treatment of coal tar. Continued distillation of the coal tar yields a variety of products, including benzene, toluene, xylene, naphthalene, anthracene, acridine, benzopyrene, chrysene, pyrene, and phenanthrene. The many coal tar distillates are central to the synthesis of dyes, drugs, explosives, flavorings, perfumes, preservatives, synthetic resins, paints, and stains. The remaining pitch left after distillation finds uses in paving, roofing, waterproofing, and insulation materials.

Exposure routes: Inhalation, ingestion, skin contact

Where found: Pesticides, roofing materials, pipe coatings, enamels, plastics, dyestuffs, synthetic fibers, synthetic rubbers, varnishes, paints, electrodes, binders used in aluminum smelting, epoxy resins, denatured alcohol, carbon brushes, graphites, road-paving materials, naphthalene, pharmaceuticals, high-temperature-resistant materials

At risk: Those at risk include workers exposed to coal tars or coal tar pitches. Additionally, patients using therapeutic levels of coal tar preparations may be at risk for skin cancer. Especially vulnerable are workers exposed to coal tar fumes found in coal gasification and coke production.

Etiology and symptoms of associated cancers: Coal tars and coal tar pitches contain several carcinogens, which include such known offenders as benzene and naphthalene. The resulting cancers include skin cancer (notably scrotal cancer), digestive tract cancers, lung cancer, bladder and kidney cancers, and leukemia. The cancer type is often associated with the workers' exposure. For example, millwrights and welders are prone to digestive tract cancers and leukemia, while workers exposed to tar distillates show an increased risk of bladder cancer, and rates of kidney cancer climb with exposure to petroleum or coal tar pitches.

History: Since 1775, when scrotal cancer was first described in chimney sweeps, industrial exposure to coal tar has been targeted as an important carcinogen. From coal tar pitch volatiles at coke ovens to pharmaceuticals used in the home, the carcinogenic potential is fully recognized.

Richard S. Spira, D.V.M.

See also: Air pollution; Carcinogens, known; Carcinogens, reasonably anticipated; Coke oven emissions; Melanomas; Photodynamic Therapy (PDT); Polycyclic aromatic hydrocarbons

▶ Coke oven emissions

Category: Carcinogens and Suspected Carcinogens
RoC status: Known human carcinogen since 1981
Also known as: 3,4- benzopyrene, benzanthracene, chrysene, phenanthrene, benzene, toluene, and xyglenes

Related cancers: Respiratory cancers including tracheal, bronchial, and lung cancers as well as cancers of the skin, prostate, scrotum, large intestine, pancreas, bladder, and kidneys

Definition: Coke oven emissions are produced when bituminous coals are heated in the absence of oxygen to produce coke, tars, and light oils. Roughly 60 percent of the coal is converted to coke; the remainder is emitted in the form of by-products including light oils and gases and vapors of methane, ethane, ethylene, propylene, formaldehyde, ammonia, nitrogen oxides, cadmium, arsenic, and carbon monoxide. Tar acids, naphthalene, creosote, and pyridine are also emitted as coke oven gas tar. These various gases and vapors fall under the category of coke oven emissions and are the source of concern as potential carcinogens.

Exposure routes: Inhalation, dermal contact

Where found: Coke oven emissions occur when coal is processed to produce coke, or when the coke is combusted as fuel for making steel and processing ores, and in the manufacturing of substances such as graphite products.

At risk: Workers in coke oven plants that produce coke from coal, at coal tar plants, and in the aluminum, steel, graphite, electrical, and construction industries are especially at risk. Residents in the immediate vicinity of coke-producing plants and coal tar industries are also at risk of higher-than-normal exposure to vapors and gases.

Etiology and symptoms of associated cancers: Coke oven emissions are related to respiratory cancers that can develop from inhalation or ingestion of toxic substances. These cancers typically interfere with speaking and breathing and often affect taste and smell. Skin cancer may result from dermal contact with toxic substances and is characterized by a tumor on or just below the skin surface, which may become red and irritated. Cancers of the prostate, scrotum, pancreas, bladder, kidney, and large intestine can develop if toxic substances are ingested and pass through the blood or urinary system. They may affect urine flow, frequency, and strength or may disable ejaculation. Pancreatic, kidney, and intestinal cancer can cause extreme abdominal discomfort as well as hinder the digestion and blood-cleansing processes.

History: Coke, or pure carbon, is used as a fuel reductant in the manufacture or synthesis of steel, iron, calcium carbide, graphite, and electrodes. The chemicals given off as coke oven emissions can be used in making plastics, solvents, dyes, drugs, paints, roads, roofing, insulation, pesticides, and sealants.

Coke production in the United States began to decrease around 1950 because of a seemingly strong relationship between exposure to coke oven emissions and cancer rates. A number of studies conducted in the United States, Japan, Sweden, and the United Kingdom have produced significant evidence linking coke oven emissions with increased cancer rates among coke oven workers, especially cancers of the skin, lungs, and prostate. One study with 15,818 cohorts showed that occupational exposure to coke oven emissions was associated with significant excess mortality from cancer of the respiratory system and of the prostate. Another study found higher rates of lung cancer among topside coke oven workers and among those working near the tops, or lids, of the ovens, where exposure rates were greatest. Additional studies have shown significant links between exposure to coke oven emissions and incidence rates of malignant skin tumors and kidney, large intestine, and pancreatic cancers.

Because of the studies confirming the relationships between coke oven emissions and cancers, numerous safety regulations are in place, including limitations on exposure levels to coke oven emissions and the use of respirators and protective clothing for coke oven workers. Still, use of coke as a fuel remains high in certain industries. Regulations require that coke oven emissions be collected, but structural defects, including loose-fitting doors and lids on coke ovens and poor engineering controls, result in continued release of varying amounts of potentially carcinogenic coke oven gases and vapors.

Dwight G. Smith, Ph.D.

See also: Air pollution; Benzene; Coal tars and coal tar pitches

▶ Cyclophosphamide

Category: Carcinogens and Suspected Carcinogens; Chemotherapy and Other Drugs

Definition: Cyclophosphamide, an alkylating agent, is a highly toxic but effective anticancer drug derived from nitrogen mustard. Since 1980, cyclophosphamide has been a known human carcinogen.

Related cancers and cardiotoxicities: Bladder cancer, myeloproliferative and lymphoproliferative malignancies (leukemias), pericarditis, myocarditis, myocardial depression

Cyclophosphamide is a cytotoxic drug that affects the growth of cancer cells. It is rapidly absorbed by the gastrointestinal tract and undergoes extensive chemical modification in the liver that converts it into two different chemicals: "phosphoramide mustard" and "acrolein." Both of these chemicals are very reactive and chemically modify deoxyribonucleic acid (DNA) within cells; producing cross-linkages between DNA strands, which interfere with DNA replication. Normal, noncancerous cells are affected as well, causing severe side effects that may include inflammation and bleeding from the bladder (hemorrhagic cystitis), bone-marrow suppression, nausea and vomiting, and hair loss (alopecia).

Although cyclophosphamide is used to treat cancer, it can cause cancer in the long term. The damage it causes to cellular DNA can generate a secondary cancer months or years after treatment, particularly at higher doses. Some people may be more susceptible than others, depending on their genetic makeup. Patients who experience hemorrhagic cystitis during treatment with cyclophosphamide have been shown to have a higher risk of bladder cancer after treatment. Patients who are treated with cyclophosphamide for primary myeloproliferative or lymphoproliferative malignancies (leukemia) are at a higher risk for a secondary hematologic malignancy (leukemia) as a long-term side effect of treatment. The symptoms of secondary acute leukemia include recurring infections, bone and joint pain, swollen lymph nodes, and shortness of breath.

Serious side effects of cyclophosphamide are not limited to cancers. It can have harmful effects on the heart, including pericarditis (inflammation of the pericardium—the heart's sac-like covering) and myocarditis (inflammation the heart muscle itself). At high doses, cyclophosphamide is associated with myocardial depression. Rarely and at high doses, the resulting myocarditis might be hemorrhagic and fatal. Risk of congestive heart failure occurs when cyclophosphamide is given to the elderly, in combination with chest radiation, and at high cumulative doses or with or after anthracyclines such as doxorubicin.

Exposure routes: Exposure occurs orally or by intravenous injection during medical treatment. Skin contact or dust inhalation is possible during the manufacturing process and in handling the drug during preparation and administration.

Where found: Cyclophosphamide is used 1) in the treatment of various cancers (including lymphoma and leukemia), 2) in bone- marrow transplant as part of a peripheral stem-cell mobilization or preparative regimen, 3) as an immune-suppressive agent following bone-marrow or solid-organ transplant, and 4) to treat autoimmune disorders such as rheumatoid arthritis.

At risk: Those most at risk for exposure to cyclophosphamide include people who have been previously treated with cyclophosphamide alone or in association with other chemotherapy drugs; health professionals (nurses, pharmacists, physicians) who handle the drug during preparation, administration, and cleanup; and workers involved in the manufacturing process. An estimated 500,000 patients are treated with cyclophosphamide annually and the general population is not considered to be at risk.

Etiology and symptoms of associated cancers: Cyclophosphamide is used to treat cancer, but studies show that it can cause a secondary cancer as a long-term side effect. It is a cytotoxic drug that affects the growth of cancer cells by interfering with the deoxyribonucleic acid (DNA) within the cells. Normal, noncancerous cells are affected as well, causing side effects that may include inflammation and bleeding from the bladder (hemorrhagic cystitis), bone-marrow suppression, nausea and vomiting, and hair loss (alopecia). Damage to cellular DNA can lead to a secondary cancer months or years after cyclophosphamide treatment. Patients who experience hemorrhagic cystitis during treatment with cyclophosphamide have been shown to be at a higher risk of bladder cancer after treatment. Signs and symptoms of bladder cancer include blood in the urine (hematuria), pelvic pain, pain during urination, and a frequent urge to urinate. Patients who are treated with cyclophosphamide for primary myeloproliferative or lymphoproliferative malignancies (leukemia) are at a higher risk for a secondary hematologic malignancy (leukemia) as a long-term side effect of treatment. The symptoms of secondary acute leukemia include recurrent infections, bone and joint pain, swollen lymph nodes, and shortness of breath.

History: Cyclophosphamide was first synthesized in 1958. The first clinical trials were published at the end of the 1950s. It has been in widespread use as a chemotherapeutic agent since the 1960s.

Melanie Hawkins, B.S.N., R.N., O.C.N.
Updated by: Jackie Dial, PhD

For Further Information

Cappello, Mary (2009). *Called Back: My reply to cancer, my return to life*. New York City, NY: Alyson Books.

Jacobs, Hollye & Messina, Elizabeth (2014). *The Silver Lining: A supportive & insightful guide to breast cancer* (Kindle edition). Retrieved from http://www.amazon.com/The-Silver-Lining-Supportive-Insightful/dp/1476743711

Mitchell, Deborah. (2012). *The Women's Pill Book: Your Complete Guide to Prescription and Over-the-Counter Medication*. New York: St. Martin's Press.

Perry, Michael Clinton, Ed. (2008). *The Chemotherapy Source Book* (4th ed.). Philadelphia, PA: Wolters Kluwer Health.

Project Inform (1998). HIV Drug Book Revised. NY: Simon & Schuster.

Other Resources

American Society of Clinical Oncology (July 2015). Long-Term Side Effects of Cancer Treatment. http://www.cancer.net/survivorship/long-term-side-effects-cancer-treatment

Chemocare (2002-2016). Cytoxan®. Retrieved from http://chemocare.com/chemotherapy/drug-info/cytoxan.aspx

Drugs.com (updated January 6, 2016). Cyclophosphamide Side Effects. Retrieved from http://www.drugs.com/sfx/cyclophosphamide-side-effects.html

Mayo Clinic (updated December 01, 2015). Cyclophosphamide (Oral Route, Intravenous Route), Side Effects. Retrieved from http://www.mayoclinic.org/drugs-supplements/cyclophosphamide-oral-route-intravenous-route/side-effects/drg-20063307

The Silver Pen (written December 26, 2010). Chemotherapy and its Side Effects. Retrieved from http://www.thesilverpen.com/breast-cancer-information-facts/breast-cancer-chemotherapy-treatment/chemotherapy-and-its-side-effects/

See also: Adrenal gland cancers; Bladder cancer; Burkitt lymphoma; Carcinoid tumors and carcinoid syndrome; Estrogen-receptor-sensitive breast cancer; Myeloproliferative disorders; Nasal cavity and paranasal sinus cancers

▶ Cyclosporin A

Category: Chemotherapy and Other Drugs; Carcinogens and Suspected Carcinogens

RoC status: Known human carcinogen since 1998

Also known as: Cyclosporin, ciclosporin, cyclosporine, CsA, CYA, Sandimmune, Neoral, Restasis, Gengraf, Cicloral

Related cancers: Lymphoma, skin cancer

Definition: Cyclosporin A is a drug approved by the U.S. Food and Drug Administration, now marketed as an immunomodulator. It is a short polypeptide with eleven amino acids, eight of which form a ring.

Exposure routes: Oral, intravenous, or topical administration

Where found: Commercially available in pharmacies

At risk: People given the drug for therapeutic immunosuppression

Etiology and symptoms of associated cancers: Cyclosporin A modifies the immune response by inhibiting calcineurin in lympocytes (primarily T cells); calcineurin is then unable to normally activate transcription of interleukin-2. It also inhibits release of the important pro-apoptotic factor cytochrome C from mitochondria. Although not important in modulating the immune response, the deficit of cytochrome C may slow or prevent normal apoptosis and act as a pro-survival factor for malignant cells.

Another mechanism by which cyclosporin A promotes cancer progression is independent of immune cell inhibition; this direct carcinogenicity involves activation of transforming growth factor beta (TGF-β). Tumors in transplant recipients may arise from the recipient's cells or from cells brought in with the transplanted organ, whereby premalignant donor cells are no longer subject to the surveillance of an intact immune system. Symptoms of lymphoma include fatigue, enlarged and painful lymph glands, and elevated white blood cell counts. Skin cancer is usually detected by visual inspection. In some patients, tumors become apparent within a few weeks of treatment initiation, and in some cases discontinuation of the drug is followed by tumor remission.

History: As part of a drug discovery effort, soil samples from Norway were tested and found to have immunosuppressive activity in the early 1970's; the active component was found to be a small peptide produced by the fungus *Tolypocladium inflatum Gams*. The drug was first administered to prevent transplanted organ rejection in 1980 and was approved for this indication in 1983. Transplant recipients were soon found through registry data to have a threefold to fivefold increased risk of cancer compared with the general population, with more aggressive malignancies and overall poorer prognosis. Despite the increased risk of cancer, cyclosporin A has since been approved for other indications, including prevention of graft-versus-host disease (GVHD), psoriasis, rheumatoid arthritis, nephrotic syndrome, and keratoconjunctivitis sicca (dry eyes). The drug continues to be widely used, and efforts to minimize post-transplant malignancies continue.

John B. Welsh, M.D., Ph.D.

See also: Aplastic anemia; Edema; Fibroadenomas; Graft-Versus-Host Disease (GVHD); Myasthenia gravis; Pancolitis; Paraneoplastic syndromes; Sjögren syndrome

▶ Di(2-ethylhexyl) phthalate (DEHP)

Category: Carcinogens and Suspected Carcinogens
RoC status: Reasonably anticipated human carcinogen since 1983; under review for removal from the *Twelfth Report on Carcinogens* (RoC)
Also known as: Diethylhexyl phthalate, bis(2-ethylhexyl) phthalate

Related cancers: DEHP does not seem to cause cancer in humans. The mechanism by which cancers are induced in experimental animals by prolonged high doses of DEHP is not relevant to humans.

Definition: DEHP is a water-insoluble organic compound, a widely used phthalate with the molecular formula of $C_{24}H_{38}P_4$. It is used as a plasticizer mainly in the plastic polyvinyl chloride (PVC) for flexibility and softness of the final product.

Exposure routes: Inhalation, ingestion, dermal contact, and medical procedures such as intravenous (IV) drug administation and blood transfusion

Where found: DEHP is mainly used in plastic products such as children's toys, vinyl upholstery, raincoats, and food packaging. Because DEHP is not chemically attached to the plastic, it can leach out. DEHP release is found in IV bags, blood bags, dialysis bags, medical tubing products, atmosphere, soil, and water. Some manufacturers have begun not to use DEHP in their products.

At risk: DEHP may cause toxicity in humans. Because of its minimum exposure to humans, however, it does not present a general risk to human health. Newborns and infants are particularly at risk for toxicity in the hospital setting. Thus, the risk of developmental and reproductive abnormalities is greater among this subpopulation.

Etiology and symptoms of associated cancers: The hepatocarcinogenicity (potential to cause liver cancer) of DEHP in rats has been proven. DEHP-induced peroxisome proliferation in rats is a phenomenon in which peroxisomes in hepatocytes (liver cells) are increased in number. Peroxisomes, also called microbodies, are intracellular respiratory organelles like mitochondria. Peroxisome proliferation protects the cell from increased oxidation. Failure to do so results in carcinogenesis—cell replication and tumor formation. No such peroxisomal route of carcinogenesis and thus no form of cancer due to DEHP have been demonstrated in humans. It may be because there are fundamental differences in metabolism between rats and humans; also, prolonged exposure of higher doses of DEHP in humans is unlikely.

History: Plasticized PVC was invented in 1926. DEHP was implicated in animal hepatocarcinogesis in 1982, which was followed by classification of DEHP as an anticipated human carcinogen. DEHP's possible removal from the twelfth *Report on Carcinogens* is based on the experts' conclusion that the chemical cannot be reasonably anticipated to cause cancer in humans. It is important to note, however, that human carcinogenicity data remain incomplete.

Arun S. Dabholkar, Ph.D.

See also: Plasticizers

▶ Diethanolamine (DEA)

Category: Carcinogens and Suspected Carcinogens
Also known as: Diethylolamine, 2,2 -dihydroxy-diethylamine, diolamine, bis-2-hydroxyethylamine, iminodiethanol

Related cancers: Liver and kidney cancer in mice

Definition: Diethanolamine (DEA) is a secondary amine in a class of organic compounds known as ethanolamines, which combine the properties of amines and alcohols. A high-production chemical, DEA is a component of metalworking fluids, pesticides, antifreeze, pharmaceuticals, and personal care products. Its fatty acid derivatives, including cocamide DEA, lauramide DEA, and oleamide DEA, are emulsifiers or foaming agents.

Exposure routes: Principally through dermal contact, inhalation of vapor and aerosols, ingestion

Where found: Intermediates in agricultural and photographic chemicals, personal care products (such as lotions, creams, shampoos, and hair dyes), textile processing, pharmaceuticals, metalworking fluids, industrial gas treatments

At risk: Workers in diethanolamine manufacturing facilities, metal industry workers exposed to lubricating liquids, consumers of personal care products and of some tobacco products

Etiology and symptoms of associated cancers: Diethanolamine increases the risk of liver cancers (hepatocellular adenoma or carcinoma) and kidney cancers (renal tubule adenoma) in mice. The cancer risk to humans has not been firmly established by adequate epidemiological studies. DEA does not damage the genetic material; rather, it perturbs cellular processes by causing a deficiency of choline, an essential nutrient in mammals. Choline depletion is known to induce changes in deoxyribonucleic acid (DNA) methylation, stimulate DNA synthesis, generate free radicals, and enhance susceptibility to oxidative damage—all events linked to tumorigenesis. Because rodents are more sensitive to choline deficiency than are humans, the relevance of the mouse tumor findings to humans is unclear.

DEA's potential carcinogenicity may stem from its ability to interact with nitrites. As contaminants or preservatives in commercial formulations, nitrites react with DEA to form nitrosodiethanolamine (NDELA), a carcinogen that induces tumors of the liver, nasal cavity, and kidney in laboratory animals. The National Toxicology Program has listed nitrosodiethanolamine as reasonably anticipated to be a human carcinogen.

History: The industrial synthesis of ethanolamines depends on the wide-scale production of the primary reactant, ethylene oxide, discovered in 1859 by the French chemist Charles Adolphe Wurtz. In 1999 at the completion of a two-year carcinogenesis study, the National Toxicology Program reported that dermal applications of DEA or cocamide DEA induced liver and kidney cancers in mice. As early as 1979 the U.S. Food and Drug Administration urged the cosmetics industry to remove DEA-derived nitrosamines from its products, but it has not strictly enforced the policy. In contrast, the European

Union has enacted legislation to reduce DEA and nitrosodiethanolamine from cosmetics and toiletries.

Anna Binda, Ph.D.

See also: 4-Aminobiphenyl; Antiperspirants and breast cancer; Carcinogens, reasonably anticipated

▶ Diethylstilbestrol (DES)

Category: Carcinogens and Suspected Carcinogens; chemotherapy and other drugs
RoC status: Known human carcinogen since 1980
Also known as: Stilbestrol

Related cancers: Breast, cervical, prostate, and vaginal cancers

Definition: Diethylstilbestrol (DES) is a synthetic form of the hormone estrogen.

Exposure routes: Patients are exposed to DES when it is used in medical therapies and in clinical trials for the treatment of prostate and breast cancer. It is typically administered orally or intravenously. Potential exposure by inhalation can occur to workers who are involved in the formulation and manufacturing of diethylstilbestrol.

Where found: DES is found at sites where it is manufactured, packaged, and supplied. It can be found at medical facilities where it is prepared and administered during cancer clinical trials and treatments. During the 1970's, it was found in cattle and sheep that were injected with diethylstilbestrol to promote their growth.

At risk: Patients who are treated with DES for prostate and breast cancers are at high risk. Workers at locations where diethylstilbestrol is manufactured, packaged, and supplied for cancer clinical trials are at risk for contamination. Health care professionals who prepare and administer DES for cancer therapy risk contamination, as do workers in labs where diethylstilbestrol is used in biochemical research.

Etiology and symptoms of associated cancers: DES behaves as a hormonal therapy. By acting as a chemical messenger in the body, it helps control the activity of cells and organs. When administered to pregnant women to help prevent miscarriages or premature deliveries, DES can cause clear-cell adenocarcinoma (CCA) of the vagina and cervix in the mother and in daughters exposed before birth. In sons exposed before birth, DES can increase the risk of testicular cancer. Since DES reduces the level of testosterone in the body, it helps slow down the growth of prostate cancer cells. Side effects of diethylstilbestrol chemotherapy include breast tenderness, lowering of sex drive, tiredness, nausea, and weight gain.

History: DES was first synthesized in 1938 at the University of Oxford. It was the first synthetic estrogen. In 1941 diethylstilbestrol was found to be effective in the treatment of gonorrheal vaginitis, menopausal symptoms, and metastatic prostate cancer. Between the 1940's and the 1980's, it was used as estrogen-replacement therapy in estrogen-deficient women. After epidemiological studies of women linked DES to vaginal and cervical cancers, the U.S. Food and Drug Administration (FDA) advised in 1971 that it no longer be given to pregnant women. To a large extent, tamoxifen has replaced the use of DES in breast cancer treatments, as has leuprolide in the treatment of prostate cancer.

Alvin K. Benson, Ph.D.

See also: Bisphenol A (BPA); Cervical cancer; Colposcopy; Gynecologic cancers; PC-SPES; Pregnancy and cancer; Testicular cancer; Vaginal cancer

▶ Dioxins

Category: Carcinogens and Suspected Carcinogens
RoC status: Under the heading "2,3,7,8-tetrachlorodibenzo-*p*-dioxin (TCDD)," known human carcinogen since 2001
Also known as: 2,3,7,8-tetrachlorodibenzo-*p*-dioxin (TCDD); polychlorinated dibenzo-*p*-dioxin (PCDD)

Related cancers: All cancers, including lung cancer and non-Hodgkin lymphoma

Definition: Dioxins are polychlorinated dibenzo-*p*-dioxins (two benzene rings bridged with two atoms of oxygen). The one in which carbons 2, 3, 7, and 8 are chlorinated is called 2,3,7,8-tetrachlorodibenzo-*p*-dioxin (TCDD). TCDD is the deadliest synthetic chemical—so much so that its toxicity is used as a benchmark by which to rate the toxicity of other chemicals through a value called a "toxic equivalency factor" (TEF).

Exposure routes: All species are exposed to dioxins through inhalation or ingestion via air, water, and food. In humans, the major source of TCDD is diet. Out of an average 120 picograms per day in food, 38 are from meat,

24 from dairy foods, 18 from milk, 13 from chicken and pork each, 8 from fish, 4 from eggs, and 2 from air.

Where found: TCDD and other dioxins are not commercial products but are formed as by-products during both organochlorine manufacturing and waste combustion and incineration operations. Dioxins contaminate the atmosphere through incineration and waste disposal; the land through manufacturing, agricultural herbicides, and incineration; and the water through effluent discharges, especially from pulp and paper plants. Residues of TCDD, because of its thermo- and bio-stability, are widely distributed in the air, soil, water, sediments, biota (flora and fauna of a region), and human food. Because it has very low solubility in water and a very high partition coefficient, it accumulates in fat, becomes concentrated in aquatic biota, and is ecomagnified through the food chain. Freshwater biota hold the highest amount of TCDD, which may also be bound to organics in sediments.

At risk: People at greatest risk for exposure to TCDD and other dioxins are those living near contaminated sites or eating contaminated foods, such as waste-incineration workers, firefighters, workers in chemical research facilities, those working in the production and use of pentachlorophenol and other chlorinated compounds, and those associated with chlorophenoxy herbicide production, use, and disposal.

Etiology and symptoms of associated cancers: TCDD has extreme potency for chronic biological effects. There is a general commonality among animal species in some of the effects of TCDD, while other effects are species-specific. For example, birth defects and lowering of male sex hormones (testicular atrophy) have been reported in several bird and mammalian species. Chronic toxicity of TCDD increases with the duration of exposure.

TCDD is regarded a both a teratogen (an agent of developmental malformations) and carcinogen (an agent of malignancy). It affects both the reproductive system (causing low sperm counts, lowering of testosterone, and testicular atrophy, among other effects) and developmental stages (leading to malformations in newborns). In humans, birth defects, termination of pregnancy, decreased fertility (lower sperm count and testosterone and testicular atrophy), endometriosis, diabetes, learning disorders, skin and lung effects, and cancer are commonly recognized.

The half-life of TCDD in humans varies from thirty days to ten years. Men cannot degrade TCDD, while women can transfer it to a fetus via the placenta and to a newborn via breast milk. TCDD causes neurobehavioral deficits and lowering of testosterone in neonates due to their exposure in utero. The U.S. federal government, for example, has had to issue warnings about the consumption of TCDD-tainted Lake Michigan fish by women who are pregnant or want to become pregnant and by children and young adults.

The carcinogenic effects of TCDD are evident in the increased rate of both benign and malignant tumors seen in those who experience significant exposures to the chemical. By binding to the "Ah receptor"—a protein ubiquitous in human and other vertebrate animal tissues that plays a major role in gene transcription—TCDD activates biological responses that can lead to carcinogenic activity. Because the chemical accumulates in fat over long periods of exposure, this carcinogenic activity increases with time, even with low chronic exposures.

History: First listed as a reasonably anticipated carcinogen in the National Toxicology Program's *Second Annual Report on Carcinogens* (1981), from the U.S. Department of Health and Human Services, TCDD underwent several subsequent studies. Some of these considered cancers in human populations occupationally exposed to TCDD, while others examined what took place at the molecular and cellular levels in human and animal tissue exposed to TCDD. The data from studies conducted through 1996 were evaluated by the International Agency for Research on Cancer (IARC), whose results were published in 1997. The IARC concluded that exposure to TCDD was linked to an overall increased risk for all cancers combined, an increased risk for lung cancer, and an increased risk for non-Hodgkin lymphoma. The U.S. government has therefore classified TCDD as a known human carcinogen since 2001.

TCDD was present in herbicides widely used in the 1960's and 1970's, including Agent Orange, used during the Vietnam War. Although TCDD no longer is used in these agents, it continues to occur as a by-product of paper and pulp bleaching (which is why some people, for example, prefer to use unbleached coffee filters and paper towels); in the incineration of municipal and hospital waste; in the production of metals; and in the combustion of both wood and fossil fuels.

M. A. Q. Khan, M.D., Ph.D.

For Further Information

Colborn, T., D. Dumanoski, and J. P. Myers. *Our Stolen Future*. New York: Dutton Press, 1995.

Committee on EPA's Exposure and Human Health Reassessment of TCDD and Related Compounds. Board on Environmental Studies and Toxicology. Division on Earth and Life Studies. National Research Council of the National Academies. *Health Risks from Dioxin and Related Compounds: Evaluation of the EPA Reassessment*. Washington, D.C.: National Academies Press, 2006.

Khan, M. A. Q., and R. H. Stanton. *Toxicology of Halogenated Hydrocarbons*. New York: Pergamon Press, 1980.

U.S. Department of Health and Human Services. Public Health Service. National Toxicology Program. *Eleventh Report on Carcinogens*. Research Triangle Park, N.C.: Author, 2005.

U.S. Environmental Protection Agency. Office of Research and Development. Office of Health and Environmental Assessment. *Health Assessment Document for 2,3,7,8-Tetrachlorodibenzo-p-dioxin (TCDD) and Related Compounds*. Washington, D.C.: Author, 1994.

Other Resources

National Academy of Sciences
http://www.nasonline.org

National Cancer Institute
http://www.cancer.gov

National Toxicology Program
http://ntp.niehs.nih.gov

See also: Agent Orange; Bile duct cancer; Curcumin; Organochlorines (OCs); Pesticides and the food chain; Sarcomas, soft-tissue; Vinyl chloride

▶ Electromagnetic radiation

Category: Carcinogens and Suspected Carcinogens
RoC status: Solar radiation, exposure to sunlamps or sunbeds, known human carcinogens since 2000; broad-spectrum ultraviolet radiation (UVR), known human carcinogen since 2002; ultraviolet A, B, and C (UVA, UVB, UVC), reasonably anticipated human carcinogens since 2002; X radiation, gamma radiation, known human carcinogens since 2004
Also known as: EM radiation, EMR

Related cancers: Skin cancers, especially melanoma; leukemia

Definition: Electromagnetic radiation is a form of energy, composed of individual oscillating photons. The amount of energy carried by each photon is proportional to its frequency. The collection of all possible frequencies of electromagnetic radiation is called the electromagnetic spectrum; this is subdivided (from highest to lowest frequency) into gamma rays, X rays, ultraviolet (UV) light, visible light, infrared light, microwaves, and radio waves. Alternatively, electromagnetic radiation can be divided into ionizing and nonionizing frequencies based on its ability to disrupt electrons.

Exposure routes: Unshielded incident radiation

Where found: Electromagnetic radiation is pervasive, and life would not be possible without it. Sunlight is the most important source of ultraviolet and visible light. Many devices also emit electromagnetic radiation.

At risk: Individuals with occupational or volitional exposure to ionizing electromagnetic radiation

Etiology and symptoms of associated cancers: When electromagnetic radiation interacts with matter, some of the photons' energy alters the structure or increases the kinetic energy of atoms. Structural alterations include ionization (loss of electrons) and breakage of covalent bonds. Deoxyribonucleic acid (DNA), ribonucleic acid (RNA), and proteins are all susceptible to damage by radiation. The skin is the primary carcinogenic target, and UV-caused skin cancers occur mostly on sun-exposed areas. Shorter wavelength electromagnetic radiation such as X rays and gamma rays penetrate the skin and can cause leukemia, lung cancer, and bone cancer. The interaction of electromagnetic radiation with DNA results in abnormal dimerization of adjacent pyrimidine bases, damage to individual bases, strand breakage, and cross-linkages between DNA and adjacent proteins. Such DNA damage contributes to cancer formation through the release of cytokines, induction of latent viruses, or mutations that cause functional changes in encoded protein molecules.

History: The biological effects of electromagnetic radiation in the form of sunlight have been known since antiquity. The understanding of visible light as part of a continuous spectrum was advanced with the discovery of radio waves in 1887 by Heinrich Hertz and of X rays in 1895 by Wilhelm Conrad Röntgen. One of the first publications on the carcinogenicity of sunlight appeared in 1907, and a causal relationship was demonstrated by study in a 1928 publication that involved induction of skin cancer in mice by exposure to ultraviolet light. Cancers were linked to penetrating electromagnetic radiation (X rays and gamma rays) shortly after the isolation and characterization of radioactive isotopes in the 1800's.

John B. Welsh, M.D., Ph.D.

See also: Cell phones; Occupational exposures and cancer; Risks for cancer; Skin cancers; Sunlamps; Sunscreens; Ultraviolet radiation and related exposures; X-ray tests

▶ Epstein-Barr Virus

Category: Carcinogens and Suspected Carcinogens
Also known as: EBV, human herpesvirus 4 (HHV-4)

Related cancers: Burkitt lymphoma, a type of non-Hodgkin lymphoma (NHL), Hodgkin lymphoma, nasopharyngeal carcinoma, gastric carcinoma

Definition: Epstein-Barr virus is one of the eight known types of human herpes viruses and is a gamma subtype in this group. Like many herpes virus species, Epstein-Barr virus appears to establish a lifelong presence in the human body, remaining quiescent for long periods of time and then inexplicably becoming active. Causally related to mononucleosis, it is also associated with a variety of human cancers, such as Burkitt lymphoma and nasopharyngeal carcinoma, and is therefore considered to be carcinogenic.

Exposure routes: Humans are the only known reservoir of Epstein-Barr virus, which is present in oropharyngeal secretions and is most commonly transmitted through saliva; transmission of the virus requires intimate contact with the saliva of an infected person, including contact with objects such as shared toothbrushes. Transmission through the air or blood does not usually occur, but transmission through blood, semen, and organ transplant has been reported. Epstein-Barr virus is causally related to infectious mononucleosis (IM), a disease characterized by the proliferation of lymphocytes (a type of white blood cell), resulting in fever, sore throat, headache, swollen lymph nodes, and, rarely, swelling of the liver or spleen. IM may be contagious for a period of weeks. However, isolation measures are not practical, since Epstein-Barr virus is frequently present in the saliva of healthy persons, who may carry and spread the virus intermittently for life. Thus, transmission of Epstein-Barr virus is virtually impossible to prevent.

Where found: The Centers for Disease Control and Prevention (CDC) estimates that 95 percent of adult Americans between the ages of thirty-five and forty have been infected by Epstein-Barr virus, but it is less prevalent in children and teenagers, a pattern observed in the developed world but not in developing regions such as Africa and Asia. In Africa, for example, most children have been infected by the virus by the age of three. Epstein-Barr virus has also been associated with nasopharyngeal cancers in Asia (especially China) and Burkitt lymphoma in equatorial Africa and Papua New Guinea. In tropical regions, Burkitt lymphoma has been shown to coexist with malaria. In the United States, Epstein-Barr virus has also been associated with nasopharyngeal cancers in immigrants from Asia. The incidence of Burkitt lymphoma has been increasing. Both Hodgkin and non-Hodgkin lymphomas are found in people whose immune systems have been compromised by drug therapy and disease. Epstein-Barr virus has also been associated with approximately 10% of gastric carcinomas.

At risk: Epstein-Barr virus has been shown to take advantage of those with weakened immune systems; Burkitt lymphoma, a non-Hodgkin lymphoma (NHL), is found in organ transplant patients undergoing immunosuppression therapy, as well as those living with human immunodeficiency virus (HIV) and acquired immunodeficiency syndrom (AIDS) who are immunocompromised by their disease. Because Burkitt lymphoma typically occurs in tropical climates where malaria is endemic, it is believed that the immune systems of those with malaria are altered, resulting in tumor production. Epstein-Barr virus is also associated with nasopharyngeal carcinoma, which is prevalent in those of Chinese and South East Asian ancestry. Environmental/occupational exposure to pesticides and organic solvents shows no significant pattern of positive association with Epstein-Barr virus and related cancers.

Etiology and symptoms of associated cancers: Occurring in nearly all regions of the world, Epstein-Barr virus is among the most ubiquitous of viruses, and most people will become infected with Epstein-Barr virus sometime during their lifetimes. In the United States, as soon as maternal antibodies dissipate, infants become vulnerable to Epstein-Barr virus infection. In adolescents, infection with the Epstein-Barr virus results in infectious mononucleosis in 35 to 50 percent of cases. Although the symptoms of infectious mononucleosis usually dissipate within weeks to several months, the Epstein-Barr virus lies dormant in a few cells in the throat and blood for the remainder of the person's life. From time to time, the virus may reactivate and is often present in the saliva, suppressing the immune system by causing repeated mutations in B cells, which may then proliferate unabated, resulting in tumors.

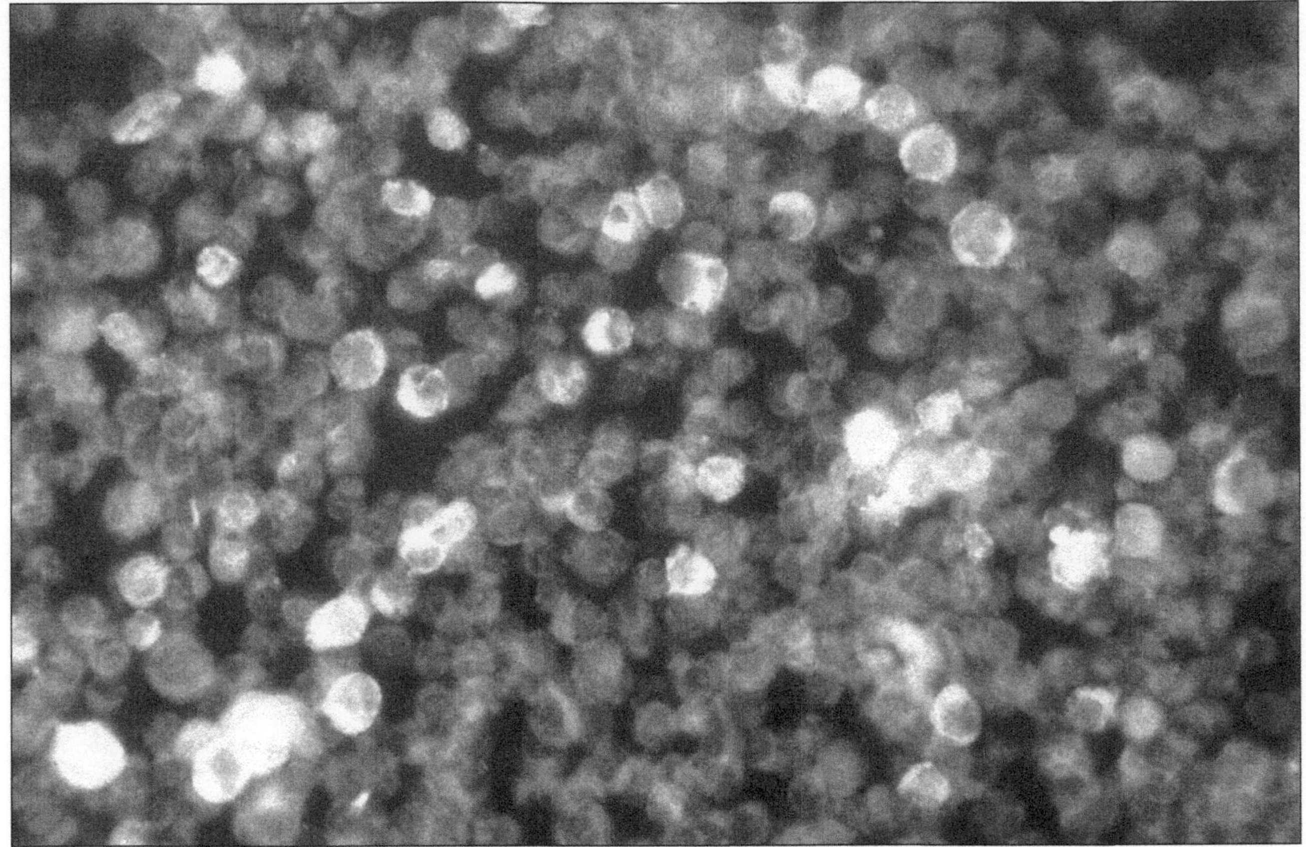

Epstein-Barr virus under the microscope. (Sol Silverman, Jr., D.D.S./Centers for Disease Control)

Epstein-Barr virus establishes a lifelong latent infection in the body's immune system that may later result in the emergence of a lymphoma or carcinoma. The initial symptoms of Burkitt lymphoma may include a swollen lymph node in the upper body or abdomen. If the tumor is found in the chest, breathing difficulties may ensue. In other patients, itching, weight loss, fever, and fatigue may be present. Burkitt lymphoma commonly results in the formation of a large tumor mass in the jawbone. Adults with AIDS often develop tumors in various parts of the body. Symptoms of nasopharyngeal cancer may include a lump in the neck or nose, numbness on the side of the face, headaches, ear pain, and difficulty speaking or breathing.

History: In the latter part of the nineteenth century and in the early part of the twentieth century, the medical community in the United States and in Europe began to report on a novel syndrome consisting of fever, sore throat, and swollen glands that was later termed mononucleosis and was later found to be causally related to Epstein-Barr virus. Epstein-Barr virus was discovered in the 1960s from a biopsy of a tumor associated with Burkitt lymphoma and was the first virus to be directly linked to human cancer; in 1964 Michael Epstein and Yvonne Barr isolated virus particles from cell lines derived from Burkitt lymphoma, hence the name, Epstein-Barr virus. Subsequently, Epstein-Barr virus was found to be the main viral cause of cancer in humans, having an etiological role in Burkitt lymphoma and other B-cell lymphomas as well as nasopharyngeal carcinoma.

Cynthia Racer, M.A., M.P.H.
Updated by: Michelle Herdman

For Further Information

Robertson, E. S. (2005). *Epstein-Barr virus.* Portand, OR: Caister Academic Press.

Tselis, A., &Jenson, H. B. (2006). Epstein-Barr virus. New York: Taylor & Francis.

U.S. Department of Health and Human Services, Public Health Service, National Toxicology Program. (2005). Eleventh Report on Carcinogens. Research Triangle Park, N.C.: Author.

Young, L. S., & Rickinson, A. B. Epstein-Barr virus: Forty years on. *Nature Reviews: Cancer*, 4(10), 757-768.

Iizasa, H., Nanbo, A., Nishikawa, J. Jinushi, M., & Yoshiyama, H. (2012). Epstein-Barr virus (EBV)-associated gastric carcinoma. *Viruses,* 4, 3420-3439.

Tsao, S., Tsang, C.M., To, K., & Lo, K. (2015). The role of Epstein-Barr virus in epithelial malignancies. *Journal of Pathology*, 235, 323-333.

See also: Blood cancers; Burkitt lymphoma; Carcinoma of Unknown Primary origin (CUP); Epidermoid cancers of mucous membranes; Gastric Carcinoma; Head and neck cancers; Hodgkin disease; Immune response to cancer; Infectious cancers; Leiomyosarcomas; Leukoplakia; Lymphomas; Non-Hodgkin lymphoma; Oncogenic viruses; Proto-oncogenes and carcinogenesis; Risks for cancer; Throat cancer; Viral oncology; Virus-related cancers

▶ Erionite

Category: Carcinogens and Suspected Carcinogens
RoC status: Known human carcinogen since 1994
Also known as: Erionit, erionita

Related cancers: Mesothelioma, lung cancer

Definition: Erionite is a colorless or white crystalline solid that forms woollike fibers and belongs to a group of minerals known as zeolites.

Exposure routes: Inhalation

Where found: Erionite is found in rock deposits in Arizona, California, Nevada, Oregon, South Dakota, and Utah in the United States and in the Faroe Islands. It is found with associated minerals that include calcite, opal, pyrite, halite, and other zeolites. Before the late 1980's, a few homes were built in the western United States with blocks that contain erionite.

At risk: Workers involved in the production and mining of erionite and its related minerals known as zeolites are at risk for contamination. As erionite occurs naturally as a mineral in outcrops of Earth's crust, residents or tourists in areas where it is found can be exposed to it. The general public is at risk for contamination from erionite that is contained within zeolites that are used in a variety of applications that include animal feed, pet litter, soil conditioners, catalysts, desiccants, oil and gas absorbents, pesticides, purification of water, and the cleanup of wastewater.

Etiology and symptoms of associated cancers: Through inhalation of erionite dust, erionite fibers can lodge in lung and mesothelial tissue. Due to the shape of the fibers, their surface reactivity, their ability to selectivity adsorb molecules from air and liquids, and their resistance to dissolution in fluids within the lung, erionite is extremely irritating and toxic to the lungs and mesothelium, producing malignant tumors in the lungs and in the thoracic and abdominal cavities.

History: Mineral ores containing erionite have been mined commercially in the United States since the early 1960's. During the 1960's and the 1970's, it was one of four commercially important zeolites. Erionite is found in many different rock types and geological settings but is rarely found in pure form. Until the late 1980's, erionite was used as a catalyst in a hydrocarbon-cracking process. During the 1980's, erionite was linked with the development of mesothelioma and lung cancer in some villages in Turkey where residents experienced chronic exposure to erionite. The use of erionite was banned in the United States by the Environmental Protection Agency in 1991.

Alvin K. Benson, Ph.D.

See also: Asbestos; Silica, crystalline

▶ Ethylene oxide

Category: Carcinogens and Suspected Carcinogens
RoC status: Known human carcinogen since 2000
Also known as: 1,2-epoxyethane, oxacyclopropane, dimethylene oxide, oxirane

Related cancers: Leukemia, stomach, lymphatic, pancreatic, and brain cancers

Definition: Ethylene oxide is a flammable, colorless gas at temperatures above 51.3 degrees Fahrenheit. It is a three-atom ring made of two carbon atoms and one oxygen atom. Each of the two carbon atoms is bonded to two hydrogen atoms.

Exposure routes: Inhalation, ingestion, skin contact

Where found: Fumigation of foodstuffs, sterilization of hospital instruments, and various synthetic chemical operations

At risk: Workers in the detergent, fungicide, and synthetic chemical fields, especially those related to ethylene glycol manufacture

Etiology and symptoms of associated cancers: The high reactivity of ethylene oxide is shown by ring opening and the introduction of new carbon groups at reactive sites in deoxyribonucleic acid (DNA). This type of reaction takes place largely at a nitrogen atom of guanosine. Such modified nucleic acid fragments have been observed in mice and are most prevalent in the liver, kidney, spleen, and testis. A variety of mutations and reverse mutations have also been found. Gene mutations and heritable translocations are common.

History: Ethylene oxide has been produced in large quantities in the United States since 1921. Annual production ranges between 2.6 million and 3.4 million metric tons. It is one of the top twenty-five chemicals in volume. Well over half of the production is consumed in the synthesis of the antifreeze, ethylene glycol.

Five studies of workers exposed to ethylene oxide, beginning in the mid-1980's, showed that exposure produces statistically significant excess tumor appearance. There are difficulties in the interpretation of each of these studies, but a causal relationship between the compound and tumor production is likely. Animal studies involving rats, mice, and hamsters clearly show its carcinogenicity.

Federal regulations exist for the control of ethylene oxide. The Department of Transportation (DOT) lists the chemical as hazardous and requires special marking, labeling, and transporting precautions. The Environmental Protection Agency (EPA) requires that the manufacture of ethylene oxide meet provisions for the control of volatile organic compounds (VOCs). Also, under the Clean Air Act, the compound is listed as one of thirty-three hazardous air pollutants that present the greatest threat to public health, and the EPA requires that as little as ten pounds of the substance must be reported. The Occupational Safety and Health Administration (OSHA) has set the permissible exposure limit at one part per million.

K. Thomas Finley, Ph.D.

See also: 1,3-Butadiene; Diethanolamine (DEA); Formaldehyde

▶ Fertility drugs and cancer

Category: Carcinogens and Suspected Carcinogens

Definition: An association between the use of fertility drugs—clomiphene citrate, follicle-stimulating hormone (FSH), human menopausal gonadotropin (MG), and gonadotropin-releasing hormone analog (GnRH)—and ovarian cancer exists if there is a statistically significant increase in the risk of cancer during the lifetime of the user of fertility drugs. Although the major concern regarding fertility drugs and cancer since the 1990's has focused on ovarian cancer, some experts have also suggested a possible relationship between fertility drugs and cancers of the breast and uterus. Because fertility drugs evoke changes in hormone levels, the potential risk should be extended to any cancer that can be triggered or modulated by hormones, as well as any indirect effects on the offspring of the user of fertility drugs.

Fertility drugs and cancer: A woman's risk of ovarian cancer is multifactorial; however, it is known that some factors increase the risk for ovarian cancer, while other factors decrease the risk. Specifically, ovarian cancer is known to increase with age, when there is a family history of ovarian cancer, and in women who have never had a child. In contrast, the risk of ovarian cancer is decreased in women who breast-feed, have at least one child, and use oral contraceptives. In considering these risk factors together, current scientific thinking is that ovarian cancer is related to the process of ovulation in most, if not all, cases. It has been suggested, but not proven, that ovarian cancer follows an abnormal repair process on the surface of the ovary following the release of the egg during ovulation. Thus, increasing the number of ovulations (incessant ovulation), either by having no interruption of ovulation due to pregnancy or by inducing ovulation with fertility drugs, would theoretically increase the risk of ovarian cancer. Conversely, inhibiting ovulation vis-à-vis pregnancy or pregnancies, breast-feeding, or through the use of oral contraceptives, would theoretically decrease the risk of ovarian cancer by decreasing the lifetime number of ovulations.

Common Fertility Drugs

Drug Name	*Brand Names*
Clomiphene citrate	Clomid Serophene Milophene
Human chorionic gonadotropin (HCG)	Pregnyl
Menotropin	Pergonal Humegon
Urofollitropin	Metrodin
Urofollitropin (highly purified)	Fertinex

Source: U.S. Food and Drug Administration

In determining the risk of fertility drugs and ovarian cancer, it is important to take into consideration confounding factors. Although some epidemiologic studies have indeed shown an increased risk of ovarian cancer in women who have used fertility drugs, when all factors are accounted for statistically, it has been concluded that it is actually infertility, rather than the fertility drugs, that has led to an increased risk of ovarian cancer. For example, in one study involving more than twelve thousand women who were followed for an average of nearly twenty years, it was found that the risk of ovarian cancer was increased twofold because of infertility alone, and there was no statistical risk of ovarian cancer due to just the fertility drugs. Because the peak onset of ovarian cancer occurs during the seventh decade of life, it will be important to continue such studies longitudinally to verify this finding.

It is noteworthy, though, that an association has been demonstrated between the use of clomiphene citrate and cancer of the uterus. Given that clomiphene citrate is chemically similar to tamoxifen (a drug routinely used to treat patients with breast cancer after surgery), which is known to be associated with cancer of the uterus, further studies are needed to verify this association.

Ovarian cancer: Approximately 25,000 women are diagnosed with ovarian cancer each year in the United States. The current lifetime incidence of ovarian cancer for any given woman is approximately 1 in 70. Unfortunately, the symptoms of ovarian cancer in its early stages are minimal to none. In advanced cases, most women with ovarian cancer complain of abdominal pain, vaginal bleeding, abdominal bloating and distension, or a change in bowel habits.

There is no accepted screening protocol for ovarian cancer, unlike cervical cancer (which can be detected by a Pap smear) or breast cancer (which can be found by self-exam, a clinical breast exam, and mammography). It is recommended by the American College of Obstetricians and Gynecologists that all women have a manual pelvic examination as part of their annual well-woman examination. During the manual pelvic examination, the examiner palpates (feels) the ovaries. Although not recommended for women at low risk for ovarian cancer, for those at high risk, a blood test (cancer antigen 125, or CA 125) and a vaginal ultrasound in which the ovarian volume is determined may be beneficial.

The standard treatment for ovarian cancer is surgical, in the form of a total abdominal hysterectomy and removal of both ovaries with postoperative chemotherapy. The five-year survival rate for patients with ovarian cancer is 50 percent, depending on the stage at the time of diagnosis and the treatment rendered. The risk of ovarian cancer can be reduced by breast-feeding, using oral contraceptives, and undergoing a tubal ligation, although the mechanism of protection for the latter is unclear. For women who are prescribed fertility drugs, when used as prescribed for less than twelve cycles with monitoring by a specially trained physician (reproductive endocrinologist), there are no convincing scientific studies that have shown an increased risk for ovarian cancer.

D. Scott Cunningham, M.D., Ph.D.

For Further Information

Althuis, M. D. "Uterine Cancer After Use of Clomiphene Citrate to Induce Ovulation." *American Journal of Epidemiology* 161 (2005): 607-615.

Ayhan, A. "Association Between Fertility Drugs and Gynecologic Cancers, Breast Cancer, and Childhood Cancers." *Acta Obstetricia et Gynecologica Scandinovica* 83 (2004): 1104-1111.

Brinton, L. "Long-Term Effects of Ovulation-Stimulating Drugs on Cancer Risk." *Reproductive BioMedicine Online* 15 (2007): 38-44.

Brinton, L. A., et al. "Ovarian Cancer Risk After the Use of Ovulation-Stimulating Drugs." *Obstetrics and Gynecology* 103 (2004): 1194-1203.

Venn, A., D. Healy, and R. McLachlan. "Cancer Risk Associated with a Diagnosis of Infertility." *Best Practice and Research Clinical Obstetrics and Gynaecology* 17 (2003): 343-367.

Other Resources

National Cancer Institute

Ovarian Cancer Prevention
http://www.cancer.gov/cancertopics/pdq/prevention/ovarian/healthprofessional

Ovarian Cancer National Alliance

Q: Do Fertility Drugs Increase Your Risk of Developing Ovarian Cancer?
http://www.ovariancancer.org/index.cfm?Fuseaction=Feature.showFeature&CategoryID=6&FeatureID=124

See also: Childbirth and cancer; Estrogen-receptor-sensitive breast cancer; Fertility issues; Gynecologic cancers; Hormone receptor tests; Hormone replacement therapy (HRT); Infertility and cancer; Ovarian cancers; Ovarian cysts; Pregnancy and cancer; Sterility

▶ Formaldehyde

Category: Carcinogens and Suspected Carcinogens
RoC status: Reasonably anticipated human carcinogen since 1981
Also known as: Formalin, formic aldehyde, methaldehyde, methanol, methyl aldehyde, methylene glycol, methylene oxide

Related cancers: Squamous cell carcinomas of the upper respiratory tract

Definition: Formaldehyde is a flammable, colorless gas at standard temperature and pressure with a strong, irritating odor. It is highly soluble in water and is most commonly encountered as a 37 percent aqueous solution known as formalin, which usually also contains 10 to 15 percent methanol to prevent formaldehyde polymerization. Because of its simple molecular structure and reactivity, formaldehyde is widely used as a starting material in plastics manufacturing. Because it irreversibly links proteins and nucleic acids to one another, it is useful as a disinfectant and a fixative/preservative in biomedical applications.

Exposure routes: Inhalation

Where found: Manufacturing plants, prefabricated dwellings, hospitals, mortuaries, smog

At risk: Workers involved in tissue fixation and in manufacturing plastics, particleboard, wood paneling, and furniture; occupants of prefabricated dwellings

Etiology and symptoms of associated cancers: When formaldehyde reacts with adjacent primary amine groups in proteins or other biomolecules, the resulting covalent bond prevents normal mobility and functioning of the joined molecules. Repeated or sustained exposure to high concentrations (greater than 15 parts per million) of inhaled formaldehyde is sufficient to cause tissue damage, mutations, and increased cell turnover, which can result in malignant transformation. Cells in the upper respiratory tract (the nasopharynx) are especially liable to formalin-induced cancers, which take the form of squamous cell carcinomas. Formaldehyde's carcinogenicity has been demonstrated only in rodents exposed to very high gas concentrations over long periods of time, and extrapolation to human carcinogenicity is speculative.

History: Formaldehyde was first described and chemically synthesized in the 1800's, although it exists in small quantities in the atmosphere naturally and is a product of amino acid metabolism in the body. Its widespread adoption in the chemical industry prompted several large studies to search for diseases associated with exposure. More than thirty epidemiologic studies have addressed formaldehyde carcinogenicity in humans, and no consistent pattern of response has been found. One expert panel concluded that no evidence existed to show a relationship between formaldehyde exposure and human cancer and if a risk did exist, it had to be very small. Because of its many other adverse health effects, formaldehyde is subject to occupational and residential monitoring, with variable exposure limits in different jurisdictions.

John B. Welsh, M.D., Ph.D.

See also: Air pollution; Artificial sweeteners; Astrocytomas; Chewing tobacco; Coke oven emissions; Lung cancers; Mineral oils; Nasal cavity and paranasal sinus cancers; Occupational exposures and cancer; Tobacco-related cancers

▶ Free radicals

Category: Carcinogens and Suspected Carcinogens
Also known as: Radicals, reactive species

Related cancers: Cancers of the skin, airways, gastrointestinal tract, liver, bladder, prostate, and kidney, as well as leukemia and other cancers

Definition: Free radicals are molecules with one or more unpaired electrons. Although there are stable radical species, the most common of which is oxygen, the presence of unpaired electrons most frequently confers high reactivity and oxidizing potential to free radicals. The most abundant free radicals in biological systems are molecules in which the unpaired electron belongs to an oxygen atom. They are known as reactive oxygen species and are mainly, but not exclusively, derived from the incomplete reduction of oxygen during mitochondrial respiration, which generates the superoxide anion radical (O_2-). Superoxide is converted to hydrogen peroxide (H_2O_2) in a reaction driven by the enzyme superoxide dismutase. Hydrogen peroxide is converted to water and detoxified by glutathione peroxidase and catalase. Hydrogen peroxide is not a free radical; however, when produced in excess (for example, in leukocytes during the respiratory burst that takes place in inflammatory processes) or when its enzymatic detoxifying mechanisms are deficient, hydrogen peroxide can be converted to hydroxyl radical (OH) in the presence of transition metals such as iron or copper.

The hydroxyl radical is the most deleterious of the reactive oxygen species because it can hydroxylate or abstract an electron from most macromolecules, including enzymes, membrane lipids, and DNA, the latter sometimes resulting in mutagenesis.

In addition to reactive oxygen species, another significant free radical in the cell is nitric oxide (NO), which is synthesized from arginine by nitric oxide synthase. Nitric oxide fills essential physiological functions but it can also act as an oxidant.

Living organisms have developed enzymatic and nonenzymatic mechanisms to neutralize free radicals. When the generation of free radicals overpowers the capacity of the natural antioxidant defense systems, however, oxidative stress occurs. Signs of oxidative stress have been found in many forms of human cancer.

Exposure routes: The pathologically related free radicals originate within the body as a product of normal aerobic metabolic processes and inflammatory reactions, but some environmental agents, such as radiation and pollutants, with diverse routes of exposure, can increase the production of free radicals.

Where found: Free-radical-generating agents are diverse, as are their sources. The most common are tobacco smoke, sunlight, X rays, and automobile exhausts. Others include the carcinogens benzene, inorganic arsenic compounds, cadmium compounds, aflatoxins, and asbestos.

At risk: Populations at highest risk are those with a low dietary intake of antioxidants or genetic deficiencies in antioxidant enzymes (for example, glutathione peroxidase) or deoxyribonucleic acid (DNA) repair mechanisms, along with tobacco smokers, people who spend a long time in areas of heavy traffic or who are directly exposed to sunlight, and those with chronic inflammatory conditions.

Etiology and symptoms of associated cancers: The carcinogenic potential of free radicals arises from their ability to damage DNA, modify proteins by oxidation, and induce lipid peroxidation. The most frequently found form of oxidative DNA damage is hydroxylation of purine and pyrimidine bases. Other consequences of free radical actions for DNA are the generation of strand brakes, deamination, and formation of etheno adducts. Oxidative modifications of proteins include nitration, nitrosylation, and acetylation, among others. In addition, one of the most damaging effects of free radicals is lipid peroxidation because of its self-propagating nature, which greatly affects the properties and functioning of cell membranes. Furthermore, lipid peroxidation products, such as the reactive aldehydes malondialdehyde and 4-hydroxynonenal, can damage DNA and proteins in the same way as free radicals.

DNA oxidative damage can cause mutations in cancer-related genes, such as tumor-suppressor genes or oncogenes, and lead to the initiation and progression of cancer. Likewise, carcinogenesis can be induced by post-translational oxidative modification of proteins involved in the regulation of cell growth, signal transduction pathways, DNA repair, or other mechanisms of cellular homeostasis. For instance, free radicals are known to induce the transcription of the proto-oncogenes *FOS* (also known as *c-fos*), *JUN* (*c-jun*), and *MYC* (*c-myc*), which stimulate cell growth. Also, posttranslational oxidative modifications of TP53 (p53), a tumor-suppressor protein, can inhibit its antiproliferative activity. Lastly, free radicals can promote not only tumor growth but also tumor migration and metastasis, by activating matrix metalloproteinases and stimulating the release of vascular endothelial growth factor. A current view of free radical actions supports the notion that these species do not act in a purely stochastic manner but are second messengers in redox-sensitive mechanisms of regulation of gene expression and enzyme activity. Aberrant and sustained redox signaling in oxidative stress situations leads to pathological changes, including cancer.

History: The relevance of free radicals in biological systems was first proposed by Denham Harman in 1956 in his classic article "Aging: A Theory Based on Free Radical and Radiation Chemistry." Harman viewed age-related diseases as the result of an accumulation of oxidative damage. In the same year, in vitro studies showing the ability of oxygen reactive species to induce chromosome fragmentation in the presence of iron suggested for the first time the hypothesis of free-radical-induced carcinogenesis. Since then, the concept has been extended and free radicals have been found to be involved in most pathological conditions.

Reyniel Cruz-Aguado, Ph.D.

For Further Information

Halliwell, B. "Oxidative Stress and Cancer: Have We Moved Forward?" *Biochemistry Journal* 401 (2007): 1-11.

Hussain, S. P., L. J. Hofseth, and C. C. Harris. "Radical Causes of Cancer." *Nature Reviews. Cancer* 3 (2003): 276-285.

Wu, W. S. "The Signaling Mechanism of ROS in Tumor Progression." *Cancer Metastasis Reviews* 25 (2006): 695-705.

Other Resources

American Cancer Society
http://www.cancer.org

National Cancer Institute
Antioxidants and Cancer Prevention: Fact Sheet
http://www.cancer.gov/cancertopics/factsheet/antioxidantsprevention

See also: Antioxidants; Beta-carotene; Bone cancers; Carotenoids; Coenzyme Q10; Curcumin; Diethanolamine (DEA); Fruits; Green tea; *Helicobacter pylori*; Herbs as antioxidants; Liver cancers; Lutein; Lycopene; Mesothelioma; Nutrition and cancer prevention; Phenolics; Resveratrol; Wine and cancer

▶ Hair dye

Category: Carcinogens and Suspected Carcinogens
RoC status: Reasonably anticipated human carcinogens include 2,4-diaminotoluene (since 1981), 2,4-diaminoanisole sulfate (since 1983), 4-chloro-*o*-phenylenediamine (since 1985), Disperse Blue 1 (since 1998)
Also known as: Hair color, coloring agent

Related cancers: Bladder, breast, endometrial, and urinary tract cancers; non-Hodgkin lymphoma; hematopoietic cancers; myelodyplasia; multiple myeloma; leukemia; preleukemia

Definition: Hair dye is a usually soluble substance for staining or coloring to change or enhance the color of hair. Synthetic hair dye falls into one of three categories: permanent, semi-permanent, and temporary. Darker hair dyes have more carcinogens than lighter dyes because more chemicals are used in the dyes.

Exposure routes: Skin contact

Where found: Hair salons, barber shops, hair dye manufacturing plants, individual residences

At risk: Hairdressers, barbers, hair dye manufacturers, individuals using hair dye either in a salon or at home. Of the three types of synthetic hair dye—permanent, semi-permanent, and temporary—carcinogens are more prevalent in permanent and semi-permanent dyes.

Etiology and symptoms of associated cancers: There appears to be an increased risk for those who use darker shades of hair color because darker shades have more chemicals than do lighter shades. In addition, the frequency and duration of use may also increase carcinogen exposure. Older versions of dyes may have a greater risk associated with them than newer versions; however, death rates from all cancers combined appear to be about the same for hair dye users and nonusers.

Most evidence does not show hair dyes to be a significant cancer risk factor, and studies indicating otherwise have been inconsistent. For example, some studies have shown an association between hair dye use and bladder or blood cancers, while others have found no association. Of all studies conducted, none has shown a direct link, only an association. Potential cancer risk relates mostly to permanent and semi-permanent dyes as opposed to temporary ones.

History: Ancient civilizations used plants to dye hair. The first synthetic dye was created in 1907. It is estimated that 45 percent of women and 6 percent of men use hair dye. Chemicals in hair dye have been shown to cause cancer in lab animals; however, these animals were fed high levels of dye over a long period, leaving the relevancy of these studies to humans unclear.

Jennifer M. Hickin, B.S.

See also: 4-Aminobiphenyl; Benzidine and dyes metabolized to benzidine; Diethanolamine (DEA); Gliomas; Occupational exposures and cancer

▶ Helicobacter pylori infection

Category: Carcinogens and Suspected Carcinogens

Definition: Helicobacter pylori is a spiral-shaped, Gram-negative bacterium that produces an enzyme called urease, which catalyzes the degradation of urea and water to carbon dioxide and ammonia (see the figure labeled Urease-Catalyzed Reaction). The ammonia generated by this reaction neutralizes stomach acid and allows this microorganism to reproduce, survive, and infect the stomach and duodenum.
Also known as: H. pylori, Campylobacter pylori, Campylobacter pyloridis

Related cancers or conditions: *Helicobacter pylori* infection confers a 1-10% risk of developing gastric or duodenal ulcers (also known as peptic ulcer disease), a 0.1-3% risk of developing gastric adenocarcinoma and a <0.1% risk of developing mucosa-associated lymphoid tissue (MALT) lymphoma. When present, *H. pylori* always induces gastritis, which can cause symptoms such as indigestion and dyspepsia. It is associated with idiopathic thrombocytopenia, iron deficiency anemia, and vitamin B12 deficiency.

Etiology and the Disease Process: Untreated bacterial infection is usually found in older adults who were infected in their younger years and who have lower socioeconomic status. Disease risk is related to the infected individual's genetic type and factors specific to the bacterial strain.

H. pylori infection is associated with developing gastric (stomach) or duodenum ulcers which are breaks in the cell lining (epithelium) penetrating deep into the muscle layer known as the muscularis mucosa. The duodenum is adjacent to the stomach in the gastrointestinal (digestive) tract, and it is the first part of the small bowel, or intestine.

H. pylori infection is associated with inflammation of the cells lining the stomach (gastritis) and the duodenum (duodenitis). This inflammation (including the extent, severity, and type of cell changes) is related to the risk of cancer development. Specific areas of the stomach (corpus) are more susceptible to gastric cancer development. Severe atrophic gastritis with or without cell changes in the stomach (corpus) is associated with high risk of developing gastric cancer. *H. pylori* is a Class I Carcinogen based on the WHO classification because there is sufficient epidemiological evidence that the bacteria cause cancers in humans.

H. pylori infection is also associated with mucosa-associated lymphoid tissue (MALT) lymphoma, most commonly in the stomach. The stomach does not contain significant lymph node tissue; however, it has been proposed that the *H. pylori*-induced gastritis leads to the formation of gastric B-cell lymphoma, marginal zone type. Similar to gastric adenocarcinoma, MALT lymphoma has been related to *H. pylori* strains that produce CagA protein as evidenced by increased antibodies against this protein in patients with this lymphoma.

The *H. pylori* induced gastritis and duodenitis are infectious diseases because of the bacterial presence. Moreover, this bacterial infection leads to chronic active inflammation with varying severity and cell lining changes in all infected individuals.

Incidence: *H. pylori* infections are the most common human bacterial infection in approximately half of the world's population. In the United States, *H. pylori* is more prevalent in lower socio-economic groups, among older adults, and in minority groups (African-Americans, and Hispanics).

Symptoms: Individuals infected with *H. pylori* may be asymptomatic (do not show symptoms).

Dyspepsia symptoms can be related to *H. pylori* infection. These include stomach discomfort, epigastric or burning pain, a feeling of early fullness or immediately after eating, heartburn, bloating, and burping. Some alarming symptoms include persistent vomiting, nausea, weight loss, abdominal mass/lump, gastrointestinal bleeding (blood in the stool), and symptoms of anemia such as feeling weak, fatigue (tiredness), pale skin color, headache, dizziness, and shortness of breath. Gastric cancer symptoms in early stages can include indigestion, loss of appetite and other dyspepsia symptoms; in advanced stages, some of the alarming symptoms may occur along with fluid accumulation in the abdomen (ascites) and yellow skin and eyes (jaundice). Patients with MALT lymphoma usually present with symptoms localized to the stomach; systemic symptoms (such as night sweats and fever) along with blood cell involvement are less common.

Screening and Diagnosis: Non-invasive methods of diagnosing *H. pylori* infection include urea breath test, serologic (blood) test, and stool antigen test. These methods are used in the "test and treat strategy" for managing *H. pylori* infection.

The urea breath test is carried-out by drinking radiolabeled ^{13}C-urea. If a patient is infected with *H. pylori*, the urease in the bacteria will convert the ^{13}C-labeled-urea to ^{13}C-labeled carbon dioxide which is then detected in the breath. This test is easy to perform and provides accurate results.

Urease-Catalyzed Reaction

$$\underset{\text{Urea}}{NH_2CONH_2} + \underset{\text{Water}}{H_2O} \xrightarrow{\text{Urease}} \underset{\text{Ammonia}}{2NH_3} + \underset{\text{Carbon dioxide}}{CO_2}$$

The serologic test detects IgG antibodies in the blood against *H. pylori*. Antibodies are glycoproteins produced by the body's immune system against infectious agents such as bacteria, and IgG is a specific type of antibody. This test needs to be validated locally to be accurate and may signify previous infection as it takes time for the antibody level to fall after successful treatment.

The stool antigen test detects *H. pylori* antigens in the stool using an enzyme-linked immunoassay.

Endoscopy of the esophagus, stomach and duodenum (EGD) is done in cases when there are alarming symptoms such as persistent vomiting, weight loss, abdominal mass, GI bleeding, and iron deficiency anemia and in patients over the age of 50 to exclude cancer. It is mandatory to obtain a biopsy of suspicious tissue samples in the stomach during this procedure. These tissues are made up of cells which are then examined in the laboratory using the microscope (histology) for pre-cancerous and cancer cells and the presence of *H. pylori*. Histologic diagnosis requires biopsy of the antrum and corpus areas of the stomach; more biopsy samples increase the probability of diagnosing precancerous cells.

A guideline called the Sydney system is followed on methods of biopsy sampling and analysis of tissue samples especially in assessing abnormalities, inflammation, gland loss and metaplasia (mature cell change from one type to another). Five areas of stomach need biopsy sampling per the Sydney system: antrum - greater and lesser curvatures, corpus - greater and lesser curvatures, and the incisura. The biopsy samples are submitted separately for the histologic analysis. For atrophic gastritis biopsy samples – Operative Link for Gastritis Assessment (OLGA) and Operative Link for Gastric Intestinal Metaplasia Assessment (OLGIM) are systems used to stratify the risk of gastric cancer.

A newer method of image-enhanced endoscopy has improved the accuracy and reproducibility of diagnosing precancerous stomach lesions. However, this method is currently in limited use and only by experienced, trained endoscopists, mainly in Japan.

Treatment and Therapy: The non-invasive methods of diagnosing *H. pylori* infection (urea breath test, serologic blood test, and stool antigen test) are used in the "test and treat strategy" for managing *H. pylori* infection. If a patient's test results are positive for *H. pylori* infection, treatment with antibiotics and acid suppressant agents will be carried-out.

All patients with symptoms are treated and this treatment provides long-term cure for gastric and duodenal ulcers not related to non-steroidal anti-inflammatory drugs (NSAIDs such as ibuprofen, naproxen, indomethacin, and meloxicam). As with all medications, treatment regimens have side-effects and discussion between clinical providers and patients is imperative. Pregnant patients should discuss the fetal side-effects of the drugs with their clinical providers.

The standard empirical triple therapy treatment includes a proton-pump inhibitor (PPI such as esomeprazole which decreases acid production by glands in the stomach lining), clarithromycin and amoxicillin for 14 days. If patients are allergic to penicillin, metronidazole is prescribed instead of amoxicillin. This treatment is used widely around the world, and its efficacy has decreased to 80% eradication of *H. pylori* infection in recent years. The decrease in efficacy is related to patients prematurely stopping their intake of prescribed antibiotics and the emergence of resistant bacteria.

In geographical areas where clarithromycin resistance is greater than 15-20%, the bismuth quadruple therapy of PPI, bismuth, metronidazole and tetracycline is recommended. In countries where bismuth is not available, non-bismuth quadruple therapy – a PPI, amoxicillin, clarithromycin and metronidazole may be used. Antibiotic resistance should be documented. Local geographic effective regimen should be used on the basis of resistant bacteria patterns.

Local surveillance of antibiotic resistance is warranted to assist clinicians on what treatment to use. Standard microbiology culture-based testing or molecular methods can be used for such testing. Molecular identification of bacteria in the biopsy sample is one molecular method; this identifies the genetic mutation in the clarithromycin resistant bacteria. Polymerase Chain Reaction (PCR)-based molecular methods are available commercially.

Prognosis, Prevention and Outcomes: *H. pylori* infections occur before the age of 12 years in developed countries through familial transmission. Screening for the infection depends on geographical locations, epidemiological factors, prevalence of infection and age-related cancer incidence.

The validated histological system risk stratification (OLGA and OLGIM) assists in the decision for need of treatment(s) and surveillance.

Gastric cancer incidence increases with age and this is associated with the time required to develop atrophic gastritis with underlying genetic changes. Eradication of *H. pylori* decreases gastric cancer risk. The degree of gastric cancer risk reduction is dependent upon the presence, severity and extent of gastric atrophy and the cellular damage at the time of eradication. The outcome of eradication should be assessed, preferably with the non-invasive tests for *H. pylori*; this is known as the test for cure. Assessment with endoscopy may be necessary in certain cases and this will need discussions between the clinical providers and patients.

Carol Ann Suda, B.S., M.T. (ASCP), S.Mt.
Updated by: Miriam E. Schwartz, M.D., M.A., Ph.D.
and Colm A. Ó'Moráin, M.A., M.D., M.Sc., D.Sc.

For Further Information

Keilberg, D. & Otterman, K. M. (2016). How *Helicobacter pylori* senses, targets, and interacts with the gastric epithelium. *Environmental Microbiology*, doi: 10.1111/1462-2920.13222. [Epub ahead of print]. This is a recent review on the mechanism of how *Helicobacter pylori* interacts with the lining of the stomach and how this bacteria affects target cells in the stomach lining. This article is available to the public and can be accessed free at http://onlinelibrary.wiley.com/doi/10.1111/1462-2920.13222/epdf

Malfertheiner, P., Megraud, F., O'Morain, C. A., Atherton, J., Axon, A. T., Bazzoli, F., ... The European Helicobacter Study Group. (2012). Management of *Helicobacter pylori* infection--the Maastricht IV/ Florence Consensus Report. *Gut,* 61(5), 646-664. This is a consensus report by 44 experts from 24 countries on the recommended management of *Helicobacter pylori* infection based on best current evidence at the time of their meeting. There were three subdivided workshops from the group's deliberations: (1) Indications and contraindications for diagnosis and treatment. (2) Diagnostic tests and treatment of infection. (3) Prevention of gastric cancer and other complications.

O'Connor, A., McNamara, D., & O'Moráin, C. A. (2013). Surveillance of gastric intestinal metaplasia for the prevention of gastric cancer. *Cochrane Database Systematic Reviews*, 9:CD009322. The authors performed a search of electronic databases to assess the utility and structure of surveillance programs for this condition and hand-searched for abstracts from relevant conferences. They found that there was lack of randomized data for this query. Given the ethical and acceptability for issues involved in randomizing surveillance, the authors recommended further non-randomized clinical studies focusing on surveillance protocols and on the role of *Helicobacter pylori* eradication that may be utilized as a more pragmatic means of preventing gastric cancer.

Smith, S. M., O'Morain, C., & McNamara, D. (2014). Antimicrobial susceptibility testing for *Helicobacter pylori* in times of increasing antibiotic resistance. *World Journal of Gastroenterology,* 20(29), 9912–9921. http://www.ncbi.nlm.nih.gov/pmc/articles/PMC4123372. This article discusses the current treatment options for *Helicobacter pylori* infection in light of the recent challenges in eradication success rapid emergence of antibiotic resistant strains of *H. pylori*. Local surveillance of *Helicobacter pylori* antibiotic resistance by susceptibility testing is also discussed as a tool to inform clinicians in their choice of therapy for treating *Helicobacter pylori* infection.This article is available to the public and can be accessed free at the web link provided.

Sugano, K., Tack, J., Kuipers, E. J., Graham, D. Y., El-Omar, E. M., Miura, S., ... Kyoto Global Consensus Conference. (2015). Kyoto global consensus report on *Helicobacter pylori* gastritis. *Gut,* 264(9), 1353–1367. http://gut.bmj.com/content/64/9/1353.long. The article contains a global consensus developed for the first time on the: (1) classification of chronic gastritis and duodenitis, (2) clinical distinction of dyspepsia caused by *Helicobacter pylori* from functional dyspepsia, (3) appropriate diagnostic assessment of gastritis and (4) when, whom and how to treat *H. pylori* gastritis. This article is available to the public and can be accessed free at the web link provided.

Other Resources

American Association for Clinical Chemistry
https://labtestsonline.org/understanding/analytes/h-pylori/tab/test

The American College of Gastroenterology (ACG)
http://www.acg.gi.org

The American Gastroenterological Association
http://www.gastro.org

Centers for Disease Control and Prevention
http://www.cdc.gov/ulcer/files/hpfacts.PDF

National Cancer Institute
http://www.cancer.gov/about-cancer/causes-prevention/risk/infectious-agents/h-pylori-fact-sheet

U.S. Department of Health and Human Services, National Institutes of Health (NIH).National Institute of Diabetes and Digestive and Kidney Diseases (NIDDK). The National Digestive Diseases Information Clearinghouse (NDDIC).Peptic Ulcer Disease and *H. pylori*. NIH Publication No. 14–4225 (August, 2014).

U.S. National Library of Medicine
https://www.nlm.nih.gov/medlineplus/helicobacterpyloriinfections.html

See also: Achlorhydria; Bacteria as causes of cancer; Gastrointestinal cancers; Hematemesis; Infectious cancers; Mucosa-Associated Lymphoid Tissue (MALT) lymphomas; Non-Hodgkin lymphoma; Pancreatic cancers; Premalignancies; Stomach cancers

▶ Hepatitis B virus (HBV)

Category: Carcinogens and Suspected Carcinogens
RoC status: Known human carcinogen since 2004

Related cancer: Liver cancer

Definition: The hepatitis B virus causes hepatitis B, a type of liver inflammation that is mainly spread through contact with blood and blood products and via sexual contact with an infected person, or carrier.

Exposure routes: Mainly spread through intimate sexual contact (50 percent) and injection drug use (15 percent), but maternal transmission (common in Asia) can occur.

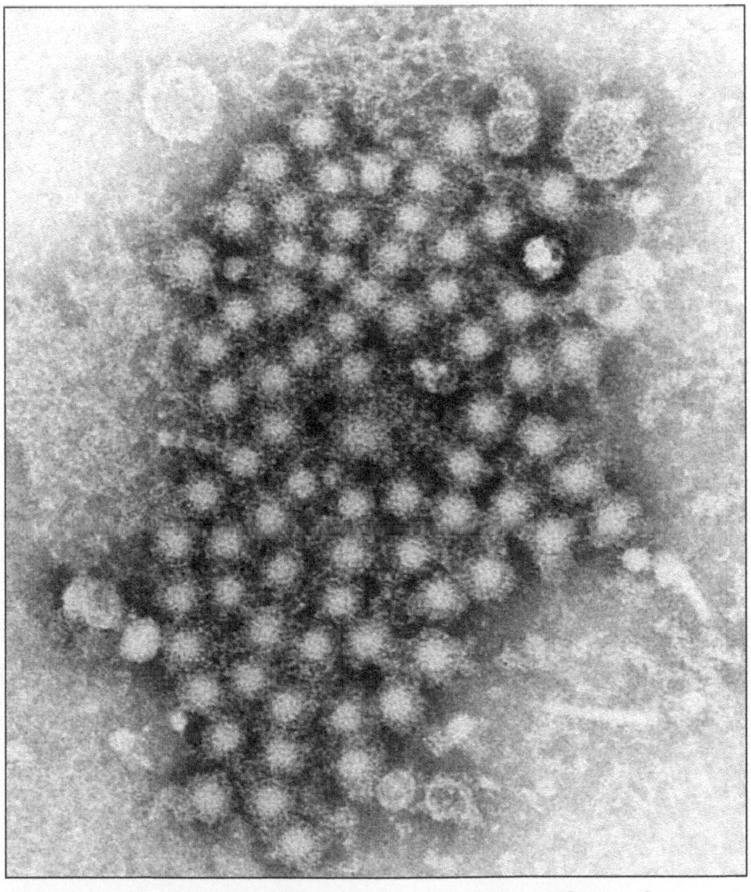

Where found: About a million people in the United States have chronic hepatitis B virus (HBV) infection. Though the incidence of chronic hepatitis B is decreasing in the United States because of a vaccine, the incidence of HBV infection has increased to 1 in 10 Americans of Asian ancestry.

At risk: Patients infected with the hepatitis B virus who are at greatest risk for liver cancer are those with cirrhosis (scarring of the liver) and a family history of liver cancer. In the United States, the highest incidence of liver cancer occurs in Asian immigrants; the frequency is lowest in whites, followed by Hispanics and African Americans. Closed environments such as prisons put people at risk. Across the globe, the vast majority of those who develop liver cancer have had the hepatitis B virus for most of their lives. However, in the United States, those with chronic hepatitis B infection mostly have contracted the infection in adulthood in association with other risk factors such as coinfection with the hepatitis C virus (HCV) or chronic alcohol abuse.

A transmission electron micrograph of hepatitis virions. (Centers for Disease Control and Prevention)

Etiology and symptoms of associated cancers: The hepatitis B virus causes hepatitis B, which can lead to chronic hepatitis B and cirrhosis, followed by liver cancer. The frequency of liver cancer can be correlated with the frequency of hepatitis B infection. It is believed that the inflammatory process involving chronic hepatitis B may be a crucial factor in the development of cancer. Most persons who are hepatitis B carriers and even those with early liver cancer may be asymptomatic. By the time symptoms do appear, liver cancer is usually inoperable. Symptoms may include jaundice, fatigue, abdominal pain and swelling, loss of appetite, nausea, vomiting, and joint pain.

History: Although hepatitis has been long known, its etiology remained a mystery until a virus found in human blood became suspect; hepatitis B virus was isolated in 1963. Discovery of a specific antigen linked to the hepatitis B virus led to development of a test to screen blood (1990), significantly reducing the incidence of post-transfusion hepatitis. A vaccine was then developed that protects against hepatitis B virus and, indirectly, against liver cancer.

Cynthia Racer, M.A., M.P.H.

See also: Aflatoxins; Ascites; Asian Americans and cancer; Bile duct cancer; CA 15-3 test; CA 19-9 test; Hepatitis C Virus (HCV); Hepatomegaly; Liver cancers; Vaccines, preventive; Viral oncology; Virus-related cancers

▶ Hepatitis C Virus (HCV)

Category: Carcinogens and Suspected Carcinogens
RoC status: Known human carcinogen since 2004
Also known as: Parenterally transmitted non-A, non-B hepatitis

Related cancers: Carcinogens known Viruses hepatitis C virus (HCV) Liver cancer (hepatocellular carcinoma) and possibly non-Hodgkin lymphoma and multiple myeloma.

Definition: The hepatitis C virus (HCV), a flavivirus, is causally related to hepatitis C, a type of liver inflammation that is mainly spread via contact with infected blood. A causal relationship has been demonstrated between HCV and liver cancer, which is usually preceded by chronic hepatitis and cirrhosis. Being a ribonucleic acid (RNA) virus, the hepatitis C virus easily mutates, making vaccine development difficult.

Exposure routes: HCV is transmitted by blood-to-blood contact with an infected individual or via blood transfusion with infected blood; rarely, maternal transmission may occur.

Where found: 150 million to 200 million people worldwide are infected with HCV. The number of acute cases of hepatitis C reported in the United States increased 20%, from 1,778 reported cases in 2012 to 2,138 reported cases in 2013.

At risk: People who have a history of injected or inhaled drug use, have been exposed to blood via sexual contact, have received a transfusion of unscreened blood, or have been exposed to contaminated instruments during tattooing, ear and body piercing, and dental procedures are at risk. People who received blood, blood products, or transplanted organs prior to 1992 (before testing of blood for hepatitis C was begun) are also at risk for HCV infection.

Health care workers are at risk from needlestick injuries. Coinfection with hepatitis D virus (HBV) or the human immunodeficiency virus (HIV) and alcohol abuse puts people at risk for chronic hepatitis C, cirrhosis (scarring of the liver), and primary liver cancer, as does having a relative with liver cancer. Much less often, HCV transmission occurs among HIV-positive persons. Also at risk are those who were ever incarcerated because of the high prevalence of hepatitis C in the prison population. Patients on long-term hemodialysis are also at risk because of the potential exposure to HCV during hemodialysis.

Etiology and symptoms of associated cancers: HCV infection causes an acute illness with a discrete onset of signs or symptoms consistent with acute viral hepatitis. Such signs and symptoms include fever, headache, malaise, anorexia, nausea, vomiting, diarrhea, and abdominal pain, and either a) jaundice, or b) elevated serum alanine aminotransferase (ALT) levels >400 IU/L. Most persons infected with HCV are asymptomatic; however, many have chronic liver disease, which can range from mild to severe.

Specific symptoms of liver cancer are usually absent until cirrhosis has occurred. Signs and symptoms of adult primary liver cancer may include a hard lump below the right side of the rib cage; right side upper abdomen discomfort; right shoulder pain, nausea, and unusual fatigue. Signs and symptoms for multiple myeloma may include bone pain and skeletal and spinal fractures; for Burkitt lymphoma, symptoms may include swollen lymph nodes, abdominal pain, tumors, weight loss, and fatigue.

History: Screening and diagnosis; Blood tests were first developed to identify the causative viruses of hepatitis B (1963) and hepatitis A (1973), but some post-transfusion blood samples proved negative for both. In the 1980's scientists identified another virus as the causative agent of "non-A, non-B hepatitis" and called it hepatitis C virus. In 1990 blood banks began screening donors for the hepatitis C virus, substantially lowering the risk of contracting post-transfusion hepatitis C.

Prognosis, prevention, and outcomes: Of every 100 people infected with hepatitis C, it is estimated that 75 to 85 will become chronically infected, liver disease will develop in 60 to 70, cirrhosis will develop in 5 to 20, and 1 to 5 will die from complications of liver disease such as cirrhosis or liver cancer. Liver cancer (hepatocellular carcinoma) is associated with cirrhosis due to chronic hepatitis C infection.

Prevention has included programs aimed at avoiding needle sharing among drug addicts. Needle exchange programs and educational interventions have reduced transmission of hepatitis C infection. However, rates of hepatitis C remain high among addicts (30% of younger users). This is primarily because the population of drug addicts is a difficult population to reach and intervene.

Among healthcare workers, safe needle-usage techniques have been introduced to reduce accidental

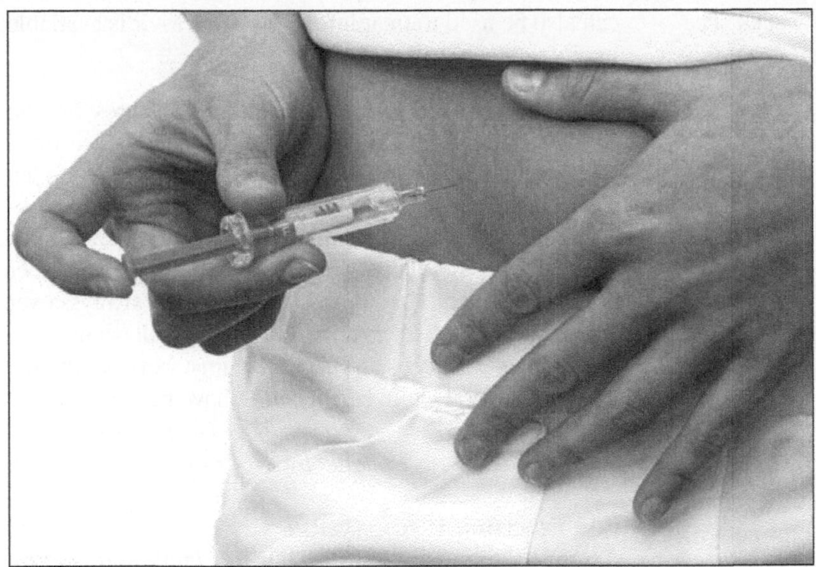

People who have a history of injected drug use are at risk for becoming infected with the hepatitis C virus. (iStock)

needle-sticks. Also newer syringes with self-capping needle systems are used to avoid the need to manually replace a cap after drawing blood which also reduces the risk of needle-sticks. There is no clear way to prevent transmission of hepatitis C from mother to child. Individuals with multiple sexual partners should use barrier precautions such as condoms to limit the risk of hepatitis C. as well as other sexually transmitted diseases. People with hepatitis C infection should avoid sharing razors or toothbrushes with others because of the possibility that these items may be contaminated with blood. Body piercing(s) or tattoo(s) should be obtained at licensed piercing and tattoo shops (facilities), while assuring the body piercing or tattoo shop uses infection-control practices. Screening tests for blood products have almost eliminated the risk of transmission of hepatitis C infection through transfusion.

Cynthia Racer, M.A., M.P.H.
Updated by: Jeffrey P. Larson PT, ATC

Other Resources

Surveillance for Viral Hepatitis – United States, 2013
CDC 1600 Clifton Road Atlanta, GA 30329-4027 USA
800-CDC-INFO (800-232-4636), TTY: 888-232-6348
Recommendations for Prevention and Control of Hepatitis C Virus (HCV) Infection and HCV-Related Chronic Disease: 2015
CDC 1600 Clifton Road Atlanta, GA 30329-4027 USA
800-CDC-INFO (800-232-4636), TTY: 888-232-6348
http://www.cdc.gov/mmwr/PDF/RR/RR4719.pdf
Hepatitis C, past or present
2012 Case Definition
CDC
1600 Clifton Road Atlanta, GA 30329-4027 USA
800-CDC-INFO (800-232-4636), TTY: 888-232-6348
http://wwwn.cdc.gov/nndss/conditions/hepatitis-c-chronic/case-definition/2012/

See also: Aflatoxins; Bile duct cancer; CA 15-3 test; CA 19-9 test; Hepatitis B virus (HBV); Hepatomegaly; Liver cancers; Viral oncology; Virus-related cancers

▶ Herpes simplex virus

Category: Carcinogens and Suspected Carcinogens; Diseases, Symptoms, and Conditions
Also known as: HSV, HSV1, HSV2
Related condition: Gingivostomatitis

Definition: Herpes simplex virus is an enveloped, double-stranded, deoxyribonucleic acid (DNA) virus that causes skin ulcers in infected persons.

Risk factors: HSV2 is sexually transmitted making sexually active adolescents and adults at risk for infection. People with weakened immune systems, such as cancer patients, are at an increased risk of recurring HSV infection and disease.

Etiology and the disease process: Herpes simplex virus 1 (HSV1), also known as oral herpes, commonly causes blisters (cold sores) and lesions on the oral mucosa (lips, throat, mouth) (herpes labialis), esophagus (herpes esophagitis), eye (herpes keratitis), face, fingers (herpes whitlow) and the central nervous system (herpes encephalitis and herpes meningitis), but it can also infect the anogenital area. Herpes simplex virus 2 (HSV2), also known as genital herpes, infects the anogenitalia area and buttocks, but can also infect the mouth and other areas.

Herpes simplex is spread through direct contact. Once a person is infected, the virus spreads to the nerve cells and remains in the body (in a latent form) for life.

The lesions in the genital area first appear red bumps but develop into watery blisters that may open, ooze fluid, and/or bleed. The lesions usually heal in seven to ten days but sometimes healing takes up to four weeks. The lesions may occasionally reappear, usually after periods of stress, fever, or overexposure to sunlight.

Cancer, human immunodeficiency virus (HIV), acquired immunodeficiency syndrome (AIDS), and the use of medications (corticosteroids) that weaken the immune system may also trigger the reappearance of symptoms.

Some studies have suggested that women infected with both herpes simplex virus and a high-risk type of human papillomavirus (HPV) have a greater likelihood of developing cervical cancer than women with HPV infection alone. However, HSV infection needs not be present for cervical cancer to develop.

Incidence: Infections with herpes simplex virus are ubiquitous and are transmitted from person to person whether or not they have symptoms. Most children will acquire an HSV1 infection during their first few years of life, usually through contact with infected saliva. In the United States, up to 90 percent of adults have antibodies to HSV1 and up to 30 percent have antibodies to HSV2.

Symptoms: HSV infections in children beyond the neonatal (newborn) period, adolescents, and adults usually have no symptoms. HSV1 may cause fever (especially during the first episode), mouth sores (fever blisters), and enlarged lymph nodes in the neck or groin. HSV2 may cause genital lesions with a burning and tingling sensation, muscle pain, vaginal discharge, and difficulty urinating.

Screening and diagnosis: HSV infections can be diagnosed by: 1) examination of the physical appearance of the skin lesions; 2) herpes culture; 3) using herpes specific antibodies [direct fluorescent antibody (DFA) test] to detect the virus; 4) screening the patient for HSV antibodies; 5) the detection of herpes DNA by the polymerase chain reaction (PCR); and 6) the Tzanck test (Tzanck smear) where the skin is scraped, fluid collected, the sample stained and microscopically examined for cells characteristic of herpes infection.

Treatment and therapy: Mild cases of the disease may not require treatment. For more severe cases, analgesics such as ibuprofen and paracetamol (acetaminophen) can be used to reduce pain and fever. Topical anesthetics including lidocaine, tetracaine, benzocaine and prilocaine can also be used to alleviate pain. Antiviral drugs such as acyclovir (Zovirax), famciclovir (Famvir), penciclovir (Denavir, Vectavir and Fenivir) and valacyclovir (Valtrex) can also be used to treat infections. Acyclovir is available in ointment and pill form.

Prognosis, prevention, and outcomes: Herpes has no cure. Recurrences, however, may be milder over time. HSV skin lesions usually heal on their own in seven to ten days, but they may take longer to heal in people with weakened immune systems. Genital HSV infection may be prevented by the use of condoms and by reducing the number of sexual partners. Condoms, however, do not always cover the whole infected area and infection may still occur.

There is no licensed vaccine against herpes simplex virus but several candidate vaccines have been studied.

Diego Pineda, M.S.

Updated by: Charles L. Vigue, Ph. D.

For Further Information

Acton, Ashton, (Ed.). (2013). *Herpes simplex virus: New insights for the healthcare professional.* Atlanta, GA: ScholarlyEditions.

Committee on Infectious Diseases, American Academy of Pediatrics. (2006). Herpes simplex. In L. K. Pickering, C. J. Baker, S. S. Long, & J. A. McMillan (Eds.), *Red Book: 2006 Report of the Committee on Infectious Diseases* (27th ed.)(pp. 361-370). Elk Grove Village, Ill.: American Academy of Pediatrics.

Diefenbach, Russell J., & Fraefel, Cornel. (Eds.). (2014). *Herpes simplex virus: Methods and protocols (Methods in molecular biology) 2014 Edition.* New York: Humana Press.

Stanberry, Lawrence. (2006). *Understanding herpes.* 2d ed. Jackson: University Press of Mississippi.

Other Resources

American Social Health Association

Herpes Resource Center.

http://www.ashastd.org/herpes/herpes_learn_treatment.cfm

Healthline

Herpes Simplex:

http://www.healthline.com/health/herpes-simplex

MedlinePlus

Herpes Simplex:

https://www.nlm.nih.gov/medlineplus/herpessimplex.html

Medscape

http://emedicine.medscape.com/article/218580-overview#a4

See also: Antifungal therapies; Cervical cancer; Epidemiology of cancer; Epidermoid cancers of mucous membranes; Gene therapy; Infection and sepsis; Vulvar cancer

▶ Herpes zoster virus

Category: Carcinogens and Suspected Carcinogens; Disease, Symptoms, and Conditions
Also known as: Varicella-zoster virus

Related conditions: chickenpox, varicella, shingles, zoster ophthalmicus

Definition: The varicella-zoster virus primary infection, which usually occurs in childhood, causes varicella or chickenpox. The virus remains dormant in nerve cells presumably held in check by the immune system. When the cell-mediated immunity wanes in later years or is impaired by disease or therapeutics, the virus re-activates and causes herpes zoster or shingles.

Risk factors: The incidence of herpes zoster increases with age (older than 50 years) and 50% of individuals living to age 85 will have experienced the disease. In the immunocompromised patient primary infection or re-activation can result in severe illness. Patients with hematologic malignancies or transplants are at high risk. Unvaccinated individuals are at risk for development of more severe varicella or herpes zoster.

Etiology and the disease process: The varicella-zoster virus is composed of an enveloped, icosahedral capsid containing double-stranded DNA. The virus is a member of the Herpesviridae family. The varicella-zoster virus produces a primary infection in childhood called varicella or chickenpox. In unvaccinated populations, 90% of children will have had chickenpox by 15 years of age. The virus then resides in sensory ganglia, particularly the trigeminal and dorsal root ganglia, in a state of latency. When age, disease, or therapeutics reduces T-cell responsiveness, the virus begins to replicate and spread.

The first signs of zoster or shingles are localized pain and increased sensation for 1 to 3 days before the vesicular rash appears in a dermatomal distribution corresponding to the area of skin supplied by the previously infected nerve. The rash never crosses the midline. The rash progresses through stages of vesicles to pustules to crusting over in about two weeks in most immunocompetent hosts. In immunocompromised patients the progression of the rash may be extended to 4 to 6 weeks. In severely compromised individuals the virus may disseminate through the bloodstream to produce a generalized rash or infect internal organs such as the liver, spleen, colon, or brain.

When the trigeminal nerve is involved, the infection can involve the eye. Vision loss is a danger and requires emergency ophthalmologic consultation for treatment. In many patients the most troublesome symptom is the pain referred to as post-herpetic neuralgia. This pain can last for months.

Symptoms: The appearance of herpes zoster is accompanied by pain in one side of the body along with tingling and a burning sensation. The skin reddens and blisters appear. The small blisters are dense and deep and later ooze and crust. Other symptoms include headache, chills, fever, abdominal pain, joint pain, lymph node swelling, hearing loss, genital lesions, vision and taste problems, and a general feeling of malaise.

In some immunocompromised patients there may be no rash. The virus rapidly invades the bloodstream spreading to internal organs. The first indication of infection may be liver failure.

Screening and diagnosis: The diagnosis of varicella-zoster virus infection is usually made clinically on the basis of a careful history and physical examination. Confirmatory tests are usually not necessary, but can be performed. Historically, the Tzanck test was used. This test involves obtaining scrapings from the base of a vesicle and after staining looking for multinucleate giant cells. Because the test has a sensitivity of only 60% and cannot distinguish between Herpes simplex and varicella-zoster viruses it has been abandoned. Vesicular scrapings can be used for direct fluorescent antibody staining and microscopic examination or PCR testing for a more accurate diagnosis. Rarely, virus may be cultured and tested for antiviral susceptibility if resistance is suspected.

Treatment and therapy: Early antiviral therapy is helpful in resolving the rash and limiting the development of post-herpetic neuralgia in the usual patient. Treatment is accomplished with oral valacyclovir (Valtrex) or famciclovir (Famvir). In the case of disseminated, more severe disease, prompt therapy with intravenous acyclovir is necessary. Rarely, resistant strains of varicella-zoster are encountered and can be treated with cidofovir or foscarnet.

Pain and itching associated with the rash are controlled with analgesics and antihistamines, respectively. Postherpetic neuralgia can be difficult to treat, but gabapentin (Neurotin) and pregabalin (Lyrica) have been used successfully.

Prognosis, prevention, and outcomes: Usually herpes zoster lesions heal within two to three weeks after the first signs appear. Patients, especially the elderly, may experience temporary or permanent weakness or paralysis or may develop a nerve pain that lasts for years. If the eyes are involved, the person may become blind if not treated. In the immunocompromised patient the illness can be more prolonged and of greater severity, but it is rarely fatal.

Patients with varicella or zoster are considered infectious until all of the skin lesions have resolved. Immunocompetent patients with herpes zoster require only contact precautions, while all other varicella-zoster infected patients require both airborne and contact precautions.

Zoster vaccine is a live, attenuated virus vaccine (Oka strain) that is recommended for children and adults without evidence of immunity in a two dose schedule. The vaccine is 75-90% effective in prevention of symptomatic illness and 95% effective in preventing severe disease. A single dose of the vaccine is recommended for all immunocompetent adults over 50 years of age. The vaccine should not be administered to any immunocompromised patients, such as patients with cancer or transplants. Antiviral drugs can be effectively used to prevent disease in immunocompromised patients exposed to varicella. Additionally, varicella immune globulin (VariZIG) may be given.

Diego Pineda, M.S.
Updated by: H. Bradford Hawley, M.D.

For Further Information

Jorgensen, J., Pfaller, M., Carroll, K., Funke, G., Landry, M., Richter, S., & Warnock, D. (Eds.). (2015). *Manual of Clinical Microbiology,* 11th ed. Washington, DC: ASM Press.

Goldman, Lee, & Schafer, Andrew L. (Eds.). (2015). *Goldman-Cecil Medicine*, 25th ed. Philadelphia, PA, Saunders.

Strasfeld, L., & Chou, S. (2010). Antiviral drug resistance: Mechanisms and clinical implications. *Infectious Disease Clinics of North America* 24(2): 413-437.

Other Resources

Centers for Disease Control - Vaccines and Immunizations; Varicella (Chickenpox) Vaccination
www.cdc.gov

See also: Paraneoplastic syndromes; Viral oncology; Virus-related cancers

▶ HER2/neu protein

Category: Carcinogens and Suspected Carcinogens
Also known as: Human epidermal growth factor receptor 2, ERBB2, ErbB2, HER-2, HER2

Related cancer: Breast cancer

Definition: HER2/neu (human epidermal growth factor receptor 2) is one of four members of the epidermal growth factor receptor family. It is a receptor that is present normally on the outer membranes of cells. Certain growth factors are responsible for activation of these receptors, triggering them to send proliferation signals to the cell. However, HER2/neu is often overexpressed in various cancers such as breast cancer. This is typically because a genetic alteration in the HER2/neu gene causes an increase in HER2/neu receptors on the cell surface. Overexpression of the receptor causes cells to divide more rapidly, increases their mobility, and increases their invasive potential. For this reason, HER2/neu overexpressing cells are more likely to form aggressive cancers.

Exposure routes: Overexpression is typically caused by a genetic alteration in the HER2/neu gene.

Where found: HER2/neu protein is a receptor tyrosine protein kinase. It is a product of the *ERBB2* (*Erb-B2*) gene which is also referred to as *HER2* (human epidermal growth factor receptor 2), *NEU* (named for a rodent neural tumor), and *HER2/neu*. The protein is found in normal cells of the human body.

At risk: Overexpression of *HER2* (*ERBB2*) occurs in about 15 to 30 percent of breast cancers. It also commonly occurs in uterine, ovarian, and stomach cancers.

Etiology and symptoms of associated cancers: HER2/neu-positive breast cancers are characteristically more aggressive, have poorer prognosis, poorer response to chemotherapy and higher recurrence. Several targeted treatments have been developed for breast cancers with HER2/neu overexpression and have been shown to increase survival rates when combined with chemotherapy. These treatments include Herceptin (trastuzumab), Kadcyla (ado-trastuzumab emtansine), and Perjeta (pertuzumab). They can also significantly reduce the risk of recurrence in women with HER2/neu-positive tumors.

Symptoms of breast cancer include any change in the size or shape of the breast, change in the look or feel of the breast or nipple, or any lumps or thickening in or near the breast or underarm area. Other more obvious changes include nipple discharge, tenderness, inverted nipple, ridges, or pitting of the breast.

History: Epidermal growth factor receptors were first identified as potential oncogenes in the early 1980's. A mutated form of the receptor was shown by researchers to link cell-growth signals to cancer. Discovery of similar oncogenes led to identification of *HER2/neu*, which was quickly found to be overexpressed in breast cancer patients and correlated with metastatic and aggressive forms of the disease. Testing for *HER2/neu* overexpression is standard for any newly diagnosed invasive carcinoma. One test is fluorescence in situ hybridization (FISH, sometimes referred to as in situ hybridization ISH) which functions to measure the number of genes that code for HER2/neu. Another test is immunohistochemistry (IHC), which measures the amount of HER2/neu protein expressed on the surfaces of cancer cells.

Terry J. Shackleford, Ph.D.
Updated by: Charles L. Vigue, Ph. D.

For Further Information

Bazell, Robert. (1998). *Her-2: The Making of Herceptin, a Revolutionary Treatment for Breast Cancer*. New York: Random House.

Yu L, Wang Y, Yao Y, Li W, Lai Q, Li J, … Yang J. (2014). Eradication of growth of HER2-positive ovarian cancer with trastuzumab-DM1, an antibody-cytotoxic drug conjugate in mouse xenograft model. *International Journal of Gynecological Cancer,* 24(7): 1158-1164.

Other Resources

V-ERB-B2 Avian Erythroblastic Leukemia Viral Oncogene Homolog 2; ERBB2. Online Mendelian Inheritance of Man.
http://www.omim.org/entry/164870.

ERBB2. Genetics Home Reference.
http://ghr.nlm.nih.gov/gene/ERBB2.

See also: Breast cancers; Carcinomas; Endometrial cancer; Family history and risk assessment; Immune response to cancer; Monoclonal antibodies; Neuroendocrine tumors; Oncogenes; Pathology; Proto-oncogenes and carcinogenesis; Receptor analysis; Tubular carcinomas; Tumor markers

▶ HIV/AIDS-related cancers

Category: Diseases, Symptoms, and Conditions; Carcinogens and Suspected Carcinogens
Also known as: AIDS-associated Kaposi sarcoma

Related conditions: Kaposi sarcoma (KS), lymphoma, progressive multifocal leukoencephalopathy (PML)

Definition: The immunodeficiency associated with advanced human immunodeficiency virus (HIV) disease can give rise to a variety of cancers. HIV infection does not appear to cause cancer directly, though some researchers have suggested HIV is capable of altering the regulation of certain types of oncogenes.

The most common cancer related to acquired immunodeficiency syndrome (AIDS) is Kaposi sarcoma, a form of the disease that arises from cells of mucous membranes or tissues lining lymphatic vessels. Other types of cancers observed more frequently among HIV-positive individuals include progressive multifocal leukoencephalopathy (PML), which results from the activation of a human papovavirus; non-Hodgkin lymphoma; and squamous cell carcinomas. A variety of other forms of tissue-specific cancers, including those of the liver and lung, are also observed with greater frequency among AIDS patients.

Risk factors: Intravenous drug users and hemophiliacs, as well as those who engage in unprotected sex (especially with multiple partners), are at high risk of contracting HIV. The form of cancer that is likely to develop as a result of HIV infection is a function of the means of transmission of the virus. Kaposi sarcoma is associated with transmission through sex and is found primarily in gay men. Other forms of AIDS-related cancers are the result of immunosuppression, in particular the reduced level of CD4+ T-lymphocyte helper cells, and are not limited to those who became infected with HIV through sexual means.

Etiology and the disease process: Both Kaposi sarcoma and progressive multifocal leukoencephalopathy have a

A Snapshot of AIDS Worldwide, 2007

HIV-Infected People	
Total	33.2 million
Adults	30.8 million
Women	15.4 million
Children under age 15	2.5 million
Deaths	
Adults	1.7 million
Children under age 15	330,000
New Cases	
Total	2.5 million
Adults	2.1 million
Children under age 15	420,000

Source: AIDS Epidemic Update, World Health Organization, December, 2007

viral etiology. Since Kaposi sarcoma is most commonly found in gay men rather than among HIV-positive hemophiliacs or in populations of intravenous drug abusers, HIV researchers long suspected it was a sexually transmitted disease with a viral etiology. In 1994, a newly discovered agent, later termed human herpesvirus 8 (HHV-8), was determined to be the cause of HIV-related Kaposi sarcoma. While the virus is relatively common, it appears to replicate in the white cell population of immunosuppressed individuals, eventually triggering the development of Kaposi sarcoma. The increased diagnosis of Kaposi sarcoma in people with an immune system weakened by mechanisms other than AIDS lends support to the hypothesis.

The induction of Kaposi sarcoma in AIDS patients appears to result from an interaction between the two viruses, HIV and HHV-8. Among the gene products produced by HIV is a transactivation protein, TAT, which acts to induce endothelial cell growth. HHV-8 in turn encodes a number of cytokines that likewise stimulate cell division within the skin. At the same time, angiogenesis factors are produced that induce blood-vessel production within the developing tumor. The result is a substantial blood supply that produces the purplish lesions common in Kaposi sarcoma. The fact that Kaposi sarcoma is more common in men than in women suggests that hormonal factors may also play a role in the process.

Several forms of lymphomas, either non-Hodgkin lymphomas (NHL) or, less commonly, Hodgkin disease, as a group represent the second most common type of AIDS-related cancers. Although a viral etiology is suspected for some lymphomas, including Hodgkin disease, the actual cause of these illnesses has yet to be firmly established. In some cases, the underlying cause has been shown to be mutations of certain oncogenes.

Progressive multifocal leukoencephalopathy is caused by a member of the human papovavirus family, the Jamestown Canyon virus, carried by many individuals within the central nervous system. Disease associated with the virus is rare, limited almost entirely to persons with a defective immune system. The means of activation of this virus is unclear.

Incidence: Approximately 40 percent of persons with advanced HIV disease will develop cancer. The most common form is Kaposi sarcoma, developing in some 20 percent of HIV-infected persons. Before the onset of the AIDS epidemic in the 1970's, the incidence of Kaposi sarcoma within the population of the United States was about 0.3 per 100,000 people. The incidence peaked nationally at 8.9 per 100,000 by the end of the 1980's, with the incidence as high as 32 per 100,000 in cities such as San Francisco. Since then, Kaposi sarcoma numbers have decreased, the result of the introduction of antiretroviral therapy as well as in the decrease in numbers of individuals newly infected with HIV. In San Francisco, for example, the incidence of Kaposi sarcoma had dropped to a level of 2.8 per 100,000 by the year 2000. The number of people affected by Kaposi sarcoma remains high in areas of the world such as Africa and Asia, where HIV infection remains common and treatment is minimal.

As with Kaposi sarcoma, the incidence of lymphomas showed a significant increase in the 1980's as a result of the AIDS epidemic. The incidence of non-Hodgkin lymphomas rose from a level of 10.7 per 100,000 in the mid-1970's to a peak of 31.4 per 100,000 in the mid-1990's. The introduction of antiretroviral therapy as well as a leveling and reduction in the numbers of new cases of HIV infection resulted in a decline of such lymphomas to 21.6 per 100,000 by the end of the twentieth century.

About 5 percent of HIV-positive persons are estimated to develop progressive multifocal leukoencephalopathy. The actual incidence is unclear because diagnosis is often made during autopsy, resulting in a likely underreporting of the precise number.

Symptoms: Kaposi sarcoma associated with AIDS is a particularly aggressive form of the disease. A spreading purplish lesion is often the first indication of Kaposi sarcoma, particularly if the individual has been determined to be HIV-positive. Lymphomas usually begin as lumps or tumors in lymph nodes, with confirmation based on biopsy. Evidence for progressive multifocal leukoencephalopathy is symptomatic, based on evidence of neurological deterioration: mental disturbances, ataxia, and loss of speech, sight, and other senses.

Screening and diagnosis: A preliminary diagnosis of Kaposi sarcoma is most commonly based on the appearance of purplish lesions. A histological examination of biopsy material is used to confirm the diagnosis. The staging system for Kaposi sarcoma differs from that for other cancers that define a stage based on the size or metastasis of the cancer. Staging of Kaposi sarcoma attempts to take into account the extent of immunosuppression as well as the characteristics of the sarcoma by using three criteria: the size or extent of the tumor (T), the level of CD4 cells (I), and the extent of illness (S). Each category has two subgroups, defined as 0 (good risk) or 1 (poor risk).

Diagnosis of the type of non-Hodgkin lymphoma is based on identification of the "appropriate" cell from biopsy material. Staging is based on the Ann Arbor system:

- Stage I: Cancer is limited to a single site or organ and has not spread.
- Stage II: Cancer is limited to two lymph node groups or organ in the same region but has begun to spread.
- Stage III: Cancer is in two lymph node groups with possible involvement of an organ.
- Stage IV: Cancer has spread beyond the initial site.

Treatment and therapy: Since development of AIDS-related cancer is the result of the immunosuppression that follows HIV infection, any form of chemical treatment is carried out in conjunction with reversal, even if temporary, of the immunosuppressive state. Treatment of the immunosuppressive state involves a combination of drug cocktails—highly active antiretroviral therapy (HAART)—that do not cure the disease but may inhibit replication of the virus for varying periods of time.

Treatment of Kaposi sarcoma depends on the extent of the cancer, including whether metastasis has taken place. If the cancer is localized, radiation or surgery may be sufficient, such as Kaposi sarcoma localized to the skin or mouth. However, Kaposi sarcoma frequently develops at multiple sites or has already spread by the time of diagnosis, requiring the use of anticancer chemotherapeutic agents such as doxorubicin, daunorubicin, or paclitaxel. Among the more promising forms of chemotherapy are those that inhibit angiogenesis, the formation of blood vessels. Combinations of therapy that include drugs to enhance the immune response are also being tested.

Treatment of non-Hodgkin lymphoma also depends on reducing the viral load and restoring a level of immune function. Following HAART, radiation or chemotherapy is the preferred treatment. Generally chemotherapy uses a combination of drugs—cyclophosphamide, hydroxydoxorubicin/doxorubicin, vincristine (Oncovin), and prednisone (CHOP protocol)—as well as selective combinations. Other treatments have adapted forms of immunotherapy in conjunction with chemotherapy, including the use of monoclonal antibodies.

Treatment of progressive multifocal leukoencephalopathy is problematic and historically has involved the direct infusion of drugs into the brain. However, HAART treatment, if successful, frequently results in the spontaneous remission of the disease.

Prognosis, prevention, and outcomes: The prognosis for AIDS-related Kaposi sarcoma patients is a function of the extent of spread. If the tumor has been caught early and immune function has improved, the recovery rate is high. Once the disease has spread, however, the chances for recovery become increasingly poor.

The likely prognosis of non-Hodgkin lymphoma is based on the International Prognostic Index, which takes into account factors such as age, the stage of the disease, and the extent of overall general health, including the state of immunosuppression. If all factors are optimal, especially the level of immune function, approximately 75 percent of patients survive five years or more.

Prognosis in progressive multifocal leukoencephalopathy patients remains poor. Before the development of HAART, 90 percent of patients died within three months of diagnosis. Even in the presence of therapy, the mortality rate remains approximately 50 percent within several months of diagnosis.

Richard Adler, Ph.D.

For Further Information

Cockerell, Clay, and Alvin Friedman-Kien. *Color Atlas of AIDS*. Philadelphia: W. B. Saunders, 1996.

Feigal, Ellen, et al., eds. *AIDS-Related Cancers and Their Treatment*. New York: Marcel Dekker, 2000.

Pelengaris, Stella, and Michael Khan, eds. *The Molecular Biology of Cancer*. Malden, Mass.: Blackwell, 2006.

Stine, Gerald. *AIDS Update: 2007*. New York: McGraw-Hill, 2007.

Other Resources

The Body: The Complete HIV/AIDS Resource
Cancer in the HIV-Infected Population
http://www.thebody.com/content/art16834.html

National Cancer Institute
Kaposi Sarcoma Treatment
http://www.cancer.gov/cancertopics/pdq/treatment/kaposis/patient

National Organization for Rare Diseases
Progressive Multifocal Leukoencephalopathy
http://www.rarediseases.org/search/rdbdetail_ abstract.html?disname=Progressive%20Multifocal%20 Leukoencephalopathy

See also: Africans and cancer; Anal cancer; Anoscopy; Antiviral therapies; Blood cancers; Bone cancers; Castleman disease; Cervical cancer; Developing nations and cancer; Dry mouth; Epstein-Barr Virus; Gastrointestinal cancers; Hepatitis C virus (HCV); Herpes simplex virus; Hodgkin disease; Immunoelectrophoresis (IEP); Infectious cancers; Kaposi sarcoma; Leiomyosarcomas; Leukoplakia; Lymphomas; Medical marijuana; Merkel cell carcinomas (MCC); Moles; Night sweats; Oncogenic viruses; Organ transplantation and cancer; Pneumonia; Poverty and cancer; Proteasome inhibitors; Proto-oncogenes and carcinogenesis; Risks for cancer; Squamous cell carcinomas; Statistics of cancer; Viral oncology; Virus-related cancers

▶ Hormone Replacement Therapy (HRT)

Category: Carcinogens and Suspected Carcinogens
RoC status: Some forms of estrogen have been known human carcinogens since 1985, while other forms have been known human carcinogens since 2002; progesterone has been a reasonably anticipated human carcinogen since 1985.
Also known as: Menopausal hormone therapy, estrogen replacement therapy

Related cancers: Breast and uterine cancers, possibly ovarian, testicular, and prostate gland cancers

Definition: Hormone replacement therapy (HRT) involves administration of estrogen alone or estrogen in combination with progesterone. Estrogen is a general term for any number of sex hormones, including estradiol, the main estrogen produced by the body, and estriol and estrone, which are products of estradiol metabolism. Progesterone is another sex hormone, which often opposes estrogen in action. Progestin is a general term for progesterone or other substances that have the same effect as progesterone.

Exposure routes: Estrogen and progesterone, whether naturally occurring in the body or inhaled, ingested, injected, or absorbed through the skin, travel through the bloodstream. They are then absorbed by estrogen-dependent cells or metabolized by the liver for final excretion in urine and stool.

Where found: Estrogen and progesterone are found in many animal fluids and tissues, including milk and meat, as well as many plants, including palm kernel oil. The estrogen most often used in HRT is extracted from the urine of pregnant mares. Estrogens and progesterones are also used commercially in skin and hair products in low concentrations. The most likely route of excessive exposure is use of prescribed HRT in oral, dermal, or vaginal preparations.

At risk: Women who use HRT are at greatest risk. Workers in facilities where prescription estrogen and progesterone products are made can be also exposed through inhalation or skin contact.

Etiology and symptoms of associated cancers: Prolonged or excessive estrogen exposure causes estrogen-dependent cells to divide more rapidly than normal. Overexposure to estrogen can damage chromosomes or alter gene expression in estrogen receptor cells. Estrogen receptors are proteins within cells that bind to estrogen and stimulate production of certain tissue cells, including breast, ovarian, and uterine lining cells. Overexpression of estrogen receptors causes increased cell division and deoxyribonucleic acid (DNA) replication, which increases the chance for mutations and causes tumor growth. The mechanism by which progesterone is associated with cancer is not known, but many studies have shown that injection of progesterone in animals causes tissue overgrowth and tumor formation in the uterine lining, the breast, and other reproductive tissues.

The cancers that are known to result from HRT include breast cancer (lobular more than ductal) and endometrial, or uterine, cancer. At least one study has shown a causal relationship between HRT and ovarian cancer, but other studies have had conflicting results. The most common symptom of breast cancer is a lump or mass in the breast. Some breast cancers present as calcifications in breast ducts, with no mass. These are usually discovered on mammography. Uterine cancer is slow growing and is often found on imaging studies of the abdomen ordered for vaginal bleeding in a postmenopausal woman or for other symptoms not related to the cancer.

History: Estrogen is a hormone naturally produced by the ovaries, placenta, testes, and adrenal glands. It regulates development of secondary sex characteristics, such as breast development and body hair distribution, and is important in the growth and functioning of all reproductive organs as well as bones. It regulates brain processes associated with reproduction, including mood and interest in sex. One of its most important functions is maintaining the lining of the uterus and preparing the body for pregnancy.

Progesterone is produced by the ovaries in adult women and by the placenta during pregnancy. It is also produced by the adrenal glands and, like estrogen, is found in many body tissues and fluids. Progesterone is essential in the thickening and vascularity of the uterine lining that allow the fertilized ovum to implant and grow during pregnancy. Both hormones are used in oral contraceptives.

Estrogen, alone or with progestin, has been prescribed for menopausal women to relieve unpleasant side effects of menopause and was once thought to prevent heart attacks and retard aging. Progestins are prescribed, among other reasons, to regulate the menstrual cycle and prevent miscarriage.

HRT use flourished in the 1960's and 1970's until researchers started noticing a marked increase in the incidence of endometrial, or uterine lining, cancer in women treated with estrogen replacement therapy. The results of one of the first studies to make the connection were published in 1975 in the *New England Journal of Medicine* by D. C. Smith and colleagues, who found a 4.5 times greater risk of endometrial adenocarcinoma in postmenopausal women being treated with estrogen alone. Many other studies followed, and conjugated estrogen, a mixture of naturally occurring estrogens, was listed as a known carcinogen in 1985. Other studies, including a Swedish study by I. Persson and colleagues published in the *British Medical Journal* in 1989, found that estrogen therapy in combination with progestins did not increase the risk of endometrial cancer, so combination therapy came into common use, with an estimated 40 million prescriptions in the United States in 1992. By 1999, studies were showing an increased risk for breast cancer in patients using estrogen alone or combination (estrogen-progestin) therapy.

The definitive study for the association of breast cancer and HRT was the 1991 Women's Health Initiative, a U.S. government-sponsored research study consisting of clinical trials and an observational study, which included trials on more than 16,000 postmenopausal women using estrogen alone or combination therapy. The combination therapy part of the study was stopped in 2002, after nearly six years of research, because the findings showed the risks of combined HRT to be greater than the benefits. The study found that the incidence of breast cancer increased and that the risk increased with the duration of HRT. The estrogen-alone part of the study was stopped in 2004 because data indicated an increased risk of stroke in patients taking estrogen supplements. Estrogen-alone therapy did not increase the risk of breast cancer in the study population.

Use of HRT dropped significantly after the Women's Health Initiative results were published, as did the incidence of breast cancer. Some researchers thought the drop was a direct result of less use of HRT. Other studies concluded that the decrease in the incidence of breast cancer began four years before the Women's Health Initiative results were announced and that the decrease in the incidence of breast cancer was more likely to be a result of fewer women getting mammograms. Mammograms were part of the required follow-up for women getting HRT, and it is ironic that many women may have stopped getting mammograms because of decreased medical care that resulted from stopping HRT. This could have delayed detection of breast cancers.

Studies of HRT continue, but the consensus seems to be that women who need HRT for relief of menopausal symptoms should receive therapy in the lowest effective dose for the shortest period of time needed. Estrogen therapy was shown in the Women's Health Initiative to be effective in treatment of osteoporosis, or thinning of bone tissue, but its use is recommended only for patients who are not candidates for other treatments. HRT is no longer recommended for prevention of coronary artery disease. The benefits of HRT include a decreased risk of colorectal cancer and osteoporosis and relief of troublesome menopausal symptoms. Patients in need of HRT should discuss options with their physicians, who will weigh the benefits and risks of treatment for each patient.

Cathy Anderson, R.N., B.A.

For Further Information

Lacey, J. V., et al. "Menopausal Hormone Therapy and Ovarian Cancer Risk in the NIH-AARP Diet and Health Study Cohort." *Journal of the National Cancer Institute* 98, no. 19 (2006): 1397-1405.

Li, C. I., et al. "Changing Incidence Rate of Invasive Lobular Breast Carcinoma Among Older Women." *Cancer* 88, no. 11 (2000): 2561-2569.

Persson, I., et al. "Risk of Endometrial Cancer After Treatment with Oestrogens Alone or in Conjunction with Progestogens: Results of a Prospective Study." *British Medical Journal* 298, no. 6667 (January 21, 1989): 147-151.

Stefanick, M. L., et al. "Effects of Conjugated Equine Estrogens on Breast Cancer and Mammography Screening in Postmenopausal Women with Hysterectomy." *Journal of the American Medical Association* 295, no. 14 (2006): 1647-1657.

U.S. Department of Health and Human Services, Public Health Service, National Toxicology Program. *Eleventh Report on Carcinogens*. Research Triangle Park, N.C.: Author, 2005.

Other Resources

American College of Obstetrics and Gynecology
http://www.acog.org

International Agency for Research on Cancer
http://www.iarc.fr/index.html

MayoClinic.com
Hormone Therapy: Is It Right for You?
http://www.mayoclinic.com/health/hormone-therapy/WO00046

National Institutes of Health
Menopausal Hormone Therapy Information
http://www.nih.gov/PHTindex.htm

See also: Adjuvant therapy; Aging and cancer; Amenorrhea; Androgen drugs; Antiestrogens; Biological therapy; Birth control pills and cancer; Breast cancers; Diethylstilbestrol (DES); Endocrine cancers; Endometrial cancer; Estrogen Receptor Downregulator (ERD); Estrogen-receptor-sensitive breast cancer; Fertility drugs and cancer; Gynecologic cancers; Hormonal therapies; Hormone receptor tests; Hot flashes; Hypercoagulation disorders; Hysterectomy; Ovarian cancers; Phytoestrogens; Pregnancy and cancer; Progesterone receptor assay; Receptor analysis; Tumor markers

▶ Human growth factors and tumor growth

Category: Carcinogens and Suspected Carcinogens
Also known as: Mitogens, cytokines

Definition: Growth factors are naturally occurring proteins that act as signaling molecules between cells and participate in the control of cell growth and cellular differentiation. Most growth factors stimulate proliferation of different cell types, but some are involved in inhibition of cell growth or even cause target cells to undergo apoptosis.

Classification of growth factors and their receptors is as follows:

- Platelet-derived growth factor family (PDGF, CSF-1, M-CSF, SCF)
- Vascular endothelial growth factor family (VEGF)
- Epidermal growth factor family (EGF)
- Fibroblast growth factor family (FGF)
- Insulin family: Insulin-like growth factors (for example, IGF-I, IGF-II)
- Hepatocyte growth factor (HGF)
- Neurotrophin family (for example, NGF, TRK family)
- Ephrin family (EPH): a subfamily of receptor tyrosine kinases, RTK
- Agrin family
- GDNF family
- Angiopoietins
- Discoidin domain receptors
- Orphan receptors

Related cancers: Multiple endocrine neoplasia type 2, leukemias, breast cancers, colon carcinoma

Where found: Naturally in the body

At risk: No specific risk group

Etiology and symptoms of associated cancers: Binding of a growth factor to its cell-surface receptor triggers an intracellular signal transduction pathway leading to changes in gene expression. The receptors of many growth factors have intrinsic proteintyrosine kinases in their cytosolic domains, which transmit the growth signal by phosphorylating tyrosine residues on themselves or on one or more target proteins, thus initiating a cascade of events. Several types of mutations lead to overproduction of constitutively active receptors, which transmit growth signals in the absence of the normal ligands.

Tumors need nourishment by blood vessels to continue growing. Many tumors produce growth factors, called "transforming" or "tumor" growth factors (TGFs), that stimulate the growth of blood vessels (angiogenesis). Basic FGF, TGFα, and VEGF have angiogenic properties and are secreted by many tumors. Growing of the tumor increases the probability of new harmful mutations. Availability of blood vessels also facilitates metastatic processes.

Some growth factors like TGFβ have the ability to inhibit the growth of many cell types, including most epithelial and immune system cells. Loss of TGFβ-mediated growth inhibition contributes to the development and progression of a variety of tumors. The TGFβ signaling pathway is also connected to expression of extracellular matrix proteins, such as collagen, a lack of which may contribute to metastasis.

History: NGF and EGF were the first growth factors to be discovered and characterized in the beginning of the 1950's by Rita Levi-Montalcini and Stanley Cohen through the testing of growth-promoting extracts of animal tissues. In the following decades, other growth factors were isolated and characterized.

Nicola E. Wittekindt, Dr.Sc. (ETH Zürich)

See also: Angiogenesis; Angiogenesis inhibitors; Aplastic anemia; Beckwith-Wiedemann Syndrome (BWS); Breast cancers; Cancer biology; Colony-Stimulating Factors (CSFs); Craniosynostosis; Cytokines; Endometrial cancer; Gene therapy; HER2/neu protein; Immune response to cancer; Interleukins; Myelofibrosis; Neuroendocrine tumors; Obesity-associated cancers; Oncogenes; Pituitary tumors; Receptor analysis

▶ Human Papillomavirus (HPV)

Category: Carcinogens and Suspected Carcinogens
RoC status: Known human carcinogen since 2004

Related cancers: Cervical cancer, anogenital cancers (anus, vulva, vagina, penis), oropharangeal cancers

Definition: Human papillomaviruses (HPVs) are a group of more than 170 related DNA viruses. They are called papillomaviruses because some cause warts (verrucae), or papillomas, which are benign (noncancerous) tumors. HPV is spread by casual skin-to-skin contact with an infected person. HPV infection is the most commonly sexually transmitted infection (STI) where over forty HPV types are sexually transmitted. Types 6 and 11 cause about 90% of genital warts. Several HPV types are linked to cervical cancer where types 16 and 18 are thought to cause over 99% of cervical cancer. About 79 million Americans are infected with HPV. Every year, HPV causes about 470,000 cases of cervical cancer world-wide.

Exposure routes: Sexually transmitted (genital-genital contact, oral-genital contact, and sexual intercourse), skin-to-skin contact

Where found: Genitalia and skin

At risk: Sexually active people, especially those with multiple sexual partners

Etiology and symptoms of associated cancers: Most HPV infections cause no symptoms and are and are cleared by the immune system within weeks or months. Some people, however, may develop a persistent infection, which, depending on the type, may lead to genital warts or cancer. A woman with a persistent infection with high-risk types of HPV may show precancerous changes on Pap smears. These precancerous changes can lead to carcinoma in situ (localized cervical cancer), which may progress to invasive cervical cancer if not treated.

History: In the 1990's, several researchers noted that virtually all women with cervical cancer were infected with HPV.

In 2006, Gardasil (Merck and Company), a vaccine which protects against both infection and the cancer caused by HPV types 6. 11, 16 and 18, was approved by the FDA. It is recommended that all boys and girls 11 years and older be vaccinated. Gardasil 9 was approved by the FDA in 2014 and protects against 9 HPV types (6, 11, 16, 18, 31, 33, 45, 52, and 58).

In 2014, the FDA approved cobas manufactured by Roche Molecular Systems, Inc. as a primary screen for 14 HPV types associated with cervical cancer.

Diego Pineda, M.S.
Updated by: Charles L. Vigue, Ph. D

For Further Information

DeVita, Vincent. T & DeVita-Raeburn, Elizabeth. (2015). *The death of cancer: After fifty years on the front lines of medicine, a pioneering oncologist reveals why the war on cancer is winnable--and how we can get there.* New York: Sarah Crichton Books.

Dixon, Danielle. (2014). *Cervical cancer causes, symptoms, stages & treatment guide: Cure cervical cancer with a positive outlook.* Seattle, WA: Amazon Digital Services.

Löwy, Ilana. (2011). *A woman's disease: The history of cervical cancer.* New York: Oxford University Press.

Perth, Danial. (2013). *HPV and men.* Seattle, WA: Amazon Digital Services.

Other Resources

Centers for Disease Control and Prevention
Gynecologic Cancers.
http://www.cdc.gov/cancer/cervical/basic_info/risk_factors.htm.

Human Papilloma Virus (HPV).
http://www.cdc.gov/std/hpv/stdfact-hpv.htm.

National Cancer Institute
HPV and Cancer.
http://www.cancer.gov/about-cancer/causes-prevention/risk/infectious-agents/hpv-fact-sheet.

Medscape
Human Papilloma Virus.

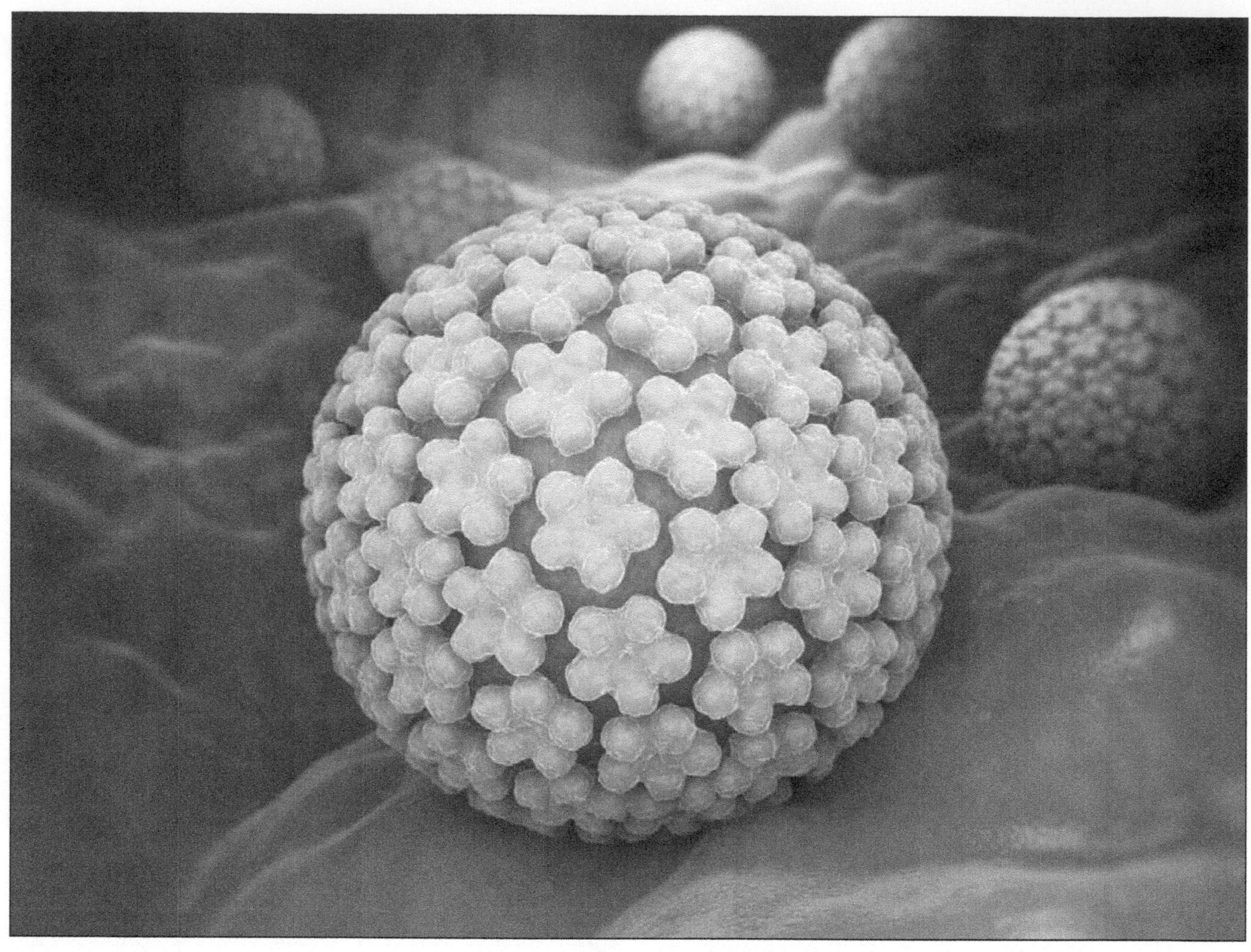

Human papillomavirus. (iStock)

http://emedicine.medscape.com/article/219110-overview.

U. S. Food and Drug Administration
Human Papilloma Virus (HPV).
http://www.fda.gov/ForConsumers/ByAudience/ForWomen/ucm118530.htm.

See also: Anal cancer; Antiviral therapies; Birth control pills and cancer; Carcinoma of Unknown Primary origin (CUP); Cervical cancer; Developing nations and cancer; Epidemiology of cancer; Epidermoid cancers of mucous membranes; Gynecologic cancers; Head and neck cancers; Herpes simplex virus; Immune response to cancer; Infectious cancers; Lip cancers; Metastatic squamous neck cancer with occult primary; Oncogenes; Oncogenic viruses; Oral and oropharyngeal cancers; Pap test; Penile cancer; Pregnancy and cancer; Prevention; Throat cancer; Urethral cancer; Urinary system cancers; Vaccines, preventive; Vaginal cancer; Viral oncology; Virus-related cancers; Vulvar cancer

▶ Human T-cell Leukemia Virus (HTLV)

Category: Carcinogens and Suspected Carcinogens
Also known as: Human T-lymphotropic virus, adult T-cell lymphoma virus; HTLV-1 may also be called human T-cell lymphotropic virus type 1 or adult T-cell lymphoma virus type 1

Related cancers: T-cell leukemia, T-cell lymphoma

Definition: Human T-lymphotropic virus is a retrovirus grouped into four separate species: Human

T-lymphotropic virus 1, 2, 3, or 4. Although HTLV-2, 3, and 4 are found in humans, they have not yet been clearly identified as the causative agent for a specific disease. However, infection with the HTLV-1 virus may result in adult T-cell lymphoma, adult T-cell leukemia, loss of spinal nerve function, eye damage that may lead to blindness, infectious dermatitis, and other inflammatory disorders.

Exposure routes: Sexual transmission, breast-feeding, blood transfusions, intravenous drug use

Where found: The HTLV-1 virus is endemic in Japan and central Africa, It is also present in South America, parts of the southeastern United States, Melanesia, Papua New Guinea, and the Caribbean basin.

At risk: Worldwide, approximately 15 million people are infected with the HTLV-1 virus. In Japan alone, more than 1 million people carry the virus, resulting in 800 leukemia cases each year. The prevalence rate in the United States is uncertain, but intravenous drug users are at special risk, with infection rates reaching an alarming 50 percent in some areas.

Etiology and symptoms of associated cancers: T cells are central to cell-mediated immunity. Originating in the bone marrow, T cells mature in the thymus, where they acquire surface markers allowing them to distinguish self from nonself. The HTLV-1 virus takes up residence by infecting a subset of the T cells called CD4+ helper cells. Once there, they grow continuously, turn on specific genes, and evolve into leukemic cells that spread throughout the body. The resulting leukemia is classified as acute, lymphomatous, chronic, or smoldering. The acute and lymphomatous forms have a poor prognosis, with survival rates averaging less than one year. There is no standardized treatment.

History: Following interspecies transmission, this virus diverged from its simian prototype about 50,000 years ago in Africa. Discovered in 1977 as the causative agent for adult T-cell leukemia, this virus was the first identified human retrovirus. In 1980 Robert C. Gallo and Bernard J. Poiesz confirmed the virus's infectivity, resulting antibody response, and presence in a patient with T-cell cancer.

Richard S. Spira, D.V.M.

See also: Acute Lymphocytic Leukemia (ALL); Acute Myelocytic Leukemia (AML); Antifungal therapies; Cutaneous T-Cell Lymphoma (CTCL); Cyclin-dependent kinase inhibitor-2A (*CDKN2A*); Genetics of cancer; Infectious cancers; Leukemias; Mycosis fungoides; Oncogenic viruses; Proto-oncogenes and carcinogenesis

▶ Ionizing radiation

Category: Carcinogens and Suspected Carcinogens
RoC status: Known human carcinogens include X radiation and gamma radiation (since 2004), neutrons (since 2004), radon (since 1994), and thorium dioxide (since 1981)
Also known as: Gamma radiation, X radiation

Related cancers: Lung, bone, bone marrow (leukemia), thyroid, breast, liver, skin

Definition: Ionizing radiation is energy released from the disintegration of unstable atomic nuclei during radioactive decay. This type of radiation may originate from X radiation or the emission of various subatomic particles from both natural and artificial sources. Some substances decay at faster rates than others and are more or less stable than others.

Exposure routes: Inhalation, ingestion, direct external exposure

Where found: Ionizing radiation is both naturally occurring and artificially produced. It is found in radon (55 percent) and in the earth. Nonnatural sources include military weapons, nuclear reactors, and electronic products. Technologically enhanced naturally occurring radioactive materials (TENORMs) concentrate ionizing radiation in solid sludge, water treatment facilities, aluminum oxide reactions, fertilizers, coal ash, concrete aggregates, diagnostic medical procedures, cable insulation, security screening equipment, and equipment used to kill microorganisms in food.

At risk: Children, pregnant women, industry workers, medical personnel, military personnel, residents in high background radiation areas

Etiology and symptoms of associated cancers: Ionizing radiation, regardless of the source, damages deoxyribonucleic acid (DNA, the genetic material) inside cells. The damage can be chromosomal breaks, cell mutations, and actual cell transformation. The consequences of this damage range from immediate cell death to transformation into cells that become malignant over time. The ability of ionizing radiation to kill cells explains its use to treat many cancers. Cancer cells divide more rapidly and are more vulnerable to radiation. Thus, ionizing radiation has the ability, when the trajectory of the beam is focused on a tumor, to shrink tumors by killing cells.

Immediate symptoms of exposure vary according to the type of particle, the dose, the length of exposure, and the route of exposure. Radiation sickness, or acute radiation syndrome, results from immediate excessive high-dose exposure. Whole body penetration damages the cardiovascular and central nervous systems. The blood pressure will drop (hypotension), and the brain will swell. Nausea, vomiting, convulsions, and confusion will follow. Death is inevitable when exposure is greater than 3,000 rads.

History: In 1896 Henri Becquerel presented his discovery of radioactivity in Paris at the Academy of Sciences. During the 1900's scientists Marie and Pierre Curie, Dmitry Mendeleyev, and Wilhelm Conrad Röntgen defined the properties of ionizing radiation. Many of the scientists working with ionizing radiation died as a result of their exposures. In 1970 the Environmental Protection Agency started regulating ionizing radiation.

Janet R. Green, M.S.P.H.

See also: Acoustic neuromas; Afterloading radiation therapy; Astrocytomas; Ataxia Telangiectasia (AT); Blood cancers; Bone cancers; Bone scan; Brain and central nervous system cancers; Brain scan; Carcinomas; Carcinomatosis; Electromagnetic radiation; Endotheliomas; Hemangiopericytomas; Hemangiosarcomas; Imaging tests; Leukemias; Magnetic Resonance Imaging (MRI); Malignant tumors; Meningiomas; Mesenchymomas, malignant; Mutagenesis and cancer; Myelodysplastic syndromes; Myelofibrosis; Nijmegen breakage syndrome; Nuclear medicine scan; Radiation oncology; Radionuclide scan; Radiopharmaceuticals; Radon; X-ray tests

▶ Melphalan

Category: Carcinogens and Suspected Carcinogens
RoC status: Known human carcinogen since 1980
Also known as: Alkeran

Related cancers: Acute leukemia

Definition: Melphalan is a highly toxic anticancer drug that belongs to a family of drugs known as alkylating agents. It is a derivative of nitrogen mustard.

Exposure routes: Orally or by intravenous injection as part of medical treatment. Skin contact or dust inhalation is possible during the manufacturing process and in handling of the drug during preparation and administration.

Where found: Used in the treatment of various cancers including multiple myeloma and ovarian and breast cancer

At risk: People who have been previously treated with melphalan alone or in association with other chemotherapy drugs; health professionals (nurses, pharmacists, physicians) who handle the drug during preparation, administration, and cleanup; workers involved in the manufacturing process. The general population is not considered to be at risk.

Etiology and symptoms of associated cancers: Melphalan is used to treat cancer but can itself cause a secondary cancer as a long-term side effect. It is a cytotoxic drug that affects the growth of cancer cells by interfering with the deoxyribonucleic acid (DNA) within the cells. It is the damage to cellular DNA that can lead to a secondary cancer months or years after treatment with melphalan. Studies of melphalan (and other alkalating agents) indicate that the risk of secondary leukemia increases with the cumulative dose and chronicity of treatment. In one study, the ten-year cumulative risk of developing acute leukemia or myeloproliferative syndrome after melphalan therapy was 19.5 percent for cumulative doses ranging from 730 to 9,652 milligrams (mg). In this same study, as well as in an additional study, the ten-year cumulative risk of developing acute leukemia or myeloproliferative syndrome after melphalan therapy was less than 2 percent for cumulative doses under 600 mg. However, there is no known cumulative dose below which there is no risk of developing a secondary malignancy. The symptoms of secondary acute leukemia include recurrent infections, bone and joint pain, swollen lymph nodes, and shortness of breath.

History: The nitrogen mustards were developed as a derivative of sulfur mustard gas, which was first used as a weapon of war in 1917. Observation of military personnel exposed to sulfur mustard showed that it lowered the white blood cell count. Drugs derived from nitrogen mustard, such as melphalan, were introduced into the clinical setting in 1946.

Melanie Hawkins, B.S.N., R.N., O.C.N.

See also: Hyperthermic perfusion; Multiple myeloma

▶ Mineral oils

Category: Carcinogens and Suspected Carcinogens
RoC status: Known human carcinogen since 1980
Also known as: Petroleum distillate, untreated and mildly refined oils

Related cancers: Skin cancers, particularly squamous skin cell cancers of the scrotum, as well as stomach, bladder, pancreatic, large intestine, rectal, mouth, throat, and lung cancers

Definition: Mineral oils include lubricant-based oils and other products derived from them. They are insoluble in water and are composed of complex mixtures of aliphatic hydrocarbons, naphthenics, and aromatics. Among those that are considered to be most carcinogenic are the polycyclic aromatic hydrocarbons (PAH), particularly benzopyrene, as well as nitrosamines, chlorinated paraffins, long-chain aliphatics, sulfur, N-phenyl-2-naphthylamine, and formaldehyde.

Exposure routes: Mineral oils can be absorbed directly through dermal contact, via inhalation, and by ingestion of substances containing or contaminated with untreated or mildly treated mineral oils.

Where found: Minerals are found at industry work sites and in the environment because about two billion liters of used (and potentially contaminated) lubricating oils are released every year. At least 750 million of these are used as road oil or in asphalt.

At risk: These commonly in contact with mildly treated or untreated mineral oils include workers in the metal, glass, newspaper printing, and automobile and airplane manufacture, and cotton and jute spinning industries.

Etiology and symptoms of associated cancers: Mineral oils generally cause skin cancers by dermal contact, resulting in red, swollen, and possibly painful marks or tumors on or beneath the skin. Stomach and pancreatic cancers often cause abdominal pain. Bladder, large intestine, and rectal cancers, often caused by ingestion of harmful levels of mineral oils, effect excretion of waste, making urination or excretion painful. Cancers of the mouth, throat, and lung are generally caused by inhalation or ingestion of toxic substances in mineral oils. First symptoms are flulike or coldlike irritation of breathing passages, which progressively increases to the point at which breathing and speaking are affected, eventually severely.

History: Mineral oils are used as a base in the manufacture of many types of refined lubricant oils. These refined oil products are then used in construction work, metalwork, manufacturing diesel oils, and mining. Nearly half of the lubricating oils are used in automobile manufacturing and operation. These include engine oils, transmission oils, lubricating oils for gears, bearing oils, and transmission fluids. Highly refined and purified white mineral oils are used for certain medicinal, food, and pharmacological purposes.

Most of the studies on mineral oils as carcinogens have involved relationships between cancers and metalworkers in the West Midlands district of the United Kingdom. Case studies revealed an excess incidence of skin cancers in these metalworkers as well as higher levels of gastrointestinal and bladder cancers. Similarly, studies of cancer incidence in printing occupations have shown increased incidence of and mortality related to a variety of respiratory cancers, including buccal cavity, pharyngeal, and lung cancers.

Results from a number of animal studies show similar relationships. For example, mice treated with repeated application of mineral oils directly to the skin had dramatically increased incidence of skin cancer. Similar applications of mineral oils to rabbits and rhesus monkeys produced tumors typically associated with the skin.

Despite these concerns, mineral oils are still widely used in the United States and elsewhere across the globe and are for sale everywhere. Roughly 85 percent of the manufactured mineral oil products are used for lubricants, another 12 to 14 percent are used as aromatic oils, and the remaining are produced for greases. Finally, refined mineral oils are still an important component of many industries in which lubricants are necessary.

Dwight G. Smith, Ph.D.

See also: Carcinogens, known; Lung cancers; Occupational exposures and cancer; Pancreatic cancers; Rectal cancer; Skin cancers; Squamous cell carcinomas; Stomach cancers; Throat cancer

▶ Mustard gas

Category: Carcinogens and Suspected Carcinogens
RoC status: Known human carcinogen since 1980
Also known as: HD, senfgas, sulfur mustard, blister gas, s-lost, lost, Kampfstoff LOST, yellow cross liquid, yperite

Related cancers: Cancers of the larynx, pharynx, upper respiratory tract, and lungs

Definition: Mustard gas is a member of the sulfur mustards, which are blister-inducing agents (vesicants). Mustard gas is actually a liquid at room temperature that is clear to yellow or brown in color and is either odorless or smells like garlic, onions, or mustard. Mustard gas was originally introduced as a chemical weapon during World War I and has been used throughout the world since then. It is a powerful irritant that damages the eyes and respiratory tract and causes large blisters on exposed skin.

Exposure routes: Inhalation and dermal contact

Where found: Used during chemical warfare attacks and in research laboratories.

At risk: Military personnel or civilians exposed to mustard gas during chemical warfare attacks, workers who manufacture it, and people who live near stockpiles of it or come into contact with unexploded ordnances loaded with it

Etiology and symptoms of associated cancers: Because mustard gas often has no odor, people are unaware that they have been exposed to it until the onset of symptoms, which usually begin two to twenty-four hours after exposure. Symptoms include redness, itching, yellow blistering of the skin, pain, swelling and tearing of the eyes, runny nose, sneezing, hoarseness, shortness of breath, sinus pain, bloody nose, cough, abdominal pain, diarrhea, fever, nausea, and vomiting. More severe exposures can cause second-to-third-degree burns of the skin, light sensitivity in the eyes or severe pain and blindness, chronic respiratory disease, and death.

Mustard gas is an alkylating agent that chemically alters the nitrogenous bases in deoxyribonucleic acid (DNA). Alkylation of DNA damages it and generates mutations but can also cause chromosome breakage. Mustard-gas-induced mutations cause either cell death or transformation into a tumor cell. Therefore, mustard gas is a confirmed carcinogen in humans and animals, and exposure to it increases a person's risk for respiratory and lung cancer.

Some 25 percent of all people who get lung cancer show no symptoms, but normally, the symptoms include cough, shortness of breath, wheezing, chest pain, and coughing up blood (hemoptysis). Nonspecific symptoms include weight loss, weakness, fatigue, depression, and mood changes. The spread of the cancer decreases lung capacity, and patients die because they are unable to inspire sufficient quantities of oxygen.

History: During World War I, the German army first used mustard gas in July, 1917, against British soldiers near the Belgian city of Ypres. Since then, mustard gas has been used globally, but sporadically, in modern warfare.

Epidemiological studies from the 1970's and 1980's established that soldiers and production workers exposed to mustard gas for longer periods of time showed an increased risk of respiratory cancers.

The Geneva Protocol of 1925, which was modified and extended the Chemical Weapons Convention of 1993, prohibits the development, production, and stockpiling of chemical weapons, which includes mustard gas.

Michael A. Buratovich, Ph.D.

See also: Alkylating agents in chemotherapy; Carcinogens, known; Chemotherapy; Laryngeal cancer; Lung cancers; Melphalan; Nasal cavity and paranasal sinus cancers; Oral and oropharyngeal cancers

▶ 2-Naphthylamine

Category: Carcinogens and Suspected Carcinogens
RoC status: Known human carcinogen since 1980
Also known as: 2-Aminonaphthalene, beta-naphthylamine

Related cancers: Bladder cancer

Definition: 2-Naphthylamine, an aromatic amine, is a yellowish crystalline solid that turns purplish-red in air and has an ammoniacal odor.

Exposure routes: For the general public, exposure to 2-naphthylamine comes from inhalation of emissions from burning organic matter that contains nitrogen. Two primary sources are coal furnaces and tobacco smoke. Occupational exposure occurs through inhalation by laboratory personnel doing research with 2-naphthylamine.

Where found: 2-Naphthylamine is used only in laboratory research. It is still found in some dyes and rubber compounds that were manufactured before 1974. It is a by-product of tobacco smoke and coal burning and is an impurity found in commercially produced 1-naphthylamine.

At risk: Scientists and laboratory technicians who work where 2-naphthylamine is used in research as a catalyst or an antioxidant have a high risk for 2-naphthylamine contamination. Because 2-naphthylamine is generated in tobacco smoke, people who smoke are at high risk for contamination. The general public is at risk for contamination from secondhand tobacco smoke and from the burning of organic matter that contains nitrogen, such as coal.

Etiology and symptoms of associated cancers: When 2-naphthylamine is metabolized, it can be activated by liver enzymes to form adducts with blood-serum proteins, such as hemoglobin. In some cases, 2-naphthylamine can undergo additional metabolism to form reactive compounds that are transported to the bladder, where they bind to deoxyribonucleic acid (DNA) molecules. In experimental laboratory animals, 2-naphthylamine DNA adducts have been found in the bladder and in the liver. In laboratory tests on cultured human cells, 2-naphthylamine caused genetic damage that involved DNA strand breaks, changes in chromosome structure or number, addition or deletion of chromosomes, and cell transformation.

History: 2-Naphthylamine was commercially produced in the United States from the early 1920's until the early 1970's. It was used in the production of sulfonic acids, red-dye stuffs, and agrochemicals, and as a catalyst and an antioxidant in the vulcanization of rubber. After the International Agency for Research on Cancer (IARC) showed its link to the increased risk of bladder cancer, its commercial production was banned in the early 1970's. There are still a few companies in the United States that manufacture 2-naphthylamine for use in laboratory research. The last time it was imported into the United States in any significant amount was in 1967.

Alvin K. Benson, Ph.D.

See also: Bladder cancer; Carcinogens, known; Carcinogens, reasonably anticipated; Cigarettes and cigars; Occupational exposures and cancer

▶ Nickel compounds and metallic nickel

Category: Carcinogens and Suspected Carcinogens
RoC status: Metallic nickel, reasonably anticipated human carcinogen since 1980; nickel compounds, known human carcinogens since 2002
Also known as: Ni

Definition: Nickel is a silvery white, hard, malleable, and ductile metal that forms complex compounds, most often with oxygen, sulfur, iron, and arsenic. Some nickel uptake is essential to humans but more concentrated amounts can be harmful. It remains unknown exactly which forms of nickel compounds are carcinogenic, but studies show that airborne and water-soluble compounds may be most associated with cancer risk, possibly because of greater exposure.

Because nickel is widely distributed in soils, water, air, detergents, tobacco, and food, everyone is exposed to varying levels of nickel and its compounds. Food, including vegetables and chocolates, often contains larger amounts of nickel, as does tobacco. Nickel fumes or contaminants released by tobacco smoking may cause an increased risk of respiratory cancers, including those of the nose, larynx, and lungs. Contaminant levels of nickel in humans have also been linked with birth defects, including heart disorders, and have been implicated in cancerous proliferation of breast cells.

In addition to being identified in the National Toxicology Program's *Report on Carinogens* as carcinogenic, nickel compounds are classified by the International Agency for Research on Cancer (IARC) as Group 1 compounds, which are "causally associated with cancer in humans." Metallic nickel is currently classified as a Group 2B compound, or "possibly carcinogenic to humans," but will most likely be changed to category A, a known human carcinogen. Nickel and its compounds have also been identified as hazardous air pollutants in the United States' Clean Air Act.

Related cancers: Nasal, throat, lung, breast, and prostate cancer

Exposure routes: Inhalation of nickel fumes from tobacco smoke and aerosols from burning of fossil fuels; ingestion of foods, especially chocolates and vegetables

Where found: Earth has a solid core of nickel but this is far within the interior. Most soils typically contain trace amounts, which can be absorbed in plants and ingested by animals, including humans. Soil nickel and nickel compounds may be leached into water systems or wind driven and carried as nickel-contaminated dust in the atmosphere. Small amounts of nickel and its compounds also occur in the world's oceans and seas, where organisms can absorb it. It is a contaminant in coal and oil and is emitted into the atmosphere by powerplants and incinerators. Nickel compounds are also found in jewelry, other metals, and in everyday household items such as detergents.

At risk: Everyone is at some risk. Workers in smelters that process ores containing nickel, in the electroplating industry, and in steel manufacturing are at risk of higher levels of exposure to nickel and its compounds. Smoking tobacco in all its forms also exposes heavy smokers to nickel contaminants that may increase the risk of cancer.

Etiology and symptoms of associated cancers: Nasal, throat, lung, breast, and prostate cancer are all related to inhalation or ingestion of nickel compounds and metallic nickel in excess amounts. Nasal, throat, and lung cancer can affect breathing, speaking, taste, and smell. Breast cancer can be present in the form of a subdermal lump that may be painful. Prostate cancer can cause severe pain, decrease urination flow, frequency, or strength, and inhibit ejaculation.

History: Nickel and its compounds are primarily used in the preparation of alloys of steel and other metal products. For example, addition of nickel to steel, copper, and other metals produces an alloy that is stronger and more resistant to heat and corrosion. Thus, nickel is important in gas turbines and rocket engines, where strength and resistance to high temperatures are factors. Nickel alloys are also used to manufacture propeller shafts of boats and piping in desalinization plants, where resistance to corrosion is important. Nickel is also used as a key ingredient in the manufacture of rechargeable nickel cadmium batteries, coinage, and in nickel plating of jewelry and other products. Nickel wire also continues to be in demand for some industrial purposes.

Nickel and its compounds are recognized and listed as carcinogenic substances, especially in occupations in which workers are routinely exposed to nickel fumes. The Environmental Protection Agency (EPA) formally determined that nickel and its compounds, especially nickel subsulfides, are human carcinogens in 1984, and in 1990 the International Agency for Research on Cancer also listed nickel as potentially carcinogenic. Further regulations are possible pending ongoing reviews at federal and state levels.

Dwight G. Smith, Ph.D.

See also: Carcinogens, known; Carcinogens, reasonably anticipated; Head and neck cancers; Laryngeal cancer; Nasal cavity and paranasal sinus cancers; Occupational exposures and cancer; Salivary gland cancer

▶ Oncogenic viruses

Category: Carcinogens and Suspected Carcinogens
Also known as: Oncoviruses

Related cancers: Cancers of the cervix, skin, uterus, penis, nasopharynx, and liver; Kaposi sarcoma; Burkitt lymphoma; non-Hodgkin lymphoma; adult T-cell leukemia; Merkel cell carcinoma (skin), also known as neuroendocrine cancer of the skin.

Definition: An oncogenic virus is a virus that infects normal cells, alters the cells' properties, and transforms them into cancer cells. Oncogenic viruses can cause cancer in a variety of animals, including humans. These viruses can have either deoxyribonucleic acid (DNA) or ribonucleic acid (RNA) as their genetic material.

Exposure routes: Viruses, suspected oncogenic Carcinogens, Sexual, blood-to-blood contact; exchange of bodily fluids

Where found: Ubiquitous

At risk: People who are in contact with others

Etiology and symptoms of associated cancers: Etiology depends on whether the genetic material is DNA or RNA. Oncogenic DNA viruses include the Epstein-Barr virus (EBV), human papillomavirus (HPV), human herpesvirus 8 (HHV-8), hepatitis B virus (HBV), and Merkel cell polyomavirus. Oncogenic RNA viruses include the human T-cell lymphotropic viruses 1 and 2 (HTLV-1 and HTLV-2), **and** hepatitis C virus (HCV).

The Epstein-Barr virus (EBV), also known as human herpesvirus 4 (HHV-4), has been strongly linked to nasopharyngeal cancer and certain forms of Burkitt lymphoma that are endemic in central Africa. EBV is also suspected of causing some cases of Hodgkin disease. Human herpesvirus 8 (HHV-8) is linked to Kaposi sarcoma. Hepatitis B virus (HBV) and Hepatitis C virus (HCV) are linked to liver cancer. HBV may increase the risk of pancreatic cancer. Human papillomavirus (HPV) can cause various conditions from benign warts to malignant cancers such as carcinomas of the vulva, cervix, uterus, penis, anus, and throat. Although there are more than one hundred recognized types of HPV, only a few are known to cause cancer.

Upon entering a cell, viral DNA may integrate into the host genome and express its viral genes, the oncogenes, which cause tumors. Sometimes the virus integrates next to a cellular gene and causes cancer by inducing an overexpression of that cellular gene.

The RNA viruses associated with human cancers are human T-cell lymphotropic viruses 1 and 2 (HTLV-1 and HTLV-2), which cause adult T-cell leukemia and hairy cell leukemia, respectively; and hepatitis C virus (HVC).

When an RNA tumor virus enters the cell, a DNA copy of its RNA is made in a process known as reverse transcription. The DNA copy may integrate into the host genome and express the viral gene that causes cancer. Alternatively, the integrated DNA can cause cancer by inducing the overexpression of a cellular gene.

History: In 1911, Peyton Rous discovered that sarcomas in chickens were caused by viruses. By the late 1970's it had become clear that certain viruses also caused cancer in humans.

Charles L. Vigue, Ph.D.

For Further Information

Crawford, D. H., Johannessen, I., & Rickinson, A. B. (2014). *Cancer virus: The discovery of the Epstein-Barr Virus*. New York: Oxford.

Damania, B., & Pipas, J. (Eds.). (2009). *DNA tumor viruses*. New York: Springer.

Gupta, S. P. (Ed.). (2014). *Cancer-causing viruses and their inhibitors*. Boca Raton, FL: CRC Press.

Ou, Jing-hsuin James, & Yen, T. S. B. (2010). *Human oncogenic viruses*. Hackensack, NJ: World Scientific.

Other Resources

Hunt, Richard C. Oncogenic Viruses: DNA Tumor Viruses and RNA Tumor Viruses (Retroviruses). Microbiology and Immunology Online.
http://www.microbiologybook.org/lecture/retro.htm

See also: Cancer biology; Oncogenes; Proto-oncogenes and carcinogenesis; Viral oncology; Virus-related cancers

▶ Organochlorines (OCs)

Category: Carcinogens and Suspected Carcinogens
Also known as: Environmental, occupational, developmental, neuro-, and reproductive toxicants

Definition: Chlorination of hydrocarbons produces organochlorines, which are chemically stable, fatty, and toxic. OCs accumulate in fat and thus are transported via the food chain to top carnivores, including fish, birds, mammals, and humans. OCs are common contaminants of food, air, water, soil, and breast milk. They comprise diverse subgroups, members of which cause various types of health effects ranging from acutely fatal to chronically toxic over generations. Many OCs cause liver hypertrophy and cancer; neurotoxic, embryotoxic, reproductive, developmental, and immunotoxic effects; and various types of cancers in the pubescent children of exposed mothers.

OCs are produced by the chlorination of some of the petroleum hydrocarbons and can remain in the environment decades after being introduced. They are used in insecticides, fungicides, herbicides, miticides, polychlorinated biphenyls (PCBs), flame retardants, metal cleaners, dry-cleaning solvents, polyvinyl chloride (PVC) and other plastics, paints, dyes, synthetic intermediates, refrigerants, rayon and cellulose manufacturing, detergents, degreasers, disinfectants, halothanes, soft PVC surgical equipment, medicines—some eleven thousand common products contain them or use them in the manufacturing process.

The manufacture, use, and disposal of OCs create environmental and health problems. For example, for only one polymer, PVC, the downstream export of products from its synthesis amounts to 1,229 million metric tons. In another example, pulp and paper industries in North America produce 100 million tons of OCs. The waste by-products that pose the most serious health and ecosystem risks of the manufacturing process include PCBs, polychlorinated dibenzodioxins (PCDDs), polychlorinated dibenzofurans (PCDFs), and polychlorinated diphenyl ethers (PCDEs). Other notorious OCs include the pesticides dichlorodiphenyltrichloroethane (DDT) and dichlorodiphenyldichloroethylene (DDE), cyclodiene insecticides, Mirex, hexachlorobenzene, hexachlorocyclohexanes, and various solvents.

PCBs are mixtures of various congeners and isomers, which are chemically stable and viscous, with low volatility. From agriculture to office buildings, automobiles, and homes, PCBs have caused widespread contamination. Major environmental sources of PCBs include manufacturing wastes, careless waste disposal, and dumping.

Related cancers: Liver and testicular cancer

Exposure routes: Food, air, water, mother's milk

Where found: Air, water, food, breast milk

At risk: Those at highest risk for cancers associated with organochlorines (OCs) include embryos, fetuses, suckling newborns, and adults who are occupationally exposed to or living in the vicinity of the sources of release.

Etiology and symptoms of associated cancers: Organochlorines constitute one of the most diverse groups of cancer-causing chemicals considering their volume, categories of use, and persistence. OCs exert both specific and broad-spectrum effects. Out of all known effects, dioxin-like effects are the most serious cause of public concern: estrogenic effect leading to breast cancer; testosterone degradation leading to male infertility; nervous system damage leading to neurobehavioral deficits in offspring of mothers exposed to OCs; immunosuppression issues; development problems (lower birth weights, shorter gestation, birth defects); and occurrence of other types of cancers.

Both U.S. and European farmworkers exposed to OC pesticides have a six-times higher risk of getting testicular cancer. Many workers involved in the manufacture of 2,6-di-tert-butyl-p-cresol (DBPC; commonly used as a food preservative) have high OC concentrations in their bodies, low sperm count, and no children. Twenty-two OCs are endocrine disruptors, mimic estrogens (xenoestrogens), and induce an enzyme that degrades testosterone. An estimated 220 million pounds of farm pesticides per year in the United States act as xenoestrogens, which can also lead to breast cancer and other hormonal effects.

In the United States, DDE residues in women's fat can be transferred to the fetus or to a baby through breast milk and cause testicular cancer in their sons. OC effects are elevated in the womb and just after birth due to fat mobilization. Nursing infants get 4 to 12 percent of their lifetime's dioxin exposure via the intake of breast milk.

The stunning rise in breast cancer since the 1950's has been suspected to be related to only a few OCs. DDE, PCBs, and DDT are suspected of being involved in human breast cancer and are found in the fat and serum of women with breast cancer. In Copenhagen the risk of breast cancer appeared to be twice as high and aggressive in women with the highest serum concentration as compared with those with the lowest concentration of dieldrin. DDT is regarded as a possible human carcinogen, while PCBs are labeled as probable human carcinogens. PCB-180 and DDE may also be linked to non-Hodgkin lymphoma.

History: Organochlorines do occur, although very rarely, in nature, and are usually associated the high-temperature events such as forest fires and volcanoes. The use and manufacture of OCs by people started in the late 1800's. They were heavily introduced into the environment with the beginning of widespread use of pesticides, particularly DDT, in 1939.

Several billion tons of OCs have been used since World War II, and their residues are present in both humans and the environment. Rachel Carson's 1962 best seller *Silent Spring* sounded the alarm for the general public about the dangers of pesticides in the environment. Production and usage of OC pesticides started declining in the 1970's, and those suspected to be carcinogens were banned in the United States and later throughout much of the world, although some countries continued to use them. Millions of tons of OCs per year were still being produced in the early twenty-first century.

Organochlorine residues remain in the environment (air, water, land) and thus in human food and breast milk for decades. Residues of pesticides banned in the 1970's were still present in the food supply in the early twenty-first century. More OCs were targeted to be banned globally in the May, 2001, Stockholm Convention on Persistent Organic Pollutants; however, the George W. Bush administration did not ratify the treaty for the United States. Although many OCs have been banned over the years, others are still registered for use.

M. A. Q. Khan, M.D., Ph.D., and
Samreen F. Khan, M.S.

For Further Information

Colborn, T., D. Dumanoski, and J. P. Myers. *Our Stolen Future*. New York: Dutton Press, 1995.

Khan, M. A. Q., S. F. Khan, and F. Shutari. "Ecotoxicology of Halogenated Hydrocarbons." In *Encyclopedia of Ecology*. Washington, D.C.: National Council of Science and Environment, 2007.

Khan, M. A. Q., and R. H. Stanton. *Toxicology of Halogenated Hydrocarbons*. New York: Pergamon Press, 1980.

Tenenbaum, D. J. "POPS in Polar Bears: Organochlorines Affect Bone Density." *Environmenal Health Perspectives* 112, no. 17 (2004): A1011.

Thornton, J. *Environmental Impacts of Polyvinyl Chloride* (PVC) Building Materials. Washington, D.C.: Healthy Building Network, 2002.

U.S. Environmental Protection Agency. *The Effects of Great Lakes Contaminants on Human Health*. Report to U.S. Congress. EPA 95-R-95-107. Chicago: Author, 1995.

Other Resources

Department of Health and Human Services
Agency for Toxic Substances and Disease Registry
http://www.atsdr.cdc.gov

International Agency for Research on Cancer
http://www.iarc.fr/index.html

U.S. Department of Labor
Occupational Safety and Health Administration (OSHA)
Hazardous and Toxic Substances

http://www.osha.gov/SLTC/hazardoustoxicsubstances/index.html

See also: Dioxins; Pesticides and the food chain

▶ Pesticides and the food chain

Category: Carcinogens and Suspected Carcinogens
RoC status: Dichlorodiphenyltrichloroethane (DDT), reasonably anticipated human carcinogen since 1985
Also known as: Insecticides—chlorinated hydrocarbons, organophosphates, carbamates, dinitrophenols, thiocyanates, growth regulators, inorganics (arsenicals and fluorides), microbials; herbicides—amides, acetamides, carbamates, thiocarbamates, phenoxy compounds, dinitrophenols, dinitroanilines; fungicides—dicarboximides, chlorinated aromatics, dithiocarbamates, mercurials; algicides—organotins; molluscicides—chlorinated hydrocarbons; nematocides—halogenated alkanes; rodenticides—anticoagulants, botanicals, fluorides, inorganics, thioureas

Related cancers: Lymphoma, brain tumors, leukemia, cancers of the breast, skin, stomach, prostate, ovaries

Definition: Pesticides refer to any substance or mixture of substances intended for preventing, destroying, repelling, or lessening the damage of any pest. A pest is any living organism that could harm crops and people or other animals, or is in an undesirable location. Pesticides may be chemical, biological, or antimicrobial. They are released into the environment primarily through the spraying of insecticides on fruits and vegetables and other crops, such as corn, wheat, rice, and cotton, and by the use of herbicides on grass. Pesticides are believed to be responsible for a number of cancers.

Exposure routes: Ingestion, inhalation, absorption

Where found: Pesticides are found in the environment, in streams, rivers, lakes, groundwater, and the soil, including fields (where chlorophenols, particularly in the form of weed killers, build up over the years) and chemically treated lawns. DDT, banned in the United States in 1972, still exists in the soil and is stored in the fatty tissues of individuals; it may also be on products imported into the United States from countries where it is allowed.

Pesticides have entered the food chain: Chemicals from pesticides get into groundwater or streams, then into the grass and other vegetation, then into carnivorous animals and then omnivorous animals such as humans. Those animals at the top of the food chain, such as humans or scavengers, fare worse than those below them, as the buildup of toxins is much greater at the top. In the aquatic food chain, chemicals from pesticides enter agricultural runoff or wastewater, then are taken up by algae and plankton, then smaller organisms, then larger fish, and finally humans. Fish containing mercury or other chemicals can be lethal to people.

At risk: People who produce or distribute pesticides, agricultural workers and people living in close proximity to fields, people who use pesticides in and around their homes, and people who eat fish or pesticide-treated fruits and vegetables

Etiology and symptoms of associated cancers: Studies have shown that human bodies contain hundreds more chemicals—including those contained in pesticides—than they did fifty years ago. Pesticides are linked to lymphoma, a cancer of the white blood cells. Of the two kinds of lymphoma, Hodgkin disease and non-Hodgkin lymphoma (NHL), the latter is most associated with pesticide carcinogens. Non-Hodgkin lymphoma begins when a blood cell (lymphocyte) becomes malignant and subsequently produces descendants of the single cell in which mutations (errors) have occurred. Although lymphoma can occur in any part of the body, tumors typically form in the lymphatic system, meaning bone marrow, lymph nodes, the spleen, and blood. The initial symptoms are usually perceived as swelling around the lymph nodes at the base of the neck, fever, fatigue, and unexplained weight loss.

Breast cancer is linked to organochlorine pesticides, which affect the endocrine system. Absorbed through ingested foods, the pesticides mimic, alter, or modulate hormonal activity and are therefore known as endocrine disruptors. Raising the activity and quality of estrogens the human body produces causes tumors to form. Pesticides are also linked to ovarian cancer, in that malignant ovarian tumors are endocrine related and hormone dependent.

Atrazine, used on 96 percent of the United States corn crop, exists in most drinking water supplies in the Midwest and has been linked to birth defects in farmers' children. Long-term exposure to atrazine has been linked to weight loss, cardiovascular damage, retina and muscle degeneration, and cancer.

Organophosphate pesticides, which have largely replaced organochlorine pesticides, are connected with skin and eye problems, headaches, dizziness, nausea, vomiting, and abdominal pain. The thirty-seven compounds that make up this group destabilize a key enzyme in the brain known as cholinesterase, causing trauma to the brain and nervous system. Studies have related pesticide risk with respiratory problems, memory disorders, dermatologic conditions, cancer, depression, neurologic deficiencies, miscarriages, and birth defects. Primarily, these pesticides affect the nervous system by disrupting the enzyme that regulates acetylcholine, a neurotransmitter.

Definitive proof that DDT is a human carcinogen is still lacking, but it has been associated with liver, lung, and thyroid tumors.

History: More than four thousand years ago, Sumerians dusted sulfur on their crops to kill insects, and more than two thousand years ago, ancient Greeks used pesticides to protect their crops. By the fifteenth century, arsenic, mercury, and lead—highly toxic chemicals—were used on crops to eliminate insects. During the seventeenth century, farmers used nicotine sulfate, derived from tobacco leaves, as an insecticide, and in the nineteenth century, pyrethrum, extracted from chrysanthemums, and rotenone, removed from roots of tropical vegetables, were used as pesticides.

In 1939 Swiss scientist Paul Müller discovered the potency of a compound made of carbon and hydrogen called dichlorodiphenyltrichloroethane (DDT), first used in World War II against typhus, plague, malaria, and dengue and yellow fevers. After the war, DDT use in the United States soared. Farmers killed pests such as boll weevils that were devastating cotton crops, and the government used low-flying crop-dusting planes to rid the forests of gypsy moths. Other parts of the world began using DDT to combat malaria; after homes and huts were sprayed in North Africa, Asia, India, and Zanzibar, the number of malaria cases declined drastically.

In 1962 Rachel Carson published *Silent Spring*, the product of more than four years of research, in which she maintained that pesticides were harming wildlife and the environment. Using meticulous documentation, Carson claimed that the government knew little about the dangers of pesticides. Although the book was criticized as well as praised, it spurred concerns about pesticides and other pollutants, leading to the beginning of the environmental movement and President Richard M. Nixon's creation of the Environmental Protection Agency (EPA) in 1970. Soon the EPA targeted DDT, eventually banning it in 1972. Although time has proven Carson's position on the harm from pesticides to wildlife correct, the idea that DDT is a human carcinogen is still being contested.

In the years since its ban, DDT has been replaced by a huge array of insecticides, herbicides, and pesticides that have been tentatively linked with tumors and cancers of the lymphatic, endocrine, neurological, respiratory, and reproductive systems but have not been proven to to be carcinogens. Although studies have shown an increase in the rates of tumors or cancers in agricultural areas where large amounts of pesticides are used, scientific proof of the connection is inconclusive. Because of the gap in time between exposure and the first symptoms of illness (frequently decades) and the inability to pinpoint a particular pesticide as the carcinogen, definite scientific proof is hard to provide.

Nevertheless, strict regulations are in effect: The EPA must approve any pesticide for sale or use in the United States, and the Food Quality Protection Act (1996) requires the oversight of the manufacture, distribution, and use of pesticides. Although the causal relationship between pesticides and cancer is hard to establish, pesticides have other proven health risks, and many people in the United States are trying to minimize or avoid their use. The EPA provides many suggestions on how to use pesticides more safely, and some people have turned to organically grown products as a way to avoid most pesticides.

Because of the carcinogenic potential of pesticides, the organic foods industry has grown. The Organic Foods Production Act (1990) authorized national standards for the production, handling, and processing of organically grown agricultural products. Essentially, organic farming is an ecological system that avoids chemical pesticides, promotes soil conservation, and integrates the parts of the farming system into an ecological whole. Although organic farming cannot guarantee that the soil does not contain pesticide residue, the practice follows methods designed to minimize contamination from air, soil, and water. Organic meat, poultry, eggs, and dairy products come from animals that are not given any antibiotics or growth hormones. Organic food is produced without using conventional pesticides or fertilizer made from synthetic ingredients or sewage sludge. Organic farms use cover crops, green manures, animal manures, and crop rotation to manage weeds, insects, and diseases and promote biological activity and long-term soil health.

Mary Hurd, M.A.

For Further Information

Beres, Samantha. *Pesticides: Critcal Thinking About Environmental Issues*. Farmington Hills, Mich.: Greenhaven Press, 2002.

Carson, Rachel. *Silent Spring*. 1962. Reprint. Boston: Mariner Books, 2007.

Dunn, Jancie. "Toxic Overload: Teflon, Pesticides on Golf Courses, Plastic Bottles—An Explosion of Research Is Investigating Environmental Links and Breast Cancer." *Vogue*, October, 2006, 326ff.

Hemingway, Jean. "An Overview of Pesticide Resistance." *Science* 5, no. 298 (October 4, 2003): 96-97.

Izakson, Orna. "Farming Infertility: Country Living May Be Hazardous to Your Potency." *E/The Environmental Magazine* 15, no. 1 (January/February, 2004): 40-41.

Levine, Marvin J. *The Toxic Time Bomb in Our Midst*. Westport, Conn.: Praeger, 2007.

National Research Council. *Carcinogens and Anticarcinogens in the Human Diet*. Washington, D.C.: National Academy Press, 1996.

_______. *Pesticides in the Diets of Infants and Children*. Washington, D.C.: National Academy Press, 1993.

Rosenberg, Tina. "What the World Needs Now Is DDT." *The New York Times*, May 23, 2004, p. 8.

U.S. Department of Health and Human Services, Public Health Service, National Toxicology Program. *Eleventh Report on Carcinogens*. Research Triangle Park, N.C.: Author, 2005.

Wright, Karen. "Testing Pesticides on Humans." *Discover* 3, no. 12 (December, 2003): 66-69.

Other Resources

National Cancer Institute

Cancer Trends Progress Report—2007 Update: Pesticides
http://progressreport.cancer.gov/doc_detail.asp?pid=1&did=2007&chid=71&coid=713&mid=

U.S. Environmental Protection Agency

Pesticides
http://www.epa.gov/pesticides/index.htm

See also: Acrylamides; Agent Orange; Aplastic anemia; Arsenic compounds; Astrocytomas; Bisphenol A (BPA); Coal tars and coal tar pitches; Coke oven emissions; Curcumin; Dietary supplements; Diethanolamine (DEA); Dioxins; Epstein-Barr Virus; Erionite; Herbs as antioxidants; Macrobiotic diet; Neuroectodermal tumors; Non-Hodgkin lymphoma; Occupational exposures and cancer; Organochlorines (OCs); Pancreatic cancers; Premalignancies; Prevention; Richter syndrome; Risks for cancer; Vinyl chloride

▶ Phenacetin

Category: Chemotherapy and Other Drugs; Carcinogens and Suspected Carcinogens
RoC status: Reasonably anticipated human carcinogen since 1980
Also known as: Saridon, Acetophenetidin

Related cancers: Urothelial neoplasms, especially transitional cell carcinoma of the renal pelvis and bladder

Definition: Phenacetin is an analgesic and antipyretic introduced in 1887. It was linked to urothelial neoplasms, especially transitional cell carcinoma of the renal pelvis and bladder, as well as interstitial nephritis in combination with renal papillary necrosis and was removed from the market in 1983.

Exposure routes: Oral ingestion

Where found: Sold as an analgesic and antipyretic (fever-reducing) medication

At risk: All who have taken medications containing phenacetin

Etiology and symptoms of associated cancers: The cause and mechanism of the nephropathic change due to phenacetin in humans is unknown, but the renal lesion sometimes seen was interstitial nephritis in combination with renal papillary necrosis.

When administered in the diet, phenacetin caused benign and malignant tumors of the urinary tract in mice and rats of both sexes and of the nasal cavity in rats of both sexes, according to studies by the International Agency for Research on Cancer (IARC). There is limited evidence for the carcinogenicity of phenacetin in humans because this medication was usually taken mixed with other drugs.

History: Phenacetin, first introduced in 1887, was used principally as an analgesic and fever reducer. Its analgesic effects are reportedly because of its actions on the sensory tracts of the spinal cord. In addition, phenacetin acts as a negative inotrope on the heart, weakening the heart's muscular action. Phenacetin also was once used as a stabilizer for hydrogen peroxide in hair-bleaching preparations. Many case reports provided evidence that abuse of analgesic mixtures containing phenacetin resulted in kidney cancer (cancer of the renal pelvis). It was implicated in kidney disease (nephropathy) and renal papillary necrosis due to abuse of analgesics and was withdrawn from the U.S. market in 1983.

Phenacetin was first listed in the *First Annual Report on Carcinogens* (RoC; 1980), and analgesic mixtures containing phenacetin were first listed in the *Fourth Annual Report on Carcinogens* (1985).

Debra B. Kessler, M.D., Ph.D.

See also: Adenocarcinomas; Bladder cancer; Gallbladder cancer; Gastrointestinal oncology; Kidney cancer; Renal pelvis tumors; Transitional cell carcinomas; Urethral cancer; Urinary system cancers

▶ Plasticizers

Category: Carcinogens and Suspected Carcinogens

Definition: Plasticizers are chemical substances that are used as additives during the manufacture of various polymers such as polyvinyl chloride (PVC), food packaging, food storage containers, children's toys, and medical devices to impart flexibility, strength, and durability.

Types of plasticizers: A large variety of chemicals are used as plasticizers. They are classified into various categories based on their chemical structure. The most widely used plasticizers are derived from the family of dicarboxylic esters and are commonly known as phthalates: Examples include di(2-ethylhexyl) phthalate (DEHP), di-n-octyl phthalate (DOP), adipates, and maleates. Chemicals from the family of organophosphates and some glycol esters are also used as plasticizers.

Uses: Phthalates such as DEHP are predominantly used in the manufacture of PVC, which is one of the oldest polymers used to make pipes and various plastic containers. Phthalates are also used as plasticizers in medical devices such as dialysis bags, intravenous bags, and tubing. They are also used in detergents, lubricating oils, flooring materials, food-packaging materials, and storage containers.

Environmental exposure: Plasticizers are not covalently bound to the plastic matrix, and they consequently leach out when in contact with oils, fats, and other greasy substances, especially at higher temperatures. This is especially true of phthalates, which are used in food wraps and containers. Plasticizers in food wraps have been shown to migrate into and contaminate fatty foods such as meat, cheese, and oily snacks. Plasticizers are also released into the environment directly during the manufacture of plastics and from discarded plastic containers, wraps, and pipes. As plastics have myriad uses, the plasticizers in them are ubiquitous contaminants of air, water, food, and medicines. Human exposure to plasticizers is mainly through ingesting water and food contaminated with them. Infants are exposed to plasticizers when they chew or suck on plastic toys or pacifiers or drink liquids out of plastic feeding bottles. Another source of exposure is through air, in which plasticizers such as DEHP adhere to aerosol particles. Animal studies have shown that phthalates can cross the placental barrier, and therefore, this can potentially cause prenatal exposure in humans.

Toxicity and metabolism: Toxicity studies on plasticizers (especially the phthalates DEHP and DOP) have been done on rodents through various exposure routes. It has been found that the rodents metabolize phthalates readily, and the liver and kidneys are common target organs for general toxicity. The major concern about the toxicity of phthalates stems from reports from the U.S. National Toxicology Program showing several of them to be carcinogenic in rodents. The mechanism of carcinogenesis in rodents or other species is as yet unclear, and there are no clear-cut studies extrapolating the animal data to humans. Many industry groups and advocacy panels have analyzed the animal data on the toxicity of plasticizers and have failed to come to a consensus because the toxicity patterns vary greatly by species and routes of exposure. Plasticizers have been detected in breast milk and children's blood samples, but there are no studies that clearly relate childhood exposure to the risk of adult human cancers, and therefore childhood exposure to plasticizers is shrouded in controversy.

There are reports in literature that indicate that plasticizers, especially the phthalates, act as hormone disrupters. Hormones are chemical messengers produced by various glands in animals and humans that travel through the bloodstream and regulate growth, reproduction, and metabolic functions in the body. This system, known as the endocrine system, is a very finely tuned mechanism in the body, and endocrine disrupters can readily throw it off balance, creating major health and cancer risks. Young animals and children are more vulnerable to exposure to such disrupters because their systems are still in the developmental stage, so there is a great concern regarding the exposure of infants and children to phthalates.

Preventive measures: Because plasticizers are widely distributed environmental contaminants, there is a great deal of concern regarding cancer and other health risks to adult human populations as a result of exposure of infants and children to environmental endocrine disrupters. The conflicting conclusions from various animal studies and the lack of data extrapolating the animal exposure studies to human infants and adults underscore the complexity of the science. More studies delineating the toxicokinetics of plasticizers, especially in vulnerable subpopulations such as pregnant and lactating women, premature infants, and children, are needed. There are many ongoing studies to assess the risk of exposure to plasticizers and evaluate the potential of early childhood exposure in increasing the risk of cancer in adults.

The European Union has recommended banning the use of certain phthalates. Toy manufacturers are funding research to develop newer plasticizers with greater biodegradability and lower toxicity, such as alkyl citrates and esters of vegetable oils. These environmentally benign plasticizers are being developed for use in food-packaging materials, medical devices, and children's toys. With all the conflicting health and cancer risk data on plasticizers, it makes perfect sense for individuals and industry and government regulatory agencies to take reasonable steps to limit exposure to plasticizers.

Lalitha Krishnan, Ph.D.

For Further Information

Huber, W. W., B. Grasl-Kraupp, and R. Schulte-Hermann. "Hepatocarcinogenic Potential of Di(2-ethylhexyl) Phthalate in Rodents and Its Implications on Human Risk." *Critical Reviews in Toxicology* 26 (1996): 365-481.

Sissell, Kara. "States, Retailers Push to Eliminate Phthalates from Toys." *Chemical Weekly* 170, no. 12 (April 14-21, 2008): 29.

_______. "Study Links Phthalates and Infant Care Products." *Chemical Weekly* 170, no. 5 (February 11-18, 2008): 29.

Voiland, Adam. "More Problems with Plastics: Like BPA, Chemicals Called Phthalates Raise Some Concern." *U.S. News & World Report*, May 19, 2008, p. 54.

Woodward, Kevin N. *Phthalate Esters: Toxicity and Metabolism*. Boca Raton, Fla.: CRC Press, 1988.

Other Resources

Canadian Cancer Society

Phthalates

http://www.cancer.ca/ccs/internet/standard/0,3182,3172_1706523966__langId-en,00.html

National Toxicology Program

http://cerhr.niehs.nih.gov

U.S. Environmental Protection Agency

Consumer Factsheet on: Di (2-ethylhexyl) Phthalate

http://www.epa.gov/OGWDW/dwh/c-soc/phthalat.html

U.S. Food and Drug Administration

FDA Public Health Notification: PVC Devices Containing the Plasticizer DEHP

http://www.fda.gov/cdrh/safety/dehp.html

See also: Bisphenol A (BPA); Carcinogens, known; Carcinogens, reasonably anticipated; Childhood cancers; Di(2-ethylhexyl) phthalate (DEHP); Organochlorines (OCs); Risks for cancer; Vinyl chloride

▶ Polycyclic aromatic hydrocarbons

Category: Carcinogens and Suspected Carcinogens
RoC status: Reasonably anticipated human carcinogen since 1981
Also known as: Polynuclear aromatic hydrocarbons, polyaromatic hydrocarbons, PAHs

Related cancers: Lung, colon, skin, and bladder cancer

Definition: Polycyclic aromatic hydrocarbons (PAHs) refer to a group of chemicals formed from burning wood, coal, oil, gas, and other carbon-containing substances.

Exposure routes: Inhalation, ingestion, skin contact

Where found: In air (from motor vehicle exhaust, burning wood and refuse, tobacco smoke, industrial emissions, smoke from fires), contaminated water and food, meat cooked by certain high-temperature methods (such as grilling), and coal tar products used to treat skin conditions

At risk: Industrial workers in coking plants; coal tar, aluminum, iron, steel, and asphalt production plants; and petroleum refineries; as well as road construction workers, smokers, and those exposed to tobacco smoke

Etiology and symptoms of associated cancers: Polycyclic aromatic hydrocarbons are procarcinogens in that they are converted by the detoxification system in the human body to substances that can cause cancer. Such substances bind to deoxyribonucleic acid (DNA), the molecules that carry a person's genetic blueprint. Studies suggest that this binding causes changes in DNA that lead to cancer.

Some symptoms of associated cancers include shortness of breath, coughing, weight loss (lung cancer); blood in urine (bladder cancer); weight loss, blood in stools, change in bowel habits (colon cancer); change in a wart or mole, or a skin growth that may exhibit redness (skin cancer).

History: Polycyclic aromatic hydrocarbons are naturally present in the environment (such as in coal, peat, and crude oil) and are also formed artificially by various burning processes. The involvement of substances containing polycyclic aromatic hydrocarbons in causing cancer was shown in 1775 when Percival Pott, a British surgeon, described scrotal cancer in chimney sweeps who had been exposed to coal soot. Coal tar was subsequently (1915) found to induce tumors when repeatedly applied to rabbits' ears. In 1933 a specific polycyclic aromatic hydrocarbon isolated from coal tar , benzo(a) pyrene, was shown to cause skin cancer in mice. Animal studies have since shown that repeated administration of this and other polycyclic aromatic hydrocarbons to animals through skin, the air, or diet causes various types of cancer, including breast, skin, stomach, lung, and bladder cancer. Human studies have shown an association between lung, bladder, colon, and skin cancer in industry workers exposed to high levels of polycyclic aromatic hydrocarbons.

Polycyclic aromatic hydrocarbon emissions are regulated by several agencies. The Occupational Safety and Health Administration (OSHA) regulates the exposure of industrial workers to polycyclic aromatic hydrocarbons. The Environmental Protection Agency regulates the amount of polycyclic aromatic hydrocarbons released into surface waters (Clean Water Act) and the air (Clean Air Act) and present in drinking water (Safe Drinking Water Act). The Food and Drug Administration regulates the amount of polycyclic aromatic hydrocarbons in bottled drinking water.

Jason J. Schwartz, Ph.D., J.D.

See also: Air pollution; Bronchial adenomas; Carcinogens, known; Carcinogens, reasonably anticipated; Chewing tobacco; Coal tars and coal tar pitches; Coughing; Lung cancers; Mineral oils; Occupational exposures and cancer; Skin cancers; Soots; Tobacco-related cancers

▶ Radon

Category: Carcinogens and Suspected Carcinogens
RoC status: Known human carcinogen since 1994

Also known as: Radon-222, thoron (radon-220), actinon (radon-219)

Related cancers: Lung cancer

Definition: Radon is an invisible, odorless, radioactive gas produced naturally from uranium in rocks and soil. Except for areas rich in uranium-ore deposits, radon is usually present at low levels in water, soil, and outdoor air. It decays spontaneously to form solid radioactive products called radon daughters that emit ionizing radiation, mostly as alpha particles and gamma radiation. Radon gas may seep into buildings from underlying soil and accumulate at dangerous levels in indoor spaces. Its levels can be measured by using radon test kits.

Exposure routes: Inhalation, ingestion

Where found: Uranium mines and mills, hard-rock mines, phosphate mines, granite formations, groundwater, soil, air, building materials

At risk: Workers in uranium mining and milling, workers in iron-ore and fluorite mining, general population exposed to indoor radon levels of 4 picoCurie per liter (pCi/L) or higher

Etiology and symptoms of associated cancers: Radon is the second leading cause of lung cancer after cigarette smoking and accounts for 15 percent of lung cancers worldwide. Most of the risk to humans is from inhaled radon daughters that can lodge in the lungs and emit energetic particles. Damage to epithelial cells in lung tissue can eventually lead to cancer. For smokers, the risk of lung cancer is even greater because of the synergistic effects of radon and smoking.

The deadliest of all cancers, lung cancer has an overall five-year survival rate of less than 15 percent. Radon-related lung cancers include squamous cell carcinoma, adenocarcinoma, and large-cell carcinoma. In its early stages, lung cancer may be asymptomatic or have nonspecific symptoms (weight loss, fatigue, and fever). By the time symptoms develop that are suggestive of the disease (chronic coughing, shortness of breath, hoarseness, bloody sputum, difficulty swallowing, wheezing, and chest pain), the cancer has usually spread to other organs.

History: Once produced commercially for use in radiotherapy, radon is used mostly in research. Scientists established radon's carcinogenicity primarily from occupational studies conducted between the 1950's and 1980's that revealed high mortality rates from lung cancer among underground uranium miners. In 1984 exposure to radon in buildings came to be recognized as a potential health hazard. In the Indoor Radon Abatement Act of 1988, the U.S. Environmental Protection Agency (EPA) recommended that indoor radon levels not exceed average levels outdoors (about 0.4 pCi/L). This standard is one tenth of the recommended safety level for homes.

Anna Binda, Ph.D.

See also: Air pollution; Benzene; Bronchoalveolar lung cancer; Carcinogens, known; Carcinogens, reasonably anticipated; Ionizing radiation; Lung cancers; Occupational exposures and cancer; Risks for cancer

▶ Report on Carcinogens (RoC)

Category: Carcinogens and Suspected Carcinogens
Also known as: RoC

Definition: The *Report on Carcinogens* (RoC) is a U.S. government document, issued by the National Toxicology Program (NTP) of the U.S. Department of Health and Human Services (DHHS), which identifies and profiles substances that are known to cause cancer or that are reasonably anticipated to cause cancer in a significant number of persons residing in the United States. It is published every two years by the Department of Health and Human Services to comply with the Public Health Service Act, Section 301(b)(4). The first edition was published in 1980.

Content: The RoC lists substances for which there is published scientific evidence establishing a relationship between exposure to the substance and the development of cancer. The substances are categorized as "known to be human carcinogens" or "reasonably anticipated to be human carcinogens" based on human and laboratory animal studies and epidemiological studies.

The report presents information on each substance. It identifies regulations and guidelines pertaining to the substance and discusses how they decrease the risk of exposure. All substances nominated for review are included in the report with explanations of why they were included in or excluded from the list.

Review process: The process begins with a substance being nominated for review. Requests for RoC nominations are published in the Federal Registry. Sources include the public, other agencies, and reviews of scientific literature.

A nomination is reviewed by several scientific committees within the Department of Health and Human Services. These committees consider background information, additional literature searches, and public comments when making their recommendations. The secretary of the department makes the final review and approval before submitting the report to Congress.

Affiliated agencies: Agencies that are involved with the nomination and review process are the Agency for Toxic Substances and Disease Registry (ATSDR), the Consumer Product Safety Commission (CPSC), the Environmental Protection Agency (EPA), the Food and Drug Administration (FDA), the National Center for Environmental Health (NCEH), the National Institute for Occupational Safety and Health (NIOSH), the Occupational Safety and Health Administration (OSHA), the National Institutes of Health (NIH), the National Cancer Institute (NCI), and the National Institute of Environmental Health Sciences/NTP (NIEHS/NTP).

Limitations: The RoC will not include a substance if exposure is limited to a small number of people. The report does not discuss the benefits of a substance versus its risk of causing cancer. It does not provide the specific conditions under which a substance will cause cancer to develop.

The focus of the report is to present technical and scientific information—the supported facts—and not to discuss the many variables involved for cancer to develop.

Carol Ann Suda, B.S., M.T. (ASCP), S.M.

See also: Air pollution; Asbestos; Carcinogens, known; Carcinogens, reasonably anticipated; Cigarettes and cigars; Dioxins; National Cancer Institute (NCI); Occupational exposures and cancer; Pesticides and the food chain

▶ Silica, crystalline

Category: Carcinogens and Suspected Carcinogens
RoC status: Reasonably anticipated human carcinogen since 1991; known human carcinogen since 2000
Also known as: Quartz, cristobalite, tridymite, sand

Related cancers: Lung cancer is related to exposure to respirable quartz and cristobalite but not to amorphous silica.

Definition: Respirable crystalline silica, primarily quartz dusts occurring in industrial and occupational settings, is known to be a human carcinogen, based on studies in humans indicating a causal relationship between exposure to respirable crystalline silica and increased lung cancer rates in workers. Respirable crystalline silica was first listed in the *Sixth Report on Carcinogens* (RoC), published in 1991 by the National Toxicology Program of the U.S. Department of Health and Human Services, as "reasonably anticipated to be a human carcinogen" based on evidence of carcinogenicity in experimental animals; however, the listing was revised to "known to be a human carcinogen" in the *Ninth Report on Carcinogens* in 2000.

Exposure route: Inhalation

Where found: Silica sand has been used in the manufacture of glass and ceramics and in foundry castings and has been used as an abrasive in sandpaper and grinding and polishing agents. It is also found in sandblasting materials, in oil and natural gas recovery, in quarries, in water filtration for sewage treatment plants, and in the production of silicon. Cristobalite is a major component of refractory silica bricks. Extremely fine grades of silica sand known as flours may be used in toothpaste, scouring powders, metal polishes, paints, rubber, paper, plastics, wood fillers, cements, road-surfacing materials, and foundry applications. Crystalline silica is also found in tobacco products.

At risk: Quarry and granite workers as well as workers involved in the ceramic, pottery, refractory brick, and diatomaceous earth industries are most at risk.

Etiology and symptoms of associated cancers: Marked and persistent inflammation, specifically inflammatory cell-derived oxidants, may provide a mechanism by which respirable crystalline silica exposure can result in lung cancer.

History: Crystalline silica is composed of silicon and oxygen. The mineral is ubiquitous in both nature and people's daily lives. Scientists have known for decades that prolonged excessive exposure to crystalline silica dust in mining environments can cause silicosis, a lung disease. During the 1980's, studies were conducted that suggested that crystalline silica also was a carcinogen. As a result of these findings, crystalline silica has been regulated under the Occupational Safety and Health Administration's Hazard Communication Standard (HCS).

Debra B. Kessler, M.D., Ph.D.

See also: Asbestos; Bronchial adenomas; Carcinogens, known; Carcinogens, reasonably anticipated; Chewing tobacco; Lung cancers; Mesothelioma; Occupational exposures and cancer; Prevention; Tobacco-related cancers

▶ Simian virus 40

Category: Carcinogens and Suspected Carcinogens
Also known as: Simian vacuolating virus 40, SV40

Related cancers: Malignant mesothelioma, osteosarcoma, choroid plexus tumors, ependymomas, non-Hodgkin lymphoma

Definition: Simian virus 40 is a polyomavirus of the family Papovaviridae and is found in several species of monkeys.

Exposure routes: The actual route of exposure of simian virus 40 in humans is under investigation. There is speculation that millions of Americans were exposed to the virus between 1955 and 1963 during the mass immunizations with the original Salk (injectable) and Sabin (oral) polio vaccines. However, some people too young to have received the original polio vaccines have tested positive for exposure to the virus. Therefore, other routes of exposure, such as person to person, may be possible.

Where found: As a latent infection in several species of macaque monkeys; also in biomedical research labs to transform human cells or be inoculated into laboratory animals for oncology studies

At risk: People who were vaccinated with the Sabin and Salk polio vaccines between 1955 and 1963; about one hundred army camp men who were inoculated with adenovirus vaccines contaminated with simian virus 40 in the 1950's and 1960's; lab researchers working with the virus

Etiology and symptoms of associated cancers: Carcinogenesis may be induced by inactivation of cellular tumor-suppressor proteins (TP53 and RB1).

History: The virus was discovered in 1960 in the rhesus macaque kidney cells used to amplify the polio virus for the original Salk and Sabin polio vaccines. In 1961, after learning that inoculated simian virus 40 caused cancer in laboratory animals, the U.S. federal government required that new stocks of polio vaccine be free of the virus. Since then, the Salk and Sabin vaccine stocks have been produced using human or African green monkey cell lines extensively screened for viral contaminants.

The National Cancer Institute has reported that forty years of epidemiological studies in the United States and Europe have not shown increased cancer risk in people who may have been exposed to simian virus 40. However, polymerase chain reaction (PCR) testing has revealed traces of simian virus 40 in many malignant mesothelioma tumors and (in one study) 42 percent of non-Hodgkin lymphomas, among others. However, association does not mean causation, and PCR testing techniques for simian virus 40 have not been standardized. Lab contamination could also be a problem. The linkage between simian virus 40 exposure and cancer in humans is still being actively investigated.

Lisa J. Shientag, V.M.D.

See also: Adenoviruses; Carcinogens, known; Carcinogens, reasonably anticipated; Ependymomas; Hodgkin disease; Human T-cell leukemia virus (HTLV); Lymphomas; Medical oncology; Mesothelioma; Non-Hodgkin lymphoma; Oncogenes; *RB1* gene; TP53 protein; Tumor-suppressor genes

▶ Sunlamps

Category: Carcinogens and Suspected Carcinogens
RoC status: Known human carcinogen since 2000
Also known as: Ultraviolet radiation (UVR), ultraviolet A (UVA), ultraviolet B (UVB), artificial ultraviolet radiation, nonsolar ultraviolet radiation

Related cancers: Skin cancer, squamous cell carcinoma, basal cell carcinoma, nonmalignant melanoma, malignant melanoma, intraocular melanoma

Definition: Sunlamps are lamps that produce ultraviolet radiation.

Exposure routes: Through skin

Where found: Sunlamps, sunbeds, tanning salons, tanning booths, home tanning lamps

At risk: People who use artificial sources of ultraviolet radiation such as sunlamps or tanning salons

Etiology and symptoms of associated cancers: Sunlamps or other artificial sources of ultraviolet radiation are used primarily for cosmetic reasons, such as to obtain a suntan, as well as for treatment of certain medical conditions. Approximately 25 million people in the United States use sunbeds each year, with 1 to 2 million people visiting tanning facilities as often as one hundred times a year. Teenagers and young adults, usually female, use sunlamps most often.

Epidemiological studies report that exposure to sunlamps increases the risk of skin cancer. A person's risk of skin cancer is related to lifetime exposure to ultraviolet (UV) radiation, with greater incidence observed with increasing duration of exposure, especially in those using sunlamps before the age of thirty and in those who readily sunburn. Ultraviolet radiation from sunlamps can affect all skin types, but people with fair skin that freckles or burns easily, a skin type generally associated with red or blond hair and light-colored eyes, are at greater risk.

Sunlamps increase the risk of skin cancer because they involve exposure to ultraviolet radiation. Although ultraviolet radiation emissions vary substantially according to the device, the radiation exposure can be similar to or greater than that from the sun. Depending on the frequency of use, commonly used sunlamps deliver several times the annual ultraviolet A dose. Newer indoor tanning units may emit ultraviolet A and ultraviolet B radiation at levels as much as fifteen times greater than solar ultraviolet radiation. Ultraviolet radiation damages deoxyribonucleic acid (DNA) in skin cells, which can lead to skin cancer.

Skin cancers that have been associated with use of a sunlamp include basal and squamous cell carcinomas as well as melanoma. Most basal cell and squamous cell skin cancers can be cured if found and treated early. Both basal and squamous cell skin cancers occur on parts of the skin frequently exposed to the sun, such as the face. Basal cell carcinoma grows slowly and rarely spreads to other parts of the body. Squamous cell carcinoma is more aggressive and sometimes spreads to lymph nodes and organs inside the body.

Although much less prevalent than other types of skin cancer, melanoma is the most serious. Melanoma occurs in pigment cells in the skin called melanocytes. When melanoma becomes cancerous, it can become invasive and spread to other parts of the body. When melanoma starts in the skin, it is called cutaneous melanoma. Melanoma may also occur in the eye and is then called ocular melanoma or intraocular melanoma.

Not all skin cancers look the same, but a change on the skin is the most common sign of skin cancer. Some skin changes that may occur include a new growth, a sore that does not heal, a change in an existing growth, or red or brown spots that are rough, dry, and scaly. Melanoma usually begins in a mole, with the first symptom typically a change in size, shape, or color of an existing mole or the appearance of a new mole. Melanomas vary in their appearance, but most melanomas have a black or blue-black area and usually appear abnormal or "ugly looking."

History: Sunlamps have been used for many years to treat a range of skin conditions, vitamin D deficiency, and neonatal jaundice. Sunlamps have also been used increasingly for cosmetic tanning in commercial salons or at home. Ultraviolet emissions from artificial tanning devices have changed over time. Before the mid-1970's, sunlamps were primarily used in the home, except for medical use, and mostly emitted ultraviolet B and with a small amount of ultraviolet C. In the early 1980's sunlamps that emitted ultraviolet A radiation were developed and used mainly at commercial tanning salons. Sunlamps in use in the twenty-first century emit mostly ultrlaviolet A radiation and some ultraviolet B radiation.

The U.S. Food and Drug Administration (FDA) Center for Devices and Radiological Health developed regulations concerning ultraviolet lamps in sunlamps that specify requirements for performance, protective eyewear, and labeling, and require tanning salons to post warnings about the dangers associated with exposure to artificial ultraviolet radiation. The American Medical Association, the American Academy of Dermatologists, and the Centers for Disease Control and Prevention have all issued statements discouraging the use of sunlamps for nonmedical purposes.

Catherine J. Walsh, Ph.D.

For Further Information

Chen, Y. T., et al. "Sunlamp Use and the Risk of Cutaneous Malignant Melanoma: A Population-Based Case-Control Study in Connecticut, USA." *International Journal of Epidemiology* 27 (1998): 759-765.

Gallagher, R. P., J. J. Spinelli, and T. K. Lee. "Tanning Beds, Sunlamps, and Risk of Cutaneous Malignant Melanoma." *Cancer Epidemiology Biomarkers and Prevention* 14, no. 3 (2005): 562-566.

Swerdlow, A. J., et al. "Fluorescent Lights, Ultraviolet Lamps, and Risk of Cutaneous Melanoma." *British Medical Journal* 297 (1988): 647-650.

U.S. Department of Health and Human Services, Public Health Service, National Toxicology Program. *Eleventh Report on Carcinogens*. Research Triangle Park, N.C.: Author, 2005.

Other Resources

American Academy of Dermatology
http://www.aad.org

Centers for Disease Control and Prevention
Skin Cancer
http://www.cdc.gov/cancer/skin/

National Cancer Institute
What You Need to Know About Skin Cancer
http://www.cancer.gov/cancertopics/wyntk/skin

National Toxicology Program
FDA Radiological Health Program
http://www.fda.gov/cdrh/radhealth/products/sunlamps.html

See also: Basal cell carcinomas; Electromagnetic radiation; Melanomas; Moles; Skin cancers; Squamous cell carcinomas; Ultraviolet radiation and related exposures; Young adult cancers

▶ Thiotepa

Category: Carcinogens and Suspected Carcinogens
RoC status: Known human carcinogen since 1998
Also known as: TESPA, triethylenethiophosphoramide, TSPA, thio-TEPA

Related cancers: Leukemia

Definition: Thiotepa is a colorless or white crystalline solid that is odorless.

Exposure routes: Some cancer patients are exposed to thiotepa when it is used as a chemotherapy treatment. It is typically administered intravenously. It may be injected into muscle tissue, directly into a tumor, or through a catheter into a body cavity. Potential exposure by direct contact can occur to workers who are involved in the formulation, packaging, preparation, and administration of thiotepa for use in chemotherapy treatments.

Where found: Thiotepa is found at sites where it is manufactured, packaged, and supplied. It can be found at medical facilities where it is prepared and administered during cancer treatments. During the 1970's it was found in some polymeric flame retardants for cotton and in some insecticides.

At risk: Patients who are treated with thiotepa for various cancers, including bladder cancer, ovarian cancer, breast cancer, bronchial cancer, mesotheliomas, and lymphomas, are at high risk. Workers at locations where thiotepa is manufactured, packaged, and supplied for chemotherapy treatments are at risk for contamination. Health care professionals who prepare and administer thiotepa for cancer therapy risk contamination.

Etiology and symptoms of associated cancers: Thiotepa is an alkylating agent that slows or stops the growth of cancer cells in the human body. It can induce deoxyribonucleic acid (DNA) damage, changes in chromosome structure or number, addition or deletion of chromosomes, and cell transformation. It can also control the accumulation of fluids in body cavities that results from various cancers. Side effects of thiotepa chemotherapy include low white and red blood cell counts, decrease in platelets, hair loss, mouth sores, loss of appetite, tightness of the throat, nausea and vomiting, hives, rash, bladder irritation, and painful urination.

History: Thiotepa was first used in cancer therapy treatment of lymphomas and malignant tumors in 1953. Between 1970 and 1978, a link was established between the secondary development of leukemia and exposure to thiotepa. In the *Second Report on Carcinogens* (RoC; 1981), it was listed as a highly probable human carcinogen. By the 1990's, it was produced only in Japan. In the *Eighth Report on Carcinogens* (1998), thiotepa was listed as a known human carcinogen. To a large extent, it has been replaced by nitrogen mustard gas derivatives for chemotherapy treatments. It is still used in combination with other chemotherapy drugs for lymphomas and for bladder, ovarian, breast, lung, and brain cancers.

Alvin K. Benson, Ph.D.

See also: Alkylating agents in chemotherapy; Antineoplastics in chemotherapy; Chemotherapy; Leukemias; Occupational exposures and cancer

▶ Ultraviolet radiation and related exposures

Category: Carcinogens and Suspected Carcinogens
RoC status: Solar radiation and exposure to sunlamps or sun beds, known carcinogens since 2000; broad-spectrum ultraviolet radiation (UVR), known carcinogen since 2002; ultraviolet A, B, and C (UVA, UVB, and UVC), reasonably anticipated carcinogens since 2002
Also known as: UV, ultraviolet light, black light, UVR, UVA, UVB, UVC

Related cancers: Melanoma and nonmelanocytic skin cancers

Definition: Ultraviolet light is electromagnetic radiation that lies between X rays and visible light in the spectrum, with wavelengths between 100 and 400 nanometers (nm). UV is divided into long-wave UVA (315-400 nn), UVB (280-315 nm), and short-wave UVC (100-280 nm).

Exposure route: Through skin

Where found: Sunlight, tanning beds

At risk: Individuals chronically exposed to sunlight or occupationally exposed to ultraviolet (UV) light sources, especially those with fair skin

Etiology and symptoms of associated cancers: The damage caused by exposure to UV radiation depends on the intensity and wavelengths of the radiation, the duration of exposure, and many other highly individual factors. Cancers caused by UV radiation are based on damage to cellular deoxyribonucleic acid (DNA) and suppression of the immune system. Since UV radiation is absorbed efficiently by the skin, this is the primary carcinogenic target, and UV radiation-caused skin cancers occur mostly on sun-exposed areas. The interaction of UV radiation with DNA results in abnormal dimerization of adjacent pyrimidine bases, damage to individual bases, strand breakage, and cross-linkages between DNA and adjacent proteins. Such DNA damage contributes to cancer formation through the release of cytokines, induction of latent viruses, or mutations that cause functional changes in encoded protein molecules. Skin cancers are typically noted and diagnosed by inspection before producing systemic illness.

History: Hippocrates, a physician in ancient Greece, recognized that depression was more common in the winter months and recommended sunbathing to treat both medical and psychological maladies. Ultraviolet light as a component of sunlight and its interactions with matter were first demonstrated in the early 1800's. Ultraviolet radiation's ability to injure the eyes was noted in 1843 in welders, and papers from 1889 confirmed that ultraviolet rays cause skin burns. An epidemiologic study published in 1907 first associated sun exposure and skin cancer. A causal relationship was demonstrated in a 1928 publication that described induction of skin cancer in mice by exposure to UV radiation. The peak carcinogenic response of UVB at 310 nm was identified in 1975. Reduction of UVB in favor of UVA rays is a current strategy to reduce the carcinogenicity of tanning beds. Liberal use of sunscreens is a current recommendation to reduce the incidence of melanoma.

John B. Welsh, M.D., Ph.D.

See also: Basal cell carcinomas; Carcinogens, known; Electromagnetic radiation; Melanomas; Merkel Cell Carcinomas (MCC); Moles; Occupational exposures and cancer; Premalignancies; Skin cancers; Squamous cell carcinomas; Sunlamps; Sunscreens

▶ Vinyl chloride

Category: Carcinogens and Suspected Carcinogens
RoC status: Known human carcinogen since 1980
Also known as: Chloroethene, chloroethylene, ethylene monochloride

Related cancers: Liver cancer, possibly brain and lung cancers

Definition: Vinyl chloride is a toxic, colorless, combustible gas that has a sweet odor.

Exposure routes: For the general public, exposure to vinyl chloride occurs through inhalation of contaminated air, ingestion of contaminated foods and drinking water, or skin contact with consumer products containing vinyl chloride. Occupational exposure occurs by inhalation or skin contact during the production or use of vinyl chloride.

Where found: More than 95 percent of all vinyl chloride is used to manufacture polyvinyl chloride (PVC) and copolymers. The rest is used in organic synthesis and miscellaneous applications. PVC, a plastic resin, is used in myriad applications, including pipes, automotive parts, furniture, electrical insulation, videodiscs, flooring, windows, toys, wrapping plastic, medical supplies, credit cards, and storage containers.

At risk: People who work where vinyl chloride is produced; where plastics, rubber, resins, PVC, furniture, or automotive parts are manufactured; or around railroad cars that carry vinyl chloride have a high risk for vinyl chloride contamination. People who live near industries that manufacture or use vinyl chloride in their products or who live near hazardous waste sites or landfills also risk exposure to vinyl chloride. Between 1958 and 1974, hair sprays contained vinyl chloride, causing beauty salon workers and hair spray users to be exposed.

Etiology and symptoms of associated cancers: Breathing high levels of vinyl chloride for short periods of time can cause dizziness, sleepiness, and unconsciousness. Extremely high levels over short periods of time can result in death. Breathing vinyl chloride over long periods of time can decrease blood flow to the hands, making hand bones brittle, and can produce permanent liver damage, nerve damage, immune reactions, and liver cancer. Exposure of the skin to vinyl chloride can produce numbness, redness, and blisters. Dioxins produced as by-products of vinyl chloride production and from burning waste PVC can suppress the immune system, cause a variety of cancers, and produce endometriosis.

History: Vinyl chloride has been in existence since at least the early part of the nineteenth century. It was first produced commercially in the 1920's. In the late 1960's vinyl chloride was definitely linked to liver cancer. It has become one of the highest-volume chemicals produced in the United States. Approximately 15 billion pounds of vinyl chloride were manufactured annually in the United States during the mid-1990's.

Alvin K. Benson, Ph.D.

See also: Bisphenol A (BPA); Brain and central nervous system cancers; Bronchial adenomas; Carcinogens, known; Carcinogens, reasonably anticipated; Di(2-ethylhexyl) phthalate (DEHP); Dioxins; Endotheliomas; Fibrosarcomas, soft-tissue; Gliomas; Hemangiosarcomas; Liver cancers; Lung cancers; Occupational exposures and cancer; Organochlorines (OCs); Plasticizers; Sarcomas, soft-tissue

▶ Wood dust

Category: Carcinogens and Suspected Carcinogens
RoC status: Known human carcinogen since 2002
Also known as: Sawdust, wood flour, sander dust

Related cancers: Cancer of the nasal cavities and the sinuses

Definition: Wood dust is composed of fine particles of the hard, fibrous substance that grows beneath the bark of trees in their trunks and branches. Woodworking tools release many lightweight specks of wood into the air. Electric and manual tools create wood dust when they chip, saw, turn, drill, sand, or carve wood. Outdoor compost piles also create visible clouds of wood dust when their layers of wood and leaves are agitated.

Exposure routes: Inhalation

Where found: Sawmills and other wood-processing mills, lumberyards, woodworking shops, furniture and cabinetmaking industry, carpentry industry, composting facilities

At risk: Woodworkers in manufacturing industries; wood products press operators; workers who handle wood compost; wood carvers

Etiology and symptoms of associated cancers: The carcinogenic actions of wood dust in the nose and sinuses are not clearly understood. Animal tests show that wood dust damages deoxyribonucleic acid (DNA) and breaks chromosomes. Human studies indicate that exposure to it is associated with nasal adenocarcinoma, sinus squamous cell carcinoma, and cancer of the nasopharynx.

The active biological components of wood dust, cellulose and lignins (substances that make wood rigid), might cause these cancers. Organic chemical components, such as resin acids, terpenes, and tannins, might also be involved. Also, the particulate nature of wood dust most likely adds to its carcinogenicity.

Symptoms of these cancers include spontaneous epistaxis (nosebleed) and chronic obstruction of the nasal or sinus passages.

History: Studies in England in the 1960's showed that rare nasal cancers occurred in woodworkers. During a 1970's National Cancer Institute study, a high percentage of woodworkers died of these cancers.

In 1995 the International Agency for Research on Cancer (IARC) classified wood dust as a Group 1 human carcinogen. In 2002 the National Toxicology Program of the Department of Health and Human Services declared wood dust to be a human carcinogen in the *Tenth Report on Carcinogens* (RoC). In 2005 the National Institutes of Health estimated that the occupations of 2 million people worldwide expose them to the carcinogenic effects of wood dust.

The Occupational Safety and Health Administration (OSHA), the National Institute for Occupational Safety and Health (NIOSH), the IARC, and the American Conference of Governmental Industrial Hygienists (ACGIH) have established exposure limits, and their recommendations include avoidance, use of dust masks, daily removal of wood dust, and ventilation.

Susan E. Ullmann, M.T. (ASCP), M.A.

See also: Air pollution; Carcinogens, known; Carcinogens, reasonably anticipated; Carcinomas; Head and neck cancers; Occupational exposures and cancer; Prevention; Throat cancer

▶ Abiraterone acetate (Zytiga)

Category: Chemotherapy and Other Drugs
Also known as: Zytiga, adrenal inhibitor

Definition: Classified as an adrenal inhibitor, abiraterone acetate (Zytiga®, a trademark of Janssen Biotech, Inc.) is a type of hormone therapy used in combination with prednisone to treat men with prostate cancer.

Cancers treated: Specifically, abiraterone acetate is used to treat castration-resistant prostate cancer that has metastasized (spread to other parts of the body) in patients who have received prior chemotherapy containing docetaxel.

Delivery routes: Oral

How it works: Male hormones, including androgens and testosterone, stimulate the growth of prostate cancer. Abiraterone acetate interferes with certain enzymes in the adrenal glands that produce androgens so they cannot be used by the tumor cells. The medication interrupts androgen production at 3 sources: the testes, the adrenal glands, and the tumor itself.

Side effects: The most common side effects include vomiting, weakness, joint swelling or pain, hot flushes, bruising, swelling in the legs or feet (edema), diarrhea, cough, urinary tract infection and shortness of breath.

Serious side effects include high blood pressure (hypertension) low blood potassium levels (hypokalemia), and fluid retention (edema). Signs and symptoms of these conditions, which should be reported to the patient's doctor immediately, include rapid or irregular heartbeat, chest pain, difficulty breathing, or inability to urinate. Other signs and symptoms, which should be reported to the patient's doctor within 24 hours, include dizziness, confusion, muscle weakness, feeling faint or lightheaded, leg pain, headache, or swelling in the hands and feet.

Patients are monitored closely with blood tests before and during treatment to evaluate the effects of the medication. Some abnormal blood test results that may occur when taking this medication include: low red blood cells (anemia), high blood sugar levels, high blood cholesterol, high triglycerides, or increased liver enzymes (ALT). Any patient with a history of heart disease or who has had a stroke should be very closely monitored, since abiraterone can greatly raise the risks of a cardiovascular event in such patients.

Abiraterone should not be used in women and men who are sexually active. They must use a barrier method of contraception, such as condoms, while being treated with abiraterone and for at least one week after treatment, since the medication can cause fetal harm.

Angela Costello, BS

For Further Information

Kluetz, P. G., Ning, Y. M., Maher, V. E., Zhang L., Tang, S., Ghosh D., … Padzur, R. (2013). Abiraterone acetate in combination with prednisone for the treatment of patients with metastatic castration-resistant prostate cancer: U.S. food and drug administration drug approval summary. *Clinical Cancer Research* 19(24): 6650-6656. http://clincancerres.aacrjournals.org/content/19/24/6650

Ryan, C. J., Smith, M. R., Fizazi K., Saad, F., Mulders, P. F. A., Sternberg, C. N., … Rathkopf, D. E. (2015). Abiraterone acetate plus prednisone versus placebo plus prednisone in chemotherapy-naive men with metastatic castration-resistant prostate cancer (COU-AA-302): Final overall survival analysis of a randomised, double-blind, placebo-controlled phase 3 study. *The Lancet Oncology* 16(2): 152-160. http://www.thelancet.com/journals/lanonc/article/PIIS1470-2045%2814%2971205-7/fulltext

Ryan, C. J., Smith, M. R., de Bono, J. S., Molina, A., Logothetis, C. J. de Souza, P., … Rathkopf, D. E. (2013). Abiraterone in metastatic prostate cancer without previous chemotherapy. *New England Journal of Medicine* 368(2): 138-148. http://dx.doi.org/10.1056/NEJMoa1209096

Other Resources

Zytiga
https://www.zytiga.com

American Cancer Society
http://www.cancer.org

CancerNet
http://www.cancer.net

Chemocare.org
http://www.chemocare.org

National Cancer Institute
http://www.cancer.gov

U.S. Food and Drug Administration
http://www.fda.gov

See also: Chemotherapy

▶ Adenoviruses

Category: Chemotherapy and Other Drugs
Also known as: *Adenoviridae* viruses

Definition: An adenovirus is a twenty-sided symmetrical icosahedron measuring between 80 and 100 nanometers in diameter with 252 capsomers forming its outside capsid (protein shell). Adenoviruses contain double-stranded, linear deoxyribonucleic acid (DNA), sometimes referred to as dsDNA. Their name is derived from lymphoid tissue in the pharynx known as adenoids. Adenoviruses were first isolated from human tonsils in the 1950's. Today, there are more than forty identified types of human viruses in the family Adenoviridae. Adenoviruses can be genetically engineered to serve as vectors that deliver targeted gene therapy to human cells.

Cancers treated: Breast, colorectal, head and neck, liver, and prostate cancers

Delivery routes: Injection

How these agents work: Adenoviruses are nonenveloped (naked) viruses, meaning that they lack a lipid and protein outer covering. Counterintuitively, viruses without this outer covering are better able to withstand environmental stressors such as acid, drying, and heat and therefore may live longer outside a host cell. Most adenoviruses cause respiratory illnesses, conjunctivitis (pinkeye), or gastroenteritis. They are transmitted through respiratory droplets or fecal-oral transmission.

Adenoviruses are well suited to gene therapy because of their environmental robustness, the ease of manipulating the adenovirus genome, and their ability to infect a number of different kinds of tissues. The DNA inside the adenovirus may one day be altered to encode up to forty genes.

For use in cancer therapy, adenoviruses are first inactivated to render them incapable of causing a sustained infection inside the body, even though such viruses can still infect particular cells. By subjecting inactivated adenoviruses to recombinant DNA technology, they can be endowed with the ability to express novel proteins that can liquidate cancer cells. Infecting cancer cells with these genetically-engineered adenoviruses might flag cancer cells for destruction by the immune system, directly break the cells apart (cell lysis), or activate genes that cause the cells to die (apoptosis), or stop replicating.

In order to infect the host cell, adenoviruses attach to a specific site, known as the Coxsackie-Adeno Receptor (CAR), which triggers the host cell to surround and engulf the viral particle. Once the virus is inside the cell, the particle makes its way to the host cell nucleus, where it completes its disassembly and releases its DNA. In a lytic cycle, replication of host cell DNA is inhibited and replication of adenovirus DNA occurs instead. Eventually the host cell breaks apart (lyses) and releases the newly created adenoviruses.

A particular strain of adenovirus, known as Ad5, has been the vector of choice in cancer chemotherapy. Ad5 is capable of infecting both replicating and non-replicating cells. The inability of the virus to integrate into the cell's chromosomes also limits its ability to transform a normal cell into a cancer cell, which is a concern with any potentially transforming viral vector. Unfortunately, loss of expression of the CAR site is common among tumor cells, limiting the efficacy of the Ad5 approach.

Since most people have been exposed to adenoviruses, the immune system can also mount an immune response to the adenoviruses before they have a chance to target the cancer cells. Initial trials involving co-administration of low-dose immunosuppressives did not prove successful. However, deleting early gene products (those expressed prior to viral DNA replication) in genetically engineered viruses has shown greater promise in avoiding the problem of immune recognition; the immune response against adenoviruses is primarily directed against early gene products.

Side effects: Adenovirus side effects include inflammation at site of injection, inappropriate immune response, fever, and cold-like symptoms.

Pamela Richardson, M.S.
Updated by Richard Adler

For Further Information

Brenner, Malcolm & Hung, Mien-Chie. (Eds.). (2014). *Cancer gene therapy by viral and non-viral vectors.* Hoboken, NY: John Wiley & Sons.

Rein, D., Breidenbach, M., & Curiel, D. T. (2006). Current developments in adenovirus-based cancer gene therapy. *Future Oncology,* 2(1), 137-143.

Vorburger, S., & Hunt, K. (2002). Adenoviral gene therapy. *The Oncologist*, 7(1), 46-59.

Wold, W.S., & Toth, K. (2013). Adenovirus vectors for gene therapy. *Current Gene Therapy*, 13(6), 421-433.

See also: Gene therapy; Oncogenes; Oncogenic viruses; Simian virus 40

▶ Alkylating agents in chemotherapy

Category: Chemotherapy and Other Drugs
ATC code: 101A

Definition: Alkylating neoplastic agents form a class of chemotherapeutic drugs, all of which consist of highly reactive compounds containing alkyl groups. They are employed as antineoplastics, drugs that kill neoplasms (cancerous tumor cells) by interfering with their deoxyribonucleic acid (DNA) and cell division.

Cancers treated: Various, especially slow-growing cancers such as solid tumors and leukemias

Subclasses of this group: Alkyl sulfonates, ethyleneimines and methylmelamines, nitrogen mustards, nitrosoureas, platinum compounds, triazenes

Delivery routes: These drugs are administered both intravenously and orally in capsule and tablet form, on an inpatient, outpatient, and at-home basis, depending on the specific drug, type of cancer, and its location and aggressiveness. When possible, these drugs are best delivered to the tumor site to limit damage to normal cells.

How these drugs work: One of the oldest classes of chemotherapeutic drugs, alkylating agents were discovered during World War II when physician Cornelius P. Rhoads drew a connection between the lowered white blood cell counts in six hundred sailors (who had been exposed to mustard gas during the sinking of the *Liberty* in 1943) and the possibility that the nitrous mustards could be adopted for use in leukemia patients.

It was later observed that alkylating agents substitute alkyl groups for the hydrogen groups in the DNA of tumor cells. The alkyl groups cross-link guanine nucleobases in the double-helix strands of DNA, which makes it impossible for the two DNA strands to uncoil and separate in preparation for replication. As a result, these drugs prevent tumor cells from dividing during mitosis, stopping the cells' growth. They may also stimulate the natural process of cell death (apoptosis). Because DNA is more actively replicated and transcribed in rapidly dividing cancer cells than in normal cells, these drugs are more toxic to tumor tissue than to normal tissue. Alkylating agents are also known to add methyl or alkyl groups onto any of the four nitrogenous bases found in DNA (adenine, guanine, cytosine, thymine), frequently altering the base-pairing relationships and leading to new mutations.

Side effects: Although alkylating agents are more toxic to cancer cells than to normal cells, these drugs are nonspecific. That is, they target normal as well as cancerous tissue, so they exhibit the "Janus effect": They kill both bad and good cells. Therefore they have toxic side effects, depending on the specific drug, its dosage, the duration of administration, and the individual patient's physical condition and attitude. Common side effects include depressed blood cell counts, tiredness and fatigue, diarrhea, alopecia (hair loss), nausea and vomiting, infertility (both amenorrhea in women and impaired spermatogenesis in men), damage to intestinal mucosa, exfoliation of the bladder epithelium resulting in fluid retention, and in extreme cases cardiotoxicity, which would mitigate the chemotherapy regimen. In addition, some alkylating agents increase the risk of future malignancies, such as acute myeloid leukemia, which may emerge years after treatment.

Christina J. Moose, M.A.

For Further Information

Chabner, Bruce A., and Dan L. Longo, eds. *Cancer Chemotherapy and Biotherapy: Principles and Practice*. Philadelphia: Lippincott Williams & Wilkins, 2006.

Fischer, David S., et al. *The Cancer Chemotherapy Handbook*. 6th ed. St. Louis: Mosby, 2003.

Panasci, Lawrence C., and Moulay A. Alaoui-Jamali, eds. *DNA Repair in Cancer Therapy*. Totowa, N.J.: Humana Press, 2004.

Podolsky, M. Lawrence. *Cures out of Chaos*. Newark, N.J.: Harwood Academic, 1997.

Skeel, Roland T. *Handbook of Cancer Chemotherapy*. 6th ed. Philadelphia: Lippincott Williams & Wilkins, 2003.

Other Resources

National Cancer Institute
Drug Information Summaries
http://www.cancer.gov/cancertopics/druginfo/alphalist

See also: Antineoplastics in chemotherapy; Bis(chloromethyl) ether and technical-grade chloromethyl methyl ether; 1,4-Butanediol dimethanesulfonate; Carcinogens, known; Carcinogens, reasonably anticipated;

Common Alkylating Agents

Drug	*Brands*	*Subclass*	*Delivery*	*Mode Cancers Treated*
Altretamine (hexamethylmelamine)	Hexalen	Ethylenimines	Oral	Ovarian cancer
Busulfan		Alkyl sulfonates	Oral, IV	Chronic myelogenous leukemia, other blood cancers
Carboplatin (CBDCA)	Paraplatin	Platinum compounds	IV	Ovarian carcinoma
Carmustine (BCNU)	BiCNU, Gliadel Wafer	Nitrosoureas	IV	Brain tumors, multiple myeloma, Hodgkin disease, non-Hodgkin lymphoma, malignant melanoma, breast cancer, gastrointestinal cancers, Ewing sarcoma, and Burkitt lymphoma; applied topically for mycosis fungoides
Chlorambucil	Leukeran	Nitrogen mustards	Oral	Chronic lymphocytic leukemia, some non-Hodgkin lymphomas, advanced Hodgkin disease
Cisplatin (CDDP)	Platinol-AQ	Platinum compounds	IV	Metastatic testicular tumors, metastatic ovarian tumors, advanced bladder carcinoma
Cyclophosphamide (CTX)	Cytoxan	Nitrogen mustards	Oral, IV	Lymphomas, multiple myelomas, leukemias, mycosis fungoides, neuroblastoma, ovarian carcinoma, retinoblastoma, breast cancer
Dacarbazine (DTIC)	DTIC-Dome	Triazenes	IV	Melanoma, Hodgkin disease
Ifosfamide (isophosphamide)	Ifex	Nitrogen mustards	IV	Germ cell testicular cancer, sarcomas
Lomustine (CCNU)	CeeNU	Nitrosoureas	Oral	Brain tumors, Hodgkin disease, bronchogenic carcinoma, non-Hodgkin lymphomas, malignant melanoma, breast cancer, renal cell carcinoma, carcinoma of the GI tract
Mechlorethamine (nitrogen mustard)	Mustargen	Nitrogen mustards	IV	Hodgkin disease, lymphosarcoma, chronic myelocytic or chronic lymphocytic leukemia; polycythemia vera; mycosis fungoides, bronchogenic carcinoma, non-Hodgkin lymphomas, malignant melanoma, breast cancer, renal cell carcinoma, carcinoma of the GI tract; applied topically for mycosis fungoides
Melphalan (L-PAM)	Alkeran	Nitrogen mustards	Oral, IV	Multiple myeloma, ovarian carcinoma
Oxaliplatin (oxalatoplatin, oxalatoplatinum)	Eloxatin, Transplatine	Platinum compounds	IV	Advanced ovarian cancer; may be effective for head and neck cancers, skin cancer, lung cancers, and non-Hodgkin lymphomas
Procarbazine	Matulane, Natulane	Hydrazine derivatives	Oral	Hodgkin disease and other lymphomas, brain tumors, skin cancer, lung cancer, multiple myeloma, mycosis fungoides
Streptozocin	Zanosar	Nitrosoureas	IV	Pancreatic islet cell cancer
Temozolomide	Temodar	Triazenes	Oral	Brain tumors (astrocytomas)
Thiotepa	Thioplex	Ethylenimines	IV, spinal injection, bladder infusion	Bladder cancer, ovarian cancer, breast cancer, lymphomas, bronchogenic carcinoma, and metastatic pleural, pericardial, and peritoneal cancers

Androgen Drugs for Breast Cancer Treatment

Drug	*Brands*	*Subclass*	*Delivery Mode*
Testolactone	Teslac	Anabolic steroid	Oral
Testosterone enanthate	Delatestryl	Testosterone ester	Intramuscular
Fluoxymesterone	Androxy, Halotestin, Ora-Testrylm Android-F, Hysterone	Alkylated androgen	Oral
Methyltestosterone	Tested, Virilon, Android-10, Methitest	Alkylated androgen	Oral

Chemotherapy; Chlorambucil; 1-(2-Chloroethyl)-3-(4-methylcyclohexyl)-1-nitrosourea (MeCCNU); Cyclophosphamide; Infertility and cancer; Mustard gas; Sterility; Thiotepa

▶ Androgen drugs

Category: Chemotherapy and Other Drugs
ATC code: G03B

Definition: Androgens are steroid hormones produced by the adrenal glands and testes or ovaries, responsible for male sex characteristics in the body. Testosterone, an endogenous androgen, is converted to estrogen by the enzyme aromatase. Androgenic agents can be used in the treatment of breast cancer.

Cancers treated: Metastatic hormone-responsive breast cancer in postmenopausal women, or in premenopausal women who have undergone ovary ablation

Subclasses of this group: Anabolic steroids, alkylated androgens, testosterone esters

Delivery routes: Administered orally as tablets or capsules, or by intramuscular injection

How these drugs work: Testosterone esters are lipophilic compounds that, when dissolved in oil, are administered via intramuscular injection. Alkylated androgens can be given orally as their metabolic deactivation is hindered by the alkyl group at the 17α position.

The mechanism of action for androgenic agents in breast cancer has not been fully established, though they are believed to block the growth of estrogen-dependent tumors by inhibiting aromatase activity.

Older drugs such as calusterone underwent clinical trials in the 1960's and 1970's, with response rates of approximately 20 percent. Androgen drugs are not considered first-line therapy for breast cancer, as they are more toxic than other hormonal agents in use and response rates remain low. Androgens, when used, are frequently given in combination with aromatase inhibitors to inhibit the production of estrogen in vivo.

Side effects: Androgens are male sex hormones and can cause masculinizing effects in women, including deepening voice, hirsutism, acne, and clitoral enlargement. Alkylated androgens are less potent than testosterone and hence possess a lower risk of these side effects, but liver toxicity, cholestatic hepatitis, and jaundice can occur at relatively low doses. Androgen therapy should be discontinued following abnormal liver function tests until the cause has been determined.

Androgen therapy in patients with preexisting cardiac, renal, or hepatic disease increases the risk of edema and progression to congestive heart failure. In such cases, dosing should be discontinued and administration of a diuretic considered.

Breast cancer patients undergoing androgen therapy are at increased risk of bone breakdown and reabsorption, leading to hypercalcemia. If this occurs, then drug therapy should be discontinued and the patient evaluated, as hypercalcemia may also indicate the progression of bone metastases.

Karen M. Nagel, Ph.D.

See also: Amenorrhea; Antiandrogens; Appetite loss; Bisphenol A (BPA); Breast cancer in men; Chemoprevention; Endocrine cancers; Fanconi anemia; Granulosa cell tumors; Hormonal therapies; Myelofibrosis; Receptor analysis; Tumor flare

▶ Angiogenesis inhibitors

Category: Chemotherapy and Other Drugs

Definition: Because cancerous tumors need blood to live and grow, they persuade the body to build vessels in a process called angiogenesis. Angiogenesis inhibitors prevent the formation of new blood vessels so that tumors starve and die.

Cancers treated: Multiple myeloma, mantle cell lymphoma, metastatic colorectal cancer, advanced renal cancer, gastrointestinal stromal tumors

Delivery routes: Delivered intravenously to patients in hospital (Velcade, Avastin) or orally to outpatients in tablet (Sutent, Nexavar) and capsule (Thalomid) form.

How these drugs work: Angiogenesis is critical to normal growth, providing a network of new blood capillaries that deliver oxygen and nutrients to developing tissues. Once formed, capillaries usually do not increase in size or number. Normal exceptions to this include wound repair, adaptation to exercise training, and monthly menstruation cycles.

Tumors require a constant supply of newly-formed blood capillaries in order to grow. Once a tumor starts to require a blood supply, it begins to secrete "growth factors," proteins that induce growth. One chemical secreted by tumors, Vascular Endothelial Growth Factor or VEGF, signals endothelial cells in the lining of blood vessels to develop blood vessels. New capillaries sprout, attach themselves to the tumor, and deliver oxygen and nutrients. This blood supply also allows tumor cells to spread to other areas of the body (metastasize), a process that is a major cause of cancer mortality.

Preventing the process of angiogenesis might be a powerful tool in preventing tumor growth, diminishing the growth of new tumor cells and causing tumors to grow more slowly or even diminish in size. In 1971, Dr. Judah Folkman, of Children's Hospital in Boston, published a significant angiogenesis paper. He hypothesized that all tumor growth is angiogenesis-dependent and asserted that interrupting its blood supply causes a tumor to die. Angiogenesis inhibitors were first discovered in 1975 and since have been detected in such diverse natural sources as tree bark, green tea, fungi, shark cartilage and muscle, sea coral, and sundry herbs.

As of 2015, the U.S. Food and Drug Administration (FDA) had approved thirteen angiogenesis inhibitors for use in cancer treatment. While all these targeted therapies work by interrupting cell-signaling pathways—particularly VEGF—needed for vessel formation, they are subdivided into three categories:

–Monoclonal antibodies are designed to target specific proteins called antigens, such as those that appear on cancer cells. Once attached, they signal other immune cells to destroy cells around the antigen—as do all antibodies.

–Tyrosine-kinase inhibitors (TKIs) block tyrosine kinase, an enzyme that activates proteins in the process of vessel formation.

–mTOR inhibitors aim for the mammalian target of rapamycin (mTOR). mTOR is a protein kinase that induces growth factors to initiate the process of angiogenesis. The mTOR pathway is more active in certain cancers such as those of brain, breast, pancreas, and kidney.

Two other anti-angiogenic agents are approved that inhibit angiogenesis, though their inhibition is not completely understood and possibly indirect. There are also anti-angiogenesis agents used for cancers of the skin.

Side effects: The side effects of angiogenesis inhibitors are often connected to their interference with the circulatory system. Some common side effects include bleeding; high blood pressure; rash and/or dry skin; tender, thickened areas on palms and soles (hand-foot syndrome); and impaired wound healing.

Problems with VEGF blockade: Any drug treatment has unintended effects, and experience has revealed adverse or unexpected effects of anti-angiogenesis. The majority of anti-angiogenesis drugs whose mechanisms are understood work by blocking VEGF so that the tumor can no longer induce angiogenesis. Ironically, some of these effects are generated by the very absence of VEGF signals.

- Some patients cannot tolerate VEGF-blocking drugs and some develop cardiotoxicity as revealed by reductions in left-ventricular ejection fraction, a measure of cardiac competency.
- Some cancers develop apparent resistance to VEGF blockers. VEGF-signal blockade seems to be the impetus of this resistance, but the precise mechanism depends on the cancer type and the particular VEGF blocker employed. When VEGF signals are blocked, tumors may seek previously unsuspected sources of vascularization using pro-angiogenic elements that eschew VEGF. VEGF-free growth factors can be unexpectedly competent.
- When VEGF blockade disrupts blood vessels serving a tumor, many tumor cells deprived of oxygen will die. However, a few may survive the challenge because they are relatively tolerant to hypoxia (oxygen depletion). Such survivors in effect become cancer stem cells (progenitors) that produce offspring less reliant on oxygen and the vessels that supply it. Although this has not been established, some suggest that when treatment consists solely of VEGF blockade, surviving the stress of hypoxia might intensify a tumor's malignancy. Even when treatment includes other drugs, what amounts to hypoxic cell

selection might yield tumors with enhanced abilities to invade and thrive.

- When VEGF blockade is suspended, some tumors seek to replace their interrupted blood supplies. Revascularization can be swift, as "empty-sleeve" scaffolding of vessels remaining after blockade can be rapidly remobilized.
- Because VEGF participates in maintenance of established vessels, VEGF blockade can injure such vessels, sometimes to the point of inducing hemorrhage or thrombosis (clots).

Beyond VEGF blockade: Although tumor angiogenesis in primarily dependent on VEGF signaling, VEGF interruption induces effective work-arounds via alternate mechanisms. But VEGF is not the only growth factor involved in angiogenesis, and researchers are exploring molecular functions that govern vessel formation. Molecular agents are being designed to inhibit other growth factors. Targeting multiple signaling pathways is not only more effective at blocking signal passage, it also impedes resistance.

As often happens in biological incursions, interfering with vessel formation to disable cancer has become much more of a labyrinthine process than originally conceived. More understanding is needed about molecular processes involved in angiogenesis, biomarkers to indicate those likely to respond, and biomarkers to directly measure response. Also crucially important, the mechanisms of tumor resistance must be better understood. Despite the complexities, the advantages of molecular targeted drugs—with minimal side effects and much-diminished toxicity over traditional "sledgehammer" chemotherapy—must not be underestimated.

Bernard Jacobson, Ph.D.
Updated by: Jackie Dial, PhD

For Further Information

Cook, K.M., & Figg, W.D. (2010). Angiogenesis inhibitors: current strategies and future prospects. *CA: A Cancer Journal for Clinicians*, 60(4): 222-243. http://dx.doi.org/10.3322%2Fcaac.20075

Davis, D. W., R. S. Herbst, and J. L. Abbruzzese. (Eds.). (2007). *Antiangiogenic cancer therapy*. New York: CRC Press.

Folkman, J. (1971). Tumor angiogenesis: Therapeutic implications. *New England Journal of Medicine*, 285: 1182-1186.

Leifer, John, and Leifer, Lori L. (2015). *After you hear it's cancer: A guide to navigating the difficult journey ahead.* Lanham, MA: Rowman & Littlefield.

Li, William. (2010). *Can we eat to starve cancer?* (TED talk). Retrieved from https://www.ted.com/talks/william_li?language=en

Other Resources

EurekAlert! (2015). Blood vessel 'doorway' lets breast cancer cells spread through blood stream. Retrieved from http://www.eurekalert.org/pub_releases/2015-08/aeco-bv080515.php

Food and Drug Administration, A to Z index (2016). http://www.fda.gov

National Cancer Institute (2011). Angiogenesis inhibitors. http://www.cancer.gov/about-cancer/treatment/types/immunotherapy/angiogenesis-inhibitors-fact-sheet

The Angiogenesis Foundation (2015). Treatments. https://www.angio.org/learn/treatments/

See also: Angiogenesis; Biological therapy; Chemotherapy; Oral and oropharyngeal cancers; Sarcomas, soft-tissue

▶ Anthraquinones

Categories: Complementary and Alternative Therapies; Chemotherapy and Other Drugs

Definition: Anthraquinones form a group of anticancer agents derived from plant products. Anthraquinones naturally occur in some plants, such as aloe, senna, rhubarb, Cascara buckthorn, and sheep sorrel. Indian rhubarb root (*Rheum palmatum*) contains several anthraquinones. Sheep sorrel (*Rumex acetosella*) contains several types of anthraquinones. Subclasses of this group are emodin, aloe emodin, and anthraquionone derivatives. A number of conventional chemotherapeutic agents, such as Adriamycin (doxorubicin), are derivatives of anthraquinones.

Cancers treated or prevented: Prostate cancer, breast cancer, non-Hodgkin lymphoma, acute leukemia

Delivery routes: Anthraquionones are typically consumed as a mixture of several botanicals, such as in a tea, although intravenous administration has been used in the past.

How these drugs work: Anthraquionones are ingredients in herbal mixtures such as Essiac or Flor-Essence that are typically consumed as a tea. The primary herbs in these botanical mixtures, rhubarb and sheep sorrel, are thought to contain anthraquionones. Such herbal extracts have been in use as a cancer treatment since the 1920's, when they were popularized by a Canadian nurse, Rene Caisse, who obtained the recipe from a woman who claimed that it cured her breast cancer. Caisse opened a clinic and treated patients for more than forty years. After her death, researchers at Memorial Sloan-Kettering in New York tested her product, with inconclusive results.

Anthraquionones are alleged to have anti-inflammatory effects and cytotoxic effects against tumor cells. Proponents claim that they strengthen the immune system, reduce tumor size, and improve and prolong the lives of people with many types of cancer. Although they have been shown to have tumor inhibition properties, they have been shown to stimulate tumor cell growth as well.

Anthraquinones have been shown to stimulate various cytokines that are important in tumor cell defense, including IL-1, IL-6, and TNF. In experimental settings, anthraquinones have been shown to potentiate the action of Adriamycin (doxorubicin), a widely used chemotherapy drug, but the clinical significance of this action is unknown. Anthraquionone derivatives, such as Adriamycin and mitoxantrone, have been shown to be effective as chemotherapeutics.

Side effects: Natural anthraquinones and their derivatives have laxative properties. Therefore, a side effect associated with anthraquionones is diarrhea as well as hyperkalemia as a result of chronic diarrhea. They have also been reported to cause nausea, vomiting, and contact dermatitis. A principal danger of this and other unconventional therapies is that they may delay diagnosis and conventional treatment of serious disease.

C. J. Walsh, Ph.D.

See also: Essiac; Green tea; Herbs as antioxidants

▶ Antiandrogens

Category: Chemotherapy and Other Drugs
ATC code: 102BB, G03HA

Definition: Antiandrogens are a class of drugs used to treat prostate cancer. They can cause tumor cell death by blocking the effect of androgens, which are hormones required for the development and survival of both normal and cancerous prostate cells.

Cancers treated: Prostate cancer

Subclasses of this group: Nonsteroidal antiandrogens and synthetic steroids

Delivery routes: Administered orally as either capsules or tablets, can be taken on an at-home basis

How these drugs work: Androgens are male hormones, which include testosterone, dehydroepiandrosterone, and dihydrotestosterone. Androgens bind to androgen receptors on the surface of prostate cells and turn on signaling pathways involved in cellular development and survival and normal prostate function. Most prostate cancers, however, are also dependent on androgen signaling. Therefore, without it, tumors may stop growing.

Nonsteroidal antiandrogens and synthetic steroids compete with natural androgens for binding sites on androgen receptors, thereby blocking the activity of the natural androgens. Synthetic steroids can also act on the hypothalamus in the brain to reduce the production of testosterone.

Although antiandrogens inhibit androgen activity, blood levels of testosterone and other androgens may still be high, which could promote cancer cell growth. Therefore, antiandrogens are commonly used in combination with other drugs that lower androgen levels, such as luteinizing hormone-releasing hormone agonists, which can stop testosterone production. Antiandrogens may also be combined with inhibitors of the 5-α reductase enzyme, which block the conversion of testosterone into dihydrotestosterone. Dihydrotestosterone is thought to be a more potent and active androgen than testosterone.

Side effects: Because antiandrogens affect the prostate, they may cause low sperm counts or reduce fertility. Other common side effects include diarrhea, hot flashes, liver toxicity, constipation, decreased appetite, nausea or vomiting, and flulike symptoms. Long-term treatment may also cause osteoporosis, in which bones become weakened.

There are also some drug-specific side effects. For example, nilutamide can temporarily cause the eyes to become light sensitive and take longer to adjust to changes in light and dark settings. Flutamide is also associated with the rare side effects of dizziness, fainting, and severe headaches.

Elizabeth A. Manning, Ph.D.

Common Antiandrogens for Prostate Cancer Treatment

Drug	*Brands*	*Subclass*	*Delivery Mode*
Bicalutamide	Casodex	Nonsteroidal antiandrogen	Oral
Cyproterone acetate	Androcur, Climen	Synthetic steroid	Oral
Flutamide	Eulexin	Nonsteroidal antiandrogen	Oral
Nilutamide	Anandron, Nilandron	Nonsteroidal antiandrogen	Oral

See also: Antiestrogens; Breast cancer in men; Breast cancers; Chemoprevention; Hormonal therapies; Immunotherapy; Tumor flare

▶ Antidiarrheal agents

Category: Chemotherapy and Other Drugs
ATC code: AO7DA

Definition: Antidiarrheal agents are a class of drugs used for the treatment or symptomatic relief of diarrhea.

Cancers treated: Antidiarrheal agents are typically used to treat diarrhea associated with carcinoid tumors, colon cancer, lymphoma, thyroid cancer, pancreatic cancer, and pheochromocytoma, as well as cancer treatment-induced diarrhea, caused by such treatments as chemotherapy, radiation therapy, surgery, and bone marrow transplantation. Other causes of diarrhea in patients with cancer include anxiety and stress associated with the diagnosis. For these patients, antidiarrheal agents may be used in combination with antianxiety drugs.

Patients who have diarrhea with a different underlying cause should receive treatment specific to the cause. For example, those who have diarrhea caused by *Clostridium difficile* should be treated with the antibiotic metronidazole. Antidiarrheal agents may be administered as adjunct therapy after the initiation of antibiotic therapy.

Subclasses of this group: Adsorbents, bulk-forming agents, opioids, piperidine derivatives, synthetic octapeptides, mucosal prostaglandin inhibitors

Delivery routes: Administered orally in tablet, caplet, capsule, suspension, and liquid form at home or in the hospital; octreotide is administered by subcutaneous injection or by continuous intravenous (IV) infusion while the patient is hospitalized

How these drugs work: Adsorbents bind with intestinal contents, increasing their density. Adsorbents such as kaolin and charcoal may inhibit the absorption of other antidiarrheals, making them ineffective. Bulk-forming agents treat diarrhea by absorbing water within the bowel and producing a formed stool.

Mucosal prostaglandin inhibitors stimulate the absorption of fluid and electrolytes through the intestinal wall. They also reduce intestinal inflammation and motility by inhibiting prostaglandin synthesis. Moreover the mucosal prostaglandin inhibitor bismuth subsalicylate is thought to have antimicrobial action against *Escherichia coli*, a bacterium that causes diarrhea. Opioids bind to receptor sites in the intestinal tract, slowing intestinal motility. Synthetic octapeptides inhibit the release of serotonin, gastrin, vasoactive intestinal peptide, secretin, motilin, and pancreatic polypeptide, slowing intestinal motility. Piperidine derivatives reduce peristolic activity by acting directly on the intestinal wall muscles. The reduction in peristolic activity delays intestinal content transit time, increases fecal density, and reduces fluid and electrolyte loss.

Side effects: Side effects vary according to the drug class. Adsorbents such as bismuth subsalicylate may cause temporary darkening of the tongue and stools. Bulk-forming agents such as polycarbophil may cause abdominal discomfort, bloating, dependence (with prolonged use), increased flatus, and intestinal blockage. Mucosal prostaglandin inhibitors such as aspirin may cause allergic reaction, bruising, gastrointestinal bleeding, hearing loss, hepatitis, itching, low platelet count, nausea, prolonged bleeding time, ringing in the ears, and rash.

Opioids such as diphenoxylate hydrochloride and atropine sulfate may cause abdominal discomfort, allergic reaction, blurred vision, confusion, dizziness, dry mouth, dry skin, euphoria, headache, inability to urinate, increased heart rate, itching, loss of appetite, nausea, pancreatitis, rash, respiratory depression, restlessness, sedation, swollen gums, and vomiting. Piperidine derivatives

Common Antidiarrheal Agents

Drug (Other Names)	*Brands*	*Subclass*	*Delivery Mode*	*Conditions Treated*
Aspirin	Bayer aspirin, Ecotrin, Empirin, Halfprin, Norwich Extra Strength	Mucosal prostaglandin inhibitor	Oral	Radiation therapy-induced diarrhea
Bismuth subsalicylate	Bismatrol, Bismatrol Extra Kaopectate, Extra strength Kaopectate, Pepto-Bismol, Pepto-Bismol Maximum Strength, Pink Bismuth	Adsorbent, mucosal prostaglandin inhibitor	Oral	Diarrhea associated with colon cancer; lymphoma; thyroid cancer; pancreatic cancer; pheochromocytoma; cancer treatment (antibiotic therapy, bone marrow transplantation, chemotherapy, radiation therapy)
Charcoal	Charcoal Plus DS, CharcoCaps	Adsorbent	Oral	Diarrhea associated with colon cancer; lymphoma; thyroid cancer; pancreatic cancer; pheochromocytoma; cancer treatment (antibiotic therapy, bone marrow transplantation, chemotherapy, radiation therapy)
Difenoxin hydrochloride and atropine sulfate	Motofen	Opioid	Oral	Diarrhea associated with colon cancer; lymphoma; thyroid cancer; pancreatic cancer; pheochromocytoma; cancer treatment (antibiotic therapy, bone marrow transplantation, chemotherapy, radiation therapy)
Diphenoxylate hydrochloride and atropine sulfate	Logen, Lomanate, Lomotil, Lonox	Opioid	Oral	Diarrhea associated with colon cancer; lymphoma; thyroid cancer; pancreatic cancer; pheochromocytoma; cancer treatment (antibiotic therapy, bone marrow transplantation, chemotherapy, radiation therapy)

(continued)

such as loperamide may cause abdominal pain, distention or discomfort; allergic reaction; constipation; dizziness; dry mouth; drowsiness; fatigue; nausea; rash; and vomiting. The synthetic octapeptide, octreotide, may cause abdominal discomfort, arrhythmias, backache, blurred vision, burning or pain at the injection site, cold symptoms, fat malabsorption, flatulence, flulike symptoms, flushing, gallbladder problems, hair loss, hyperglycemia, hypoglycemia, hypothyroidism, joint pain, low heart rate, nausea, pancreatitis, redness at the injection site, swelling, urinary tract infection, and vomiting.

Collette Bishop Hendler, R.N., M.S.

For Further Information

Drug Facts and Comparisons 2008. 62d ed. St. Louis: Wolters Kluwer Health, 2008.

Karch, Amy M. *2008 Lippincott's Nursing Drug Guide*. Philadelphia: Wolters Kluwer/Lippincott Williams & Wilkins, 2008.

Nursing 2008 Drug Handbook. Philadelphia: Lippincott Williams & Wilkins, 2008.

See also: Antinausea medications; Chemotherapy; Colorectal cancer; Crohn disease; Diarrhea; Enteritis; Gastrointestinal complications of cancer treatment;

Common Antidiarrheal Agents *(continiued)*

Drug (Other Names)	*Brands*	*Subclass*	*Delivery Mode*	*Conditions Treated*
Kaolin and pectin	Kao-Spen, Kapectolin, KP	Adsorbent	Oral	Diarrhea associated with colon cancer; lymphoma; thyroid cancer; pancreatic cancer; pheochromocytoma; cancer treatment (antibiotic therapy, bone marrow transplantation, chemotherapy, radiation therapy)
Loperamide	Imodium, Imodium A-D, Kaopectate II Caplets, Maalox Anti-Diarrheal Caplets, Pepto Diarrhea Control	Piperidine derivative	Oral	Diarrhea associated with colon cancer; lymphoma; thyroid cancer; pancreatic cancer; pheochromocytoma; cancer treatment (antibiotic therapy, bone marrow transplantation, chemotherapy, radiation therapy)
Octreotide	Sandostatin, Sandostatin LAR	Synthetic octapeptide	Subcutaneous injection, IV	Diarrhea associated with colon cancer; lymphoma; thyroid cancer; pancreatic cancer; pheochromocytoma; cancer treatment (antibiotic therapy, bone marrow transplantation, chemotherapy, radiation therapy)
Paregoric	Camphorated Tincture of Opium	Opioid	Oral	Diarrhea associated with colon cancer; lymphoma; thyroid cancer; pancreatic cancer; pheochromocytoma; cancer treatment (antibiotic therapy, bone marrow transplantation, chemotherapy, radiation therapy)
Polycarbophil	Equalactin, Fiberall, FiberCon, Fiber-Lax, Konsyl Fiber, Mitrolan, Phillips' Fibercaps	Bulk-forming agent	Oral	Diarrhea associated with colon cancer; lymphoma; thyroid cancer; pancreatic cancer; pheochromocytoma; cancer treatment (antibiotic therapy, bone marrow transplantation, chemotherapy, radiation therapy)

Inflammatory bowel disease; Laxatives; Side effects; Symptoms and cancer

▶ Antifungal therapies

Category: Chemotherapy and Other Drugs

Definition: Antifungal therapies form a class of anti-infective drugs that are effective against fungi (including molds) such as species of *Candida, Aspergillus*, and *Zygomyces*.

Cancers treated: Fungal infections may occur in cancer and transplant patients when their immune systems are impaired or when skin or mucosal barriers are breached. Vulnerability can be increased by the cancers themselves, therapies with radiation or drugs, intravascular lines, and urinary catheters. *Candida* species are normally found on skin and in the gastrointestinal tract from mouth to anus. When the opportunity is afforded, *Candida* organisms will proliferate, invade the body, and cause systemic and potentially fatal infections. Topical and oral antifungals are often used as preventative measures (prophylaxis). Systemic candidiasis requires prompt treatment with an intravenous antifungal agent.

Common Antifungal Agents

Polyenes

i. amphotericin B desoxycholate (Amphocin, Fungizone)

a) Lipid-associated formulations

- Amphotericin B cholesteryl sulfate complex (Amphotec, Amphocil)
- Amphotericin B lipid complex (Abelcet)
- Amphotericin B liposomal (AmBisome)

ii. Nystatin (Mycostatin, Milstat, Nystex)

Azoles

- Fluconazole (Diflucan)
- Ketoconazole (Nizoral)
- Itraconazole (Sporanox)
- Voriconazole (Vfend)
- Posaconazole Noxafil)
- Isavaconazole (Cresemba)

Echinocandins

- Caspofungin (Cancidas)
- Micafungin (Mycamine)
- Anidulafungin (Exacis)

Pyrimidines

- Flucytosine(Ancoba)

Aspergillus species are environmental organisms that infect immunocompromised hosts through the respiratory tract. Until recent years, *Aspergillus* has been an almost always lethal complication for lung transplant patients, stem cell transplant patients, and patients with hematologic malignancies. The development of new azoles has dramatically improved survival rates.

Zygomyces have caused invasive and often fatal disease in diabetics, transplant recipients, and cancer patients. The development of lipid-associated amphotericin B compounds has improved treatment outcomes. However, the use of voriconazole for prophylaxis has increased the incidence of zygomycosis.

Finally, there are an assortment of unusual fungi that have risen to fill the void created by prophylaxis's success treating more common fungi. *Acremonium*, *Fusarium*, *Paecilomyces*, and *Scedosporium* infections have joined *Cryptococcus* species and other endemic fungi in producing difficult-to-diagnosis and -treat infections in cancer patients.

Subclasses of this group: Polyenes, pyrimidines, azoles, echinocandins

Delivery routes: Antifungal agents can be administered orally in capsules, tablets, or liquid suspension or vaginally by vaginal tablets. They can be taken in hospital or at home. Some antifungal agents are administered by intravenous infusion while the patient is hospitalized. As the patient's condition improves, infusions may be provided at home or in an outpatient treatment center. Rarely, amphotericin B has been administered by inhalation or intrathecal injection (injection into the subarachnoid space of the spinal canal).

How these drugs work: Polyenes bind to ergosterol components of the fungal cell membrane and produce a transmembrane channel that enables ions to leak from the fungal cell which results in death of the fungal organism. Pyrimidines interact with RNA and interfere with protein synthesis and also inhibit fungal DNA synthesis. Azoles interfere with sterol synthesis leading to reduced concentrations of ergosterol (an essential component of the fungal cell membrane). Echinocandins inhibit the synthesis of glucans, which are necessary for fungal cell wall integrity, and this deficiency causes rupture of the fungal cell and death.

With increasing exposure to antifungal agents, fungi have developed resistance to treatment. Testing of fungi cultured from infected patients to determine their susceptibility to antifungals is complicated and is usually only available in reference laboratories. Combinations of antifungal agents and the development of new antifungals have been necessary to successfully treat fungal infections caused by more resistant fungal strains. These fungi are both previously common species that have become resistant and other previously rare species that were already resistant.

Side effects: Side effects vary according to the antifungal agents. Amphotericin B can cause acute infusion-related reactions with chills, fever, tachypnea, and hypotension. This agent can also cause dose-related renal and liver failure. All of these adverse effects are less frequent with the lipid-associated formulations of amphotericin B and can be ameliorated by preventative measures and careful monitoring of blood chemistries.

Azoles are relatively nontoxic, but have many drug interactions that can lead to problems. These agents are metabolized in the liver through the cytochrome P450 pathway. This can produce problems when they are administered along with other drugs metabolized using the same pathway.

The echinocandins are also infrequently associated with adverse effects. Occasionally histamine-related effects, such as flushing, urticaria, and pruritus may be encountered during intravenous infusion.

Flucytosine is likewise relatively safe when usual doses are administered. However, this drug is often given in combination with amphotericin B. If the amphotericin B impairs renal function, then flucytosine will accumulate as it is normally excreted by the kidney. The resulting high levels of flucytosine can suppress bone marrow production of red cells, white cells, and platelets.

Collette Bishop Hendler, R.N., M.S.
Updated by: H. Bradford Hawley, M.D.

For Further Information

Bennett, John E., Dolin, Raphael, & Blazer, Martin J. (Eds.). *Principles and practice of infectious diseases* (8th ed.). Philadelphia, PA.: Saunders.

Marr, Kieren A., & Subramanian, Aruna K. (Eds). (2010). Infections in transplant and oncology patients. *Infectious Disease Clinics of North America,* 24(2): 257-529.

Walsh, Thomas J., & Andes, David R. (Eds.). (2015). Advances and new directions for echinocandins. *Clinical Infectious Diseases,* 61(suppl. 6): S601-S683.

Verweij, P. E., Chowdhary, A., Melchers, W. J. G., & Meis, J. F. (2016). Azole resistance in *Aspergillus fumigatus*: Can we retain the clinical use of mold-active antifungal azoles?" *Clinical Infectious Diseases,* 62(2): 362-368.

Other resources

Infectious Disease Society of America, Practice Guidelines: Antimicrobial Agents in Neutropenic Patients, Aspergillus & Candidiasis
www.idsociety.org/IDSA_Practice_Guidelines

Centers for Disease Control and Prevention - Cancer Patients and Fungal Infections
www.cdc.gov

See also: Aflatoxins; Candidiasis; Infection and sepsis; Neutropenia; Side effects

▶ Antimetabolites in chemotherapy

Category: Chemotherapy and Other Drugs
ATC code: 101B

Definition: Antimetabolites are drugs that interfere with deoxyribonucleic acid (DNA) replication processes in cells. These agents have a structure very similar to that of some of the components involved in the synthesis of nucleotides, the structural units of DNA. This similarity causes the cell to mistake the antimetabolite for a natural component, allowing the drug to effectively inhibit nucleotide synthesis. Nucleotide synthesis and subsequent DNA replication are processes that a cell must undergo before it can divide, and therefore quickly growing tumor cells are particularly susceptible to interference with DNA replication. Further, inhibiting DNA replication triggers the activation of death-promoting pathways in these cells, causing the antimetabolite to decrease the tumor size.

Cancers treated: Many solid tumors, including breast, colon, lung (small-cell and non-small-cell), ovarian, and head and neck cancers; several leukemias and lymphomas, including acute lymphocytic leukemia, indolent B-cell lymphoma, and non-Hodgkin lymphoma

Subclasses of this group: Folic acid antagonists, pyrimidine antagonists, purine antagonists, sugar-modified analogs, ribonucleotide reductase inhibitors

Delivery routes: Intravenous (IV), oral, intra-arterial (into an artery), intrathecal (into the spinal canal)

How these drugs work: The development of antimetabolite therapy was based on the understanding of the importance of DNA replication in cell division and proliferation. Antimetabolites inhibit DNA replication through one or both of two mechanisms. First, these drugs can inhibit the synthesis of nucleotides, the structural molecules that make up the DNA strand. The four nucleotides that are used to replicate DNA are divided into two categories. The two purine nucleotides are adenine and guanine, while the two pyrimidines are cytosine and thymine. With the exception of thymine, these nucleotides also serve as the structural units for ribonucleic acid (RNA). In RNA, thymine is replaced with another nucleotide, uracil. When the synthesis of these molecules is inhibited, the cellular pool of nucleotides is reduced, limiting the ability of the cell to synthesize new DNA strands. The second mechanism of action is the actual incorporation of the antimetabolite into the DNA itself. It is known that the enzymes responsible for DNA replication can mistake the agents for DNA nucleotides, but the direct consequences of this mistaken identity are as of yet unknown. There are four main subclasses of antimetabolites: folic acid antagonists, pyrimidine and purine antagonists, sugar-modified analogs, and ribonucleotide reductase inhibitors.

Folic acid (folate) antagonists are thought to act primarily through inhibition of the dihydrofolate reductase

Common Antimetabolites

Drug (Other Names)	*Brands*	*Subclass*	*Delivery Mode*	*Conditions Treated*
Azacytidine (Aza-C, 5-AC)	Vidaza	Pyrimidine antagonist	IV	Chronic myelocytic leukemia
Capecitabine (prodrug of fluorouracil)	Xeloda	Pyrimidine antagonist	Oral	Metastatic colorectal cancer, metastatic breast cancer
Chlorodeoxyadenosine (CdA)	Cladribine, Leustatin	Purine antagonist	IV	Indolent B-cell lymphocytic leukemia (especially hairy cell leukemia); may have activity in chronic lymphocytic leukemia and non-Hodgkin lymphoma
Cytarabine (ara-C)	Cytosar-U, DepoCyt	Sugar-modified analog	IV, intrathecal, subcutaneous	Acute nonlymphocytic leukemia, advanced non-Hodgkin lymphoma, chronic myelocytic leukemia, meningeal leukemia
Fludarabine (F-ara-A)	Fludara	Sugar-modified analog	IV, oral	Refractory chronic lymphocytic leukemia, non-Hodgkin lymphoma
Fluorodeoxyuridine (FdUrd, 5-FUdR, FdUMP)	FUDR, Floxuridine	Pyrimidine antagonist	Hepatic arterial infusion	Cancer of the gastrointestinal tract, especially tumors that have metastasized to the liver
Fluorouracil (FUra, 5-FU)	Adrucil	Pyrimidine antagonist	IV	Many solid cancers, including colorectal, breast, head and neck, gastric, and pancreatic tumors
Gemcitabine	Gemzar	Pyrimidine antagonist	IV	Locally advanced or metastatic lung cancer, pancreatic cancer, ovarian cancer, metastatic breast cancer
Hydroxyurea (HU, hydroxycarbamide)	Droxia, Hydrea	Ribonucleotide reductase inhibitors	Oral	Chronic myelocytic leukemia, head and neck cancer, cervical cancer, ovarian cancer, melanoma
Mercaptopurine (MP, 6-MP)	Purinethol	Purine antagonist	Oral	Acute lymphocytic leukemia
Methotrexate (MTX, amethopterin)	Trexall, Rheumatrex	Folic acid antagonist	Oral, IV, intra-arterial, intrathecal	Breast cancer, bone cancers including osteogenic sarcoma, acute lymphocytic leukemia, head and neck cancer, bladder cancer, and several other solid tumors including lung, uterine, and cervical cancer
Pentostatin (2′-deoxycoformycin, dCF)	Nipent	Purine antagonist	IV	Indolent B-cell lymphocytic leukemia (especially hairy cell leukemia); may have activity in chronic lymphocytic leukemia
Thioguanine (TG, 6-TG)	Thioguanine Tabloid	Purine antagonist	Oral	Acute nonlymphocytic leukemia
Tiazofurin	Riboxamide	Purine antagonist	IV	Currently in clinical testing for several leukemias, especially chronic myelocytic leukemia

(DHFR) enzyme. DHFR functions to change the structure of folic acid, also known as vitamin B9, allowing it to be used in various metabolic processes that result in the formation of nucleotides. Inhibition of DHFR therefore reduces the production of many of the nucleotides essential for DNA replication. Methotrexate is the prototypical folate antagonist, and it has been successfully used as an anticancer drug in the clinic for decades. One of the reasons that methotrexate is so efficacious is that once it enters the cell, it is chemically modified in such a way that it is unable to exit the cell. This causes the intracellular concentration of methotrexate to remain very high.

Pyrimidine and purine antagonists target tumor cells via a dual mechanism of action-inhibition of nucleotide synthesis and incorporation into DNA. To inhibit nucleotide synthesis, pyrimidine antagonists can directly inhibit the thymidylate synthase protein, a critical enzyme in the formation of the thymine nucleotide. When thymidylate synthase mistakes pyrimidine antagonists for their natural substrate, the agent inhibits and traps the enzyme in the middle of the catalysis reaction. A stable complex of the enzyme and drug are formed, decreasing the number of enzymes available for the further formation of thymine. Because there is a relatively small concentration of thymine normally in the cell, reducing these pools can drastically inhibit DNA synthesis. The most common pyrimidine antagonists, fluoropyrimidines, have also been found to incorporate into DNA and RNA, replacing the nucleic acids thymine and uracil, respectively. This incorporation occurs at a relatively low level, however, and is not thought to be the primary cause for cell death. Fluoropyrimidines, especially 5-fluorouracil, are used to treat many commonly occurring cancers, including colorectal, breast, gastric, pancreatic, and head and neck tumors.

Compared with pyrimidine antagonists, purine antagonists incorporate more readily into nucleic acids. Purine antagonists also inhibit the synthesis of nucleic acids. Each purine antagonist may inhibit purine synthesis at different points along the metabolic pathway, but their effects are perhaps most notable on the enzymes PRPP amidotransferase and IMP dehydrogenase. Purine antagonists are considered to be self-limiting, meaning that the biochemical effects produced by the agent can antagonize each other. For example, when purine synthesis is inhibited, total DNA replication is reduced, thereby diminishing the potential for incorporation of the drug into the DNA. The main purine antagonists are mercaptopurine and thioguanine, and they are used primarily to treat leukemia, especially in children.

Sugar-modified analogs were discovered in screening programs established after the clinical success of pyrimidine and purine antagonists was established. Widely used in leukemia therapy, the sugar-modified analog cytarabine was isolated from a species of sponge from the Caribbean Sea. It is characterized by a modification of the sugar moiety, not the base portion, of the nucleotide analog. Unlike the other pyrimidine and purine antagonists, which can affect both DNA and RNA, cytarabine almost exclusively affects DNA. The primary mechanism of action of cytarabine is incorporation into the DNA in place of the cytosine nucleotide. The other main sugar-modified analog, fludarabine, has a modification in both the base and sugar moiety.

Hydroxyurea is the prototypical ribonucleotide reductase inhibitor. The enzyme ribonucleotide reductase has a global effect on all DNA synthesis, as it is the enzyme responsible for converting the precursor ribonucleoside diphosphates to deoxyribonucleotide diphosphates.

Side effects: In general, antimetabolites are more toxic to cells that are actively dividing, compared to cells that are not. Because tumor cells rapidly proliferate, antimetabolites can target these cells quite effectively. The drugs cannot differentiate, however, between cancer cells and rapidly dividing healthy cells, such as those that occur in the bone marrow, the lining of the gastrointestinal tract, and hair follicles. Therefore, most side effects induced by these drugs are dependent on which normal cells are affected. Methotrexate toxicity is mainly confined to the bone marrow and the gastrointestinal tissue lining. The side effects that can result in systemic therapy with pyrimidine and purine antagonists are mainly bone marrow suppression, although gastrointestinal toxicity can occur. Fluoropyrimidines, in particular, induce nausea, vomiting, anorexia, and diarrhea.

Lisa M. Cockrell, B.S.

For Further Information

Jackman, Ann L., ed. *Antifolate Drugs in Cancer Therapy*. Totowa, N.J.: Humana Press, 1999.

Kantarjian, Hagop M., et al. *The MD Anderson Manual of Medical Oncology*. New York: McGraw-Hill, 2006.

Kufe, Donald W., et al., eds. *Holland Frei Cancer Medicine 7*. 7th ed. Hamilton, Ont.: BC Decker, 2006.

Pratt, William B., et al. *The Anticancer Drugs*. 2d ed. New York: Oxford University Press, 1994.

Rustum, Youcef M., ed. *Fluoropyrimidines in Cancer Therapy*. Totowa, N.J.: Humana Press, 2003.
Skeel, Roland T. *Handbook of Cancer Chemotherapy*. 7th ed. Philadelphia: Lippincott Williams & Wilkins, 2007.

Other Resources

National Cancer Institute
Drug Information Summaries
http://www.cancer.gov/cancertopics/druginfo/alphalist

See also: Antineoplastics in chemotherapy; Chemotherapy

▶ Antinausea medications

Category: Chemotherapy and Other Drugs
ATC code: A04A

Definition: Antinausea agents, or antiemetics, encompass a range of drug classes that act on the peripheral and central nervous systems to prevent nausea and vomiting. In patients with cancer, antiemetics are used to control acute, delayed, and anticipatory nausea and vomiting that result from chemotherapy.

Cancers treated: Indirectly used in the treatment of many cancers to control nausea and vomiting associated with many chemotherapy regimens

Subclasses of this group: Serotonin-3 antagonists, substituted benzamides, corticosteroids, pheothiazines, benzodiazepines, butyrophenones, cannabinoids, neurokinin-1 antagonists

Delivery routes: Administered to inpatients and outpatients as oral tablets, capsules, or liquids; as intravenous or intramuscular solutions; or as rectal suppositories

How these drugs work: Nausea and vomiting, or emesis, are the most common chemotherapy-associated toxicities, affecting more than 75 percent of patients, especially with the development of combination regimens. The effective use of antinausea agents to improve chemotherapy tolerance is one of the most important advances of supportive cancer care. Among the first of agents to deter emesis was metoclopramide, a substituted benzamide that acts as a dopamine receptor antagonist and, at higher doses, as an additional serotonin receptor antagonist. Although the exact mechanisms of nausea and vomiting reflexes have not been determined, neurotransmitter blockade at dopaminergic, serotonergic, neurokinin-1, and other receptors in the central nervous system or peripherally in the gastrointestinal tract successfully controls the reactions. Like metoclopramide, phenothiazines such as chlorpromazine and butyrophenones such as haloperidol also prevent nausea and vomiting by dopaminergic blockade. Dopamine antagonism from these three subclasses provides relief of moderate emesis.

The more newly developed serotonin-3 (5HT-3) receptor antagonists work peripherally, especially in the small intestine, and are extremely effective for the treatment and prevention of acute emesis. Ondansetron, granisetron, and dolasetron are equivalent in efficacy and may provide total receptor blockade, as evidenced by their dose-related efficacy plateaus. Palonsetron, a newer agent, is longer acting than others in the subclass. Because acute emesis is associated with peripheral control and delayed emesis is associated with central control, 5HT-3 antagonists are more effective in treating acute nausea and vomiting, which occurs in the first twenty-four hours after chemotherapy is administered.

Benzodiazepines such as lorazepam have some antiemetic activity by blocking cortical input to the emetic center but are more useful for their sedative and anxiolytic effects, which make the agents ideal for combination regimens. In addition, these drugs induce retrograde amnesia, which is successful in preventing anticipatory nausea and vomiting that may occur with repeat chemotherapy administration.

Neurokinin-1 (NK-1) receptors are more recently studied targets of nausea mechanisms; the only currently approved agent in the NK-1 antagonist class is aprepitant. Because NK-1 mediates substance P activation of NK-1 receptors in the brainstem, aprepitant's NK-1 receptor antagonism is useful for the treatment of delayed emesis, which is more centrally mediated. Although its efficacy alone is not yet confirmed, aprepitant successfully prevents acute and delayed nausea and vomiting when combined with serotonin antagonists and corticosteroids.

Corticosteroids, especially dexamethasone, methylprednisolone, and prednisone, have a confirmed effect, alone or in combination, against moderate nausea and vomiting, despite an unknown mechanism of action and a lack of receptor blockade. Corticosteroids are often the second drug in a combination regimen with dopamine, serotonin, or NK-1 receptor antagonists.

Lastly, cannabinoids such as dronabinol act centrally with psychotropic activity to provide limited but affirmed antinausea activity. They can be used for patients with

Common Antinausea Agents

Drug	*Brands*	*Subclass*	*Delivery Mode*	*Type of Nausea Treated*
Aprepitant	Emend	Neurokinin-1 receptor antagonist	Oral	Delayed prophylaxis, primarily (combined with corticosteroid)
Chlorpromazine, prochlorperazine, promethazine	Thorazine, Compazine, Phenergan	Phenothiazines	Oral, IV, rectal	Mild-to-moderate acute (combined with corticosteroid or 5HT-3 antagonist); breakthrough
Dexamethasone, methylprednisolone	Decadron, Medrol, MethaPred	Corticosteroids	Oral, IV	ild-to-moderate acute as monotherapy; moderate-to-severe acute when combined with 5HT-3 antagonist; delayed prophylaxis when combined with NK-1 inhibitor; delayed postchemotherapy when combined with substituted benzamide; anticipatory
Dronabinol		Cannabinoids	Oral	Anticipatory, breakthrough, or refractory nausea and vomiting
Haolperidol, droperidol	Haldol, Inapsine	Butyrophenones	Oral, IV, intramuscular	Mild-to-moderate acute (not recommended agents because of toxicities)
Lorazepam	Ativan	Benzodiazepine	Oral, IV, intramuscular	Anticipatory or breakthrough
Metoclopramide	Reglan	Substituted benzamide	Oral, IV	Acute or anticipatory (not as first-line agent); delayed when combined with corticosteroid
Ondansetron, granisetron, dolasetron, palonosetron	Zofran, Kytril, Anzemet,	Serotonin-3 receptor antagonists	Oral, IV	Uncontrolled mild, moderate, or severe acute; Moderate-to-severe acute (combined with corticosteroid); Delayed (less effective than NK-1 inhibitor)

moderate emesis and poor tolerance or response to other agents or for patients who need control of breakthrough pain.

Side effects: Each subclass of antinausea agents is associated with different side effects; successful combination regimens provide greater efficacy without overlapping drug toxicities. Metoclopramide side effects are primarily related to dopamine antagonism and include extrapyramidal reactions, including acute dystonic reactions. Akathisia, or restlessness, is common and may persist for hours. Drowsiness and diarrhea are also possible. Phenothiazines and butyrophenones also cause dopamine-related drowsiness, diarrhea, and extrapyramidal reactions. In addition, constipation, dizziness, and hypotension have been noted. Lorazepam is associated with sedation in addition to amnesia, confusion, transient enuresis, and blurred vision. Serotonin antagonists all have similar side effects of mild to moderate headache in 20 to 30 percent of patients and mild, uncommon occurrences of constipation or diarrhea. Corticosteroids may cause insomnia, hyperglycemia, gastrointestinal upset, and, rarely, psychosis. NK-1 antagonism leads to fatigue, dizziness, headache, and gastrointestinal disturbances. Side effects of dronabinol include dysphoria, hallucinations, dizziness, dry mouth, sedation, and disorientation.

Nicole M. Van Hoey, Pharm.D.

For Further Information

Grunberg, S. M. "Antiemetic Activity of Corticosteroids in Patients Receiving Cancer Chemotherapy: Dosing, Efficacy, and Tolerability Analysis." *Annals of Oncology* 18, no. 2 (February, 2007): 233-240.

Jordan, K., H. J. Schmoll, and M. S. Aapro. "Comparative Activity of Antiemetic Drugs." *Critical Reviews in Oncology/Hematology* 61, no. 2 (February, 2007): 162-175.

Roila, F., S. Fatigoni, and G. Ciccarese. "Daily Challenges in Oncology Practice: What Do We Need to Know About Antiemetics?" *Annals of Oncology* 17, suppl. 10 (September, 2006): 90-94.

See also: Chemotherapy; Gastrointestinal complications of cancer treatment; Nausea and vomiting; Topoisomerase inhibitors

▶ Antineoplastics in chemotherapy

Category: Chemotherapy and Other Drugs
ATC code: 101
Also known as: Chemotherapeutic agents, antitumor compounds, cytotoxic antibiotics

Definition: Antineoplastics are anticancer drugs used to treat malignancies and cancerous growths.

Cancers treated: Various types of cancers

Subclasses of this group: Alkylating agents, antimetabolites, mitotic inhibitors, topoisomerase inhibitors, cytotoxic antibiotics

Delivery routes: Oral, intravenous, intramuscular, or subcutaneous injection

How these drugs work: Antineoplastics are chemicals used to treat cancer and inhibit tumor cell growth. Since the term "neoplastic" refers to cancer cells, "antineoplastic" literally means "anticancer cells." Antineoplastic agents are used to stop tumor development or prevent the spread of cancer and to relieve some symptoms associated with cancer or prolong patient survival. Antineoplastics are also sometimes referred to as chemotherapeutic agents, antitumor compounds, or cytotoxic antibiotics.

The first antineoplastic agents were used in the 1940's and were either made from synthetic chemicals or derived from natural plants. More than fifty antineoplastic agents are approved by the Food and Drug Administration (FDA) for use in the United States. There are several major categories of antineoplastic agents based on their origins, chemical structures, and how they work. These classifications include alkylating agents, antimetabolites, cytotoxic antibiotics, mitotic inhibitors, and topoisomerase inhibitors. Antineoplastic agents inhibit tumor cell growth using different mechanisms, with many affecting deoxyribonucleic acid (DNA) synthesis and interfering with cell division. Others work by altering immune function or affecting hormonal status of tumors. Antineoplastic drugs are either cell-cycle specific or non-cell-cycle specific, with cell cycle-specific drugs acting only during certain phases of the cell cycle while non-cell cycle-specific drugs may act during any cell cycle phase.

The largest group of antineoplastic compounds is the alkylating agents, which were among the first anticancer drugs used. These compounds are the most commonly used agents in chemotherapy. Alkylating agents work by directly damaging DNA and preventing the cell from reproducing. These drugs work in all phases of the cell cycle. Alkylating agents work by cross-linking DNA and preventing DNA bases from pairing up correctly, which interferes with DNA synthesis. Categories of alkylating agents include busulfans, alkylating-like drugs, nitrogen mustards, ethylenimines, and nitrosureas. Nitrogen mustards comprise the largest group of alkylating drugs and are particularly useful for treating neoplasms that increase white blood cells, such as lymphomas and leukemias, because they result in leukopenia. Unlike most other types of antineoplastic agents, nitrosureas can cross the blood-brain barrier and thus are useful for treating brain tumors. Also included among the alkylating agents are the metal salts, such as carboplatin and cisplatin. Other examples of alkylating agents include chlorambucil, cyclophosamide, and thiotepa.

Antimetabolites in chemotherapy work by interfering with cancer cell metabolism. Antimetabolites are analogs of normal metabolites (nucleic acids) and act by replacing natural substances. Since these compounds structurally resemble DNA base pairs, they become incorporated into DNA, thus interfering with DNA synthesis. Antimetabolites are cell-cycle specific and attack cells only during certain cell cycle phases. Most antimetabolites are preferentially effective against cells that are actively synthesizing DNA. Antimetabolites are classified by the metabolite that they affect and include folic acid, purine, and pyrimidine analogs. All these compounds function by interfering with DNA synthesis in some way, either by directly inhibiting important enzymes or by being converted into substances that impair DNA synthesis. Methotrexate, a folic acid analog, inhibits an enzyme necessary for regeneration of intermediates required for DNA synthesis. Pyrimidine and purine analogs are converted into compounds that inhibit enzymes involved in DNA synthesis. 5-Fluorouracil and cytarabine are examples of pyrimidine analogs. Purine analogs include 6-mercaptopurine and pentostatin.

Some antineoplastic drugs are considered antimitotics or mitotic inhibitors and bind to tubulin, preventing polymerization of microtubules necessary for mitotic spindle formation. This prevents mitosis and arrests cells during metaphase. Many of the vinca alkaloids function as mitotic inhibitors. Topoisomerase inhibitors interfere with DNA synthesis by disrupting the function of the enzymes topoisomerases I and II, which are important in tubulin formation. Topoisomerases control the structure of DNA necessary for replication, and compounds that inhibit these enzymes work by preventing DNA from being unwound, a step required for DNA synthesis. Topoisomerase inhibitors include ironotecan, topotecan, etoposide, and teniposide.

Many antineoplastic compounds are derived from plants and are known as natural products. They vary mechanistically, with some functioning as alkylating agents, some inhibiting mitosis, and some affecting enzymes important in DNA synthesis. The Vinca alkaloids, made from the periwinkle plant (*Catharanthus rosea*), and the taxanes, made from the Pacific yew tree (*Taxus*), work as mitotic inhibitors by disrupting microtubule formation. Podophyllotoxins, derived from the mayapple plant (*Podophyllum peltatum*), and camptothecans, from the Asian "Happy Tree" (*Camptotheca acuminate*), function as topoisomerase inhibitors. Most of these compounds are effective against tumor cells during various cell cycle phases.

Another category of antineoplastics includes the antitumor or cytotoxic antibiotics, many of which are produced by species of the soil fungus Streptomyces. There are several cytotoxic antibiotics, such as Dactinomycin (actinomycin D), bleomycin, and doxorubicin. Cytotoxic antibiotics generally act during various phases of the cell cycle. Dactinomycin works by binding to DNA and preventing ribonucleic acid (RNA) synthesis, an important step in making proteins. Doxorubicin works by causing DNA to uncoil, which prevents the cell from reproducing. Bleomycin acts by fragmenting DNA.

There are also many compounds that do not fit into these categories but are still useful antineoplastic agents, such as hormones, enzymes, and reagents used in immunotherapy. Immunotherapy hormones work by altering the cellular environment, making it unfavorable for tumor growth. Enzymes, such as L-asparaginase, break down substances such as asparagine that tumor cells need for survival. Mitotane is a chemical related to the insecticide dichloro-diphenyl-trichloroethane (DDT) and interferes with the formation of adrenocortical steroids, with selective cytotoxic effects toward cells of the adrenal cortex. Other compounds include retinoids, such as bexarotene and tretinoid.

Side effects: Antineoplastic compounds can destroy normal cells as well as neoplastic cells, although generally antineoplastic agents have greater effects on tumor cells because they grow rapidly. Many side effects associated with antineoplastic agents occur because of their effects on normal cells, especially those that divide rapidly, such as the cells of hair follicles, ovaries, testes, and blood-forming organs. Hair loss is common as a result of effects on hair follicles. Anemia, immune system impairment, and clotting problems result from adverse effects on blood-forming organs, which lead to decreased red blood cell, white blood cell, and platelet numbers. Nausea and vomiting are among the most common adverse side effects. Other side effects may include blood in the urine, diarrhea, fever or chills, cough, wheezing, shortness of breath, unusual bruising, problems with urination, dizziness, irregular heartbeat, skin rash, fatigue, loss of taste, headache, swelling, allergic reactions, or body aches.

C. J. Walsh, Ph.D.

For Further Information

Eckman, Margaret & Labus, Diana. (Eds.). (2008). Clinical pharmacology made incredibly easy (3rd ed.). Philadelphia: Lippincott Williams & Wilkins. This book provides clear descriptions of mechanisms of action of drugs and their interactions in treatment and disease.

Skidmore-Roth, Linda. (2016). Mosby's 2016 nursing drugs reference. St. Louis: C. V. Mosby. This is the newest edition of a reference that has been valuable for over 30 years. More than 5,000 drugs are profiled, with an emphasis on patient safety.

Vardanyan, Ruben, & Hruby, Victor. (2006). Synthesis of essential drugs. Philadelphia: Elsevier. Provides descriptions of mechanism of action, implementation, and synthesis of medicinal drugs.

Trendowski, Matthew. (2015). Recent advances in the development of antineoplastic agents derived from natural products. Drugs, 75(17):1993-2016. A review journal article that covers recent advances in natural product based drug discovery and examines mechanisms of action and current clinical data.

Other Resources

Cancer Backup
General Information on Chemotherapy. http://www.cancerbackup.org.uk/Treatments/Chemotherapy

MedlinePlus
http://www.nlm.nih.gov/medlineplus/druginformation.html

American Cancer Society
www.cancer.org

Chemotherapy Drugs: How They Work
http://www.cancer.org/treatment/treatmentsandsideeffects/treatmenttypes/chemotherapyprinciplesanindepth

National Cancer Institute
Drug Information Summaries.
http://www.cancer.gov/cancertopics/druginfo/alphalist

See also: Alkylating agents in chemotherapy; Chemotherapy; Immunotherapy; Proteasome inhibitors

▶ Antiviral therapies

Category: Chemotherapy and Other Drugs
ATC code: J05

Definition: Antiviral agents are used to treat infections caused by viruses. In patients with cancer, they are also used in combination with other medications to treat human papillomavirus (HPV)-positive cervical cancer and head and neck squamous cell cancer. Antiviral agents known as protease inhibitors, nucleoside reverse transcriptase inhibitors, and nonnucleoside reverse transcriptase inhibitors are indicated for human immunodeficiency virus (HIV) infection.

Cancers treated: Cervical cancer, head and neck cancers, HIV infection and opportunistic viral infections associated with all types of cancer.

Subclasses of this group: Nucleotide analogs, purine nucleoside analogs, acyclic guanine derivatives, pyrophosphate analogs, purine nucleoside guanine derivatives, protease inhibitors, nucleoside reverse transcriptase inhibitors, nonnucleoside reverse transcriptase inhibitors

Delivery routes: Administered orally in the form of capsules, tablets, and solutions at home or in the hospital; some also administered in the hospital by intravenous (IV) infusion or subcutaneous injection

How these drugs work: The first successful antiviral drug, acyclovir, was discovered in the 1960's for the treatment of herpesvirus infection. The increased incidence of HIV infection in the 1980's initiated the development of a variety of antiviral agents that are available today. Antiviral agents work in a variety of ways depending on the drug type. Some competitively inhibit an enzyme located on the viral deoxyribonucleic acid (DNA) chain, halting growth of the viral DNA. Some work on viral ribonucleic acid (RNA), preventing the virus from penetrating healthy cells. Others inhibit viral nucleic acid synthesis by interacting directly with the DNA enzymes. Protease inhibitors inhibit the enzyme needed for viral replication. Reverse transcriptase inhibitors also inhibit viral replication after incorporating themselves into the viral DNA.

Side effects: The most common side effects associated with antiviral therapy include gastrointestinal symptoms such as anorexia, abdominal pain, diarrhea, dyspepsia, flatulence, nausea, and vomiting. Other side effects that may occur with antiviral therapy include headache, dizziness, insomnia, depression, suicidal ideation, peripheral neuropathy, weakness, rash, sweating, back pain, chest pain, fever, muscle ache, pneumonia, weight loss, anxiety, elevated or decreased blood pressure, pancreatitis, tremor, cough, shortness of breath, chills, low white blood cell count, low platelet count, anemia, hypoglycemia, seizures, hepatitis, and liver toxicity.

Collette Bishop Hendler, R.N., M.S.

For Further Information

Drug Facts and Comparisons 2008. St. Louis: Wolters Kluwer Health, 2008.
Lorigan, Paul, ed. *Lung Cancer*. Dana-Farber Cancer Institute Handbook. New York: Mosby Elsevier, 2007.
Nursing 2008 Drug Handbook. Philadelphia: Lippincott Williams & Wilkins 2008.

See also: Antidiarrheal agents; Antifungal therapies; Aplastic anemia; Herpes simplex virus; Herpes zoster virus; Infection and sepsis; Leukoencephalopathy; Viral oncology; Virus-related cancers

Common Antiviral Agents

Drug (Other Names)	*Brands*	*Subclass*	*Delivery Mode*	*Conditions Treated*
Abacavir sulfate	Ziagen	Nucleoside reverse transcriptase inhibitor	Oral	Human immunodeficiency (HIV) infection in patients with Kaposi sarcoma, other opportunistic cancers
Acyclovir, acyclovir sodium	Zovirax	Synthetic purine nucleoside	Oral, IV	Varicella and herpes zoster in cancer patients
Adefovir dipivoxil	Hepsera	Acyclic nucleotide analog	Oral	Chronic hepatitis in cancer patients
Amantadine hydrochloride	Symmetrel	Synthetic cyclic primary amine	Oral	Prevention or treatment of influenza A in cancer patients
Amprenavir	Agenerase	Protease inhibitor	Oral	Kaposi sarcoma for treatment of HIV infection
Atazanavir sulfate	Reyataz	Protease inhibitor	Oral	HIV infection in patients with Kaposi sarcoma, other opportunistic cancers
Cidofovir	Vistide	Nucleotide analog	IV	Cytomegalovirus (CMV) retinitis
Darunavir ethanolate	Prezista	Protease inhibitor	Oral	Kaposi sarcoma for treatment of HIV infection
Delavirdine mesylate	Resciptor	Nonnucleoside reverse transcriptase inhibitor	Oral	Kaposi sarcoma for treatment of HIV infection
Didanosine (ddl)	Videx, Videx EC	Nucleoside reverse transcriptase inhibitor	Oral	HIV infection in patients with Kaposi sarcoma, other opportunistic cancers
Efavirenz	Sustiva	Nonnucleoside reverse transcriptase inhibitor	Oral	HIV infection in patients with Kaposi sarcoma, other opportunistic cancers
Emtricitabine	Emtriva	Nucleoside reverse transcriptase inhibitor	Oral	HIV infection in patients with Kaposi sarcoma, other opportunistic cancers
Enfuvirtide	Fuzeon	Fusion inhibitor	Subcutaneous injection	HIV infection in patients with Kaposi sarcoma, other opportunistic cancers
Entecavir	Baraclude	Guanosine nucleoside analog	Oral	Chronic hepatitis B in patients with cancer
Famciclovir	Famvir	Synthetic acyclic guanine derivative	Oral	Acute herpes zoster infection and recurrent genital herpes in patients with cancer
Fosamprenavir calcium	Lexiva	Protease inhibitor	Oral	HIV infection in patients with Kaposi sarcoma, other opportunistic cancers
Foscarnet sodium (phosphonoformic acid)	Foscavir	Pyrophosphate analog	IV	CMV retinitis in patients with cancer

(continued)

Common Antiviral Agents *(continiued)*

Gangciclovir	Cytovene	Synthetic purine nucleoside guanine analog	Oral, IV	CMV retinitis in patients with cancer
Indinavir sulfate	Crixivan	Protease inhibitor	Oral	HIV infection in patients with Kaposi sarcoma, other opportunistic cancers
Lamivudine	Epivir	Nucleoside reverse transcriptase inhibitor	Oral	HIV infection in patients with Kaposi sarcoma and other opportunistic cancers; chronic hepatitis B infection in cancer patients
Lopinavir and ritonavir	Kaletra	Protease inhibitor	Oral	HIV infection in patients with Kaposi sarcoma, other opportunistic cancers
Nelfinavir mesylate	Viracept	Protease inhibitor	Oral	HIV infection in patients with Kaposi sarcoma, other opportunistic cancers
Nevirapine	Viramune	Nonnucleoside reverse transcriptase inhibitor	Oral	HIV infection in patients with Kaposi sarcoma, other opportunistic cancers
Oseltamivir phosphate	Tamiflu	Selective neuraminidase inhibitor	Oral	Prevention and treatment of influenza infection
Ribavirin	Copegus, Rebetol, Ribaspheres, Virazole	Synthetic nucleoside	Oral, inhalation	Chronic hepatitis infection
Ritonavir	Norvir	Protease inhibitor	Oral	HIV infection in patients with Kaposi sarcoma, other opportunistic cancers
Saquinavir mesylate	Invirase	Protease inhibitor	Oral	HIV infection in patients with Kaposi sarcoma, other opportunistic cancers
Stavudine (2,3 didehydro-3deoxythymidine, d4T)	Zerit, Zerit XR	Nucleoside reverse transcriptase inhibitor	Oral	HIV infection in patients with Kaposi sarcoma, other opportunistic cancers
Tenofovir disoproxil fumarate	Viread	Nucleoside reverse transcriptase inhibitor	Oral	HIV infection in patients with Kaposi sarcoma, other opportunistic cancers
Tipranavir	Aptivus	Protease inhibitor	Oral	HIV infection in patients with Kaposi sarcoma, other opportunistic cancers
Valacyclovir hydrochloride	Valtrex	Synthetic purine nucleoside	Oral	Herpes zoster and genital herpes in cancer patients
Valganciclovir	Valcyte	Synthetic nucleoside	Oral	CMV retinitis in cancer patients
Zanamivir	Relenza	Selective neuraminidase inhibitor	Inhalation	Prevention and treatment of influenza virus A and B
Zidovudine (azidothymidine, AZT)	Retrovir	Nucleoside reverse transcriptase inhibitor	Oral, IV	HIV infection in patients with Kaposi sarcoma, other opportunistic cancers

▶ Bacillus Calmette Guérin (BCG)

Category: Chemotherapy and Other Drugs
ATC code: 103AX03
Also known as: BCG Live, Pacis BCG Live, TICE BCG

Definition: Bacillus or bacille Calmette Guérin (BCG) solution is an immunotherapeutic agent containing live, weakened bacteria. It is currently approved by the U.S. Food and Drug Administration (FDA) as a primary therapy for carcinoma in situ of the urinary bladder. The BCG solution for bladder cancer contains water, saline, and a freeze-dried and live (but avirulent) strain of *Mycobacterium bovis*, an organism that causes tuberculosis in cattle.

The BCG vaccine is used throughout the world to immunize humans against tuberculosis, with varying rates of efficacy; the BCG vaccine is not routinely administered in the United States. BCG is named for the two Pasteur Institute researchers who discovered the vaccine against human tuberculosis: physician Léon Charles Albert Calmette (1863-1933) and bacteriologist Jean-Marie Camille Guérin (1872-1961).

Cancers treated: Superficial or early-stage bladder cancer in which tumors have not entered the muscle layer of the bladder wall

Delivery routes: Instillation

How this substance works: Generally BCG treatment follows surgery to remove tumors from the surface (epithelium) of the inside of the bladder (lumen). A health care provider inserts a catheter to deliver the BCG solution to the bladder. The solution remains in the bladder for at least two hours. The millions of *M. bovis* bacteria in BCG solution stimulate the immune system to seek out and destroy cancer cells. Patients usually have a series of weekly instillations over a number of months followed by maintenance instillations, depending on the treatment plan.

The exact mechanism of action of the BCG solution is unknown. It is thought that certain proteins in the bacteria adhere to the urothelium or lining of the bladder wall. The urothelium then releases a number of cytokines or inflammatory substances that alert the immune system that a pathogen is present. The bacteria may also enter the cancer cells and break down proteins to display on the cancer cell surface, thus flagging it for destruction by the immune system.

Approximately 70 percent of patients respond to initial treatment, and 75 percent of those patients remain free of bladder cancer for more than five years. Because BCG contains live bacteria, patients with compromised immune systems should not be treated with BCG solution. Patients should also not take antibiotics, which would kill the live bacteria and prevent effective treatment.

Side effects: Most patients (80 to 90 percent) who receive successive treatments with BCG solution experience one or more side effects, including the urgent need to urinate, blood in the urine, pain during urination, fatigue, nausea, chills, and a low-grade fever that lasts twenty-four to seventy-two hours.

Pamela Richardson, M.S.

See also: Biological therapy; Bladder cancer; Immunocytochemistry and immunohistochemistry; Immunotherapy

▶ BCR-ABL kinase and inhibitors

Category: Chemotherapy and Other Drugs
Also known as: Imatinib (trade names Gleevec in the United States, Canada and South Africa and Glivec in Europe, Australia and Latin America), dasatinib (trade name Sprycel), nilotinib (trade name Tasigna), bosutinib (trade name Bosulif), ponatinib (trade name Iclusig).

Definition: BCR-ABL is a fusion tyrosine kinase formed when the *ABL1* gene on chromosome 9 is translocated to the *BCR* gene on chromosome 22. The constitutively active fusion BCR-ABL kinase is directly related to chronic myelogenous leukemia (CML). BCR-ABL inhibitors bind to the BCR-ABL kinase and inhibit its activity.

Cancers treated: The BCR-ABL protein is a fusion tyrosine kinase resulting from the translocation of the *ABL1* [ABL (Abelson) proto-oncogene 1, non-receptor tyrosine kinase] gene from region q34 of chromosome 9 to the *BCR* (breakpoint cluster region) gene on region q11 of chromosome 22. The translocated chromosome, officially designated t(9;22) (q34.1;q11.2), is referred to as the Philadelphia chromosome (Ph1) and is characteristic of chronic myelogenous leukemia (CML). Imatinib, dasatinib, nilotinib, bosutinib, and ponatinib are drugs effective against Ph1 positive CML. Imatinib is also used to treat acute lymphoblastic leukemia, aggressive systemic mastocytosis, gastrointestinal stromal tumors (GIST), skin cancer, bone marrow disorders, and certain other malignancies.

Delivery routes: Gleevec (imatinib mesylate, the mesylate salt of imatinib) and its derivatives are easily absorbed and delivered orally as film-coated tablets (100 mg and 400 mg) with food and 8 ounces of water. The dose varies and depends on the disease and the age and weight of the patient.

How these drugs work/history of development: ABL and BCR are an ATP requiring tyrosine kinase and a serine/threonine kinase, respectively. The two kinases transfer a phosphate group from ATP to its protein targets. The fusion of ABL tyrosine kinase with a relatively small portion of BCR confers constitutive tyrosine kinase activity on the ABL part of the enzyme. This causes unregulated cell division and inhibition of DNA repair, which leads to cancer, especially CML.

In the mid to late 1980s, Ciba-Geigy established a program to develop a drug that would selectively target and specifically inhibit the BCR-ABL tyrosine kinase. By 1990, Ciba-Geigy had developed a compound called CGP-57148B that inhibits BCR-ABL activity by binding near the ATP-binding site of the BCR-ABL fusion enzyme and stabilizing it in an inactive conformation. The compound inhibits downstream BCR-ABL-activated pathways, leading to the cessation of cell growth and division and the induction of apoptosis. The compound effectively eliminated Ph^1 –positive cells in CML patients. Just before phase I clinical trials began in 1998, Ciba-Geigy and Sandoz merged and was renamed Novartis. CGP-57148B was renamed Signal Transduction Inhibitor-571 (STI-571).

Novartis began phase II trials in August 1999 and phase III trials by late 2000. On February 27, 2001, Novartis filed an application with the US Food and Drug Administration (FDA) for accelerated review and approval of STI-571. With the application, Novartis submitted the generic name of imatinib mesylate and the trade name of Glivec (pronounced GLEE-vek). The FDA required Novartis to change the name of the drug to avoid confusion with other drugs in use for unrelated disorders. Novartis chose Gleevec although the drug is marketed in Europe, Australia, and Latin America as Glivec. Approval was granted on May 10, 2001.

Point mutations in the *abl-bcr* fusion gene that replace a threonine at position 315 with an isoleucine (T315I) affect a critical fold in the enzyme and prevent a tight fit between imatinib and the kinase, which renders the enzyme resistant to imatinib. Third-generation drugs such as bosutinib (Bosulif) developed by Pfizer and ponatinib (Iclusig) developed by Ariad are effective against T315I-resistant cells. Other resistant mutations cause overexpression of the *abl-bcr* fusion gene, resulting in overproduction of so much BCR-ABL kinase that the normal dose of the drug is not inhibitory. Other resistance-conferring mutations have also been discovered. Some of these mutations preexist in resistant patients and other mutations develop during the treatment.

Imatinib and its relatives are also effective against other tyrosine kinases such as KIT and PDGF-R (platelet derived growth factor receptor).

CML, especially Ph^1-negative, is also treated with other drugs such as busulfan, hydroxyurea, and cytosine arabinoside (ara-C) that do not inhibit BCR-ABL kinase.

Side Effects: The side effects of imatinib and its derivatives are usually benign and include but are not limited to flu-like symptoms, nausea, diarrhea, rash, infections, loss of appetite, weight gain, edema (lungs and other tissues), headache, leg cramps, itchy rash, easy bruising, unusual bleeding (nose, mouth, vagina, or rectum), bloody stools and urine, mouth and skin sores, rapid heart rate, shortness of breath, fatigue, dry skin, muscle weakness, purple or red pinpoint spots under the skin; dizziness, drowsiness, and blurred vision. Serious side effects occur less frequently and can include signs of an allergic reaction (hives, difficulty breathing, and swelling of the face, lips, tongue, or throat), severe edema, hemorrhage, and liver toxicity. Side effects may be more serious in the elderly. Women who are pregnant, who may become pregnant or are breast feeding should not take or handle imatinib or its derivatives. Imatinib can interact with certain other drugs and should not be used in combination with other drugs without consulting a pharmacist and/or a physician.

Charles L. Vigue, PhD

For Further Information

Hughes, Timothy P., David M. Ross & Melo, Junia V. (2014). *Handbook of chronic myeloid leukemia*. New York: Springer.

Shokat, Kevan M., (Ed.). (2014). *Methods in enzymology: Protein kinase inhibitors in research and medicine* (Vol. 548). Waltham, MA: Academic Press.

Wapner, Jessica. (2013). *The Philadelphia chromosome: A mutant gene and the quest to cure cancer at the genetic level.* New York: The Experiment.

Other Resources

National Cancer Institute: *BCR-ABL fusion gene*
http://www.cancer.gov/publications/dictionaries/cancer-terms?cdrid=561237

Medscape: Mechanisms of BCR-ABL in the Pathogenesis of Chronic Myelogenous Leukemia
http://www.medscape.com/viewarticle/500691
American Cancer Society: Do we know what causes chronic myeloid leukemia?
http://www.cancer.org/cancer/leukemia-chronic myeloidcml/detailedguide/leukemia-chronic-myeloid-myelogenous-what-causes

See also: Chemotherapy

▶ Benzodiazepines

Category: Chemotherapy and Other Drugs
ATC code: N05BA
Also known as: Alprazolam (Xanax), diazepam (Valium), lorazepam (Ativan)

Definition: Benzodiazepines are a class of drugs with antianxiety, sedative, and muscle-relaxing properties.

Cancers treated: Adjuvant therapy for many types of cancer

Delivery routes: Orally by capsule or tablet, intramuscularly by injection

How these drugs work: Benzodiazepines are a class of medications that act primarily on the gamma aminobutyric acid-α (GABA-A) receptors in the brain. Medications within the class vary according to their rapidness of onset, potency, frequency of dosing, length of effect, and half-life. They are typically used in the general medical population to alleviate anxiety or treat insomnia. Benzodiazepines are put to similar uses with cancer patients, as well as directed toward disease-specific conditions.

When choosing among benzodiazepines, physicians consider the unique properties of specific medications (such as speed of onset, duration of effect, side effects), as well as patient characteristics (age, vigor, pain tolerance, coping skills) and the types of cancer and treatments involved. Short-acting medications with rapid onset are often employed to treat acute anxiety, panic, and phobic responses to therapy. Longer-acting medications may be selected to assist patients engaging in painful or aversive cancer treatments (such as chemotherapy) to promote relaxation, reduce anticipatory anxiety, suppress recall of treatment, and alleviate nausea and restlessness (akisthisia). Long-acting benzodiazepines may also be employed to treat generalized anxiety and grief reactions stemming from cancer. Highly sedating benzodiazepines are often used to treat anxiety-related insomnia.

Side effects: A number of side effects are associated with benzodiazepines. Long-term use can lead to drowsincss and deficits in memory, concentration, and motor coordination. Though safe for most in recommended dosages, benzodiazepines can potentially cause respiratory depression, and patients should be monitored closely as they initiate treatment. All benzodiazepines, especially those with rapid onsets and short durations of action, have the potential to cause dependence and, in rare cases in the cancer patient population, abuse. Consequently, physicians must closely supervise patients' use of these medications. Abrupt discontinuation of benzodiazepines may cause withdrawal symptoms that, while severe, are usually managed with appropriate medical intervention. These symptoms include "rebound" anxiety, confusion, agitation, seizures, and, rarely, death.

Paul F. Bell, Ph.D.

See also: Antinausea medications; Anxiety; Pain management medications

Common Benzodiazepines

The following common benzodiazepines are used to treat acute mania, alcohol dependence, seizures, anxiety, insomnia, and muscular disorders.

Trade Name	*Generic Name*
Ativan	lorazepam
Dalman	flurazepam
Dormicum	midazolam
Halcion	triazolam
Klonopin	clonazepam
Lexotanil	bromazepam
Librium	chlordiazepoxide
Loramet	lormetazepam
Mogadon	nitrazepam
ProSom	estazolam
Restoril	temazepam
Rohypnol	flunitrazepam
Sedoxil	mexazolam
Serax	oxazepam
Valium	diazepam
Xanax	alprazolam

▶ BET inhibitors

Category: Chemotherapy and Other Drugs

Definition: Small molecules that reversibly bind to members of the bromodomain-extraterminal family of proteins and prevent them from activating the expression of particular genes.

Cancers treated: Being tested as treatments against several different types of cancer.

Delivery routes: oral, subcutaneous, intravenous, and to be determined.

How these drugs work: Human DNA is assembled into a tight, compact structure called chromatin. The basic structural subunit of chromatin consists of approximately 147 bases of double-stranded DNA wrapped around an eight-subunit protein complex. This octameric complex consists of two copies of four different histone proteins; histone 2A (H2A), histone 2B (H2B), histone 3 (H3), and histone 4 (H4). The histone octamer plus its associated DNA constitutes a so-called "nucleosome." The front or amino termini of histone proteins are very positively charged, which causes histones to bind tightly, albeit non-specifically, to negatively charged DNA.

Gene regulation in cells is largely controlled by the reversible modification of histone proteins. Enzymes called "histone acetyl transferases" attach acetyl groups (CH_3-COO^-) to the amino termini of histone proteins, which neutralize the positive charge of histones and diminish their affinity for DNA. The loosening of the structure of chromatin facilitates the activity of the gene expression machinery.

BET Inhibitor	Company	Clinical Trial
FT-1101	Forma Therapeutics	NCT02543879 - Phase I Relapsed/Refractory Acute Leukemia or High-Risk Myelodysplastic Syndrome (MDS)
CPI-0610	Constellation Pharmaceuticals	NCT01949883 – Phase I Progressive Lymphoma
CPI-0610	Constellation Pharmaceuticals	NCT02157636 – Phase I Previously Treated Multiple Myeloma
CPI-0610	Constellation Pharmaceuticals	NCT02158858 – Phase I Acute Leukemia, MDS, or Myelodysplastic/Myeloproliferative Neoplasms
GSK525762 (formerly I-BET762)	GlaxoSmithKline	NCT01943851 – Phase I Relapsed, Refractory Hematologic Malignancies
GSK525762	GlaxoSmithKline	NCT01587703 – Phase I NMC and Other Cancers
GSK2820151	GlaxoSmithKline	NCT02630251 – Phase I Advanced Recurrent Solid Tumors
OTX015	Oncoethix GmbH – subsidiary of Merck	NCT02259114 – Phase I Advanced Solid Tumors
BMS-986158	Bristol-Meyers-Squibb	NCT02419417 – Phase I/II Advanced Solid Tumors
INCB054329	Incyte Corporation	NCT02431260 – Phase I/II Advanced Malignancies
BAY1238097	Bayer	NCT02369029 – Phase I Advanced Malignancies
TEN-010	Tensha Therapeutics	NCT02308761 – Phase I Acute Myeloid Leukemia MDS
TEN-010	Tensha Therapeutics	NCT01987362 – Phase I Solid Tumors

Histone acetylation has an additional function with respect to activating gene expression. Cells contain proteins that possess a specific protein substructure (domain) called a "bromodomain." Bromodomain-containing proteins bind to acetylated amino acids (specifically acetyl-lysine) in histone proteins and activate gene expression or further modify the structure of chromatin.

One particular class of bromodomain-containing proteins, the BET or bromodomain- extraterminal family of proteins, regulate gene expression through their interaction with other proteins. They recruit elements of the gene expression machinery to specific spots on chromosomes to stimulate gene expression. In humans, BET family members include BRD2, BRD3, BRD4, and BRDT. Abnormalities of BRD protein function have been linked to several different types of cancers.

Small molecules called BET inhibitors reversibly bind to the acetyl-lysine-binding pocket of bromodomain-containing proteins and prevent them from associating with acetylated histones. BET inhibitors can ameliorate the abnormal gene expression patterns caused by BRD protein dysfunction. Because many different types of cancers show BRD-dependent gene expression abnormalities, BET inhibitors have the potential to treat a wide range of different cancers.

As an example, NUT midline carcinoma (NMC) is a rare, aggressive epithelial cancer characterized by chromosomal rearrangements that involve specific regions of chromosome 15 (15q14). In the vast majority of cases, the particular chromosome rearrangements found in NMC cells produce a fusion between the NUT gene and the BRD3 or BRD4 genes. In cell culture and in laboratory animals transplanted with NMC cells, the BET inhibitor JQ1 induces the differentiation of NMC cells and arrests their growth. Unfortunately, the body breaks down JQ1 too quickly for it to be therapeutically useful.

However, other BET inhibitors have entered clinical trials and are presently being tested for efficacy against several different types of cancer (see table).

The therapeutic capabilities of BET inhibitors are only beginning to be realized.

Side Effects: Remain to be determined.

Michael Buratovich, PhD

For Further Information

Egger, Gerda & Arimondo, Paola. (Eds.). (2016). *Drug discovery in cancer epigenetics*. Waltham, MA: Academic Press.

Filippakopoulos, Panagis. (2012). "Histone recognition and large-scale structural analysis of the human bromodomain family." *Cell* 149(1): 214-231.

Huang, Suming, Litt, Michael D., & Blakey, C. A. (Eds.). (2015). *Epigenetic gene expression and regulation*. Waltham, MA: Academic Press.

Shi, Junwei, & Vakoc, Christopher R. (2014). "The mechanisms behind the therapeutic activity of BET bromodomain inhibition." *Molecular Cell* 54(5): 728-736.

Other Resources

Structural Genomic Consortium:
http://www.thesgc.org/groupprofile/9493

See also: Histone acetylation/deacetylation; Cognitive effects of cancer and chemotherapy

▶ Biological therapy

Category: Chemotherapy and Other Drugs

Also known as: Immunotherapy, biological response modifier therapy, biotherapy, biologic agents, biologic therapies, biologicals

Definition: Biological therapy is an emerging, growing class of cancer drugs that work to help optimize the ability of the body's immune system to fight cancer or other diseases, or to help lessen side effects from other cancer treatments such as chemotherapy.

Cancers treated: A number of cancers, including melanoma, leukemia, breast, ovarian, colon, lung, and kidney cancers

Subclasses of this group: Cytokines, monoclonal antibodies, colony-stimulating factors, antiangiogenesis agents, cancer vaccines

Delivery routes: The delivery route varies depending on which biological therapy is being used. Various biological therapies may be given by mouth, by intravenous (IV) drip (infusion), by subcutaneous or intramuscular injection, or by delivery directly into a body cavity to treat a specific site.

How these drugs work: The cells, antibodies, and organs of the immune system work to protect and defend the body against foreign invaders, such as bacteria or viruses. The immune system is a complex network of cells and organs that work together in a variety of ways. White blood cells are a very important part of the immune system. Lymphocytes are a type of white blood cell found in the blood and many other parts of the body that are intimately involved with the way that most biologic agents work. Types of lymphocytes include B cells, T cells, and natural killer (NK) cells. B cells mature into plasma cells that secrete proteins called antibodies, which recognize and attach to foreign substances known as antigens. Each type of B cell makes one specific antibody that recognizes one specific antigen. T cells produce proteins called cytokines, which include interferons, interleukins, and colony-stimulating factors. Cytokines are proteins that activate the immune system and that play an important role in communication between immune system cells. NK cells produce powerful cytokines that attach to and kill many foreign invaders, infected cells, and cancerous cells.

Advances in techniques of molecular biology since the 1980's have brought about a revolution in the understanding of many biological processes at a molecular level, including mechanisms involved in immunity and the pathogenesis of many diseases. In many cases, it has become possible to identify discrete specific molecular targets for therapeutic intervention and to design therapies to block or interact with those targets. At the same time, technological advances have made it possible to engineer and to produce these targeted therapeutic molecules for medical use.

Physicians and researchers have found that, in addition to protecting the body against foreign invaders, the immune system might be able to differentiate between healthy cells and cancer cells in the body and to eliminate cancerous ones. Biological therapies are designed to repair, stimulate, or enhance the immune system, either directly or indirectly, by assisting in the following ways: making cancer cells more recognizable by the immune system, boosting the killing power of immune system cells, changing the way in which cancer cells grow such that they act more like healthy cells, stopping the process that changes a normal cell into a cancerous cell, enhancing the body's ability to repair or replace normal cells damaged or destroyed by other forms of cancer treatment such as chemotherapy or radiation, and preventing cancer cells from spreading to other parts of the body.

Biological therapies involve molecules that the body normally produces in small amounts in response to infection and disease and the use of modern recombinant deoxyribonucleic acid (DNA) technology to produce these molecules in large amounts for use in the treatment of cancers and other diseases. Molecular splicing of genes or portions of genes of interest to form DNA sequences that code for recombinant or fusion proteins is performed. These recombinant DNA sequences are spliced into plasmid vector molecules that can be introduced into host cells, which can be used in scaled-up production of large amounts of the purified recombinant or fusion protein.

Important types of biological therapies are cytokines (interferons and interleukins), monoclonal antibodies, growth factors, colony-stimulating factors, antiangiogenesis agents, and cancer vaccines.

Interferons were the first cytokines to be produced in the laboratory for use as biological therapies. Several types of inferons occur naturally in the body, of which interferon alpha is the most widely used in cancer treatment. Interferons can improve the immune system function against cancer cells and may in addition directly slow the growth of cancer cells or promote their development into cells with more normal behavior. There is some evidence that interferons may also stimulate NK cells and T cells, thereby boosting the immune system's function against cancer cells. Intron A (interferon alpha) has been approved by the Food and Drug Administration (FDA) for cancer treatment; it is used for the treatment of hairy cell leukemia, melanoma, chronic myeloid leukemia, and AIDS-related Kaposi sarcoma and non-Hodgkin lymphoma.

Interleukins are also cytokines that occur naturally in the body. Many types have been identified. Interleukin-2, which stimulates the growth and activity of many immune cells which can destroy cancer cells, has been the most widely studied in cancer treatment. Proleukin (interleukin-2) has been approved for use in the treatment of metastatic melanoma and metastatic renal cell carcinoma.

Monoclonal antibodies are a single species of antibody that is produced in the laboratory from a single type of cell and is specific for a particular antigen. The production of monoclonal antibodies involves the creation of a hybrid cell line specific for that antibody molecule, called a hybridoma. Once produced, a hybridoma can be perpetuated in the laboratory to produce as much of the pure monoclonal antibody as desired. Monoclonal antibodies may be used in several ways. They may be used to boost the immune response to cancer cells, they may be designed to act against growth factors to inhibit the growth of cancer cells, and they may be linked to anticancer drugs, radioactive substances, or toxins to act as a vector to deliver these toxic agents directly to cancer cells. Rituxan (rituxamab) and Herceptin (trastuzumab) are examples of monoclonal antibodies that have been approved by the FDA, Rituxan for the treatment of non-Hodgkin lymphoma and Herceptin to treat metastatic breast cancer.

Common Biological Therapies

Drug (Other Names)	*Brands*	*Subclass*	*Delivery Mode*	*Cancers Treated*
Aldesleukin (interleukin-2)	Proleukin	Cytokine	Subcutaneous	Kidney cancer, melanoma
Alemtuzumab	Campath	Monoclonal antibody	IV	Chronic lymphocytic leukemia
Bacillus Calmette-Guérin vaccine	TheraCys BCG, TICE BCG	Vaccine	Introduction into bladder	Bladder cancer
Bevacizumab	Avastin	Monoclonal antibody	IV	Lung cancer, colorectal cancer
Cetuximab	Erbitux	Monoclonal antibody	IV	Head and neck cancers, colorectal cancer
Epoetin alfa, erythropoietin	Procrit	Colony-stimulating factor	Subcutaneous	Boosts red blood cell level during chemotherapy
Epratuzumab	LymphoCide	Monoclonal antibody	IV	B-cell leukemia
Filgrastim, granulocyte colony-stimulating factor	Neupogen	Colony-stimulating factor	Subcutaneous, IV	Boosts white blood cell level during chemotherapy
Gemtuzumab ozogamicin	Mylotarg	Monoclonal antibody	IV	Acute myclogcnous leukemia
Ibritumomab tiuxetan	Zevalin	Monoclonal antibody	IV	B-cell lymphoma
Interferon alpha-2a	Roferon-A	Cytokine	Subcutaneous	Hairy cell leukemia
Interferon alpha-2b	Intron-A	Cytokine	Subcutaneous	Melanoma, hairy cell leukemia, non-Hodgkin lymphoma, Kaposi sarcoma
Lym-1	Oncolym	Monoclonal antibody	IV	Lymphoma
Oprelvekin (interleukin-11)	Neumega	Cytokine	Subcutaneous	Boosts platelet level during chemotherapy
Panitumumab	Vectibix	Human monoclonal antibody	IV	Colorectal cancer
Quadrivalent human papillomavirus recombinant vaccine	Gardasil	Vaccine	Intramuscular	Cervical cancer
Rituximab	Rituxan	Monoclonal antibody	IV	Non-Hodgkin lymphoma
Tositumomab	Bexxar	Monoclonal antibody	IV	B-cell lymphoma
Trastuzumab	Herceptin	Monoclonal antibody	IV	Breast cancer

Colony-stimulating factors (CSFs) stimulate bone marrow cells to divide and develop into white blood cells, red blood cells, and platelets. CSFs may be helpful for some patients undergoing treatment for cancer because many anticancer drugs used in chemotherapy can damage the body's ability to make these important cells in the bone marrow. Thus patients receiving chemotherapy have an increased risk of developing infections, anemia, and bleeding more easily. The dose of chemotherapy that a patient receives, and therefore the chemotherapy regimen's effectiveness in fighting cancer, can sometimes be increased by using CSFs to eliminate or reduce the risk of infection or the need for transfusions. Neupogen (filgrastim) and Procrit (epoetin alfa) are colony-stimulating factors that the FDA has approved for use in cancer patients, Neupogen to boost the number of white blood cells during chemotherapy and Procrit to boost the number of red blood cells during chemotherapy.

Antiangiogenesis agents, also called angiogenesis inhibitors, are an emerging type of biological therapy that show promise in fighting cancer. Cancer cells are rapidly dividing cells that depend on a rich network of small blood vessels to supply them with oxygen and nutrients. Tumors must generate this network of new blood vessels, a process called angiogenesis. Several types of molecules and antibodies have been shown to prevent angiogenesis and shrink tumors. Avastin (bevacizumab) is an antiangiogenic monoclonal antibody that has been approved for the treatment of lung and colorectal cancers.

Cancer vaccines are another type of biological therapy being studied. Vaccines for infectious diseases work by exposing an uninfected individual to a weakened form of the infectious agent. The vaccine stimulates the immune system to mount an immune response to the agent but cannot cause the disease. The immune system produces antibodies specific to antigens present on the surface of the infectious agent. The immune system is also stimulated to produce certain types of T cells, which remember the exposure to the antigen. If the individual is subsequently challenged with the same infectious agent, then these T cells will orchestrate a quick and effective immune response, protecting the individual from contracting the disease. Cancer vaccines to treat existing cancers (therapeutic vaccines) or to protect healthy individuals from developing cancer (prophylactic vaccines) are being studied. Therapeutic vaccines may be effective in stopping the growth of existing cancer cells, in preventing cancer from recurring, or in killing existing cancer cells. Prophylactic vaccines are administered to healthy individuals to protect against cancers that are caused by viruses. Gardisil (quadrivalent human papillomavirus recombinant vaccine) is a prophylactic vaccine that has been approved by the FDA for the prevention of cervical cancer caused by human papillomavirus.

Some biological therapies have been approved by the FDA for certain types of cancer, while many, still in development, are offered in clinical research studies to measure the effects of the treatment. In these cases, study results are often used as part of the FDA evaluation of the drug's efficacy and safety.

Side effects: The side effects of biological therapy regimens are variable from patient to patient. The most common side effects are a result of stimulation of the immune system and are similar to flulike symptoms, including fever, chills, body aches, nausea, vomiting, loss of appetite, and fatigue. Some patients may experience a rash or swelling at the injection site. Most side effects diminish one to two days after treatment. For patients who receive multiple doses of a biological therapy, the side effects usually lessen over time.

Jill Ferguson, Ph.D.

For Further Information

Kimura, F. "Molecular Target Drug Discovery." *Internal Medicine* 46 (2007): 87-89.

Old, L. J. "Immunotherapy for Cancer." *Scientific American* 275 (1996): 136-143.

Reang, P., M. Gupta, and K. Kohli. "Biological Response Modifiers in Cancer." *Medscape General Medicine* 14 (2006): 33.

Rosenberg, Steven A., ed. *Principles and Practice of the Biologic Therapy of Cancer*. 3d ed. Philadelphia: Lippincott Williams & Wilkins, 2000.

Sorscher, S. M. "Biological Therapy Update in Colorectal Cancer." *Expert Opinion on Biological Therapy* 7 (2007): 509-519.

Zafir-Lavie, I., Y. Michaeli, and Y. Reiter. "Novel Antibodies as Anticancer Agents." *Oncogene* 28 (2007): 3714-3733.

Other Resources

American Cancer Society
Immunotherapy
http://www.cancer.org/docroot/CRI/content/CRI_2_4_4X_Biological_Therapy_Immunotherapy_50.asp?sitearea=

Emory Healthcare
Biologic Therapies for Cancer Care
http://healthlibrary.epnet.com/GetContent.aspx?token=8482e079-8512-47c2-960c-a403c77a5e4c&chunkiid=32583

National Cancer Institute
Biological Therapy
http://www.cancer.gov/cancertopics/biologicaltherapy

Stanford Comprehensive Cancer Center
Biological Therapy for Cancer Treatment
http://www.cancer.gov/cancertopics/biologicaltherapy

See also: Anthrax; Antineoplastics in chemotherapy; Bacillus Calmette Guérin (BCG); Cancer biology; Chemotherapy; Cytokines; Gene therapy; Immune response to cancer; Immunotherapy; Medical oncology; Metastasis; Monoclonal antibodies; Nutrition and cancer treatment; Stem cell transplantation; Tumor necrosis factor (TNF); Tyrosine kinase inhibitors; Vaccines, therapeutic

▶ Bisphosphonates

Category: Chemotherapy and Other Drugs
ATC code: M05BA

Definition: Bisphosphonates are medications that act primarily on bone to inhibit resorption or bone destruction resulting from cell-induced bone breakdown. They treat various bone-degenerating conditions.

Cancers treated: Breast cancer, hypercalcemia of malignancy (HCM), metastatic bone cancer, multiple myeloma, bone pain, osteoporotic bone loss from cancer treatments

Subclasses of this group: Aminobisphosphonates, nonaminobisphosphonates

Delivery routes: Bisphosphonates are administered as oral tablets and as intravenous (IV) solutions to outpatients and inpatients. Bisphosphonates in any form are best administered without food to avoid decreased bioavailability.

How these drugs work: Bone resorption is part of normal bone regeneration mediated by osteoclasts, or bone breakdown cells. Abnormal osteoclast activity results from lytic bone lesions of multiple myeloma, metastatic bone tumors from breast cancer or other solid tumors, or osteoporosis from glucocorticoids in chemotherapy regimens and from breast-cancer-induced menopause.

Bisphosphonates inhibit resorption by decreasing osteoclast activity. This mechanism reduces further bone loss and fracture, minimizes pain associated with osteoclast lesions and weakened bone, and reverses hypercalcemia of malignancy (HCM), which can result when bone breakdown releases calcium to the blood. Monthly bisphosphonate administration has been shown to reduce the incidence of bone metastases in women with breast cancer as well, and these drugs have substantially reduced the risk of bone loss and fracture in spinal vertebrae and the hip.

Side effects: A major side effect of this drug class is irritation of the esophageal mucosa, which can be reduced by taking the drug with a full glass of water and by remaining in an upright position directly after drug ingestion. This side effect may occur even with IV administration.

Other side effects include constipation, diarrhea, dyspnea, myalgia, fever, decreased calcium and phosphate, and altered magnesium. Impaired kidney function and renal failure are possible. IV administration causes fever, flulike syndrome, and local injection site reactions. Other side effects noted in trials of patients with cancer include anxiety, headache, insomnia, anorexia, and abdominal pain.

Nicole M. Van Hoey, Pharm.D.

See also: Bone scan; Hypercalcemia; Paget disease of bone

Common Bisphosphonate Agents

Drug	*Brands*	*Delivery Mode*	*Cancers/Conditions Treated*
Alendronate	Fosamax	Oral	Glucocorticoid-induced osteoporosis
Etidronate	Didronel	Oral, IV	Hypercalcemia of malignancy (HCM)
Ibandronate	Boniva	Oral, IV	Breast cancer bone metastases; menopause-induced osteoporosis
Pamidronate	Aredia	IV	HCM malignancy with or without bone metastases; breast cancer and multiple myeloma; off-label for pain associated with prostatic carcinoma; possible prevention of breast cancer-related bone loss
Risedronate	Actonel	Oral	Glucocorticoid-induced osteoporosis; possible prevention of breast cancer-related bone loss
Tiludronate	Skelid	Oral	Bone metastases
Zoledronic acid	Reclast, Zometa	IV	Multiple myeloma; solid tumor bone metastases; HCM

▶ Bortezomib (Velcade)

Category: Chemotherapy and Other Drugs
Also known as: Velcade®; [(1R)-3-methyl-1-[[(2S)-1-oxo-3-phenyl-2-[(pyrazinylcarbonyl) amino]propyl] amino]butyl] boronic acid; PS-341.

Definition: Bortezomib is a chemotherapeutic agent, specifically a modified dipeptidyl boronic acid whose molecular formula is $C19H25BN4O4$.

Cancers treated: Bortezomib is currently approved by the Food and Drug Administration to treat multiple myeloma and mantle cell lymphoma.

Mantle cell lymphoma (MCL) begins in a type of lymphocyte (white blood cell of the immune system) known as a B-lymphocyte. Most cases of MCL involve B-lymphocytes in a specific area of a lymph node known as the mantle zone. Lymph nodes are responsible for filtering foreign bodies or other harmful substances from the body.

In multiple myeloma, the affected cell is a B-lymphocyte that has developed into a plasma cell. Plasma cells specialize in the production of antibodies, proteins that identify and neutralize pathogens. Multiple myeloma primarily affects bone marrow (the soft tissue center of most bones).

Delivery routes: Subcutaneous or intravenous routes.

How these drugs work: Bortezomib is the first in a class of drugs called proteasome inhibitors. A proteasome is a cellular, multiprotein complex involved in degrading or processing intracellular proteins. Such proteins may be degraded for various reasons, such as when they are damaged or no longer needed.

Bortezomib has been found to affect several intracellular proteins involved in mediating various cell regulatory pathways, including cell proliferation and programmed cell death (apoptosis). Apoptosis is a normal and controlled physiological process that degrades a cell into small, membrane-bound bodies (apoptotic bodies) that are removed by the immune system. The process is necessary, for example, during embryonic development, and to remove old, damaged or virus-infected cells, and cancer cells. Bortezomib treatment can activate particular intracellular proteins, prevent the activation of others, or positively or negatively affect the production of still other proteins. Although a wide variety of intracellular proteins may be affected by bortezomib treatment and subsequent proteasome inhibition, examples of such proteins include, nuclear factor-kappa β (NF-κβ), c-Jun amino-terminal kinase, p53 and gp130 (a glycoprotein, or a protein to which short sugar chains are attached).

NF-κβ, whose activation is prevented by bortezomib treatment, is a transcription factor, a protein that promotes the production of other proteins. NF-κβ promotes production of proteins that block apoptosis and others that promote cell growth, cell division, and ultimately cell survival. Conversely, bortezomib activates c-Jun amino-terminal kinase, a protein that activates certain enzymes called "caspases," such as caspase-3 and caspase-8. Caspases are a family of proteases, proteins that cleave proteins at defined sites, and induce apoptosis.

Bortezomib treatment increases production of p53, a tumor suppressor protein. This protein has a variety of anticancer functions, including promoting apoptosis and preventing cell division. Conversely, bortezomib treatment decreases production of gp130. This glycoprotein is necessary for the activity of various cytokines, small proteins involved in various cellular processes, including cellular proliferation (eg, tumor cell proliferation) and differentiation (conversion of one cell type into another).

Side effects: The most common side effects include nausea, vomiting, diarrhea, fatigue, tingling or numbness in the hands, arms, legs or feet, constipation, decreased levels of red blood cells, rash, fever, decreased quantities of platelets, and decreased levels of white blood cells.

Jason J. Schwartz, PhD, JD

For Further Information

Accardi, F., Toscani, D., Bolzoni, M., Dalla Palma, B., Aversa, F. & Giuliani, N. (2015). Mechanism of action of bortezomib and the new proteasome inhibitors on myeloma cells and the bone microenvironment: Impact on myeloma-induced alterations of bone remodeling. *Biomed Research International*, v. 2015, Article ID 172458, 13 pages.

Ping Dou, Q. & Zonder, J. A. (2014). Overview of proteasome inhibitor-based anti-cancer therapies: Perspective on bortezomib and second generation proteasome inhibitors versus future generation inhibitors of ubiquitin-proteasome system. *Current Cancer Drug Targets*, 14(6), 517-536.

Vanneman, M., & Dranoff, G. (2012). Combining immunotherapy and targeted therapies in cancer treatment. *Nature Reviews Cancer*, 12(4): 237-251.

Chen, D., Frezza, M, Schmitt, S, Kanwar, J. & Dou, Q.P. (2011). Bortezomib as the first proteasome inhibitor anticancer drug: Current status and future perspectives. *Current Cancer Drug Targets*, 11(3): 239-253.

Richardson, P. G., Mitsiades, C., Hideshima, T. & Anderson, K. C. (2006). Bortezomib: Proteasome inhibition as an effective anticancer therapy. *Annual Review of Medicine*, 57, 33-47.

Chauhan, D., Hideshima, T., & Anderson, K. C. (2005). Proteasome inhibition in multiple myeloma: Therapeutic implication. *Annual Reviews of Pharmacology and Toxicology*, 45, 465-476.

Other Resources

Millennium Pharmaceuticals, Inc.
http://www.velcade.com

Multiple Myeloma Research Foundation
http://www.themmrf.org

Lymphoma Research Foundation
http://www.lymphoma.org

US Food and Drug Administration
Questions and Answers on Velcade®
http://www.fda.gov/Drugs/DrugSafety/PostmarketDrugSafetyInformationforPatientsandProviders/ucm106502.htm

See also: Chemotherapy

▶ Brompton cocktail

Category: Chemotherapy and Other Drugs
Also known as: Brompton's mixture, hospice mix

Definition: Brompton cocktail is a palliative elixir containing morphine, cocaine, ethanol, and other ingredients to lessen or prevent the pain and distress associated with terminal illness, especially advanced cancer. It is no longer part of standard care.

Cancers treated: Previously used for advanced, painful tumors in patients near death

Delivery routes: Oral as a liquid

How this substance works: Elixirs of morphine and cocaine were first described in 1896 as treatments for the pain associated with advanced cancer by the English surgeon Herbert Snow. A specific mixture was published under the auspices of the Royal Brompton Hospital in London in 1952; the ingredients included morphine hydrochloride, cocaine hydrochloride, alcohol, and chloroform water. Several different formulations calling for heroin (diacetylmorphine), cannabis, antiemetics, distilled spirits, and sedatives have been promoted over the years. Flavoring syrup is sometimes added. It was widely used in the early 1970's, mostly in hospice care. Two of its main proponents were Cicely Saunders, founder of the modern hospice movement, and Elisabeth Kübler-Ross, a psychiatrist and authority on end-of-life care. The active ingredients are intended to provide a welcome combination of analgesia, disinhibition, and stimulation. Cough suppression was an important effect in patients with lung or airway malignancies (or end-stage tuberculosis). The mixture was promoted as more cost effective at treating intractable cancer pain than parenteral narcotics.

Several significant liabilities have contributed to the disappearance of the Brompton cocktail from modern oncology practice. In 1979, controlled trials showed that oral morphine alone gave pain relief equivalent to the cocktail, that oral morphine and oral heroin were equally effective, and that oral cocaine had no effect on patients' alertness or sociability. One study concluded that "the Brompton Cocktail is no more than a traditional British way of administering oral morphine to cancer patients in pain." The potential for diversion and abuse was illustrated by a case report in which an individual obtained the mixture illicitly and injected it in lieu of heroin. Each of the cocktail's active ingredients has addictive and tolerization potential, making discontinuation difficult. Even though terminal cancer patients often require multiple drugs for symptom management, the convenience of an "all-in-one" mixture of drugs such as the Brompton cocktail is outweighed by the benefits obtained by monitoring and adjusting analgesics, antineoplastics, antiemetics, and psychoactive drugs individually.

Side effects: The side effects include sedation, confusion, constipation, decreased breathing, tolerization, and addiction.

John B. Welsh, M.D., Ph.D.

See also: Do-Not-Resuscitate (DNR) order; End-of-life care; Home health services; Hospice care; Pain management medications; Palliative treatment

▶ Capecitabine

Category: Chemotherapy and Other Drugs
Also known as: Xeloda

Cancers treated: Capecitabine is approved to treat breast, colon, and other cancers that have spread (metastasized).

Delivery routes: Capecitabine is given in pill form. The pills are taken within 30 minutes after eating. Two to 3 quarts of water should be consumed every 24 hours.

How drug works: Capecitabine is activated by enzymes in the body and converted to 5-fluorouracil (5'-FU) which inhibits production or repair of DNA, eventually causing death of that cell. Capecitabine (5'-deoxy-5-fluorouridine, 5'-DFUr) is converted to 5'-deoxy-5-fluorocytidine (5'-DFCyd) by the enzyme carboxylesterase which is found in liver and some types of tumor cells. Next 5'-DFCyd is metabolized to 5'-deoxy-fluorouridine (5'-DFUrd) by cytidine deaminase found in high concentrations in liver and tumor tissues. 5'-DFUrd is then acted on by thymidine phosphorylase, abundant in tumors, to produce active 5'-fluorouracil. Normal and tumor cells convert 5'-fluorouracil to 5'-fluoro-2'-deoxyuridine monophosphate and 5'-fluorouridine triphosphate. 5'-fluorouridine triphosphate and the folate cofactor N^{5-10}-methylene tetrahydrofolate covalently bind to thymidine synthase and inhibit formation of thymidylate from 2'-deoxyuridate. Thymidylate is a precursor for thymidine phosphate, which is required for DNA synthesis. Its absence inhibits cell division. Also nuclear transcription enzymes may incorporate 5'-fluorouridine triphosphate into RNA synthesis, which interferes with RNA processing and protein synthesis. Rapidly dividing cells, such as blood cells, mouth, stomach, and bowel cells, are more sensitive to 5'-fluorouracil. Capecitabine is not very toxic to cancer cells, but the resulting 5'-fluorouracil is effective in killing cancer cells.

Side effects: Patients generally do not experience every side effect. Side effects of capecitabine include reduction in hemoglobin, decrease in number of red blood cells, lymphocytes and neutrophils, elevation of liver enzymes alanine transaminase and aspartate transaminase, fatigue, numbness/tingling in hands and feet, and palmar-plantar erythrodysesthesia (hand-foot syndrome), in which the hands and feet become red and swollen. In severe cases cracking and peeling of skin on hands and feet occurs. Cracks can become sites for infection. To reduce hand-foot syndrome symptoms, avoid high water temperatures, friction on hands (such as scrubbing dishes), wearing rubber gloves that would cause hands to overheat, and frequently apply creams such as Udderly Smooth™ and Aquaphor™ to affected areas.

Susan J. Karcher, PhD

For Further Information

McLellan, B. (2013). How to recognize and manage hand-foot syndrome due to capecitabine or doxorubicin. *ASCO Post,* 4(10). http://www.ascopost.com/issues/june-25,-2013/how-to-recognize-and-manage-hand-foot-syndrome-due-to-capecitabine-or-doxorubicin.aspx

Miwa, M., Ura, M., Nishida, M., Sawada, N., Ishikawa, T., Mori, K., … Ishitsuka, H. (1998). Design of a novel oral fluoropyrimidine carbamate, capecitabine, which generates 5-fluorouracil selectively in tumours by enzymes concentrated in human liver and cancer tissue. *European Journal of Cancer.* 34(8): 1274-1278.

Gómez, H. L., Neciosup, S., Tosello, C., Mano, M., Bines, J., Ismael, G., (2016). A phase II randomized study of lapatinib combined with capecitabine, vinorelbine, or gemcitabine in patients with HER2-positive metastatic breast cancer with progression after a taxane. *Clinical Breast Cancer,* 16(1): 38–44.

Walko, C. M. and Lindley, C. (2005). Capecitabine: A review. *Clinical Therapeutics,* 27(1): 23–44. http://www.sciencedirect.com/science/article/pii/S0149291805000068

Other Resources

Cancer.Net
http://www.cancer.net/navigating-cancer-care/side-effects/hand-foot-syndrome

RxList
http://www.rxlist.com/xeloda-drug/clinical-pharmacology.htm

▶ Cetuximab

Category: Chemotherapy and Other Drugs
Also known as: Erbitux

Definition: Cetuximab (Erbitux) is a chimeric (mouse/human) monoclonal antibody used to treat several cancers.

Cancers treated: Cetuximab is approved for the treatment of KRAS wild-type epidermal growth factor receptor (EGFR)-expressing metastatic colorectal cancer, and in squamous cell head and neck cancer (SCCHN). It is used off-label to treat advanced EGFR-expressing non-small cell lung cancer. It is most commonly given in combination with irinotecan for colorectal cancer, and with radiation and platinum-based therapy for SCCHN. In either case, 5-fluorouracil is typically included. The drug may also be given alone, particularly in cases where the patient has failed irinotecan or platinum therapy or is intolerant to irinotecan. A number of other combination therapies are currently being studied.

Delivery routes: Cetuximab is given by intravenous infusion.

How these drugs work: EGFR, also known as HER1 (human epidermal growth factor receptor 1) or ErbB-1 (name derived from a viral oncogene to which these receptors are homologous), a transmembrane glycoprotein in the type I receptor tyrosine kinase family along with HER2/neu (ErbB-2), HER3 (ErbB-3), and HER4 (ErbB-4), is expressed in several human cancers, including those of the head and neck, colon, and rectum. Cetuximab binds EGFR with higher-affinity than its natural ligands. The antibody-receptor complex is then internalized without activating the intrinsic tyrosine kinase. Signal transduction though this cell pathway is blocked, tumor growth is inhibited, and apoptosis or cell death occurs. Genomic testing for the KRAS gene (which encodes for a small protein in the EGFR pathway) is routine as patients with wild-type KRAS tumors have a response rate of over 60% to cetuximab. Patients with mutated KRAS genes are unlikely to benefit from treatment with cetuximab or other anti-EGFR drugs such as panitumumab.

Side effects: Severe infusion reactions occur in approximately 3% of patients, typically with the first infusion. The drug has a boxed warning for this side effect and premedication with an H1-histamine receptor antagonist such as intravenous diphenhydramine is required to minimize the degree of reaction, which can include rapid onset of airway obstruction, urticarial (hives), hypotension, shock, myocardial, and/or cardiac arrest. Severe diarrhea may result if the drug is given in combination with irinotecan. Other serious side effects include dehydration, kidney failure, interstitial lung disease, pulmonary embolism, and dermatologic toxicities. Low magnesium levels (hypomagnesemia) and accompanying electrolyte abnormalities ranged from 14% to 55% in clinical trials, and onset can occur days to months after initiation of Cetuximab; periodic monitoring of electrolytes is essential during and for at least 8 weeks following completion of therapy. The most common adverse effects are rash and other cutaneous reactions, headache, infection, and diarrhea.

Karen Nagel Edwards, PhD

For Further Information

Pazdur, R. (July 2, 2103). *FDA Approval for Cetuximab.* Retrieved from http://www.cancer.gov/about-cancer/treatment/drugs/fda-cetuximab

United States Food and Drug Administration. (July 9, 2015). *Information on Cetuximab (marketed as Erbitux).* Retrieved from http://www.fda.gov/Drugs/DrugSafety/PostmarketDrugSafetyInformationforPatientsandProviders/ucm113714.htm

Other Resources

National Comprehensive Cancer Network
http://www.nccn.org/patients/

American Cancer Society
http://www.cancer.org/

▶ Chemotherapy

Category: Chemotherapy and Other Drugs

Definition: Chemotherapy is the treatment of cancer with medications that have a certain toxic effect on cancer cells. Chemotherapy drugs are used to slow the growth of cancer cells, shrink tumors prior to other treatments such as surgery or radiation, prevent cancer cells from spreading, relieve cancer symptoms, or cure a specific cancer by destroying cancer cells.

- First-line or standard chemotherapy: Given to destroy cancerous cells before disease progression or recurrence; first-line chemotherapy has been determined, through research studies and clinical trials, to have the greatest probability of treating a certain type of cancer
- Second-line chemotherapy: Given to destroy cancerous cells when the disease has not responded to first-line chemotherapy or has recurred after first-line chemotherapy
- Neo-adjuvant chemotherapy: Given to reduce the size of a cancerous tumor prior to surgery or radiation therapy

Adjuvant chemotherapy: Given to destroy cancerous cells that may remain after a known cancerous tumor has been surgically removed or after radiation therapy

• Consolidation or intensification chemotherapy: Given once a remission is achieved with the goal of sustaining a remission
• Induction chemotherapy: Given to induce a remission
• Maintenance chemotherapy: Given in lower doses to help prolong a remission
• Palliative chemotherapy: Given to ease the symptoms of cancer and improve a patient's quality of life

Cancers treated: All

Subclasses of this group: Chemotherapy drugs are divided into subclasses based on their chemical structure, function and relationship to other drugs. Subclasses of chemotherapy include: alkylating agents, anthracyclines, angiogenesis inhibitors (antiangiogenics), antimetabolites, anti-tumor antibiotics, aromatase inhibitors, biologic response modifiers, corticosteroids, hormonal therapy, mitotic inhibitors (antimitotics), monoclonal antibodies, nitrosoureas, platinum derivatives, and topoisomerase inhibitors. Some chemotherapy drugs do not fit into these classifications.

Delivery routes: Chemotherapy drugs are most commonly administered intravenously (through an IV or port) or orally (by mouth) as pills, capsules, or liquid. They may also be administered topically (applied to the skin) as creams or lotions or injected directly into a tumor (intratumorally or intralesionally), into the muscle (intramuscularly), or under the skin (subcutaneously). The administration method is dependent on the drug's specific action, dose, and potential side effects. In some cases, two or more administration methods may be used at once.

Intravenous chemotherapy medications may be infused through a percutaneous central catheter (a thin, flexible tube, also called a PICC line) inserted under the skin into a vein in the arm or hand; through a central venous catheter, also called a vascular access device; or through a port implanted into a large vein in the neck, chest, or arm. A central venous catheter is used to deliver chemotherapy when several drugs need to be administered at the same time, when continuous infusion chemotherapy is being given, or when long-term therapy is needed. A catheter may also be placed in an artery (intra-arterial), in the cerebrospinal fluid (intrathecal), in the chest (intrapleural), in the abdomen (intraperitoneal), or in the bladder (intravesical) to deliver the medication. A medication infusion pump may be used with a catheter to deliver a preprogrammed dose of medication. Pumps can be internal (implanted under the skin during a surgical procedure) or external (worn outside the body).

Chemotherapy can also be delivered via liposomal therapy, a method that uses liposomes (microscopic synthetic capsules) to deliver chemotherapy drugs. The coating on the liposome capsules allows the medication to remain in the circulation for a longer period of time, so that the drugs selectively target cancer cells and, in turn, decrease the side effect profile on healthy tissues. Some liposomal medications currently available include cytarabine liposome (DepoCyt), doxorubicin hydrochloride liposome (Doxil, Evacet, Lipo-Dox, Dox-SL), irinotecan hydrochloride liposome (Onivyde), vincristine sulfate liposome (Marqibo), and daunorubicin lipid complex injection (DaunoXome).

Chemotherapy can be administered on an inpatient, outpatient, or at-home basis, depending on the specific drug and the type of cancer, its location, and its aggressiveness. Where chemotherapy is administered depends upon the type of medication, the patient's insurance requirements, as well as the physician's and patient's personal preferences.

Chemotherapy drug dosages are based on a patient's body weight in kilograms or a patient's body surface area expressed in meters squared, which is calculated using the patient's height and weight. Chemotherapy is given at regular intervals, or cycles, depending on the type and stage of cancer and how many chemotherapy drugs are being given at the same time. Rest periods between doses allow healthy, non-cancerous cells to recover from the effects of the medication. It is important for patients to receive the full recommended course of therapy to achieve the maximum therapeutic benefit. In some cases, the physician may adjust the course of treatment based on the incidence of certain side effects.

How these drugs work: Chemotherapy is a systemic treatment; the medicines travel throughout the body and are not confined to one specific treatment area. Therefore, chemotherapy drugs can reach cancer cells that have traveled from the main tumor, through the circulatory or lymph systems, and to other parts of the body. Chemotherapy drugs may be given as a monotherapy or in combination with other drugs or treatments, such as radiation therapy or surgery.

Targeted cancer therapies block the growth and spread of cancerous cells by interfering with cancer cell development, growth, and division. Some targeted therapies interfere with the proteins that are involved in the process that signals normal cells to turn into cancerous cells. Targeted therapy is available with several chemotherapy drugs. In some cases, molecularly targeted drugs can be used to interrupt specific processes vital to the survival and growth of cancer cells.

The type of chemotherapy prescribed is different for each patient and is based on the type of cancer, the stage of the disease, the patient's age and overall health, the presence of coexisting medical conditions, and other cancer treatments that may have been given previously.

A few hundred chemotherapy drugs are now available, with many more being investigated for safety and efficacy. The chemical composition, action, and side effects of chemotherapy drugs vary. Chemotherapy drugs are classified according to how they affect cancer cells' molecular context, cellular activities or processes, and specific phases of the cancer cell cycle.

In the 1940s, nitrogen mustard became the first chemotherapy agent used to treat cancer. The use of chemotherapy for cancer treatment was discovered accidentally during World War II when a group of soldiers exposed to sulfur mustard gas, a chemical warfare agent, were later found to have very low white blood cell counts. Scientists hypothesized that this agent would have a similar effect on cancer. An IV injection of nitrogen mustard was given to several patients with advanced lymphomas. These patients' cancers were all successfully treated with nitrogen mustard.

Nitrogen mustard is one of several mustard gas derivatives (including mechlorethamine, cyclophosphamide, chlorambucil and others) in a class of drugs called alkylating agents, which damage DNA and stop cell division. Drugs classified as alkylating agents (including nitrosoureas) can attack cancer cells during any phase of the cell cycle.

Natural metal derivatives, also called platinums, are similar to alkylating agents because they kill cancer cells by damaging their DNA. These types of drugs consist of platinum-based compounds that inhibit DNA replication in cancer cells by directly binding the DNA. Platinum-based compounds include cisplatin, carboplatin, and oxaliplatin. Liposomal therapy has been an effective delivery method for these drugs to reduce drug toxicity.

Antimetabolites also work by interfering with DNA and RNA, stopping cell division. Some examples include 5-fluorouracil, 6-mercaptopurine, cytarabine, floxuridine, methotrexate and others.

Anti-tumor antibiotics and anthracyclines (such as daunorubicin, doxorubicin and epirubicin) as well as topoisomerase inhibitors (such as etoposide, teniposide and mitoxantrone) work by interfering with certain enzymes that are needed for cellular DNA to replicate. Mitotic inhibitors (antimitotics, such as paclitaxel and vinblastine), plant alkaloids, and other drugs derived from natural substances have a similar mechanism of action.

Angiogenesis inhibitor drugs (antiangiogenics) may prevent the growth of blood vessels that supply oxygen from surrounding tissue to cancerous cells or tumors, thereby starving the cells of oxygen.

Monoclonal antibodies are synthetic forms of protein that can help guide chemotherapy drugs directly into a tumor. Monoclonal antibodies are used only for certain types of cancer in which cancer-specific antigens have been identified and antibodies that bind these antigens have been manufactured. Some types of breast cancer and lymphomas have been successfully treated with commercially available monoclonal antibodies.

Hormonal therapy drugs (including anti-estrogens, aromatase inhibitors, anti-androgens and others) are used to slow the growth of certain male or female cancers, such as prostate cancer or breast cancer, by interfering with the hormone needed by cancer cells to replicate.

Immunotherapy drugs (biologic response modifiers) may be used in conjunction with chemotherapy to help the patient's immune system recognize and attack cancer cells.

Side effects: Because chemotherapy drugs are systemic, they target cancerous as well as normal tissue and can have toxic side effects, depending on the specific drug, its dosage, the duration of administration, and the patient's physical condition.

One of the most common side effects of chemotherapy is fatigue, which may be the result of anemia (a decrease in oxygen-carrying red blood cells). Alternatively, chemotherapy-induced fatigue may result from the increased energy required to recover from the effects of the chemotherapy drugs. Other factors contributing to fatigue include poor appetite, lack of sleep, and emotional distress.

Depressed blood cell counts may increase the patient's risk of infection and anemia. In addition, reduced platelets can cause easy bruising or bleeding including nosebleeds, bleeding gums, blood in the urine or stool, and unusually heavy menstrual flow.

Other common side effects include nausea and vomiting, loss of appetite, diarrhea, and fluid retention. A registered dietitian can provide nutritional therapy to help the patient develop an eating plan that meets dietary requirements while reducing these side effects and making treatment more tolerable. In some cases, antinausea or antidiarrheal medications may be prescribed to prevent these side effects. It is important for patients to consult their physician(s) before taking over-the-counter remedies, as they could interact with the chemotherapy drugs.

Since many chemotherapy drugs kill fast-growing cancer cells, they also target fast-growing normal cells in the hair follicles, which can lead to alopecia (hair loss). Some chemotherapy drugs may only cause hair thinning, while others may cause complete hair loss, including body hair and eyebrows. Hair loss is temporary, and hair growth will resume after the cancer treatments are completed.

Emotional or mood changes, such as depression or anxiety, may occur. Patients should discuss their concerns about these side effects with their physician. Support groups are available to help patients cope with these feelings and antidepressant medications can be prescribed when necessary.

In some cases, chemotherapy can cause certain side effects that are painful, such as burning or pain in the fingers and toes. Pain medications may be prescribed to alleviate these side effects.

Some chemotherapy drugs may lead to infertility (both amenorrhea in women and impaired spermatogenesis in men). In extreme cases, chemotherapy can lead to heart muscle damage (cardiotoxicity), which would mitigate the clinical usefulness of such chemotherapy regimens.

There are several lifestyle changes a patient can make to manage certain side effects, such as fatigue; and mouth, gum, and throat problems. The National Cancer Institute offers a publication, Chemotherapy and You, which provides several techniques for managing side effects.

The time it takes to recover from chemotherapy side effects varies, depending on the patient's physical condition and the type of chemotherapy drug, dosage, and duration of medication administration. Chemotherapy side effects are usually short term and often go away once treatment is finished. Patients should ask their doctor about the risk of short and long term side effects, and about the risk of more serious side effects.

Angela M. Costello, B.S.

For Further Information

Chabner, B. A., & Longo, D. L. (Eds.). (2010). Cancer chemotherapy and biotherapy: Principles and practice (5th ed.). Philadelphia: Lippincott Williams & Wilkin.

Chu, E., & DeVita, V. T. (2014). Physicians' cancer chemotherapy drug manual (15th ed.). Burlington, MA: Jones & Bartlett Learning.

National Cancer Institute. (2011). Chemotherapy and you: Support for people with cancer. NIH Publication No. 11-7156. Bethesda, Md.: National Institutes of Health, U.S. Department of Health and Human Services, Rev. June 2011. Available at http://www.cancer.gov/publications/patient-education/chemo-and-you.

Skeel, R. T. & Khlief, S. N. (2011). Handbook of cancer chemotherapy (8th ed.). Philadelphia: Lippincott Williams & Wilkins.

Other Resources

American Cancer Society
http://www.cancer.org

CancerCare
http://www.cancercare.org

CancerNet
http://www.cancer.net

Chemocare.org
http://www.chemocare.org

National Cancer Institute
http://www.cancer.gov

Oncolink
http://www.oncolink.org

See also: Alkylating agents in chemotherapy; Androgen drugs; Angiogenesis inhibitors; Antiandrogens; Antiestrogens; Antimetabolites in chemotherapy; Antineoplastics in chemotherapy; Antiviral therapies; Benzodiazepines; Biological therapy; Chlorambucil; Cyclophosphamide; Cyclosporine A; Cytokines; Drug resistance and multidrug resistance (MDR); Immunotherapy; Interferon; Interleukins; Matrix metalloproteinase inhibitors; Monoclonal antibodies; Plant alkaloids and terpenoids in chemotherapy; Proteasome inhibitors; Topoisomerase inhibitors; Tyrosine kinase inhibitors; Vaccines, therapeutic

▶ Chimeric Antigen Receptor T-cell treatment

Category: Chemotherapy and Other Drugs
Also known as: CAR T-cells

Definition: An experimental treatment for blood-based cancers that utilizes T-lymphocytes collected from the blood of a cancer patient that have been genetically engineered to synthesize specialized receptors called chimeric antigen receptors (CARs) and display them on their cell surfaces. The CAR proteins endow the T-lymphocytes with the ability to specifically recognize cancer-cell proteins and destroy the cancer cells that bear them.

Cancers treated: The CAR T-cells have been used to treat **acute** lymphoblastic leukemia (ALL), non-Hodgkin lymphoma (NHL) and chronic lymphocytic leukemia (CLL), and are being tested as a treatment of several other types of cancer as well.

Delivery routes: CAR T-cells are delivered intravenously.

How these drugs work: In the preparatory stages of the treatment, T-lymphocytes (T-cells) are isolated from the patient's blood. A procedure called "apheresis" slowly removes relatively large volumes of blood from the patient over an extended period time. The T-cells are isolated from the blood and the remaining cells and plasma returned to the patient's bloodstream.

In the laboratory, genetic engineering techniques endow the patient's isolated T-cells with the ability to express CARs on their surfaces. CAR proteins impart to any cells that express them the capability to bind specific molecules on the surfaces of other cells. Molecules recognized by the immune system as foreign are referred to as "antigens." Therefore, CARs are specially engineered proteins that can specifically bind cancer cell-specific surface antigens. Once the T-cells stably express the genetically engineered CARs on their surfaces, they are known as chimeric antigen receptor T-cells (CAR T-cells).

In the laboratory, technicians employ cell culture techniques to expand the CAR T-cells from the few cells originally isolated from the patient's blood to hundreds of millions of CAR T-cells. Once the CAR T-cells grow to sufficient numbers, the technicians concentrate them and ship them to the hospital for intravenous infusion back into the patient's bloodstream.

Once inside the patient's body, the CAR T-cells recognize and attach to the cancer-specific antigen they were engineered to bind. This marks the cancer cells as foreign interlopers that must be destroyed and the CAR T-cells inject a toxic cocktail of chemicals into the nearby cancer cell that kills it by inducing programmed cell death (apoptosis).

After the CAR T-cells have killed all the available cancer cells, some of them remain in circulating blood as so-called "memory cells" that can expand if they encounter new cancer cells that express the same surface antigens. In this regard, CAR T-cells have the capability to counter cancer recurrence.

Currently, CAR T-cell therapies are only available to those patients who participate in clinical trials. However, the performance of CAR T-cells in several clinical trials has been astounding. For example, in December, 2014, the biotechnology company, Juno Therapeutics, reported that their CAR T-cell treatment, JCAR015, had put 24 of 27 adult patients with refractory ALL into remission. Six of these patients remained disease free for more than a year. Given that ALL is a very difficult disease to treat, and that most ALL patients die within a few months, such response levels were unprecedented. In another clinical trial with Novartis' CTL019 CAR T-cell therapy, 90% of patients with relapsed ALL that resisted other treatments achieved total remission, and 78% were still living 2 years later. In response to these results, the US Food and Drug Administration awarded "breakthrough status" to CTL019. The breakthrough status designation expedites the development and review of novel treatments that can potentially meet a presently unmet medical need. Other clinical trials are in progress, and CAR T-cell technology is evolving rapidly. Clearly, CAR T-cell treatments represent a new and potentially potent weapon in the war against cancer.

Side effects: Three different side effects typically accompany CAR T-cell treatments: 1) cytokine release syndrome; 2) B-cell aplasia; and 3) tumor lysis syndrome (TLS). The severity of these side effects varies between patients.

Cytokine release syndrome (CRS), the most common and potentially severe side effect of CAR T-cell treatments, results from rapid activation of the re-infused CAR T-cells. These activated CAR T-lymphocytes release large quantities of "cytokines," or small proteins that cells secrete to direct the behavior of other cells. Such large quantities of cytokines can produce low blood pressure, high fevers, confusion, or delirium, and can compromise lung function. In most patients, corticosteroid administration can relieve the effects of CRS. In severe cases, administration of tocilizumab (Actemra®), an antibody against a cytokine called interleukin-6, can quell symptoms.

B-cell aplasia refers to low levels or absence of B-lymphocytes in the blood of patients. This side effect most commonly affects CAR T-cell-treated patients who suffer from B-lymphocyte-based cancers, since CAR T-cells destroy normal B-cells as well as cancerous B-cells. Treatment with intravenous immunoglobulins can keep patients healthy while their B-cell levels recover.

Since CAR T-cells vigorously attack and destroy cancer cells, CAR T-cell treatments can cause large-scale release of tumor cell components and metabolites into the patient's bloodstream. The sudden accumulation of the flotsam and jetsam of dead cancer cells can cause TLS. Clinically, the signs of TLS usually appear 24 to 48 hours after treatment, and are characterized by excessively high blood levels of uric acid (hyperuricemia) and phosphate (hyperphosphatemia), low blood calcium levels (hypocalcemia), and acute kidney failure. Severe cases of TLS can be treated with dialysis or agents that decrease uric acid levels, such as allopurinol or probenecid.

Michael Buratovich, PhD

For Further Information

Brower, V. (2015, April 1). The CAR T-cell race. *The Scientist*, 29(4). Retrieved from http://www.the-scientist.com/?articles.view/articleNo/42462/title/The-CAR-T-Cell-Race/.

Maude, S. L., Frey, N., Shaw, P. A., Aplenc, R., Barrett, D. M., Bunin, N. J., ... Grupp, S. A. (2014). Chimeric antigen receptor T cells for sustained remissions in leukemia. *New England Journal of Medicine*, 371, 1507-1517.

McLaughlin, L., Cruz, C. R., & Bollard, C. M. (2015). Adoptive T-cell therapies for refractory/relapsed leukemia and lymphoma: current strategies and recent advances. *Therapeutic Advances in Hematology*, 6(6), 295-307.

Other Resources

Leukemia and Lymphoma Society – chimeric antigen receptor (CAR) T-cell therapy
https://www.lls.org/treatment/types-of-treatment/immunotherapy/chimeric-antigen-receptor-car-t-cell-therapy

Lymphomation.org – CAR T-cells
http://www.lymphomation.org/programing-t-cells.htm

Marketwatch—Novartis highlights research on investigational, personalized T cell therapy CTL019 in patients with forms of acute and chronic leukemia
http://www.marketwatch.com/story/novartis-highlights-research-on-investigational-personalized-t-cell-therapy-ctl019-in-patients-with-forms-of-acute-and-chronic-leukemia-2013-12-07-9183150?reflink=MW_news_stmp

National Cancer Institute – CAR T-cell therapy: engineering patients' immune cells to treat their cancers
http://www.cancer.gov/about-cancer/treatment/research/car-t-cells

See also: T-lymphocytes

▶ Colony-Stimulating Factors (CSFs)

Category: Chemotherapy and Other Drugs
ATC code: BO3XA01-erythropoietin, BO3XA02-darbepoetin alfa, LO3AA02-filgrastim, LO3AA03-molgramostim, LO3AA09-sargramostim, LO3AA10-lenograstim, LO3AA12-ancestim, LO3AA134-pegfilgrastim
Also known as: Hematopoietic growth factors

Definition: Colony-stimulating factors (CSFs) are glycoproteins that stimulate the production of blood cells. Several recombinant CSFs have achieved widespread clinical use. Others have been identified but have not been assessed in clinical trials or have not been approved for use by the Food and Drug Administration (FDA).

Cancers treated: Colony-stimulating factors are not used to treat cancers per se. Rather, they are used as supportive care to increase red blood cell, white blood cell, and hematopoietic stem cell counts that are depleted during some forms of chemotherapy or radiation therapy. CSFs generally are administered only to patients with non-myeloid malignancies and usually as primary prophylaxis to prevent febrile neutropenia or to allow dose intensity with specific chemotherapy regimens. CSFs are administered after chemotherapy or radiation therapy. They also may be used before bone marrow or stem cell transplantation to increase the number of cells available for transplant or after transplantation to assist in bone marrow recovery.

Delivery routes: Colony-stimulating factors are proteins and are subject to degradation in the stomach. Therefore, they are administered either as intravenous (IV) infusions or subcutaneous injections, depending on the specific formulation used. Some CSFs are presented in prefilled syringes, allowing patients to inject themselves at home without the need to go to a hospital or doctor's office.

How these drugs work: Hematopoiesis, the formation of blood cells, is the process by which early hematopoietic stem cells in the bone marrow with potential for renewal, proliferation, and differentiation give rise to large numbers of mature cells through a series of intermediate cells. As the stem cells mature, they lose their ability to self-renew and become specialized. Stem cells produce cells that belong to one of two lineages: lymphoid cells (white blood cells, including T-cells and B-cells), and myeloid cells (white blood cells such as granulocytes and macrophages, and platelets, or thrombocytes, and red blood cells, or erythrocytes). The process of proliferation, differentiation, and maturation is complex, with many interacting steps, and is controlled by CSFs, alone or in combination. To date, more than twenty CSFs have been identified. They are active in very small amounts.

Once CSFs were discovered in experimental models, the genes for them were identified and cloned. Some of the endogenous CSFs have been produced as recombinant human forms and have received marketing approval from the FDA.

The recombinant human forms of CSFs can be used to replace or supplement the endogenous proteins after chemotherapy or radiation therapy or in the case of anemia caused by kidney failure or the anemia of chronic disease, which includes cancer.

Erythropoietin or epoetin alfa (Epogen, Procrit) and darbepoetin alfa (Aranesp) increase the number of red blood cells by causing committed erythroid progenitor cells to proliferate and differentiate.

Filgrastim (Neupogen) and pegfilgrastim (Neulasta) are granulocyte CSFs that increase the number of neutrophils, white blood cells specific to fighting infection. Another white cell factor, lenograstim (Granocyte), is available in Europe and other countries. The granulocyte CSFs increase the circulating half-life of neutrophils and enhance their ability to attack bacteria.

Sargramostim (Leukine) is a granulocyte-macrophage CSF used to increase production of several types of white blood cells; molgramostim (Leucomax) is another version that is available in Europe. Granulocyte-macrophage CSFs are also locally active and remain at the site of infection to recruit and activate neutrophils.

Ancestim (Stemgen) is a CSF that promotes the development of stem cells, which can differentiate into all other types of blood cells; it is not available in the United States.

Interleukin-11 (oprelvekin, Neumega; L03AC02) is not a CSF but is used to increase platelet counts in patients with cancer who are receiving myelosuppressive chemotherapy.

Side effects: All drugs and biologic products that are effective have side effects, and each type of CSF has side effects specific to it. Patients who are receiving CSFs should consult their health care professionals and the package insert for specific information concerning side effects. In general, however, the side effects from use of CSFs are much less intense than those from chemotherapy or radiation therapy. Common side effects are bone pain, flulike symptoms, fever, fatigue, and loss of appetite. Colony-stimulating factors (CSFs)

MaryAnn Foote, M.S., Ph.D.
Updated by Michelle Herdman

For Further Information

Molineux, G., Foote, M. A., & Elliott, S. G. (Eds.). (2003). Erythropoietins and erythropoiesis: Molecular, cellular, preclinical, and clinical biology. Basel, Switzerland: Birkhäuser Verlag.

Morstyn, G., Foote, M. A., & Lieschke, G. J. (Eds.). (2004). *Hematopoietic growth factors in oncology: Basic science and clinical therapeutics*. Totowa, N.J.: Humana Press.

Welte, K., Gabrilove, J., Bronchud, M. H., Platzer, E., & Morstyn, G. (1996). Filgrastim (r-metHuG-CSF): The first ten years. *Blood*, 88(6), 1907-1929.

Yang, B.B., Savin, M.A., & Green, M. (2012). Prevention of chemotherapy-induced neutropenia with pegfilgrastim: Pharmakokinetics and patient outcomes. *Chemotherapy*, 58, 387-98.

Other Resources

Epogen
http://www.epogen.com

Leukine
http://www.leukine.com

Neulasta
http://www.neulasta.com

Neupogen
http://www.neupogen.com

Procrit
http://www.procrit.com

Neumega
http://www.pfizer.com/products/product-detail/neumega

See also: Biological therapy; Bone Marrow Transplantation (BMT); Cytokines; 5Q minus syndrome; Gene therapy; Immunotherapy; Interleukins; Leukopenia; Myelofibrosis; Myeloproliferative disorders; Neutropenia; Stem cell transplantation; Thrombocytopenia; Umbilical cord blood transplantation

▶ Corticosteroids

Category: Chemotherapy and Other Drugs
ATC code: H02-systemic, D07-dermatological, S02-sensory organs, M01-musculoskeletal

Definition: Corticosteroids are synthetic forms of the naturally occurring hormones produced by the cortex of the adrenal gland.

Cancers treated: Brain cancer, lymphomas, leukemias, lung cancer, renal cancer, bone cancer

Subclasses of this group: Systemic-short-acting, systemic-intermediate-acting, systemic-long-acting, inhaled, topical, intranasal, ophthalmic, intra-articular (into a joint)

Delivery routes: These drugs can be taken orally as tablets. There are solutions that may be administered intravenously. They can also be inhaled from metered dose or disk inhalers, instilled into the nostrils, applied to the skin, or dropped into the eyes. In addition, steroids may be injected into inflamed joints in the body.

How these drugs work: Corticosteroids are used primarily to suppress the immune response of the body in instances when this response is causing troublesome symptoms and/or damaging the tissues of the body. They accomplish this by decreasing the activity of white blood cells and the production of the chemicals that are involved in the symptoms of inflammation. By decreasing inflammation, corticosteroids can often decrease the symptoms of cancer and chemotherapy.

Side effects: Systemic corticosteroids have many side effects, including increased appetite, weight gain, insomnia, mood swings, muscle weakness, increased growth of body hair, easy bruising, swollen face, acne, stomach irritation, restlessness, cataracts, glaucoma, and water retention. They can cause medical problems such as osteoporosis, worsening of diabetes, and high blood pressure, as well as psychiatric problems such as depression and anxiety. Because they depress the immune response,

Common Corticosteroids

Drug	*Brands*	*Subclass*	*Delivery Mode*	*Cancers Treated*
Beclomethasone	Vanceril, QVAR	Inhaled	Inhalation	Lung cancer
Betamethasone	Celestone	Long-acting	Oral, IV	Lymphomas; leukemia; multiple myeloma; gastrointestinal, ovarian, bone, liver, and renal cancers
Dexamethasone	Decadrol, Decadron	Long-acting	Oral, IV	Brain tumors
Fluticasone	Flovent	Inhaled	Inhalation	Lung cancer
Hydrocortisone	Solu-Cortef, Cortef, Hydrocortone	Short-acting	IV	Lymphomas; leukemia; multiple myeloma; gastrointestinal, ovarian, bone, liver, and renal cancers
Methylprednisolone	Medrol, Solu-medrol	Intermediate-acting	Oral, IV	Lymphomas; leukemia; multiple myeloma; gastrointestinal, ovarian, bone, liver, and renal cancers
Prednisolone	Delta-cortef, Hydeltrasol, Predacort, Prednisol	Intermediate-acting	Oral, IV	Lymphomas; leukemia; multiplemyeloma; gastrointestinal, ovarian, bone, liver, and renal cancers
Prednisone	Deltasone	Intermediate-acting	Oral	Lymphomas; leukemia; multiple myeloma; gastrointestinal, ovarian, bone, liver, and renal cancers
Triamcinolone	Azmacort	Inhaled	Inhalation	Lung cancer

corticosteroids can increase a patient's susceptibility to infections.

Christine M. Carroll, R.N., B.S.N., M.B.A.

See also: Antinausea medications; Chemotherapy; Pain management medications

▶ Cycloastragenol

Category: Chemotherapy and Other Drugs
Also known as: *Astragalus*, TA-65

Definition: Cycloastragenol is extracted from the dried root of *Astragalus membranaceus*, a perennial flowering shrub of the Fabaceae family that is commonly used in traditional Chinese medicine. In 2001, Geron Corporation researchers isolated a molecule called TA-65 from the herb *Astragalus*, which reportedly boosted telomerase activity. Geron later licensed the product to T.A. Sciences in New York City for development as a commercially available anti-aging nutritional supplement.

Cancers treated: There is not enough clinical evidence to demonstrate the effectiveness of cycloastragenol in treating, curing, or preventing any specific disease or condition.

Delivery routes: Cycloastragenol can be taken by mouth in pill form or used as a topical formulation.

How this drug works: Cycloastragenol is thought to activate telomerase, a naturally occurring enzyme resulting in increased telomere length. The telomere is the protective cap at the end of a linear chromosome containing highly repetitive DNA that functions as a disposable buffer.

Each time a cell divides, some of the telomere is lost, causing the telomeres to gradually shorten over time. When the telomere becomes too short, the chromosome can no longer replicate, thereby causing cellular aging and deterioration. Animal studies suggest that this mechanism is responsible for accelerated cellular aging – each time the cell divides, errors in duplication accumulate, eventually resulting in cellular dysfunction and aging.

In activated T cells, select research studies have shown that telomerase activity increases telomere length. Like other kinds of cells, immune cells lose their ability to divide over time as the telomeres on their chromosomes become progressively shorter with each cell division. As a result, the disease-fighting ability of immune cells diminishes with age. In a 2008 study published in *The Journal of Immunology*, a team of researchers at UCLA found that *cycloastragenol* can prevent or slow the progressive loss of telomeres in key immune cells, potentially making it a key weapon in the fight against HIV and other viral diseases.

Some researchers suggest that the development of an effective telomerase therapy, such as cycloastragenol, could help to extend human life by re-lengthening telomeres, thereby resetting the genetic "clock" in healthy cells, while also interrupting uncontrolled cell division in cancer cells.

Side effects: There are no reported negative side effects of cycloastragenol. However, additional clinical studies in humans are needed to demonstrate the supplement's safety and effectiveness.

Precautions: Clinical study results in humans have not been published in peer-reviewed journals, suggesting the need for additional research before the supplement's safety and efficacy can be established. Nicotine is strongly contraindicated with the use of cycloastragenol, as it has been shown to increase the risk of cancer.

Angela M. Costello, BS

For Further Information

Bernardes de Jesus, B., Schneeberger, K., Vera, E., Tejera, A., Harley, C. B., & Blasco, M. A. (2011). The telomerase activator TA-65 elongates short telomeres and increases health span of adult/old mice without increasing cancer incidence. *Aging Cell* 10(4): 604–621.

Fauce, S. R., Jamieson, B. D., Chin, A. C., Mitsuyasu, R. T., Parish, S. T., Ng, S. T., ... Effros, R. B. (2008). Telomerase-based pharmacologic enhancement of antiviral function of human CD8+ T lymphocytes." *Journal of Immunology* 181(10): 7400-7406.

Molgora, B., Bateman, R., Sweeney, G., Finger, D., Dimler, T., Rita B. Effros. R. B., & Hector F. Valenzuela. (2013). Functional assessment of pharmacological telomerase activators in human T cells. *Cells* 2(1): 57-66.

Valenzuela H. F., Fuller, T., Edwards, J., Finger, D., & Molgora, B. (2009). Cycloastragenol extends T cell proliferation by increasing telomerase activity. *Journal of Immunology* 182: 90.30.

Other Resources

Nutrition.gov
http://www.nutrition.gov/dietary-supplements

▶ Cyclooxygenase 2 (COX-2) inhibitors

Category: Chemotherapy and Other Drugs
ATC code: 101XX, M01AH

Definition: Cyclooxygenase 2 (COX-2) inhibitors are nonsteroidal anti-inflammatory drugs (NSAID) that inhibit the COX-2 enzyme, which is involved in inflammation and cancer.

Cancers treated: Primarily colorectal cancers, such as familial adenomatous polyposis (FAP); others under investigation, including breast, cervical, head and neck, lung, and pancreatic cancers

Delivery routes: These drugs are administered orally as either capsules or tablets and can be taken on an outpatient basis.

How these drugs work: COX enzymes catalyze the first-step in the biosynthesis of a class of signaling molecules called prostanoids, which includes thromboxanes and prostaglandins. Specifically, COX catalyzes the conversion of the fatty acid arachidonic acid (a component of cell membrane phospholipids) into prostaglandin H_2. Prostaglandin H_2 serves as the branch point for the synthesis of other prostaglandins or thromboxanes.

Prostaglandins act locally to induce the widening of blood vessels and prevent the aggregation (clumping) of platelets, and promote inflammation. Endothelial cells, which compose the innermost walls of blood vessels, synthesize a particular prostaglandin known as prostacyclin that prevents potentially damaging blood clots from forming within blood vessels. Thromboxanes are made by platelets and promote platelet aggregation and blood clots.

Humans make three different types (isozymes) of COX enzymes: COX-1, COX-2, and COX-3. COX-1 is constantly expressed by the majority of cells at low levels. It serves various "housekeeping functions" in the body, such as protecting the stomach lining from gastric acid and maintaining kidney function. Consequently, COX-1 inhibition can cause serious gastrointestinal and renal side effects. COX-3 is a brain-specific COX encoded by the same gene as COX-1. However, the mRNA transcribed from this gene is subjected to brain-specific processing, which results in a slightly different protein. COX-3 is the target of pain relievers like acetaminophen. COX-2 is induced by inflammatory stimuli, hormones, growth factors, and cancer, and only in specific cells. COX-2 is overexpressed, however, in several cancers, including a variety of digestive cancers, and lung, breast, bladder, cervical, head and neck, and brain tumors. High levels of COX-2 expression are found in early to advanced cancers and increased regulation is particularly strong in patients with cancers that have metastasized and have a poor prognosis. Consequently, COX-2 inhibitors are being investigated for the treatment and prevention of cancer.

COX-2 enhances tumor cell proliferation and survival, inhibits the body's immune response to cancer, and induces the development of new blood vessels that feed a tumor and help it spread to other parts of the body. Because the active sites of the different COX enzymes differ, COX-2 inhibitors can form tight complexes with COX-2 that dissociate slowly, thereby blocking enzyme activity. These inhibitors only weakly and reversibly bind to COX-1, however, with no effect on its activity. Blocking only COX-2 may reduce tumor cell growth and survival and improve immune responses against tumor cells without the risk of severe gastrointestinal and renal complications observed with COX-1 inhibition. Unfortunately clinical studies of COX-2 inhibitors in cancer patients have produced mixed results, and more work is necessary in order to demonstrate the efficacy of these drugs in cancer patients.

Side effects: The major side effects of COX-2 inhibitors are cardiovascular, such as increased risks of blood clots, heart attack, stroke, and high blood pressure. This has led to two drugs, Vioxx (rofecoxib) and Bextra (valdecoxib), being removed from the market by the Food and Drug Administration (FDA). The FDA also denied approval for another COX-2 inhibitor, etoricoxib, on the basis of similar concerns, even though etoricoxib has been approved in many other countries. COX-2 inhibitors may also cause indigestion, stomach bleeding, ulcers, and perforation of the stomach or intestines. Long-term administration may result in kidney toxicity and (rarely) liver toxicity. Allergic skin rashes may also occur with celecoxib (Celebrex).

Elizabeth A. Manning, Ph.D.
Updated by: Michael Buratovich, Ph.D.

See also: Angiogenesis; Bone pain; Desmoid tumors; Hereditary polyposis syndromes; Nonsteroidal Anti-Inflammatory Drugs (NSAIDs); Pain management medications; Premalignancies

▶ Chemoprevention

Category: Chemotherapy and Other Drugs; Lifestyle and Prevention

Definition: Chemoprevention is a pharmacological approach to preventing or delaying the development of cancer. The process includes using one or several natural or laboratory-made substances (such as drugs, vitamins, dietary supplements, or foods) that interfere with carcinogenesis (the transformation of normal living cells into cancer cells) or progression of premalignant cells to cancer.

Discussion: Cancer affects people of all ages in the United States. The incidence rates of some forms of cancer have declined over the past few years while those of others have increased. Many financial and human resources have been spent on the prevention, diagnosis, and treatment of cancer. Most cancer prevention research has confirmed that certain lifestyle choices play a significant role in the development of cancer. In fact, an estimated one-third of all cancers could be eliminated through healthy lifestyle choices. Exercise and diet are primary ways to diminish the chance of developing cancer.

Chemoprevention is the result of studies directed toward the prevention of cancer rather than its treatment. These studies are designed to evaluate the effectiveness and usefulness of potential chemoprevention substances. Historically, chemoprevention research has been fruitful in developing pharmacologic approaches with certain cancers including breast, prostate, and colorectal. The value of these chemoprevention compounds in human subjects is now the focus of numerous cancer prevention clinical trials.

How chemoprevention works: Chemoprevention research has focused on ways to arrest or even reverse the process of carcinogenesis (the transformation of normal living cells into abnormal or cancer cells). Studies show that certain substances can stop the formation of cancer tumors. This is accomplished by several means, including 1) preventing mutations (genetic cellular changes) that often lead to cancer or 2) stopping the duplication of damaged cells that can result in malignant tumors. Substances can interact at various points along the process of carcinogenesis: the beginning (initiation), middle (promotion), and end (progression). These substances may inactivate the cancer-causing agent, suppress tumor growth, induce useful enzymes, or act as antioxidants.

An optimal chemoprevention agent is nontoxic, safe for long-term use, easy to administer, inexpensive, well tolerated, and effective. Chemoprevention compounds may be natural dietary products or synthetic compounds.

Examples of Chemoprevention

Over the past few decades, chemoprevention has gained increased interest with successful outcomes. Significant impact from chemoprevention can be seen in the prevention of breast, prostate, and colorectal cancer. Also, ongoing studies support potential for chemoprevention on other forms of cancer.

Breast cancer is the most common non-skin cancer among women in the United States, with an average lifetime risk of 12.4 percent, or affecting 1 in 8 women. Chemoprevention may be effective in preventing breast cancer in women who are at high risk or in preventing cancer in the second breast of women who have been diagnosed with breast cancer. From 1992 through 1997 the National Cancer Institute (NCI) funded and administered the Breast Cancer Prevention Trial (BCPT), a study featuring the antiestrogen drug tamoxifen. Results showed 49 percent fewer diagnoses of invasive and noninvasive cancer in the group that took the drug. Another study of breast cancer prevention in high-risk women compared outcomes using the chemoprevention drugs tamoxifen and raloxifene. Both tamoxifen and roloxifen, selective estrogen receptor modulators (SERMS), are used as chemoprevention to reduce the risk of breast cancer. However, they may have side effects such as fatigue, mood swings, increased risk of blood clots, stroke, and endometrial cancer. Other drugs may be used, in specific circumstances, as breast cancer chemoprevention including aromatase inhibitors (that stop the production of estrogen) and inactivators. They also come with the possibility of side effects.

Natural dietary substances have been studied for their possible chemoprevention properties. Some breast cancer epidemiologic studies have established chemoprevention properties of natural dietary phenolic compounds. Examples of high phenolic foods are fruits (such as berries) and vegetables (such as broccoli). Other areas of study in natural chemoprevention for breast cancer include turmeric/curcumin, vitamin D, flaxseed, and Omega-3 fatty acids.

Prostate cancer is the most common non-skin cancer in men and the second leading cause of cancer-related deaths in American men. The National Cancer Institute has conducted ongoing cancer prevention clinical trials assessing if certain antiandrogens and antiestrogens can prevent prostate cancer. One clinical trial used the drug finasteride to reduce dihydrotestosterone, a metabolite of testosterone associated with prostate cancer. The Prostate Cancer Prevention Trial (PCPT)'s long term results showed a reduction in the incidence of low-grade prostate cancer with regular use of this drug for seven years. However, there were side effects such as decreased libido (sexual drive), increased erectile dysfunction, and gynecomastia (excessive breast development in males). Another chemoprevention drug shown to reduce the risk of prostate cancer is dutasteride.

Natural dietary substances and supplements have produced mixed impact on prostate cancer. A study of Vitamin E and selenium failed to produce positive results. In fact, the use of Vitamin E alone demonstrated a statistically significant increase in the risk of prostate cancer. Other studies show that natural dietary substances such as green tea, lycopene, modified citrus pectin, pomegranate, and soy may offer some chemoprevention effects with prostate cancer. Side effects of these dietary substances may include gastrointestinal symptoms such as diarrhea, nausea, vomiting, bloating, or stomach irritation. More studies are needed to determine effectiveness of these natural dietary substances as chemoprevention for prostate cancer.

Colorectal cancer is the third most common non-skin cancer in the United States for women and men and also ranks second in cancer-related deaths. The National Cancer Institute (NCI) has a commitment to develop and validate possible ways to prevent colon cancer. NCI partners with the PREVENT Cancer Drug Development Program to bring new cancer prevention methods through clinical trials to practice. The literature contains chemoprevention studies focused on the use of non-steroidal anti-inflammatory drugs (NSAIDS) such as aspirin and cyclo-oxgenase-2 (COX-2) inhibitors. The use of aspirin as a chemoprevention has shown promise but carries with it the risk of side effects of gastrointestinal and hemorrhagic issues. Also under study are natural anti-inflammatory substances like omega-3 polyunsaturated fatty acids, resveratrol, and curcumin (a common spice used in Indian curries).

Increased consumption of fruits and vegetables seems to provide some protection against colorectal cancer. Possible natural dietary substances and supplements under study for chemoprevention for colon cancer include antioxidants, calcium, and vitamin D. Additional studies are indicated to assess the effectiveness of these natural dietary substances as chemoprevention for colorectal cancer.

Studies in China indicate that green tea may be chemoprotective against stomach and colon cancer.

The incidence of cervical cancer (cancer of the organ that connects the vagina to the uterus) has declined over the last 40 years. However, about $1.3 billion was predicted to be spent on cervical cancer care in 2014. The Center for Disease and Prevention (CDC)'s 2012 statistics on cervical cancer show 12,042 new cases and 4074 deaths. More than 100 viruses are strains of HPV, and more than 40 are transmitted sexually and can affect the male and female genital areas, mouth, and throat. Some produce genital warts or benign tumors, and some place women at high risk for cervical cancer. Research shows that persistent exposure to the human papillomavirus (HPV) is responsible for about 95% of cervical cancer development. In 2006, the United States Food and Drug Administration approved new vaccines (Gardasil and Cervarix) that target the HPV strains most commonly responsible for cervical cancer. Gardasil vaccine is effective against HPV-16 and 18, two high-risk HPVs that cause about 70 percent of cervical cancers. Vaccines given to young women before they become sexually active serve as chemoprevention for cervical cancer. Women may take the vaccines after they become sexually active, but they provide less protection because infection may already have occurred. As with most drugs, some side effects may occur.

Chemoprevention is being viewed as a key to cancer prevention in various types of cancers. Some studies have shown that green tea and green tea extract as well as green tea polyphenols and epigallocatechin gallate (EGCG) can serve as natural chemoprevention for cervical cancer. However, these same substances have also shown possibility in chemoprevention of cancer of the skin, colon, liver, lung, duodenum, esophagus, large intestine, and mammary glands. The use of vaccines for the hepatitis B virus may also protect against liver cancer.

Benefits and risks of chemoprevention: Over 1.6 million people are diagnosed annually with cancer in the United States. The goal of chemoprevention is to reduce the incidence of new cancers, which will improve the quality of life for many Americans and keep the workforce in place. In one study, cancer was associated with the highest loss of work days because of illness or impairment. The cost of cancer to the workers themselves and to their employers reinforces the need for measures and interventions such as chemoprevention to reduce the incidence of cancer.

Chemoprevention targets only high-risk populations because chemoprevention medications are not seen as useful or applicable for the general public and can have unpleasant side effects. However, the general public can focus on diet and food choice, as these factors may affect the incidence of certain cancers. For example, many authorities do not recommend taking vitamins and supplements but rather endorse eating a well-balanced diet that is low in unhealthy fat and includes fruits and vegetables. This is commonsense cancer prevention.

The success of diet change is not seen quickly but rather may become visible over extended periods of time. In fact, one study — called the Alpha-Tocopherol, Beta-Carotene Lung Cancer Prevention Study — demonstrated an 18 percent increase in lung cancer in the beta-carotene group. Judicious use of supplements is advised because negative outcomes as well as positive ones can occur.

People considering a change in diet should check with their health care providers, since some vitamins and supplements can interact adversely with some prescription medications.

Summary: The research involving chemoprevention is encouraging and warrants more study and research funding. Studies show that simple changes in lifestyle and eating habits can make a sizable impact on the incidence of cancer in the United States. Chemoprevention may some day prevent many forms of cancer in high risk individuals and keep cancer away in those in remission. The already burdened health care system could use its limited resources in trying to prevent other chronic diseases. Chemoprevention may not be the answer, but maybe it can be an answer to cancer in the United States.

Marylane Wade Koch, M.S.N., R.N.

For Further Information

About the Chemopreventive Agent Development Research Group. National Cancer Institute: Division of Cancer Prevention. Retrieved from http://prevention.cancer.gov/research-groups/chemopreventive-agent-development/about-chemopreventive

Mayo Clinic Staff (2014, Feb 12). *Breast cancer chemoprevention: Medicines that reduce breast cancer risk.* Mayo Clinic. Retrieved from http://www.mayoclinic.org/diseases-conditions/breast-cancer/in-depth/breast-cancer/art-20045353

Petrou, I. M.D. (2012, April 1). Individualized melanoma chemoprevention may be possible in future. *Dermatology Times.* Retrieved from http://dermatologytimes.modernmedicine.com/dermatology-times/news/modernmedicine/modern-medicine-feature-articles/individualized-melanoma-chemo?page=full

PREVENT Cancer Preclinical Drug Development Program (PREVENT). National Cancer Institute Division of Cancer Prevention. Retrieved from http://prevention.cancer.gov/major-programs/prevent-cancer-preclinical

Steward, W.P. & Brown, K. (2013, May 9). Cancer chemoprevention: A rapidly evolving field. *British Journal of Cancer*, 109: 1-7. Retrieved from http://www.nature.com/bjc/journal/v109/n1/full/bjc2013280a.html

Other Resources

Centers for Disease Control and Prevention
http://www.cdc.gov/

HPV Vaccine Questions and Answers
http://www.cdc.gov/hpv/parents/questions-answers.html

Chemopreventive Agent Development Research Group
http://prevention.cancer.gov/research-groups/chemopreventive-agent-development/about-chemopreventive

Chemoprevention: Cancer. Net
http://www.cancer.net/navigating-cancer-care/prevention-and-healthy-living/chemoprevention

National Cancer Institute: Prevention
http://www.cancer.gov

See also: Antioxidants; Beta-carotene; Bioflavonoids; Calcium; Carotenoids; Cartilage supplements; Coenzyme Q10; Dietary supplements; Fiber; Folic acid; Garlic and allicin; Ginseng, panax; Glutamine; Green tea; Herbs as antioxidants; Indoles; Isoflavones; Lutein; Lycopene; Nutrition and cancer prevention; Omega-3 fatty acids; Phytoestrogens; Prevention; Resveratrol; Saw palmetto; Soy foods; Sun's soup

▶ Decitabine/5-Azacytidine

Category: Chemotherapy and Other Drugs

Also known as: Decitabine: 5-aza-2'-deoxycytidine; chemical name is 2'-deoxy-5-azacytidine, 4-amino-1-(2-deoxy-beta-d-erythro-pentofuranosyl)-1,3,5-triazin-2(1H)-one; Dacogen®. 5-Azacytidine: azacitidine; chemical name is 4-amino-1-beta-d-ribofuranosyl-1,3,5-triazin-2(1H)-one; Vidaza®; Ladakamycin; Mylosar.

Definition: Analogues of cytidine ribonucleoside (5-Azacytidine) and cytidine 2'-deoxyribonucleoside or 5-aza-2'-deoxycytidine (Decitabine). Both are DNA hypomethylating agents and DNA methyltransferase inhibitors; they are also called antineoplastic, antimetabolite, and cytotoxic agents.

Cancers treated:

1) Myelodysplastic syndromes (MDS) – problems with production of abnormal blood components, often seen in older patients; it is a problem with the bone marrow, the area where blood components are made.

2) Acute myeloid leukemia (AML) – cancer of the blood involving the production and accumulation of abnormal cells from the "myeloid" line which includes red blood cells, platelets, and white blood cells. AML is an "acute" leukemia that tends to progress quickly without treatment and cause accumulation of immature cells.

3) Chronic myeloid anemia (CML) – cancer of the blood involving the production of abnormal "myeloid" cells that grow into mature-appearing cells but do not function properly. It is "chronic" which means it progresses at a slower pace than AML. CML can, however, transform into AML.

Delivery routes: Decitabine-intravenous (IV) only, as an infusion (a slow drip, usually lasting 1 to 3 hours at a time, over several days in a "cycle"). The infusion usually requires several cycles of 5-Azacytidine-IV or subcutaneous (SC), which is injected under the skin.

How these drugs work: The addition of multiple methyl groups (hypermethylation) to a portion of the DNA (genetic material) can shutdown genes that control normal cell processes like growth, division and apoptosis, or natural cell death. In certain cancers, like MDS, this hypermethylation leads to switching off tumor suppressor genes that suppress abnormal cell division, which leads to cancer development (uncontrolled division of abnormal cells). Thus, DNA hypermethylation of particular genes is associated with cancer cells.

Drugs like decitabine are called DNA methyltransferase inhibitors because they inhibit an enzyme called methyltransferase that catalyzes the transfer of a methyl group to cytosine bases in DNA; this inhibition leads to DNA hypomethylation. This decreased DNA "methylation" in the tumor suppressor genes of a cell (through the action of decitabine) can restore normal function in a previously rapidly dividing, cancerous cell. This allows the bone marrow, where blood components are made, to produce normal blood cells and does not harm nonactively dividing cells. Thus, DNA hypomethylation is associated with normal cells.

5-Azacytidine (5-AC) has a similar mechanism of action to Decitabine. 5-AC is both a DNA and RNA hypomethylating agent (interfering with tRNA cytosine-5-methyltransferase) because of its structure. RNA carries information from the DNA for protein production and, thus, 5-AC also affects protein synthesis. 5-AC is recommended as the treatment for elderly individuals with MDS and patients who are at high risk for MDS based on an International Prognosis Scoring System.

Both chemotherapy drugs also act as cytotoxic and antimetabolite agents, which are substances similar to normal cell components but cause cell death when incorporated into cancer cells.

Side effects: Both drugs decrease blood components (white blood cells, red blood cells, and platelets). A decrease in white blood cells can lead to infections. Fatigue can be caused by a decrease in red blood cells. Low platelets can lead to increased bleeding, bruising, and development of petechiae (small red dots on the skin).

These drugs can also cause "constitutional" symptoms such as generalized fatigue, fever, insomnia, headache, and dizziness. Approximately 40% of people experience lung-related symptoms in the form of a chronic cough, and some people will experience nausea, vomiting, diarrhea, and abdominal discomfort. Increased blood sugar and low levels of substances such as potassium and magnesium in the body can result from these drugs.

Magda Lenartowicz, MD, BA Hons (Gerontology)
Miriam E. Schwartz, MD,MA, PhD

For Further Information

Cabrero, M., Jabbour, E., Ravandi, F., Bohannan, Z., Pierce, S., Kantarjian, H. M., & Garcia-Manero, G. (2015). Discontinuation of hypomethylating agent therapy in patients with myelodysplastic syndromes or acute myelogenous leukemia in complete remission or partial response: Retrospective analysis of survival after long-term follow-up. *Leukemia Research*, 39(5):520-524.

Garcia-Manero, G. (2015). Myelodysplastic syndromes: 2015 update on diagnosis, risk-stratification and management. *American Journal of Hematology*, 90(9): 831-841.

Xie, M., Jiang, Q. & Xie, Y. (2015). Comparison between decitabine and azacitidine for the treatment of myelodysplastic syndrome: A meta-analysis with 1392 participants. *Clinical Lymphoma, Myeloma & Leukemia*, 15(1):22-28.

Other Resources

The Myelodysplastic Syndromes Foundation
http://www.mds-foundation.org/what-is-mds

U.S. National Library of Medicine—Myelodysplastic Syndromes
https://www.nlm.nih.gov/medlineplus/myelodysplasticsyndromes.html

National Cancer Institute—Azacitidine
http://www.cancer.gov/about-cancer/treatment/drugs/azacitidine

U.S. National Library of Medicine—Decitabine
https://www.nlm.nih.gov/medlineplus/druginfo/meds/a608009.html

▶ Delta-9-tetrahydrocannabinol

Category: Complementary and Alternative Therapies

Also known as: THC, dronabinol (Marinol), nabilone (Cesamet), *Cannabis sativa*, medical marijuana; slang terms include bud, ganja, grass, hemp, herb, pot, reefer, sinsemilla, weed; there are also many names signifying different growing regions and qualities of marijuana

Definition: Delta-9-tetrahydrocannabinol is the most well-known psychoactive substance in the plant *Cannabis sativa* (marijuana) that is an active ingredient. It is often called THC, for the three components in its name: tetra, hydro, and cannabinol.

Cancers treated or prevented: Delta-9-tetrahydrocannabinol is the major psychoactive ingredient in the plant *Cannabis sativa* (marijuana). It is debated as a viable medical treatment for a variety of conditions. Cancer patients usually use substances containing THC and its synthetic and derivative forms to relieve nausea and vomiting and to improve appetite. Some animal studies have also demonstrated some utility for THC to potentially decrease the incidence of some liver adenoma and carcinoma, as well as lung adenocarcinoma cells. Similarly in animals, some ability to decrease the incidence of benign tumors of the mammary gland, uterus, pituitary, testis, and pancreas has been demonstrated. THC also may enhance the effects of some standard chemotherapy agents in animal models of treatment. Extension of these findings to humans, however, is not yet clear.

Delivery routes: Drugs such as Marinol capsules and Cesamet pills are taken orally. Dried forms of marijuana, including buds of flowers and leaves, pieces of leaves, seeds, and stems, are smoked in marijuana cigarettes or pipes; burned and vaporized using other means; or ingested in foods such as baked cookies or teas. *Cannabis sativa* also may be used to produce the drug hashish, or hash, a resinous substance typically found in either block or oil form, or other forms of oils. Hash can be smoked or consumed orally; more liquid forms of oil often are consumed orally.

Individuals often use oral forms to mitigate nausea, which may accompany all forms of cancer and the chemotherapeutic drugs used to treat them. Non-oral forms (such as smoking) may be contraindicated for some types of cancer, such as lung cancers. Use also may be contraindicated in the presence of other medical and psychiatric conditions.

Animal studies may use these same methods of substance delivery. Some studies examining tumor incidence or progression also use other methods. One for example is gavage, or a device like a feeding tube. This may be used because the animal will not self-administrate the drug and/or to improve control over the dose received.

How this compound works: The human body has a cannabinoid system including receptors called CB receptors. The most studied receptors are CB1 and CB2 receptors. Other CB receptors are hypothesized to exist, but are not well understood.

CB1 receptors are located in the central nervous system (CNS) and peripherally. CB2 receptors are located primarily in the peripheral areas of the body and only in low amounts in the CNS. Both CB1 and CB2 receptors are involved in nausea and vomiting, interacting with other neurotransmitters affecting both the central nervous system (CNS) and gastrointestinal system. Products containing THC, its derivatives, and synthetic forms affect the cannabinoid system as a whole and via these CB1 and CB2 receptors.

Side effects: Current research is examining THC relative to other cannabinoids within marijuana. Some suggest that THC itself may be responsible for the psychoactive effects, while other substances, such as cannabidiol (CBD) is responsible for healing effects. Research is still pending; however, it is well known that THC side-effects may vary by user both in the short-term and long-term. This is because the drug may interact with other substances the person may be taking, as well as other conditions they may have mentally or physically. Broad short-term effects may include things such as changes in sensory experiences, increases in appetite, relaxation, increased feelings of pleasure, decreases in feelings of nausea. Less desirable effects that we might think of as side-effects may include memory and learning difficulties, panic, anxiety, coordination problems, and impaired problem solving. Long-term side-effects may include problems related to addiction, such substance use disorders, motivational problems, daily cough, phlegm problems, respiratory problems, and negative impact to the immune system. It is noteworthy that these effects are what would be observed in normal users that is, individuals without other significant physical or mental health problems who are not using any other substances. In individuals with other characteristics, such as other physical or psychiatric problems, the effects might differ in important ways, such as becoming more pronounced and or more disruptive to overall functioning.

For many years, marijuana use was thought to be associated with cancers as well, particularly those of the head, neck, and lungs, such as those commonly associated with tobacco products. This is because smoked marijuana and tobacco contain many of the same carcinogens. Contemporary scientific reviews suggest, however, that such assertions are more tentative and inconclusive. Studies controlling for co-occurring tobacco use often find that the risk often stays with the tobacco smoking habit. However, ever having used cannabis has been associated with increased risk for prostate cancer and oropharyngeal cancers, but a potentially decreased risk for bladder cancer in men. The influence of human papilloma virus and other risk factors complicate the ability of scientists to draw conclusions about these findings as well. As such, these mixed results suggest caution regarding any marijuana use without careful review of ones health profile and risks and the availability of other evidence-based treatments.

Nancy A. Piotrowski, Ph.D.

For Further Information

Grotenhermen, Franjo, & Russo, Ethan (Eds.). (2002). *Cannabis and Cannabinoids: Pharmacology, Toxicology, and Therapeutic Potential*. Binghamton, N.Y.: Haworth Press. A pharmacologic examination of marijuana and its derivatives; how they work, side-effects, and potential therapeutic uses.

Meyer, Jerrold S., & Quenzer, Linda F. (2013). *Psycho pharmacology: Drugs, the Brain, and Behavior, 2nd Ed.* Sunderland, MA: Sinauer Associations, Inc. Provides an overview of psychopharmacology, mechanisms of action for various drugs and their effects on behavior, and a chapter focused on cannabinoids and the endocannabinoid system.

Rosen, Winifred, & Weil, Andrew T. (2004). *From Chocolate to Morphine: Everything You Need to Know About Mind-Altering Drugs.* Rev. ed. Boston: Houghton Mifflin. Easy to read discussion about common every day drugs to a range of illicit substances and how they affect the body.

Other Resources

Drug and Alcohol Dependence
www.drugandalcoholdependence.com

National Cancer Institute
http://www.cancer.gov/about-cancer/treatment/cam/hp/cannabis-pdq

National Institute on Drug Abuse
www.nih.nida.gov

Psychiatric Times
www.psychiatrictimes.com

U.S. Food and Drug Administration
www.fda.gov

***See also*:** Antinausea medications; Appetite loss; Medical marijuana; Nausea and vomiting; Social and personal issues

▶ Doxorubicin

Category: Chemotherapy and Other Drugs

Definition: Doxorubicin is one of the most commonly used chemotherapeutic drugs in the anthracycline class.

Examples of anthracyclines

1. Daunorubicin
2. Doxorubicin (Adriamycin®)
3. Epirubicin
4. Idarubicin
5. Mitoxantrone

Anthracyclines were developed in the 1960s from *Streptomyces*, an aerobic bacterium that produces such antibacterial agents as streptomycin. Unlike antibiotics that treat infections, anti-tumor antibiotics alter the DNA in cancer cells to prevent replication. The anthracycline class of antineoplastics effectively treats more cancers than any other, but its success is not unblemished.

Cancers treated: Doxorubicin has a broad range of antitumor activity. Tumors most commonly responsive to doxorubicin (used alone or with other antineoplastics) include breast and esophageal cancers, sarcomas, Hodgkin's and non-Hodgkin's lymphomas, and, usually in children, Wilms' tumor. Because of its overall efficacy, doxorubicin also treats other less-responsive cancers.

Delivery: Doxorubicin is given by intravenous injection into a vein or central port over several minutes or by continuous infusion; rarely, it is injected arterially.

How anthracyclines work: Anthracyclines work in multiple ways, interfering with cell replication, damaging DNA, and promoting cell death. They target cancer cells, which tend to grow quickly, as well as other replicating cells in the body such as hair, mucosa, and bone marrow. Aromatic polyketides with an arresting red hue, anthracyclines work throughout the cell cycle.

Doxorubicin side effects: Side effects generally occur around the time of treatment. Doxorubicin's acute side effects include nausea and vomiting; sores in mouth and throat; weight changes; stomach pain; increased thirst; diarrhea; fatigue or weakness; dizziness; hair loss; separation of nails from their beds; itchy, watery, irritated, or painful eyes; burning, tingling, or painful appendages; and, briefly, red-hued urine. Doxorubicin causes temporary bone-marrow myelosuppression with declines in blood cells and platelets. Serious side effects include severe itching, hives, skin rash, difficulty in breathing or swallowing, or seizures.

Cardiotoxicity: Doxorubicin cardiotoxicity can occur during or soon after treatment (acute or subacute dysfunction)—or much later (chronic dysfunction). Early onset cardiotoxicity is usually felt as chest pain or palpitations and may be caused by heart-muscle edema, which can be reversed with treatment. A rare early onset effect is ventricular failure, but this too is reversible.

Chronic cardiomyopathy: Although results of cardiac examination after anthracycline chemotherapy may be normal, cardiomyopathy (damage to the heart muscle) may progress silently until six to 10 or more years after treatment, when symptoms may be abrupt and catastrophic. Cardiomyopathy comprises disturbances in rhythm or blood pressure, pericardial thickening, and cardiac dilation, which may progress to heart failure or death. Possibly, acute and chronic cardiomyopathies are distinct.

Incidence and risk: Incidence of early-onset doxorubicin cardiotoxicity is approximately 11% while late-onset incidence is 2% to 5% (estimates vary). Incidence increases with dose; thus, lifetime doxorubicin limits are imposed. Cardiotoxic risk is higher in those treated by doxorubicin in childhood or advanced age, and in people with preexisting heart disease. Risk increases when therapy includes other cardiotoxic drugs (especially cyclophosphamide), and with radiotherapy to the mediastinum (mid-chest). But risk factors aren't perfectly predictive; cardiomyopathy can occur at doses below doxorubicin's lifetime limit.

Cardiomyopathy mechanisms: The heart is a pump requiring abundant energy, much of it produced by mitochondria in the nuclei of myocytes (heart muscle). Although anthracycline damage to the heart is multifaceted, oxidative stress is pivotal. Doxorubicin's chemical structure breeds abundant free radicals, and cardiac cells, with their low levels of antioxidant enzymes, are uniquely vulnerable to oxidative stress. Free radicals damage DNA, inhibit DNA and protein synthesis, and trigger changes that induce apoptosis (death) of mitochondria and myocytes, which have scant ability to regenerate. Doxorubicin and its major metabolite doxorubicinol persist for some time in cardiac cells; their assaults progressively cripple the muscle, decreasing the contractility of surviving cells.

Preventive strategies: Attempts to combat doxorubicin's cardiotoxicity with antioxidants or chelation have failed, although in animal studies sulforaphane from cruciferous vegetables shows signs of protecting against oxidative stress. Doxorubicin analogues, including epirubicin, idarubicin, and mitoxantrone are engineered to decrease cardiotoxicity while retaining comparable anti-tumor efficacy. Encapsulating doxorubicin in vesicles impedes its breach of tight cardiac capillary junctions without impairing its ability to permeate tumors. Instances of fatal cardiomyopathy decline when doxorubicin is given over 48 to 96 hours, although the inconvenience of prolonged infusion generally precludes it. Currently the one FDA-approved agent that reduces anthracycline-induced cardiotoxicity is dexrazoxane.

Because it can produce secondary tumors and interfere with doxorubicin's efficacy, however, dexrazoxane treatment is limited. For those whose cardiomyopathy develops long after treatment, no effective remedy besides heart transplant is known; animal studies offer evidence that the antidepressant paroxetine may help repair the heart, although this has yet to be demonstrated in humans.

Jackie Dial, PhD

For Further Information

HemOnc Today. (2009, July 10). Phasing out anthracyclines in breast cancer: Is it time? *Healio*, http://www.healio.com/hematology-oncology/breast-cancer/news/print/hemonc-today/%7Bb-ccf5629-277b-4591-b4d1-65320a4063e9%7D/phasing-out-anthracyclines-in-breast-cancer-is-it-time

Florescu, Maria, et al. (2013) Chemotherapy-induced cardiotoxicity. Maedica (Buchar). 2013; 8(1): 59-67. http://www.ncbi.nlm.nih.gov/pmc/articles/PMC3749765

Perry, Michael Clinton. (Ed.) (2008). *The Chemotherapy Source Book* (4th ed.). Philadelphia, PA: Wolters Kluwer Health.

Strashun, Arnold. (1992). Editorial: Adriamycin, Congestive Cardiomyopathy, and Metaiodobenzylguanidine. *The Journal of Nuclear Medicine* 33(2): 215-222. http://jnm.snmjournals.org/content/33/2/215.full.pdf

Other Resources

American Association for Cancer Research (AACR). "Survivor Journeys."
https://www.aacrfoundation.org/SURVIVORS/PAGES/SURVIVOR-STORIES.ASPX?utm_source=-googlegr&utm_medium=searchad&utm_term=foundation&utm_content=mainpage&utm_campaign=survivorjourneys

BreastCancer.org. "Use of Anthracyclines to Treat Breast Cancer Has Gone Down."
http://www.breastcancer.org/research-news/20120914

Drugs.com. "Adriamycin."
http://www.drugs.com/pro/adriamycin.html

Ped-Onc Resource Center. "Late Effects: Heart."
http://www.ped-onc.org/survivors/cardio.htm

See also: Chemotherapy

▶ Drug Resistance and Multidrug Resistance (MDR)

Category: Chemotherapy and Other Drugs

Definition: Drug resistance (DR) is the loss of effectiveness of a drug used to destroy or weaken cancer cells. DR may be intrinsic (active in the cancer cell before treatment) or acquired (developed after treatment). Multidrug resistance (MDR) is the acquired adaptation of cancer cells to resist numerous structurally and functionally unrelated drugs (chemotherapy) designed to destroy cancer cells.

Resistance Development: DR and MDR are possible causes of treatment failure in cancer patients. When exposed to chemotherapeutic agents, cancer cells activate processes or synthesize molecules that can inactivate or eliminate the treatment drugs. Cancer cells have many alternative pathways at their disposal to overcome the effects of chemotherapeutic drugs. Most of these mechanisms have origins in the normal cell itself. Oncologists understand the phenomenon of DR and MDR and have developed treatment programs to delay or overcome resistance. Chemotherapy can consist of treatment with single or a combination of drugs and is commonly combined with radiation, surgery, and immunotherapy. Research is ongoing to develop drugs that specifically target DR and MDR when it develops.

Anticancer drugs have to overcome many challenges before they can accomplish a therapeutic purpose. Tumors are rapidly growing with a poorly developed vascular system. As cancer cells develop, they have difficulty receiving adequate oxygen and nutrients and therefore adapt to a hypoxic (low-oxygen) environment. This hypoxic environment can influence cancer cell resistance to therapeutic drugs, which have difficulty navigating the cancer tumor's poor vascular system. Therapeutic drugs must pass a cancer cell membrane, navigate the cytoplasm, and reach the nucleus (where they exert their effects). Also, they are required to accumulate in high enough concentrations in their active form and sustain these concentrations long enough to destroy the cancer cell.

Chemotherapeutic Drugs acting against DR and MDR proteins: A major research focus is to develop drugs that counteract DR and MDR proteins (drug efflux pumps) that transport drugs out of cancer cells. These proteins belong to a family of proteins called the adenosine triphosphate (ATP) binding cassette proteins (ABCs). The ABC proteins are overexpressed (increase greatly) when exposed to therapeutic chemotherapeutic drugs. These proteins reside in the cell membrane and consist of an embedded portion that forms a space for transport of drugs and an internal portion that binds to the ATP molecule. When the ATP molecule is bound and broken down, energy is released to drive the process.

P-glycoprotein is the main DR and MDR protein that has been studied, and it remains of primary interest. Intensive research has resulted in the developed of first-, second-, and third-generation P-glycoprotein inhibitors, with each generation improving on the previous generation. Researchers have begun development of inhibitors that bind to the ABC protein and inhibit its activity. The inhibitors have diverse chemical structures and origins. Additionally, multidrug resistance-associated protein (MRP1) is a major target of drug research. Several additional MRP proteins with structural similarities to MRP1 have been identified. Other MDR proteins have also been identified, including breast cancer-resistant protein, mitoxantrone-resistant protein, and others less well characterized.

Cellular changes associated with DR and MDR: DR and MDR are commonly associated with changes in the intracellular distribution of the therapeutic or nuclear enzymes. When DR and MDR develop, there is a redistribution of drug from the nucleus into cellular vesicles (e.g., Golgi bodies, endosomes, and lysosomes). The drugs are then transported toward the plasma membrane and excreted from the cell by the process of exocytosis. This process of elimination is considered passive and is different from the MDR efflux pumps, which require energy input to proceed (see above). The expression of MDR pumps is also associated with altered drug distribution within cancer cells.

Most chemotherapeutic drugs are mildly alkaline and have no charge. MDR cells have a more acidic pH inside subcellular vesicles than that of drug-sensitive cells. When drugs diffuse into the vesicles of MDR cells they take on a charge. The drugs are then trapped in the vesicles and cannot reach the nucleus to exert their effect. They can then be excreted from the cell by the process of exocytosis.

Glutathione and its associated enzyme, glutathionone-S-transferase (GST), are commonly found in the body and serve as a natural detoxification mechanism. GST can increase in the presence of a chemotherapeutic drug in the cancer cell. GST catalyzes the binding of glutathione to the drug. The drug becomes more water soluble, less toxic to the cell, and more readily excreted. Research is under way to develop drugs that inhibit GST and thus restore the cancer cell's sensitivity to the drug.

Chemotherapeutic Drugs that inhibit topoisomerase enzymes: Because cancer cells divide rapidly, topoisomerase inhibitor drugs are attractive treatments. The topoisomerase enzymes control the process of unwinding the DNA double helix during transcription or replication of the DNA molecule. To function, the drug must form a three-way complex with DNA and the enzyme. Conditions in the cell that interfere with this formation will lead to resistance. Mutations in the topoisomerase enzymes also cause resistance. Most topoisomerase inhibitors that have been the subject of clinical trials are derivatives of the plant extract camptothecin, although a semisynthetic derivative has also been developed.

Chemotherapeutic Drugs that inhibit DNA synthesis: Rapidly dividing cancer cells have a need for DNA synthesis to survive/thrive, so anticancer drugs (such as methotrexate and 5-fluorouracil) have been used to block pathways to its synthesis. Methotrexate inhibits the enzyme dihydrofolate reductase, while 5-fluorouracil blocks the enzyme thymidylate synthase. Both of these enzymes are required for the synthesis of nucleotides, the building blocks of DNA. Methotrexate was introduced in the mid-twentieth century for the treatment of acute lymphoblastic anemia, but resistance occurs rapidly. Resistance to the drugs can be due to increased production of the target enzymes, defective transport of the drugs, or increased excretion by efflux pumps.

A number of chloroethyl- and methyl-nitrosourea therapeutic drugs attack the guanine unit of DNA in cancer cells to exert their toxic effect. The cancer cell acquires resistance to the drug by activating the enzyme O^6-alkylguanine DNA alkyltransferase (AGT) to repair the damage. O^6-benzylguanine inhibits the action of AGT and is used clinically in combination with nitrosourea drugs to reverse the resistance. Toxicity problems can occur when these drugs are used at levels needed to attain maximum effectiveness. Protein kinase C is an enzyme that occupies a key role in the transfer of growth factor signals that result in DNA synthesis and cell division. This enzyme directly affects the expression of several proteins involved in drug resistance. These activities make protein kinase C an attractive target for therapeutic drugs.

Drugs that stimulate apoptosis: Most cancer drugs act by stimulating the process of apoptosis (programmed cell death). The susceptibility of a cancer cell to apoptosis depends on the balance between pro- and antiapoptotic proteins in the cell. When the TP53 protein (the primary proapoptotic protein) discovers genetic damage to the DNA molecule, it summons other proteins to halt cell division, and if necessary, to initiate apoptosis. Most cancers contain mutations in the *TP53* gene that not only prevent the protein it encodes (p53) from arresting the growth of potential cancer cells, but transform it into a cancer-promoting factor that favors the growth, spread, and drug resistance of tumors. Antiapoptotic proteins, particularly the Bcl-2 family, become more active during chemotherapy, leading to resistance to apoptosis.

Drugs that stimulate ceramide synthesis: Ceramide is the basic unit of sphingomyelin, a lipid structural element of cell membranes. Various stress stimuli, including radiation and chemotherapy, result in the formation of ceramide through the breakdown of sphingomyelin, or through synthesis from other molecules. Ceramide then acts as a second messenger relaying a signal to initiate apoptosis or other biological processes. DR/MDR can result in a reduction in ceramide concentration through conversion to an inactive molecule. This reduces the effectiveness of chemotherapy, since many chemotherapeutic drugs exert their effect through apoptosis. Drugs are under development that increase ceramide levels in tumor cells by promoting ceramide synthesis or by blocking the conversion of ceramide to inactive compounds.

Side effects: Depending on the chemotherapeutic drug administered, a variety of side effects can occur. These can include nausea, vomiting, diarrhea, anemia, malnutrition, memory loss, depression of the immune system, and toxicity to certain body organs. Additionally, cognitive side effects such as clinical depression or dysthymia are common.

David A. Oelle
Updated by Daniel L. Yazak, D.E.D.

For Further Information

Beeran, A.A., Maliyakkal, N., Rao, C.M., & Udupa, N. (2015). The enriched fraction of *Elephantopus scaber* triggers apoptosis and inhibits multidrug resistance transporters n human epithelial cancer cells. *Pharmacognosy Magazine,* 11(42). doi: 10.4103/0973-1296.153077.

Jandu, H., Aluzaite, K., Fogh, L., Thrdane, S.W., Noer, J.B., Proszek, J., … Stenvang, J. (2016). Molecular characterization of iriotecan (SN-38) resistant breast cancer cell lines. *BioMedCentral,* 16(34). doi: 10.1186/s12885-016-2071-1.

Klimaszewska-Wisniewska, A., Halas-Wisniewska, M., Tadrowski, T., Gagat, M., Grazaka, D., & Granka, A. (2016). Paclitaxel and dietary floavonoid fisetin: A synergistic combination that induces mitotic catastrophe and autophagic cell death in A549 non-small cell lung cancer cells. *Cancer Cell International,* 16(10). doi: 10.1186/s12935-016-0288-3.

Micsik, T., Lorincz, A., Gal, J., Schwab, R., & Petak. (2015). MDR-1 and MRP-1 activity in peripheral blood leukocytes of rheumatoid arthritis patients. *Diagnostic Pathology,* 10(216). doi: 10.1186/s13000-015-0447-1.

Montanari, F., Zdrazil, B., Digles, D., & Ecker, G.F. (2016). Selectivity profiling of BCRP versus P-gp inhibition: From automated collection of polypharmacology data to multi-label learning. *Journal of Chemiformatics,* 8(7). doi: 10.1186/s13321-016-0121-y.

Perazzoli, G., Prados, J., Ortiz, R. Caba, O., Cabeza, M.B., … Melguizo, C. (2015). Temozolomide resistance in Gliopastoma cell lines: Implication of MGMT, MMR, P-Glycoprdotein and CD 133 expression. *PLOS ONE,* 10(10). doi: 10.1371/journalpone.0140131.

Sun, K.-X., Jiao, J.-W., Chen, S., Liu, B.-L., & Zhao, Y. (2015). MicroRNA-186 induces sensitivity of ovarian cancer cells to paclitaxel and cisplatin by targeting ABCB1. *Journal of Ovarian Research,* 8(80). doi: 10.1186/s13048-015-0207-6.

Tao, K., Yin, Y., Shen, Q., Chen, Y., Li, R., Chang, W., … Zhang, P. (2016). Akt inhibitor MK-2206 enhances the effect of cisplatin in gastric cancer cells. *Biomedical Reports,* 4: 365-368. doi: 10.3892/br.2016.594.

Tian, X., Shivapurkar, N., Zheng, W., Hwang, J.J., Pishvaian, M.J., Weiner, L.M., …He, A.R. (2016). Circulating microRHA profile predicts disease progression in patients receiving second-line treatment of lapatinib and capecitabine for metastatic pancreatic cancer. *Oncology Letters,* 11: 1645-1650. doi: 10.3891/ol.2016.4101.

Xu, J.-H., Hu, S.-L., Shen, G.-D., & Shen, G. (2016). Tumor suppressor genes and their underlying interactions in paclitaxel resistance in cancer therapy. *Cancer Cell International,* 16(13). doi: 10.1186/s12935-016-0290-9.

Other Resources

National Cancer Institute
http://www.cancer.gov/

American Cancer Society
http://www.cancer.org/

Journal of the National Cancer Institute
http://jnci.oxfordjournals.org/

National Cancer Institute/Center for Cancer Research
https://ccr.cancer.gov/

Cancer Drug Resistance
http://www.ncbi.nlm.nih.gov/pubmed/11818492

See also: Alkylating agents in chemotherapy; Androgen drugs; Angiogenesis inhibitors; Antiandrogens; Antiestrogens; Antimetabolites in chemotherapy; Antineoplastics in chemotherapy; Biological therapy; Chemotherapy; Immunotherapy; Matrix metalloproteinase inhibitors; Plant alkaloids and terpenoids in chemotherapy; Proteasome inhibitors; Topoisomerase inhibitors; Tyrosine kinase inhibitors

▶ Erlotinib (Tarceva)

Category: Chemotherapy and Other Drugs
Also known as: Tarceva

Definition: Erlotinib hydrochloride is a tyrosine kinase inhibitor, which provides cytotoxic activity by blocking proteins and factors important to cell growth. Erlotinib was originally developed by OSI Pharmaceuticals and is approved to treat multiple types of cancers.

Cancers treated: In November 2005, erlotinib was approved as part of a combination therapy (with gemcitabine) to treat local advanced but unresected *metastatic* pancreatic cancer. In November 2004, erlotinib was approved for the treatment of localized or metastasized non-small-cell lung cancer (NSCLC). This approval occurred after the failure of at least one other chemotherapy regimen. In April 2010, erlotinib was approved for treatment of pancreatic adenocarcinoma and metastatic NSCLC. This approval was specified for maintenance treatment, second-line treatment, or third-line treatment after 4 cycles of platinum therapy. In May 2013, erlotinib was approved as a *first-line treatment* of NSCLC in patients with EGFR deletion or exon 21D mutations. Erlotinib was marketed to NSCLC patients by Astellas Pharma, Inc. to use concurrently with a cobas® epidermal growth factor receptor (EGFR) mutation test (Roche).

Delivery routes: Erlotinib is available as an oral tablet in 25-, 100-, and 150-mg sizes and is taken once daily. Erlotinib must not be taken with food and must not be crushed, chewed, or broken. A 100-mg once-daily dosage is approved as monotherapy for pancreatic cancer and 150-mg once-daily dosage is approved as monotherapy for NSCLC. Patients should take erlotinib at least 1 hour before or 2 hours after any meal or food intake.

How these drugs work: Tyrosine kinase inhibitors are potent blockers on the cell surface. They function to block the tyrosine kinase–epidermal growth factor signal transduction pathway at its receptor (eg, EGFR). The EGFR is essential to tumor (and other) cell growth. Inhibition of other tyrosine kinase receptors by erlotinib is still unclear. Erlotinib is approved for use only with a simultaneous test that identifies EGFR mutations that are targeted by this tyrosine kinase inhibitor.

Side effects: Rash, a major side effect of erlotinib treatment, may occur during the first week but can occur any time during treatment with a tyrosine kinase inhibitor. This rash resembles acne and can worsen with sun exposure. Other skin and nail changes are also common (such as dark or dry skin, and eye irritation). Additionally, hair changes are possible (including changes to eyelashes). Other frequent side effects that occur in over one quarter of patients include diarrhea, dyspnea (difficulty breathing), and decreased appetite. Nausea, fatigue, and vomiting are also likely.

In addition to side effects, erlotinib interacts with several different medicines, particularly those processed through the CYP3A4 and CYP1A2 enzyme systems of the liver. Medicines that inhibit CYP3A4 and CYP1A2 enzyme systems (such as several anti-fungal drugs, some antibiotics, including macrolides and ciprofloxacin, and anti-HIV medicines) increase the effects of erlotinib. Conversely, cigarette smoking or medicines that enhance these enzyme systems (such as some anti-seizure medicines, the antibiotic rifampin, and the herbal remedy St. John's Wort) decrease the activity of erlotinib.

Nicole Van Hoey, PharmD

For Further Information

Burotto, M., Ali, S. A., & O'Sullivan Coyne, G. (2014). Class act: safety comparison of approved tyrosine kinase inhibitors for non-small-cell lung carcinoma. *Expert Opinion on Drug Safety*, 14(1): 97-110.

OSI Pharmaceuticals, LLC. (2015). Tarceva (erlotinib hydrochloride) prescribing information. Retrieved from http://www.gene.com/download/pdf/tarceva_prescribing.pdf

National Cancer Institute (2013). FDA Approval for Erlotinib Hydrochloride. Retrieved from http://www.cancer.gov/about-cancer/treatment/drugs/fda-erlotinib-hydrochloride

Other Resources

ChemoCare—Erlotinib fact sheet
http://chemocare.com/chemotherapy/drug-info/erlotinib.aspx

National Cancer Institute Physician Data Query—Pancreatic Cancer Treatment
http://www.ncbi.nlm.nih.gov/pubmedhealth/PMH0032662

PubChem Open Chemistry Database: Erlotinib
http://pubchem.ncbi.nlm.nih.gov/compound/Erlotinib#section=Drug-and-Medication-Information

See also: Pancreatic cancers

▶ Glutamine

Category: Chemotherapy and Other Drugs; Lifestyle and Prevention

Definition: Glutamine is the most abundant amino acid in the body and is found in most proteins. Glutamine is considered a nonessential amino acid since the body is normally able to synthesize an adequate amount for its needs.

Cancers treated or prevented: All cancers currently treated with chemotherapy or radiation

Delivery routes: Glutamine can be taken orally by capsules, powder, or tablets. In the clinical setting, glutamine can be part of an enteral liquid formula given by feeding tube through the nose, stomach, or small intestine. Glutamine can also be given intravenously.

How this compound works: Although glutamine is found largely as a component of proteins (skeletal muscle in particular), it serves a variety of functions in the body. Stress conditions such as injury, burns, critical illness, or high-intensity exercise cause a greatly increased need for glutamine. Glutamine is considered a conditionally essential amino acid under these stress conditions, since dietary supplementation of glutamine is necessary. The gastrointestinal tract is the largest user of glutamine, particularly as a source of energy. Glutamine is important in wound healing and helps to mobilize components of the immune system. It also helps to maintain the integrity of the intestinal lining to prevent entry of bacteria and fungi.

Cancer cells have a great demand for glutamine as an energy source, which can deplete glutamine stores in muscle and other body tissues. Laboratory studies indicate that glutamine is necessary for the functioning of T lymphocytes and natural killer cells, which are components of the immune system. The depletion of body glutamine, therefore, could compromise the role of the immune system in the protection against cancer. Some researchers were concerned about supplementing cancer patients with glutamine, thinking that supplementation could increase tumor growth. Such supplementation has been found, however, to increase glutamine stores in the body and to improve intestinal and immune function.

In addition, studies have indicated that glutamine may alleviate the side effects of chemotherapy and radiation therapy. Glutamine supplementation has resulted in decreased intestinal mucosa ulceration and mouth inflammation. Peripheral neuropathy (numbness in extremities, motor weakness) often limits chemotherapeutic dosages. Glutamine may reduce the severity of neurological disorders, thereby permitting more effective dosages. Researchers believe that glutamine may work by restoring cellular levels of glutathione, a molecule that contains a sulfur group which binds to drugs and carcinogens. Glutamine supplementation increases the glutathione level in the body, thereby helping to reduce toxic drug levels. Glutamine supplementation has been shown to increase the accumulation of the chemotherapeutic drug methotrexate inside tumor cells, thereby increasing its killing effect.

Side effects: Since glutamine is so abundant in the body, even doses of up to 21 grams daily are well tolerated. Side effects are mainly gastrointestinal and include constipation and bloating.

David A. Olle, M.S.

See also: Antimetabolites in chemotherapy; Antinausea medications; Antineoplastics in chemotherapy

▶ Hepatitis C drug treatments

Category: Chemotherapy and Other Drugs
Also known as: HCV treatments; Hep C treatments

Definition: Hepatitis C is a disease that primarily affects the liver. It is caused by an infection of the hepatitis C virus. Hepatitis C may be treated in many ways, including interferon or peginterferon monotherapy, Interferon/

ribavirin combination therapy, and sofosbuvir/ledipasvir (Harvoni).

Hepatitis C infection was first discovered in 1989 by scientists at the Centers for Disease Control and Prevention (CDC), the National Institutes of Health (NIH), and the Pharmaceutical Industry.

The hepatitis C virus can be transmitted through blood products. The most common ways that infection occurs are through unsafe injection practices, such as intravenous drug users sharing needles, medical equipment that is not appropriately sterilized, and blood transfusions.

Hepatitis C infection may be either acute or chronic. Acute hepatitis C infection is most accurately described as the case in which the infected human body is able to get rid of the virus on its own. Chronic hepatitis C infection can also occur over time. According to the CDC, approximately 70% to 80% of individuals who are initially infected with hepatitis C will go on to develop the chronic form of hepatitis C infection. According to the World Health Organization (WHO), "130 to 150 million people globally have chronic hepatitis C infection. A significant number of those who are chronically infected will develop liver cirrhosis or liver cancer."

Hepatitis C-associated liver disease that develops over time is the most common cause of death of individuals infected with hepatitis C. Approximately 500,000 people die each year from hepatitis C-related liver diseases. Antiviral medicines can cure approximately 90% of persons with hepatitis C infection, thereby reducing the risk of death from liver cancer and cirrhosis, but access to diagnosis and treatment has been historically low.

There is currently no vaccine for hepatitis C; however, research in this area is ongoing.

The approach to treatment of hepatitis C infection is driven primarily by whether the infection is acute or chronic. The vast majority of patients diagnosed with acute hepatitis C infection can be successfully treated with standard therapy.

Treatments for Acute Hepatitis C Infection: Interferons are naturally occurring proteins that are released by animal cells, usually in response to the entry of a virus into the body. Interferons inhibit viruses from replicating. Interferon drugs are human interferons that are manufactured using recombinant DNA technology. Interferons do not directly kill viral or cancerous cells; they boost the immune system response and reduce the growth of malignant cells by regulating the action of several genes.

The 2 most frequently used interferon preparations in clinical trials have been IFN alfa-2b (Intron-A) and IFN alfa-2a (Roferon-A).

Some side effects that have been reported with interferon treatment are: Flu-like syndrome (i.e., fever, chills, generalized aches and pains, headache, poor appetite), fatigue, drowsiness, and low blood counts.

The addition of polyethylene glycol (PEG) molecules to interferon preparations has led to the development of long-lasting interferons that have better sustained absorption, a lower rate of clearance, and a longer half-life than unmodified interferon preparations. Two peginterferon preparations are available: PEG-IFN alfa-2b (PEG-Intron) and PEG-IFN alfa-2a (Pegasys).

Interferon therapy alone is often successfully used in treating acute hepatitis C infection. For example, Jaeckel et al., in 2001, found that treatment with interferon alfa-2b prevented 98% of patients with acute hepatitis C infection from developing chronic hepatitis C. Interferon is usually administered subcutaneously (under the skin). The dosing and duration of the therapy varies as hepatitis C infections often resolve spontaneously. However, experts recommend continuing treatment for at least 2 to 4 months after the onset of symptoms (or confirmed diagnosis) in most cases.

In several studies, peginterferon treatment has been shown to improve rates of sustained response against the hepatitis C virus, particularly for patients who have more developed progression of the disease. For example, in a trial of hepatitis C patients who had subsequently developed cirrhosis (fatty liver), Heathcote and others, in 2000, reported a sustained virologic response rate of 30% after 72 weeks of therapy with PEG-INF alfa-2a, compared with only 8% for patients treated with standard interferon alfa. Like standard interferon therapy, peginterferon is usually administered subcutaneously.

Some side effects that have been reported with peginterferon treatment are: vomiting, upset stomach, loss of appetite, mild diarrhea, weight changes, feeling very hot or cold, headache, muscle or joint pain, sleep problems (insomnia), temporary hair loss, mild skin rash, itching, redness, dryness, or swelling in the spot where the medicine was administered.

Treatment for Chronic Hepatitis C Infection: Interferon and ribavirin combination therapy helps to prevent the hepatitis C virus from reproducing in the body and is usually prescribed for people who have chronic hepatitis C infection. It may be given to people who have never had treatment or when the first set of medicines has failed to cure the infection.

Many studies have shown a higher response rate in patients taking the interferon and ribavirin combination therapy compared with those taking interferon (or peginterferon) alone. Studies have also shown that combination therapy can successfully treat some patients who have either relapsed after interferon alone or did not respond at all.

Treatment with interferon and ribavirin combination therapy is not recommended for pregnant women or women who choose not to use appropriate contraception during treatment. Female patients who have received this therapy themselves or who have been active sexual partners to men who have received this therapy should delay pregnancy for at least 6 months after the treatment is concluded.

A New Treatment for Chronic Hepatitis C Infection: In 2014, the FDA approved a new medication that cures chronic hepatitis C without any of the undesirable side effects of more traditional therapies like interferon and ribavirin combination treatment. Harvoni is a proprietary drug that is an oral combination of sofosbuvir and ledipasvir. In addition to its lack of side effects, Harvoni is much less intrusive as it is taken as a once-per-day pill.

The biggest downside of sofobuvir/ledipasvir therapy is its prohibitive price and the reluctance of insurance companies to cover the medication in most cases. As of December 2015, the price for a 12-week course of treatment with Harvoni is $95,000.

Jeremy W. Dugosh, PhD

For Further Information

Heathcote, E.J., Shiffman, M.L., Cooksley, W.G., Dusheiko, G.M., Lee, S.S., Balart, L., Reindollar, R., Reddy, R.K., Wright, T.L., Lin, A., Hoffman, J., De Pamphilis, J. (2000). Peginterferon alfa-2a in patients with chronic hepatitis C and cirrhosis. *New England Journal of Medicine,* 343(23): 1673-1680.

Jaeckel, E., Cornberg, M., Wedemeyer, H., Santantonio, T., Mayer, J., Zankel, M., Pastore, G., Dietrich, M., Trautwein, C., Manns, M.P.; German Acute Hepatitis CTherapy Group. (2001). Treatment of acute hepatitis C with interferon alfa-2b. *New England Journal of Medicine*, 345(20): 1452-1457.

Other Resources

Hepatitis C Information from the CDC
http://www.cdc.gov/hepatitis/hcv/

Hepatitis C Information from the NIH
https://www.nlm.nih.gov/medlineplus/hepatitisc.html

WHOs Guide to Hepatitis C
http://www.who.int/csr/disease/hepatitis/Hepc.pdf

Hepatitis Central Pages on living with Hep C
http://www.hepatitiscentral.com/

Financial Support for Patients
http://hepatitiscnewdrugresearch.com/hcv-drugs-financial-support.html

▶ Histamine 2 receptor antagonists

Category: Chemotherapy and Other Drugs
ATC code: A02BA

Definition: Histamine 2 antagonists are drugs that block acid production in the stomach.

Cancers treated: Multiple endocrine neoplasia (MEN), Zollinger-Ellison syndrome, Barrett esophagus

Delivery routes: These drugs are administered intravenously, or orally as tablets, capsules, chewable tablets, or liquids.

How these drugs work: Fluids in the stomach, composed primarily of hydrochloric acid and enzymes that break down proteins, aid in the digestion of food. Hydrochloric acid secretion can be triggered when histamine binds to one of its receptors, the H2 receptor, located in the cells lining the stomach (known as parietal cells). If the lower esophogeal sphincter (the muscle between the stomach and the esophagus) is not working correctly, then stomach acids may flow into the esophagus, resulting in heartburn and esophageal cell damage. Prolonged exposure to stomach acid in the esophagus can lead to gastroesophageal reflux disease (GERD).

Histamine 2 antagonists are competitive and reversible inhibitors of histamine, blocking its ability to bind to the H2 receptor and therefore decreasing stomach acid production, reducing the risk of acid reflux, and helping prevent ulcers in the stomach and small intestine.

Histamine 2 antagonists may be used to treat multiple endocrine neoplasia (MEN) and Zollinger-Ellison syndrome, which are conditions in which tumors within the digestive tract stimulate excess stomach acid production. Barrett esophagus, a precancerous condition in which normal cells lining the esophagus are damaged as a result of GERD and replaced with abnormal or cancerous cells, may also be treated with histamine 2 antagonists. Additionally, histamine 2 antagonists may be administered prior to chemotherapy to help manage gastrointestinal side effects.

Histamine 2 Receptor Antagonists

Drug	Brands	Delivery Mode	Cancers Treated
Cimetidine	Tagamet	Oral	Multiple endocrine neoplasia (MEN), Zollinger-Ellison syndrome, Barrett esophagus
Famotidine	Pepcid	Oral	MEN, Zollinger-Ellison syndrome, Barrett esophagus
Nizatidine	Axid	Oral	MEN, Zollinger-Ellison syndrome, Barrett esophagus
Ranitidine	Zantac	Oral, IV	MEN, Zollinger-Ellison syndrome, Barrett esophagus

Side effects: Common side effects of histamine 2 antagonists include mild diarrhea, allergic reactions, flulike symptoms, and bruising or bleeding easily. Intravenous (IV) administration of histamine 2 antagonists has been associated with rare cases of irregular heartbeat and elevated blood pressure. Histamine 2 antagonists may also reduce the body's ability to absorb drugs that require an acidic setting in the stomach in order to function.

Studies have shown that histamine can also promote the growth of certain colorectal cancer cell lines, with histamine 2 antagonists abrogating these effects and inducing tumor cell death. The mechanism behind these observations, however, is not yet understood.

Elizabeth A. Manning, Ph.D.

See also: Barrett esophagus; Endocrine cancers; Esophageal cancer; Esophagectomy; Esophagitis; Gastrinomas; Gastrointestinal cancers; Human growth factors and tumor growth; Hypercalcemia; Islet cell tumors; Multiple endocrine neoplasia type 1 (MEN 1); Multiple endocrine neoplasia type 2 (MEN 2); Neuroendocrine tumors; Pheochromocytomas; Pituitary tumors; Premalignancies; Thyroid cancer; Upper Gastrointestinal (GI) endoscopy; Zollinger-Ellison syndrome

▶ Histone deacetylase inhibitors

Category: Chemotherapy and Other Drugs
Also known as: HDACIs

Definition: Small molecules that inhibit enzymes called histone deacetylases, and subsequently disrupt gene expression and induce cell death in cancer cells.

Cancers treated: Cutaneous and peripheral T-cell lymphomas, multiple myeloma, and non-Hodgkin lymphoma, but being tested for efficacy against other types of cancer.

Delivery routes: Romidepsin and belinostat—injection or intravenous infusion; vorinostat and panobinostat—oral.

How these drugs work: Cells use the molecule deoxyribonucleic acid (DNA) to store genetic information. Eukaryotic organisms house their DNA in a membrane-bound structure called a nucleus that contains linear DNA molecules known as "chromosomes." Since eukaryotic cells must store large amounts of DNA in tiny spaces, they package their DNA into a compact structure known as "chromatin."

The basic structural units of chromatin, the nucleosome, consists of approximately 147 base pairs of DNA tightly wound about protein spools composed of an octamer of 4 different types of histone proteins. Nucleosomes are compacted into solenoid-type assemblages that form fibers 30 nm in diameter called 30 nm chromatin fibers. The heavily positively charged front ends (amino-termini) of histone proteins bind tightly, but nonspecifically, to the heavily negatively charged sugar-phosphate backbone of DNA.

For the purposes of gene expression, cells must loosen the interaction between histones and DNA. Cells accomplish this by chemically modifying the positively charged amino termini of histones. In particular, enzymes called "histone acetyl transferases" attach acetyl groups (CH_3-COO^-) to some of the positively charged lysine residues in the amino-termini of histone proteins. This neutralizes the positive charge of the histone and diminishes its affinity for DNA, which makes the DNA more accessible to the gene expression machinery. Conversely, enzymes called "histone deacetylases," or HDACs, remove acetyl groups from histones, which reestablishes the strong association between DNA and histones, and, typically, shuts down gene expression.

Eighteen different HDACs have been identified in humans that fall into 4 classes. All of these HDACs have distinct targets and influence the expression of specific genes that affect particular biological processes. For example, deficiencies in HDAC2, HDAC5, and HDAC9 cause heart defects, loss of function of HDAC7 affects the integrity of blood vessels, and HDAC4 deficits adversely affect cartilage formation.

Many different types of cancers show elevation of HDAC activity, and experimental attenuation of HDAC activity in such cancer cells decreases cancer cell growth, viability, and survival.

Small molecules called HDAC inhibitors (HDACIs) inhibit the catalytic activity of HDACs and selectively alter the expression of specific genes in tumor cells. Several studies have established that HDACIs only affect the expression of a subset of all expressed genes in cancer cells. In several cancer cell lines, HDACIs can inhibit the tumor-induced development of new blood vessels (angiogenesis), tumor cell invasion and migration, and induce tumor cell differentiation and cell-cycle arrest. HDACIs show antitumor activity in animal models of cancer and in human patients. Normal cells are relatively resistant to HDACI-induced cell death (apoptosis) compared to cancer cells.

Approximately 12 different HDACIs are currently being evaluated in clinical trials to treat a variety of cancers. Four HDACIs have been approved for clinical use. Vorinostat (Zolinza), the first FDA-approved HDACI, is indicated for the treatment of cutaneous T-cell lymphoma. Romidepsin (Istodax) is indicated for treatment of cutaneous T-cell lymphoma and peripheral T-cell lymphoma. Two other HDACIs have been granted accelerated FDA approval: Belinostat (Beleodaq) for the treatment of rare and fast-growing non-Hodgkin lymphoma, and panobinostat (Farydak) as part of a combination treatment for relapsed multiple myeloma. In 2013, the FDA designated another HDACI, entinostat, as a breakthrough therapy for certain types of breast cancers.

Side Effects: The most common side effects caused by romidepsin are low white blood cell counts (leukopenia), low platelet counts (thrombocytopenia), infections, nausea, fatigue, vomiting, anorexia, anemia, and electrocardiographic changes. For vorinostat, the most common side effects are diarrhea, fatigue, nausea, thrombocytopenia, and a bad taste in the mouth (dysgeusia). The most common side effects in belinostat-treated patients are nausea, fatigue, fever, anemia, and vomiting. Patients given the panobinostat-containing drug combination most commonly experience diarrhea, fatigue, nausea, peripheral edema, decreased appetite, fever, vomiting, blood chemistry anomalies, and low white and red blood cell counts.

Michael Buratovich, PhD

For Further Information

Carey, Nessa. (2013). *The epigenetics revolution: How modern biology is rewriting our understanding of genetics, disease, and inheritance*. NY: Columbia University Press.

Gray, S. G. (2001). "Targeting Huntington's disease through histone deacetylases." *Clinical Epigenetics* 2: 257-277.

West, Alison C. & Johnstone, Ricky W. (2014). "New and emerging HDAC inhibitors for cancer treatment." *Journal of Clinical Investigation* 124(1): 30-39.

Other Resources

HDAC database
http://www.hdacis.com

Huntington Outreach Project for Education at Stanford (HOPES)
http://web.stanford.edu/group/hopes/cgi-bin/hopes_test/hdac-inhibitors

See also: Chromatin; Histone acetylation/deacetylation; Cell cycle control

▶ Hormonal therapies

Category: Chemotherapy and Other Drugs
Also known as: Hormone therapy, endocrine therapy, antiestrogen therapy

Definition: Hormonal therapy is the use of exogenous hormones or hormone antagonists in the medical treatment of cancer. It removes hormones or prevents their growth and survival-promoting action in hormone-responsive cancer cells. Hormonal therapy should not be confused with hormone replacement therapy.

Cancers treated: Hormonal therapy most often refers to hormone-sensitive or hormone-receptor-positive breast cancer, but it also refers to several other types of cancers resulting from hormone-responsive tissues, including the prostate, endometrium, and adrenal cortex. Hormonal therapy may also be used to treat paraneoplastic syndromes, which arise from substances produced by tumors, or to alleviate certain chemotherapy-induced symptoms, such as anorexia (appetite loss).

Delivery routes: Oral

How these drugs work: Gonadal hormones, including estrogens and androgens, activate hormone receptors in hormone-responsive cells that, in turn, stimulate gene expression and may activate cell-signaling pathways to induce tumor growth. Hormone therapies prevent a specific hormone receptor from the activation of cell-signaling pathways that would induce tumor growth. There are two main effective strategies for starving hormone-responsive tumor cells. One strategy is to block a particular hormone's ability to activate cell-signaling pathways, and the other approach is to introduce drugs that inhibit the production of the specific hormones responsible for tumor-cell growth.

In particular, 80 percent of breast cancer needs the hormone estrogen to grow. The metabolism of estrogen starts with the synthesis of cholesterol into androgens. Then androgens, such as testosterone, are converted into estrogens via the aromatase enzyme. Primarily, estrogen is produced in the ovaries, but other tissues, including the liver, adrenal glands, and breasts, also produce estrogens. Although estrogen production in the ovaries ceases during menopause, the adrenal glands and other tissues continue to produce estrogen via the enzyme aromatase. Every year, approximately 23,000 postmenopausal women are diagnosed with estrogen-receptor-positive early breast cancer.

One type of hormonal therapy for breast cancer patients prevents estrogen from binding to estrogen receptors in order to halt the growth of cancerous cells. This strategy has led to the development of tamoxifen (Nolvadex), which is a selective estrogen-response modulator (SERM) and an estrogen receptor antagonist. Tamoxifen used to be the gold standard of hormonal medicine for patients with hormone-receptor-positive breast cancer; it is currently used for the treatment and chemoprevention of breast cancer. Tamoxifen binds to estrogen receptors to prevent their activation, therefore blocking a tumor's ability to use estrogen. Raloxifene (Evista) is another SERM commonly used for chemoprevention of breast cancer in high-risk patients, and it also prevents osteoporosis, a common side effect of hormonal therapy. Toremifene (Fareston) and fulvestrant (Faslodex) are SERMs used for the treatment of metastatic breast cancer. In particular, fulvestrant is an estrogen-receptor downregulator (ERD) that is an option for postmenopausal women with metastatic breast cancer that has stopped responding to antiestrogen therapy.

Similar to other hormone antagonists, tamoxifen is also a weak agonist, or weak estrogen. As a result, in patients who develop resistance to estrogen agonists, the best alternative treatments are the use of aromatase inhibitors, which prevent the production of estrogens. As a result, estrogen levels drop, which in turns induces apoptosis (cell death), thus halting the growth of hormone-responsive cancer cells. Several international clinical trials have shown evidence that aromatase inhibitors—Arimidex (anastrozole), Aromasin (exemestane), and Femara (letrozole)—work more effectively than tamoxifen in postmenopausal women in treating breast cancer. Therefore, aromatase inhibitors have become the standard of care for postmenopausal women with hormone-receptor-positive breast cancer. For premenopausal women, however, tamoxifen remains the choice of hormonal treatment.

Typically, tamoxifen is used as adjuvant therapy following primary treatment for early-stage breast cancer. In the case of breast cancers in postmenopausal women, the first line of breast cancer treatment tends to be the use of aromatase inhibitors, such as letrozole and anastrozole. Exemestane has been shown to be superior to megestrol in the treatment of tamoxifen-refractory breast cancer. Aminoglutethimide is a nonselective inhibitor that blocks aromatase and other enzymes that promote steroid hormone synthesis. Since it is nonselective to estrogen, it is not preferred to treat breast cancer; however, it may also be prescribed for the treatment of hyperadrenocortical syndromes, such as Cushing syndrome and adrenocortical carcinoma.

One of the most common cancers among men in the United States is prostate cancer. Antiandrogens (antitestosterone-like drugs), such as flutamide, bicalutamide, nilutamide, and cyproterone acetate, block the growth- and survival-promoting effects of testosterone and dihydrotestosterone in prostate cancer cells.

Another form of hormonal therapy is orchidectomy and ovariectomy (oophorectomy), which are surgical removal of male or female endocrine organs, respectively. In particular, removal of the Fallopian tubes and ovaries reduces the risk for or prevents breast and ovarian cancer in women at high risk because of mutations in the *BRCA1* or *BRCA2* gene. As an alternative to surgical castration, gonadotropin-releasing hormone (GnRH) analogs, such as leuprolide and goserelin, are used for chemical castration. GnRH suppresses the production of estrogen and progesterone in the ovaries and the production of testosterone by the testes.

While most hormonal therapies block hormone-induced signals to cancer cells, in some therapies the hormone supplementation has a cytotoxic effect on tumor cells. Progestins (progesterone-like drugs), androgens, and estrogens are among these hormones.

Side effects: The side effects of hormonal therapy vary among treatments. Side effects may be brief, mild, and manageable, or they may be serious. In women, side effects of hormonal therapy that are common to all treatments are mood swings, depression, weight gain, hot flashes, vaginal dryness, early start of menopause, and, in metastatic cancer, burning pain in the bones. Tamoxifen promotes a less than 1 percent increased risk of uterine cancer, blood clots, cataracts, stroke, and fertility issues. Hormone therapy with tamoxifen or estrogens may increase the chance of developing endometrial cancer; therefore, women taking tamoxifen should have a pelvic examination every year to look for any signs of cancer. In particular, abnormal vaginal bleeding (other than menstrual bleeding) while taking estrogen-like medication should be reported to a doctor as soon as possible. The benefits of tamoxifen, however, far outweigh the potential risks. Aromatase inhibitors may induce osteoporosis and cause upset stomach and sweating, and they can increase cholesterol levels and the risk of blood clotting. Unlike other aromatase inhibitors, exemestane does not appear to have ostcoporosis-promoting side effects. Similar to aromatase inhibitors, ERDs may weaken bones and cause upset stomach. In addition, ERDs may also cause swelling at the injection site. Ovariectomy weakens the bones and results in infertility.

Research has showed that tamoxifen used for early-stage breast cancer reduces the risk of recurrence of the primary cancer and the risk of developing new cancers in the other breast. Taking tamoxifen for longer than five years, however, is no more effective than five years of therapy. Many women develop resistance to the hormonal therapy over time, leading to cancer recurrence. After tamoxifen treatment, breast cancer recurs in about one-quarter of patients after five years. In large-scale clinical trials, both steroidal and nonsteroidal aromatase inhibitors have been shown to be superior to tamoxifen in extending survival in postmenopausal women with metastatic disease and in preventing recurrence when used as primary adjuvant therapy.

Anita Nagypál, Ph.D.

For Further Information

Adamo, V., et al. "Overview and New Strategies in Metastatic Breast Cancer (MBC) for Treatment of Tamoxifen-Resistant Patients." *Annals of Oncology* 18, suppl. 6 (June, 2007): 53-57.

"Adjuvant Therapy for Breast Cancer." *NIH Consensus Statement* 17, no. 4 (November 1-3, 2000): 1-35.

Arnal, J. F., et al. "Understanding the Controversy About Hormonal Replacement Therapy: Insights from Estrogen Effects on Experimental and Clinical Atherosclerosis." *Archives des maladies du coeur et des vaisseaux* 100, nos. 6/7 (June/July, 2007): 554-562.

Garrett, Andrea, and Michael A. Quinn. "Hormonal Therapies and Gynaecological Cancers." *Best Practice & Research Clinical Obstetrics & Gynaecology* 22, no. 2 (April, 2008): 407-421.

Hind, D., et al. "Hormonal Therapies for Early Breast Cancer: Systematic Review and Economic Evaluation." *Health Technology Assessment* 11, no. 26 (July, 2007).

Lethaby, Anne E., and Beverley J. Vollenhoven. "An Evidence-Based Approach to Hormonal Therapies for Premenopausal Women with Fibroids." *Best Practice & Research Clinical Obstetrics & Gynaecology* 22, no. 2 (April, 2008): 307-331.

Other Resources

American Cancer Society
Detailed Guide: Breast Cancer—Hormone Therapy
http://www.cancer.org/docroot/CRI/content/CRI_2_4_4X_Hormone_Therapy_5.asp

BreastCancer.org
Hormonal Therapy
http://www.breastcancer.org/treatment/hormonal/

National Cancer Institute
Treatment Option Overview
http://www.cancer.gov/cancertopics/pdq/treatment/breast/Patient/page5#Keypoint17

See also: Androgen drugs; Antiandrogens; Antiestrogens; Antimetabolites in chemotherapy; Antineoplastics in che motherapy; Biological therapy; Cancer biology; Chemotherapy; Corticosteroids; Cytokines; Diethylstilbestrol (DES); Estrogen Receptor Downregulator (ERD); Immune response to cancer; Immunotherapy; Interferon; Interleukins; Vaccines, therapeutic

▶ IDH1 inhibitor AG-120

Category: Chemotherapy and Other Drugs
Also known as: (no proprietary name)

Definition: A chemotherapeutic agent acting by inhibiting mutant forms of isocitrate dehydrogenase (IDH).

Cancers Treated: IDH1 inhibitors AG-120, and the clinically similar IDH2 inhibitor AG-221, are being tested in patients with advanced mutant positive hematologic malignancies who are in second or later relapse, refractory to second-line induction treatment, or who have relapsed after allogeneic transplantation. There is also a clinical trial involving glioblastoma. AG-120 is potentially useful in any cancer- containing mutant IDH1, but research efforts have so far focused on the most lethal and treatment-resistant types.

Delivery Routes: Oral. The optimum frequency and dosage have not been determined.

How this Drug Works: IDH1 and IDH2 inhibitors interfere with the production of the "oncometabolite" 2-hydroxyglutarate, and by selectively slowing the growth and proliferation of cells carrying mutant IDH. An oncometabolite is a small molecule made as a result of normal cellular metabolism, but whose accumulation affects the regulation of metabolism and primes cells for future progression to cancer. In a study of 57 patients with acute myeloid leukemia, over a period of 11 months, 31% showed a positive response. The drugs do not affect noncancerous cells; a requisite for a drug that targets a fundamental metabolic process and would interfere with cellular functioning even in nondividing cells. It is also ineffective against cancer cells that do not carry the mutation. This makes it critical to know whether the mutation is present before commencing therapy, and also limits long-term effectiveness, because even in malignancies where the IDH1 mutant predominates, some of the cells have the wild-type allele, and treatment selects for them. In surveys of astrocytomas (a type of aggressive brain cancer) the mean survival time of patients with the mutation was longer than for patients without it.

Agios, the company responsible for AG-120, is also investigating a compound, AG-881, an orally available IDH1/IDH2 inhibitor capable of fully penetrating the blood-brain barrier. This represents a significant advance in the treatment of gliomas (solid tissue brain tumors). At this time, brain tumors have proven particularly difficult to treat with chemotherapeutic agents because these do not penetrate into the malignancy when administered orally or intravenously.

Side Effects: The majority of the effects reported in the preliminary clinical study were mild to moderate, with the most common being fatigue, diarrhea, pyrexia (fever), and nausea. Thirty-five serious adverse events (including 13 deaths) were reported, including 4 cases of leukocytosis possibly related to AG-120.

Martha A. Sherwood, PhD

For Further Information

Dimitrov, L., Hong, C. S., Yang, C., Zhuang, Z., & Heiss, J. D. (2015). New developments in the pathogenesis and therapeutic targeting of the IDH1 mutation in glioma. *International Journal of Medical Sciences*, 12(3): 201-213.

Leck, Renee. (2015, June 12). Agios announces new data from ongoing phase 1 trial of AG-120 showing durable clinical activity in patients with advanced hematologic malignancies. http://investor.agios.com/phoenix.zhtml?c=251862&p=irol-newsArticle&ID=2058807

ClinicalTrials.gov. (2015). Study of orally administered AG-120 in subjects with advanced solid tumors, including glioma, with an IDH1 mutation. https://clinicaltrials.gov/ct2/show/NCT02073994

Other Resources

PubMed (online access to research papers on cancer biology)
http://www.ncbi.nlm.nih.gov/pubmed

Astrocytoma Options
http://astrocytomaoptions.com/exploring-strategies-for-idh1-mutated-gliomas/

American Brain Tumor Association—Glioblastoma
http://www.abta.org/brain-tumor-information/types-of-tumors/glioblastoma.html

▶ Imetelstat

Category: Chemotherapy and Other Drugs
Also known as: GRN163L, telomerase inhibitor GRN163L

Definition: A 13-based synthetic oligonucleotide attached to a lipid group that inhibits the enzyme telomerase and kills cancer cells.

Cancers treated: Myelodysplastic syndrome, Myelofibrosis, Essential Thrombocythemia, Non-small-cell lung cancer (all experimental).

Delivery routes: Intravenous infusion.

How these drugs work: Cells use the molecule deoxyribonucleic acid (DNA) to store genetic information. DNA consists of a polymer of "nucleotides," and since nucleotides have a front (5′ end) and back side (3′ end), DNA molecules do as well. DNA polymerases, the enzymes that synthesize DNA, only polymerize it from front to back (5′→3′ direction). DNA is a double-stranded molecule that consists of 2 nucleotide polymers, one of which lies from front to back and the other of which lies in the opposite direction. Therefore, the synthesis of molecules of DNA requires that one strand is made continuously and the other strand, discontinuously. Consequently, linear DNA molecules will always have a 3′ single-stranded overhang every time the molecule is replicated, and each time the DNA molecule is replicated, part of the molecule is lost.

To solve this problem, cells with linear chromosomes use an enzyme called "telomerase" to synthesize a repeated sequence multiple times at the ends of chromosomes to prevent chromosomal loss. These repeated sequences at the ends of linear chromosomes are known as "telomeres." The telomere-specific sequence at the ends of chromosomes is species-specific and the number of times it is repeated varies between cells of the same organism.

Telomerase consists of a protein and RNA component. The RNA component, known as the "guide RNA" (gRNA), provides the template for the synthesis of the telomeric repeat, and the sequence of the telomeric repeat is complementary to a portion of the gRNA.

Telomerase is highly active during embryonic and fetal development, but its activity fades with aging. Tissues with high levels of turnover, such as the bone marrow, gut and skin, can transiently increase their levels of telomerase. Overall the loss of telomerase activity causes telomeres to shorten and cell replication and healing to diminish.

Cancer cells, however, have high levels of telomerase, but they have short telomeres. Therefore, inhibition of telomerase can shorten the chromosomes of cancer cells and induce cell death. Imetelstat interferes with the gRNA component of telomerase and inhibits telomerase activity, thus ushering cancer cells into programmed cell death.

Side effects: In small clinical trials, 22% of patients had low levels of particular white blood cells (neutropenia), and 11% had anemia, headache, and fainting spells (syncope). Liver toxicity, however, affected every patient, which led the US Food and Drug Administration to place a full clinical hold on imetelstat on March 11, 2014. However, follow-up examinations of those patients showed that this liver damage was transient, and on October 31, 2014, the USFDA lifted the clinical hold.

Michael Buratovich, PhD

For Further Information

Ferrandon, S., Malleval, C., El Hamdani, B., Batties-ton-Montagne, P., Bolbos, R., Langlois. J-P., ... Poncet, D. (2015). Telomerase inhibition improves tumor response to radiotherapy in a murine orthotopic model of human glioblastoma. *Molecular Cancer*, 14: 134.

Nitta, R., Ning, G., Avilion, A. A., & Joseph, I. (2012). Inhibition of telomerase with imetelstat causes depletion of cancer stem cells. In M. A. Hayat (Eds.), *Stem cells and cancer stem cells: Therapeutic applications in disease and injury* (pp. 13-24). New York City, NY: Springer.

Other Resources

Geron – Imetelstat
http://www.geron.com/imetelstat

See also: Chemotherapy

▶ Immunotherapy

Category: Chemotherapy and Other Drugs
ATC code: 101, 103
Also known as: Biological therapy, biotherapy

Definition: Immunotherapy is a treatment that stimulates the immune system to fight cancer and reduce related side effects of disease. Agents come from biological sources and may be given alone or combined with chemotherapy. Immunotherapies boost the patient's immune system to fight cancer cells, while chemotherapy drugs attack the cancer cells directly.

Cancers treated: Breast cancer, lung cancer, melanoma, cervical cancer, leukemias, lymphomas, myelomas, prostate cancer, colorectal cancer, and ovarian cancer; others under investigation

Subclasses of this group: Cytokines, including interferons, interleukins, and hematopoietic growth factors; monoclonal antibodies, which can be developed from mouse antibodies (murine), a combination of mouse and human antibodies (chimeric), human antibodies combined with a small amount of mouse antibody (humanized) or only human antibodies (human), antibodies fused with a toxin or radioactive material, or cells; vaccines developed from cells, parts of cells, or antigens

Delivery routes: Agents may be administered by mouth (orally), injection (subcutaneously-intramuscularly or intravenously). Some vaccines are given into the skin (intradermal) or may be placed into the bladder in a liquid form (instillation). Agents may be taken at home or may require a visit to the physician's office or hospital. The schedule of administration varies with the agent.

How these drugs work: Cancer develops when normal cells change their genetic makeup over some period of time. As these changes occur, proteins are moved to the cell surface that the body does not recognize. An antigen is any substance that causes the immune system to produce antibodies. The body's activation of the immune system against these unrecognized substances is called an immune response and is the principle of immunotherapy. Antibodies developed outside the body or substances given to encourage the body to develop antibodies against antigens are the foundation for immunotherapy. The immune system includes lymph nodes, the spleen, tonsils, bone marrow, and white blood cells. Some of the goals of immunotherapy include: 1) increasing the immune system's sensitivity to cancer cells in order to improve the ability of the immune system to attack and kill such cells; 2) preventing normal cells from becoming malignant; 3) preventing the spread of cancer cells; 4) encouraging the body to repair damaged cells; 5) and changing the activity of normal cells around tumors.

Cytokines are used more frequently than any other type of immunotherapy, as they are employed at some point in most cancers. Because cancer treatments can cause serious side effects and complications, an important part of therapy is side effect control. White blood cells fight infection in the body and are decreased by chemotherapy drugs, leading to neutropenia. Anemia, which is a decrease in red blood cells responsible for carrying oxygen to cells, can be life-threatening in cancer patients. Erythropoietin stimulates the release of mature red blood cells and may be used as an important part of cancer therapy. Colony-stimulating factors encourage the bone marrow to convert immune cells into neutrophils, critical to fighting infection. Cytokines are naturally produced in the body but can be developed in the laboratory using a system called recombinant deoxyribonucleic acid (DNA) technology. Cytokines can be developed to interact with receptors on immune cells to stimulate, for example, red blood cells to be produced or inhibit or slow cancer cell growth. While some cytokines are not therapeutic for cancer, they are needed to allow patients to receive their full doses of both immunotherapy and chemotherapy.

A group of cytokines called interleukins are therapeutic for cancer. In 1992, interleukin-2 (IL-2) was the first immunotherapy approved for use alone in treating cancer. IL-2 is used for advanced kidney cancer and melanoma, either alone or in combination with other chemotherapies or immunotherapies. Interleukin stimulates T cells and natural killer cells in the immune system. Interferons, which are also cytokines, are thought to work by slowing the growth of cancer cells and the blood vessels that supply the tumor. It is also thought that interferons may increase the production of antigens in the cancer cell, making it more visible to antibodies. Natural killer cells may also be boosted by the administration of interferon.

Monoclonal antibodies generally interrupt signals in the cell that cause it to become cancerous. They can be developed to be attracted to the antigen secreted by the cell in order to block its function. Each monoclonal antibody is designed to bind to a specific antigen on the cell. Some monoclonal antibodies attracting significant interest are those that cause the immune system to attack the blood supply of the tumor, called antiangiogenesis. Monoclonal antibodies are known as passive immunotherapy because they use antibodies made outside the body in large numbers. Active immunotherapy is when the patient's own body makes antibodies against antigens, such as seen in vaccine therapy. There are approximately ten monoclonal antibodies approved for use in cancer treatment.

Vaccines are able to trigger the immune system to attack cancer cells with a specific antigen developed in the patient's body. Most vaccines are experimental in nature and available only as part of a research study. However, a few cancer vaccines are currently approved by the FDA for use in the United States. Some forms of active immunotherapy are not vaccines but may try to have an impact on specific locations within the immune system. Most of these therapies are not approved by the FDA and are available only in a clinical research study. Lymphokine-activated killer cell (LAK) therapy involves T cells made in the laboratory and treated with IL-2, and researchers are testing ways to make the cells more active against cancer. Tumor infiltrating lymphocyte (TIL) vaccine is composed of cells found inside tumors removed with surgery, treated with IL-2 in the laboratory, and then injected back into the patient. TIL is being tested in a variety of cancers.

Side effects: Immunotherapy may cause flulike symptoms, including fever, chills, nausea, vomiting, fatigue, headache, low blood count (anemia), inability to fight infection, bone pain, and muscle aches. If the agent is injected, then a rash or swelling may be noted at the site.

Blood pressure can drop during administration. More serious but less common side effects include bleeding, difficulty breathing, edema leading to congestive heart failure, heart damage, and severe and potentially life-threatening reactions (such as anaphylaxis).

Patricia Stanfill Edens, R.N., Ph.D., FACHE
Updated by Catherine J. Walsh

For Further Information

Chabner, Bruce A., and Dan L. Longo, (Eds.). (2006). Cancer chemotherapy and biotherapy: Principles and practice. Philadelphia: Lippincott Williams & Wilkins.

Gullatte, M. M. (2005). *Clinical guide to antineoplastic therapy: A chemotherapy handbook*. Philadelphia, PA: Oncology Nursing Society.

National Cancer Institute. (2003). Biological therapy: Treatments that use your immune system to fight cancer. *NIH Publication 03-5406*. Bethesda, MD.: National Institutes of Health. Also available at http:// www .cancer.gov.

Polovich, M., White, J. M., & Kelleher, L. O. (Eds.). (2005). *Chemotherapy and biotherapy guidelines* (2nd ed.). Pittsburgh, PA: Oncology Nursing Society.

Predergast, G. C., & Jaffee, E. M. (2013). *Cancer immunotherapy* 2nd ed). Waltham, MA: Academic Press. This book discusses the role of the immune system in suppressing tumor development and provides basic and clinical cancer researchers with an overview of immunotherapy and chemotherapy in fight against cancer.

Yamaguchi, Y. (Ed.). (2016). *Immunotherapy of cancer: An innovative treatment comes of age*. New York: Springer. A new book that summarizes present status and future for cancer immunotherapy.

Wang, X. Y., & Fisher, P. B. (Eds.). (2015). *Immunotherapy of cancer*, (Advances in Cancer Research), (Vol. 128). Waltham, MA: Academic Press, 2015. This book provides information on cancer research with expert reviews and is directed towards students and researchers.

Other Resources

American Cancer Society
Cancer Immunotherapy
http://www.cancer.org/treatment/treatmentsand-sideeffects/treatmenttypes/immunotherapy/immunotherapy-toc
This website provides introductory information for patients on Cancer Immunotherapy.

National Cancer Institute
Biological Therapies for Cancer.
www.cancer.gov/about-cancer/treatment/types/immunotherapy/bio-therapies-fact-sheet
This website provides overview and introductorhy information about biological therapies used in cancer.

Medscape
http://www.medscape.com

National Cancer Institute
Drug Dictionary. http://www.cancer.gov/drugdictionary

National Cancer Institute
Immunotherapy: Using the Immune System to Treat Cancer
www.cancer.gov/research/areas/treatment/immunotherapy-using-immune-system
This website provides information on how immunotherapy uses the body's own defense to defend against cancer and includes links to current research at NCI and recent advances in immunotherapy.

See also: Angiogenesis inhibitors; Biological therapy; Cytokines; Gene therapy; HIV/AIDS-related cancers; Immune response to cancer; Infectious cancers; Interferon; Interleukins; Lymphomas; Medical oncology; Monoclonal antibodies; Neutropenia; Radiation therapies; Vaccines, preventive; Vaccines, therapeutic

▶ Interferon

Category: Chemotherapy and Other Drugs
ATC code: 103AB (interferons); LO3AB01 (interferon alfa natural, Alferon-N, Roferon-A); LO3AB02 (interferon beta natural); LO3AB03 (interferon gamma, Actimmune); LO3AB04 (interferon alfa-2a, Roferon-A, Pegasys); LO3AB05 (interferon alfa-2b, Rebetron, Pegintron, Intron-A); LO3AB06 (interferon alfa-n1); LO3AB07 (interferon beta-1a, Avonex, Rebif); LO3AB08 (interferon beta-1b, Betaseron); LO3AB09 (interferon alfacon-1, Infergen); SO1AD05 (interferons)

Definition: Interferons are cytokines, naturally occurring proteins produced by leukocytes or fibroblasts. When a foreign agent such as a virus or cancer enters the cell, interferon is released into the body fluids to induce healthy cells to manufacture an enzyme to counter the invasion. The interferons are described as alpha, beta, and gamma according to their amino acid sequence and structure.

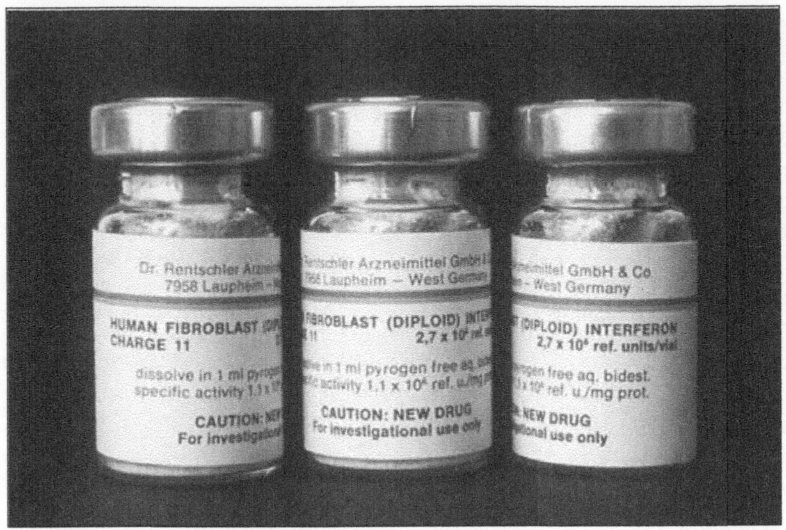

Interferon. (National Cancer Institute)

The naturally occurring interferons were first described in the 1950's. Then in 1980 scientists inserted the interferon gene into the bacteria *Esherichia coli* (*E. coli*) using recombinant DNA technology. The resulting bacterial culture allowed the recovery and purification of a quantity of interferon sufficient for therapeutic use. Today, interferon is used to fight viral infections and in conjunction with chemotherapy as an anticancer drug.

Cancers treated or prevented: Kidney cancer, malignant melanoma, multiple myeloma, carcinoid tumors, some types of lymphoma and leukemia

Delivery routes: Intramuscular, subcutaneous, or intravenous injection; also available as a nasal spray to protect against rhinoviruses

How this substance works: Interferons, both naturally and therapeutically, work by stimulating the body's own immune system by slowing, blocking, or changing the growth or function of the replication of foreign invaders such as viruses, bacteria, parasites, or tumor cells.

- Alpha interferons: Various alpha interferons have been approved to treat approximately twenty cancers and more than ten infections—interferon alfa natural for treating kidney cancer, malignant melanoma, multiple myeloma, carcinoid tumors, some types of lymphoma and leukemia, and genital warts; and interferon alfa-2a for treating viral hepatitis B and C.
- Beta interferons: Interferon beta-1a and -1b are being investigated for treating multiple sclerosis.
- Gamma interferons: Interferon gamma-1b treats granulomatous disease.

Side effects: Flulike symptoms such as fever, chills, headache, muscle aches and pains, and malaise are expected with all interferons. Life-threatening neuropsychiatric disorders such as depression and suicide have been reported, but the link between interferon and these psychiatric developments remains unclear. Fatigue, diarrhea, nausea, vomiting, abdominal pain, joint aches, back pain, and dizziness have been reported. Other possible side effects include anorexia, congestion, increased heart rate, confusion, low white blood cell count, low platelet count, low red blood cell count, increase in liver enzymes, increase in triglycerides, temporary skin rashes, hair loss or thinning, swelling, cough, and difficulty breathing.

Jane Adrian, M.P.H., Ed.M., M.T. (ASCP)

See also: Biological therapy; Bone cancers; Carcinoid tumors and carcinoid syndrome; Cardiomyopathy in cancer patients; Cytokines; Eosinophilic leukemia; Exercise and cancer; Fever; Gene therapy; Hairy cell leukemia; Immune response to cancer; Immunotherapy; Kaposi sarcoma; Kidney cancer; Liver cancers; Mantle Cell Lymphoma (MCL); Mesothelioma; Mycosis fungoides; Myelofibrosis; Myeloproliferative disorders; Non-Hodgkin lymphoma; Polycythemia vera; Waldenström Macroglobulinemia (WM)

▶ Interleukins

Category: Chemotherapy and Other Drugs
ATC code: 103AC

Definition: Interleukins are cytokines (hormones of the immune system) that are produced naturally in the body. Interleukins are an important part of the body's response to infection and disease, and they help the immune system fight cancer. They can be made in the laboratory for use in therapeutic applications.

Cancers treated: Melanoma, renal cell cancer, colorectal cancer Subclasses of this group: Biological response modifiers, immunostimulants, growth factors, colony-stimulating factors

Delivery routes: These drugs are administered through either high-dose or low-dose regimens. High-dose regimens include intravenous (IV) infusion. A lower-dose regimen is administered through subcutaneous injection.

How these drugs work: Interleukins and other biological response modifiers use the body's immune defenses to enhance or restore immune function. Interleukins can directly target tumor cells, enhance the immune response to cancer cells, or reduce side effects from other cancer treatments. Interleukins can be used alone or in combination with cancer chemotherapeutic agents.

Several interleukins are in various phases of clinical trials, but interleukin-2 (IL-2) and interleukin-11 (IL-11) have been the most widely studied and utilized. IL-2 stimulates the growth and activity of many immune cells, such as lymphocytes, which function in destroying tumor cells. IL-2 also directly interferes with cancer cell growth. Cancers currently treated with IL-2 include melanoma and renal cell carcinoma, a type of cancer that originates in the kidney. A commercial name for IL-2 used in cancer therapy is Aldesleukin or Proleukine®. Other interleukins, such as IL-11, also known as opreleukin, function as support medications by reducing side effects that result from cancer treatment, such as low platelet count or low levels of other blood components. IL-11 is beneficial to patients who are being treated with chemotherapy by decreasing the need for platelet transfusions. Such interleukins, also called growth factors or colony-stimulating factors, stimulate bone marrow cells to divide and develop into white blood cells, platelets, or red blood cells. Specifically, IL-11 stimulates the production of platelets to increase their numbers to normal levels and thus reduce the need for platelet transfusions. Research scientists continue to investigate how interleukins might be useful in treating other types of cancers, such as leukemia, lymphoma, brain, colorectal, ovarian, breast, and prostate cancers.

Side effects: Side effects resulting from the use of interleukins vary widely depending on interleukin type, dosage, and the patient. Common side effects include flulike symptoms such as fever, chills, weakness, muscle and joint aches, diarrhea, nausea, and vomiting. Treatment can also result in increased heart rate, skin rash, low white blood cell count, low platelet count, anemia, and appetite loss. Swelling, primarily in the hands, feet, and ankles, can also occur. A serious, but uncommon side effect, is capillary leak syndrome, which results in low blood pressure and poor blood flow.

Catherine J. Walsh, Ph.D.

See also: Angiogenesis; Appetite loss; Biological therapy; Castleman disease; Colony-stimulating factors (CSFs); Cyclosporin A; Cytokines; Fever; 5Q minus syndrome; Gene therapy; Helicobacter pylori; Hemangiosarcomas; Histiocytosis X; Immune response to cancer; Immunotherapy; Liver cancers; Melanomas; Mistletoe; Myelosuppression; Thrombocytopenia; Urinary system cancers

▶ Laxatives

Category: Chemotherapy and Other Drugs
Also known as: Bowel stimulants

Definition: Laxatives are drugs, food, or compounds that promote a bowel movement. They can be used to prepare the bowel for diagnostic examination or to prevent or treat constipation.

Cancers treated: All

Subclasses of this group: Bulk-producing agents, stool softeners, lubricants and emollients, hydrating agents, stimulants

Delivery routes: Laxatives are taken orally or in a suppository form.

Description: Cancer patients experience constipation for various reasons. Cancer treatments may render patients less active or mobile, which increases the risk of constipation. Depression or anxiety as a result of cancer treatments or pain can result in constipation. Repeated use of pain medications, decreased intake of fluids, or chemotherapy may lead to constipation in cancer patients. Intestinal tumors or scar tissue from intestinal surgeries for cancer can have an impact on the body's ability to empty waste material.

How these agents work: Laxatives work in diverse ways. Bulk-producing agents combine with water to increase the mass of the stool and stimulate the intestinal muscles. Common bulk-producing laxatives include psyllium husk, dietary fiber, and apples. These gentle agents enhance peristalsis within twelve to seventy-two hours.

Stool softeners or surfactants also produce bowel movements in twelve to seventy-two hours. By drawing water into the stool, these laxatives soften the stool, which is useful for cancer patients who experience pain when passing a firm stool. Stool softeners can build a tolerance, however, making the laxative ineffective for some cancer patients. Docusate (Colace) is a stool softener.

Lubricants or emollients make the stool slippery and act in the colon within six to eight hours. They work by making the stool slide more easily through the colon. An example of a lubricant laxative is mineral oil. One concern is that mineral oil can cause decreased absorption of the fat-soluble vitamins, such as A, D, E, and K.

Hydrating agents or osmotics are laxatives that draw water into the colon to soften the stool. These laxatives produce desired results within thirty minutes to six hours. Examples of hyperosmotic laxatives include milk of magnesia (magnesium hydroxide), Epsom salts (magnesium sulfate), and glycerin suppositories. GoLYTELY, a solution of polyethylene glycol (PEG) 3350 and electrolytes, is often used as a preparatory agent for colon procedures such as colonoscopy.

Another form of laxative is a stimulant or irritant, such as cascara, senna, aloe vera, biscodyl (Ducolax), or castor oil. These agents stimulate movement in the colon and are the most severe of all laxatives; they should not be the cancer patient's laxative of choice.

Side effects: The side effects of laxatives may include diarrhea and dependency. Overuse can result in the inability to have a bowel movement and lead to constipation or impaction. Because laxatives can lessen the effectiveness of some medications, a health care provider should be consulted before their use.

Marylane Wade Koch, M.S.N., R.N.

See also: Antidiarrheal agents; Antinausea medications; Chemotherapy; Crohn disease; Diarrhea; Diverticulosis and diverticulitis; Gastrointestinal cancers; Gastrointestinal complications of cancer treatment; Hemorrhoids; Inflammatory bowel disease; Rectal cancer; Side effects; Symptoms and cancer; Weight loss

▶ Lenalidomide (Revlimid)

Category: Chemotherapy and Other Drugs
Also known as: Revlimid

Definition: A thalidomide analogue used to treat several different types of blood-based cancers.

Cancers treated: Lenalidomide is used to treat multiple myeloma, myelodysplastic syndromes, and mantle cell lymphoma. Also, it is in clinical trials for several different types of lymphomas and leukemias.

Delivery routes: Oral

How this drug works: Cells dispose of broken, damaged or unnecessary proteins by degrading them. In order to properly distinguish between proteins that should be degraded and those that should not, cells utilize a tagging system that marks particular proteins for destruction. These pro-degradation tags come in the form of a 76-amino-acid polypeptide called ubiquitin. The attachment of ubiquitin multimers to proteins marks them for destruction by a large protein degradation complex called the proteasome.

Ubiquitin attachment occurs in a step-wise process that requires adenosine triphosphate (ATP) and 3 different enzymes: E1 (the ubiquitin-activating enzyme), E2 (the ubiquitin-conjugating enzyme), and E3 (the ubiquitin ligase). E1 uses the energy expended by the hydrolysis of ATP to form an energy-rich thioester bond with ubiquitin. E2 accepts the ubiquitin from E1 and forms a complex with E3 and the target protein, after which E3 attaches the ubiquitin to the target protein. Cells contain approximately 2 different types of E1s, about 60 E2s, and hundreds of different E3s. The E3s interact with specific types of E2s and only attach ubiquitin to specific target proteins. Thus, the proteasome-ubiquitin system is very tightly regulated.

Lenalidomide and related compounds bind to a specific E3 called cereblon. Cereblon works in a complex with 3 other proteins (DDB1, CUL4A, and ROC1). When bound by lenalidomide, the cereblon complex changes its target specificity and tags the transcription factors Ikaros (IKZF1) and Aiolos (IKZF3) for destruction. Typically, Ikaros and Aiolos activate the expression of tumor promoting proteins and suppress the expression of T-lymphocyte-promoting proteins. The destruction of Ikaros and Aiolos in tumor cells induces tumor cell death, and simultaneously helps the immune system fight the cancer.

Side effects: The most commonly reported mild or mod erate side effects in patients treated with lenalidomide include diarrhea, anemia (low red blood cell count), constipation, peripheral edema (swelling), neutropenia (low numbers of neutrophils, a specific type of white blood cell), fatigue, back pain, nausea, asthenia (physical weakness or lack of energy), rash, and insomnia. The most frequently reported severe or life-threatening adverse reactions include bone marrow suppression and low blood cell counts, pneumonia, hypokalemia (low blood potassium), cataract, dyspnea (difficulty breathing), disseminated vascular thrombosis (blood clot in a blood vessel), and hyperglycemia (high blood sugar).

Lenalidomide is toxic to developing babies and should never be used in pregnant women. It is also toxic to the liver and can cause liver failure in some patients.

Michael Buratovich, PhD

For Further Information

Bashey, A., Abonour, R., & Huston, J. A. (2012). *100 questions & answers about myeloma*. Burlington, MA: Jones & Bartlett Learning.

Stewart, K. A. (2014). How thalidomide works against cancer. *Science* 343(6168): 256-257.

Other Resources

Official Revlimid site
http://www.revlimid.com

See also: Proteasome inhibitors

▶ Matrix metalloproteinase inhibitors

Category: Chemotherapy and Other Drugs

Definition: Matrix metalloproteinase inhibitors suppress the enzymatic activity of extracellular matrix metalloproteinases secreted by cancer cells.

Cancers treated: Several matrix metalloproteinase inhibitors are currently in clinical trials. Their efficacies in treating cancers are unknown at this time.

Delivery routes: Oral, intraperitoneal, intrapleural

How these drugs work: Matrix metalloproteinases are a family of enzymes normally secreted by connective tissue cells and inflammatory cells (phagocytes). They are called *metallo*proteinases because they contain a zinc atom at their catalytic (active) site. These enzymes play a role in several normal physiologic processes, including embryo implantation and normal angiogenesis associated with tissue growth and wound healing.

Malignant tumors undergo invasive growth and metastasis. The viscous connective tissue matrix, composed of collagens, laminins, fibronectins, elastins, and proteoglycans, forms the scaffolding for cellular organization in tissues and provides a barrier to cancer cell migration. Cancer cells, however, can also secrete matrix metalloproteinases, which allows metastasis to proceed by breaking down the connective tissue extracellular matrix. Matrix metalloproteinases are also important contributors to abnormal angiogenesis, the process by which cancer cells stimulate the production of new blood capillaries that deliver nutrients to the tumor cells and are essential for their continued growth.

Researchers identified compounds in tissues that inhibited the activity of the matrix metalloproteinases and have developed new inhibitors by chemical synthesis. The inverse relation between matrix metalloproteinase activity and clinical outcome in cancer has led to the development and testing of these inhibitors in pancreatic, colon, and liver tumor model systems. Since 1993, matrix metalloproteinase inhibitors have undergone rapid clinical development for efficacy in treating colon, ovarian, pancreatic, prostate, gastric, skin, and both non-small-cell and small-cell lung cancers. The most promising inhibitors are those that can be administered orally, making them suitable for chronic administration, which appears to be necessary for optimal effect.

Targeting matrix metalloproteinases in cancer is complicated by the fact that they are absolutely necessary for normal physiological processes; thus researchers must find a delicate balance between disease treatment and the progression of these processes. Unfortunately, clinical trials conducted on synthetic broad-spectrum inhibitors (those targeting several matrix metalloproteinases) have yielded disappointing results in cancer pathology. Nevertheless, researchers are making intensive efforts to find new classes of matrix metalloproteinase inhibitors that have high (rather than broad) selectivity against specific metalloproteinases.

Side effects: Reported side effects from matrix metalloproteinase inhibitors include abdominal pain, fever, elevated liver enzymes, musculoskeletal pain and stiffness, mild thrombocytopenia, skin rash, and cutaneous phototoxicity.

Bernard Jacobson, Ph.D.

See also: Angiogenesis; Cancer biology; Carcinomatosis; Malignant tumors; Metastasis

▶ Monoclonal antibodies

Category: Chemotherapy and Other Drugs

Definition: Monoclonal antibodies are antibodies that recognize only one antigen and that are mass-produced in the laboratory from a single clone of a B cell, the type of immune system cell that makes antibodies.

Common Monoclonal Antibodies

Drug	*Brands*	*Subclass*	*Delivery Mode*	*Cancers Treated*
Alemtuzumab	Campath	Humanized	IV	Chronic lymphocytic leukemia
Bevacizumab	Avastin	Humanized	IV	Lung cancer, colorectal cancer
Cetuximab	Erbitux	Chimeric	IV	Head and neck cancers, colorectal cancer
Epratuzumab	LymphoCide	Humanized	IV	B-cell leukemia
Gemtuzumab ozogamicin	Mylotarg	Humanized	IV	Acute myelogenous leukemia
Ibritumomab tiuxetan	Zevalin	Murine	IV	B-cell lymphoma
Lym-1	Oncolym	Murine	IV	Lymphoma
Panitumumab	Vectibix	Human	IV	Colorectal cancer
Rituximab	Rituxan	Chimeric	IV	B-cell lymphoma
Tositumomab	Bexxar	Murine	IV	B-cell lymphoma
Trastuzumab	Herceptin	Humanized	IV	Breast cancer

Cancers treated: Lymphoma, leukemia, breast cancer, head and neck cancers, colorectal cancer, lung cancer

Subclasses of this group: Murine (composed entirely of mouse sequences), chimeric (composed of approximately one-third mouse and two-thirds human sequences), humanized (composed of at least 90 percent human sequences), and human (antibodies that are fully human in composition)

Delivery routes: As a result of their molecular size and susceptibility to enzymatic digestion in the gut if administered orally, monoclonal antibodies must usually be administered by intravenous (IV) infusion.

How these drugs work: Antibodies are proteins that bind to a specific site, or epitope, on a specific target molecule. In response to infection or immunization with a foreign agent, the immune system generates many different antibodies that bind to the foreign molecules. This pool of polyclonal antibodies contains a mixture of different antibody molecules, each of which binds to a specific epitope. Isolation of a single antibody from a polyclonal antibody pool would yield a highly specific molecular tool with the ability to bind to a single epitope. Georges Köhler, César Milstein, and Niels Kaj Jerne invented the process of producing monoclonal antibodies in 1975 and shared the 1984 Nobel Prize in Physiology or Medicine for their discovery. Since then, monoclonal antibodies have become an important tool in biological research and in medicine.

The process of producing monoclonal antibodies involves fusing an individual B cell, which produces a single antibody with a single specificity but which has a finite life span, with a long-lived myeloma tumor cell. The B cell is taken from the spleen or lymph nodes of an animal that has been challenged with the antigen of interest. The combination of the B cell and the myeloma cell produces a hybridoma cell, a kind of perpetual antibody-producing factory. The hybridoma cell produces the single specific antibody and can be grown in culture indefinitely, allowing the production of large amounts of the monoclonal antibodies. Monoclonal antibodies are potentially more effective than conventional drugs in treating cancer, since conventional drugs attack not only cancer cells but also normal cells. Monoclonal antibodies attach only to the specific target molecule. Since monoclonal antibodies are specific for a particular antigen, one designed to bind to ovarian cancer cells, for instance, will not bind to colorectal cancer cells.

The first monoclonal antibodies were made from mouse B cells. When administered into humans, mouse antibodies are recognized by the human immune system as foreign (because they are from a different species) and can elicit an immune response against them, causing allergic-type reactions. Researchers have since learned how to replace some portions of the mouse antibody sequences with human antibody sequences. The application of genetic engineering techniques has allowed the production of chimeric, humanized, and, more recently, fully human monoclonal antibodies.

An antibody molecule is composed of two heavy polypeptide chains and two light polypeptide chains. Both heavy and light chains are composed of a region that varies from antibody to antibody, the variable region, and a constant region that is conserved. By combining human sequences for the constant region with murine sequences for portions of the variable region, the amount of murine sequence can be decreased. Depending on how much murine sequence is left, the result is either a chimeric (with approximately one-third murine and two-thirds human sequence) or a humanized (with at least 90 percent human sequence) monoclonal antibody. Genetically engineered mice strains are now available that contain a large portion of human deoxyribonucleic acid (DNA) that codes for the antibody heavy and light chains, with the mouse's own heavy and light chain genes inactivated. Using these mice to produce B cells for the construction of hybridomas allows the generation of fully human antibodies, which are likely to be safer and may be more effective than the previous generation of monoclonal antibodies.

One potential treatment for cancer involves using monoclonal antibodies that bind only to a cancer cell-specific component of interest and induce an immunological response against the target cancer cell (referred to as "naked" monoclonal antibodies). Monoclonal antibodies can also be designed for the delivery of another (nonspecific) agent, such as a toxin, radioisotope, or cytokine, to the cancer cell for the purpose of killing it (referred to as "conjugated" monoclonal antibodies).

Some naked monoclonal antibodies bind to cancer cells and exert their action by marking the cells to help the body's immune system destroy them. Rituxan (rituximab) and Campath (alemtuzumab) are examples of this type of monoclonal antibody. Rituximab binds to the CD20 antigen, a protein found on B cells, and is used to treat B-cell non-Hodgkin lymphoma. Alemtuzumab binds to the CD52 antigen, another protein present on B and T cells, and is used to treat some patients with B-cell chronic lymphocytic leukemia.

Some naked monoclonal antibodies bind to functional parts of cancer cells or other cells that help cancer cells grow and act by interfering with the cancer cells' ability to grow. Herceptin (trastuzumab), Erbitux (cetuximab), and Avastin (bevacizumab) are examples of this type of monoclonal antibody. Trastuzumab binds to the HER2/neu protein, a protein present in large numbers on tumor cells in some cancers that, when activated, helps these cells grow. Trastuzumab acts by inactivating these proteins. It is used to treat some breast cancers. Cetuximab binds to the epidermal growth factor receptor (EGFR) protein, which when present in high levels on cancer cells helps them grow. Cetuximab blocks the activation of EGFR and is used to treat some advanced colorectal cancers and some head and neck cancers. Bevacizumab binds to the vascular endothelial growth factor (VEGF), a protein that cancer cells produce to attract the new blood vessels they need for growth. Bevacizumab prevents VEGF from functioning and is used to treat some colorectal, lung, and breast cancers.

Some of these monoclonal antibodies have been used in cancer treatment for many years. At first they were used mainly after other treatments had failed, but as more studies have been done the trend is to use them earlier in the course of cancer treatment.

Conjugated monoclonal antibodies (also called "tagged" or "loaded" monoclonal antibodies) are attached to anticancer (chemotherapy) drugs, toxins, or radioactive substances and used as vehicles to deliver these toxic agents directly to cancer cells. Radiolabeled monoclonal antibodies are attached to radioactive substances; treatment with such agents is called radioimmunotherapy. Chemolabeled monoclonal antibodies are attached to anticancer drugs, and immunotoxins are monoclonal antibodies attached to toxins. Zevalin (ibritumomab tiuxetan) and Bexxar (tositumomab) are examples of radiolabeled monoclonal antibodies. Both bind to an antigen on cancerous B lymphocytes and are used to treat some B cell non-Hodgkin lymphomas. Mylotarg (gentuzumab ozogamicin) is an example of an immunotoxin. It contains the toxin calicheamicin attached to a monoclonal antibody that binds to the CD33, a protein antigen present on most leukemia cells, and is used to treat some acute myelogenous leukemias.

Clinical trials of monoclonal antibody therapy are in progress for patients with almost every type of cancer. As more cancer-associated antigens have been identified and studied, it has been possible for researchers to make monoclonal antibodies against more types of cancer.

Side effects: Antibodies that contain murine sequences can be recognized by the human immune system as foreign, causing systemic inflammatory effects such as fever, chills, weakness, headaches, nausea, vomiting, and diarrhea. Some monoclonal antibodies also have side effects associated with the antigen that they target. For example, some monoclonal antibodies can affect the bone marrow's ability to produce blood cells, which can result in an increased risk of bleeding or infection in some patients.

Jill Ferguson, Ph.D.

For Further Information

George, Andrew J. T., and Catherine E. Urch, eds. *Diagnostic and Therapeutic Antibodies.* Totowa, N.J.: Humana Press, 2000.

Melero, I., et al. "Immunostimulatory Monoclonal Antibodies for Cancer Therapy." *Nature Reviews Cancer* 7 (2007): 95-106.

Reichert, J. M., and V. E. Valge-Archer. "Development Trends for Monoclonal Antibody Cancer Therapeutics." *Nature Reviews Drug Discovery* 6 (2007): 349-356.

Zafir-Lavie, I., Y. Michaeli, and Y. Reiter. "Novel Antibodies as Anticancer Agents." *Oncogene* 28 (2007): 3714-3733.

Other Resources

Access Excellence
Monoclonal Antibody Technology: The Basics
http://www.accessexcellence.org/RC/AB/IE/Monoclonal_Antibody.html

American Cancer Society
Monoclonal Antibodies
http://www.cancer.org/docroot/ETO/content/ETO_1_4X_Monoclonal_Antibody_Therapy_Passive_Immunotherapy.asp

Lymphoma Information Network
Monoclonal Antibody Therapy
http://www.lymphomainfo.net/therapy/immunotherapy/mab.html

See also: Biological therapy; CA 15-3 test; CA 19-9 test; CA 27-29 test; Carcinoembryonic Antigen Antibody (CEA) test; Carcinomas; Chemotherapy; Chronic Lymphocytic Leukemia (CLL); Colorectal cancer; Flow cytometry; Immunotherapy; Non-Hodgkin lymphoma; Oral and oropharyngeal cancers; Polyps; Radiation oncology; Radiopharmaceuticals; Receptor analysis; Richter syndrome

▶ Nonsteroidal Anti-Inflammatory Drugs (NSAIDs)

Category: Chemotherapy and Other Drugs
ATC code: M01A

Definition: Nonsteroidal anti-inflammatory drugs, or NSAIDs, are a large, heterogeneous group of medications intended to treat pain, fever, and inflammation.

Cancers treated: NSAIDs are used to treat all types of pain and discomfort associated with cancer, arthritis, gout, and dysmenorrhea (painful or difficult menstruation).

Nonsteroidal Anti-inflammatory Drugs (NSAIDs)

Drug	*Brands*	*Subclass*	*Delivery Mode*
Aspirin	Anacin, Bayer, Excedrin, Bufferin	Acetylsalicylic acid	Oral
Beclomethasone	Celebrex	Sulfonamide pyrazole	Oral
Diclofenac/misoprostol	Arthrotec	Carboxylic acid	Oral
Diclofenac sodium	Voltaren	Phenylacetic acid	Oral
Difunisal	Dolobid	Salicylic acid derivative	Oral, topical ointment
Etodolac	Lodine	Acetic acid derivative	Oral
Flurbiprofen	Ansaid	Difluoro-propionic acid	Oral
Ibuprofen	Motrin, Advil, Nuprin	Phenylpropionic acid	Oral, IV
Indomethacin	Indocin	Indole acetic acid	Oral, ophthalmic, epidural
Ketorolac	Toradol	Pyrrolizine-carboxylate	Oral, IV, intramuscular, ophthalmic
Meclofenamate sodium	Meclomen	Meclofenamic acid	Oral
Meloxicam	Mobic	Enolic acid	Oral
Nabumetone	Relafen	Naphthylalkanone (only nonacid NSAID)	Oral
Naproxen	Anaprox, Naprosyn, Aleve	Naphthylpropionic acid	Oral, topical, ophthalmic
Piroxicam	Feldene	Oxicam	Oral
Sulindac	Clinoril	Sulfinyl acetic acid	Oral
Tolmetin sodium	Tolectin	Pyrrolealkanoic acid	Oral

They have an inhibitory effect on bone tumor growth and may promote centrally mediated analgesia.

Subclasses of this group: NSAIDs are weak organic acids. Subclasses include salicylates, propionic acids, pyrrolealkonic acid derivatives, phenylalkanones, indolic acids, pyrazolone derivatives, and phenyl-naphthyl-acetic acids.

Delivery routes: These drugs are generally administered orally as a suspension in a liquid or in capsule or tablet form. Certain drugs can be given intravenously, as an intramuscular injection, as a rectal suppository, as a topical ointment, or in an ophthalmic solution.

How these drugs work: NSAIDs inhibit cyclooxygenase enzyme activity, resulting in decreased synthesis of prostaglandins (hormones that produce inflammation and pain). Cyclooxygenase 2 (COX-2) inhibitors perform the same function but mediate the metabolic pathway by selectively blocking the COX-2 enzyme.

Side effects: Common complaints from NSAID use include headache, dizziness, gastrointestinal symptoms (nausea, stomach cramps, gastric ulceration, and diarrhea), tremor, insomnia, skin rash, and platelet dysfunction. An anaphylactic (allergic) response to a particular NSAID can present as hives, rash, intense itching, and respiratory difficulties. This condition can be life threatening, and immediate emergency treatment is required.

The COX-2 inhibitors Vioxx and Bextra were pulled from the U.S. market by the Food and Drug Administration (FDA) in the early 2000's. Over an extended period of use (more than eighteen months), they place patients at significantly increased risk for heart attack and stroke. Only Celebrex remains on the market, but with significant warnings attached to its use and potential risks.

John L. Zeller, M.D., Ph.D.

See also: Breakthrough pain; Cyclooxygenase 2 (COX-2) inhibitors; Opioids; Pain management medications; Phenacetin

▶ Opioids

Category: Chemotherapy and Other Drugs
Also known as: Narcotics

Definition: Opioids are controlled drugs prescribed for the management of moderate to severe pain. Opioids include natural alkaloids (opiates) such as morphine and codeine, which are extracted from the seedpod of the poppy plant, as well as semisynthetic derivatives and fully synthetic forms.
ATC code: N02A

Cancers treated: Various

Subclasses of this group: Phenanthrenes, phenylpiperidines, diphenylheptanes, benzomorphans

Delivery routes: Oral administration is preferred because it is the least invasive and least costly route. If a patient has difficulty swallowing or suffers from nausea or vomiting, then other options may include rectal, transdermal, and transmucosal administration or injection under the skin or into the vein or spinal area. Patient-controlled access pumps that deliver opioids to these areas are also available. Opioids are produced in both long-acting and immediate-release forms and are often used with other pain medications for enhanced analgesia.

How these drugs work: Opioids mimic the body's natural painkillers (for example, endorphins) by binding to receptors on the surfaces of cells in the central nervous system and gastrointestinal tract. Full agonists, the largest group of opioids, stimulate the receptors, blocking the release of neurotransmitters and interfering with the transmission of pain signals to the brain. They also alter the perception of pain. Partial agonists produce weaker effects and may also block the analgesic action of other opioids.

Side effects: Adverse events are common across opioids and include sedation, nausea and vomiting, constipation, respiratory depression, dry mouth, itching, sexual dysfunction, and urinary retention. Because of the wealth of opioid receptor sites in the central nervous system, cognitive effects such as hallucinations, euphoria, and depression may also occur. Tolerance and physical dependence may develop, although psychological addiction is rarely associated with opioid use by cancer patients.

Judy Majewski, M.S.

See also: Acupuncture and acupressure for cancer patients; Bone pain; Breakthrough pain; Brief Pain Inventory (BPI); Brompton cocktail; Cordotomy; Do-Not-Resuscitate (DNR) order; End-of-life care; Hospice care; Medical marijuana; Nonsteroidal Anti-Inflammatory Drugs (NSAIDs); Pain management medications; Palliative treatment

Common Opioids

Drug	*Brands*	*Subclass*	*Delivery Mode*
Codeine	Tylenol Codeine, Empirin	Phenanthrenes	Oral
Fentanyl	Actiq, Duragesic, Fentora, Sublimaze	Phenylpiperidines	Oral, transmucosal, buccal, transdermal
Hydrocodone	Vicodin, Vicodin ES, Norco, Lorcet, Anexsia	Phenanthrenes	Oral
Hydromorphone	Dilaudid, Hydrostat	Phenanthrenes	Oral, rectal, IV, subcutaneous
Levorphanol	Levo-Dromoran	Phenanthrenes	Oral, IV, subcutaneous
Methadone	Dolophine, Methadose	Diphenylheptanes	Oral, rectal, IV, subcutaneous
Morphine	MS Contin, Avinza, MSIR, Duramorph, Roxanol IR, Kadian, Oramorph SR	Phenanthrenes	Oral, IV, epidural, intrathecal, intraventricular
Oxycodone	Oxycontin, OxyIR, OxyNorm, Percocet, Percodan, Roxicodone	Phenanthrenes	Oral
Oxymorphone	Numorphan, Opana, Opana ER	Phenanthrenes	Oral, rectal, IV, subcutaneous

▶ Oxaliplatin (Eloxatin)

Category: Chemotherapy and Other Drugs
Also known as: Eloxatin

Definition: Oxaliplatin (Eloxatin™, a trademark of Sanofi) is a type of platinum anti-cancer drug that is used to treat colorectal (colon or rectal) cancer that has spread (metastasized). It may also be used as adjuvant therapy to treat colorectal cancer after surgical tumor removal. Oxaliplatin is often used in combination with 5'-fluorouracil and leucovorin.

Oxaliplatin is currently being studied in the treatment of other types of cancer. It was first approved by the US Food and Drug Administration in 2002.

Cancers treated: Oxaliplatin is used to treat advanced or recurring colorectal cancer and stage III colon cancer. It is not for patients with newly diagnosed colorectal cancer.

Delivery routes: Oxaliplatin is a solution given by intravenous infusion for about two hours, and is administered by a doctor or nurse. It is usually given once every two weeks, as directed by a physician. The dosage and schedule is determined by the person's size and type of cancer.

How this drug works: Oxaliplatin works by attaching to the strands of DNA within cells, including cancer cells. This prevents cancer cells from multiplying, which can stop the growth and spread of the cancer.

Side effects: The most common side effects of oxaliplatin include numbness and tingling or cramping of the hands or feet (often triggered by exposure to cold air or objects), nausea and vomiting, diarrhea, mouth sores, low blood counts, fatigue, and loss of appetite.

Allergic reactions to oxaliplatin can occur and are potentially quite serious. For this reason, patients should be monitored closely for the following developments: rash, hives, itching, reddening of the skin, difficulty breathing or swallowing, hoarseness, feeling of the throat closing, swelling of the lips and tongue, dizziness, lightheadness, and fainting. These are all signs of an allergic reaction and should be reported to the patient's doctor immediately

Patients are monitored closely with blood tests before and during treatment to evaluate the effects of the medication. Oxaliplatin may cause a decrease in white blood cell count, which can increase the risk of infection. Patients should call their doctor immediately if they experience possible signs of infection, including: fever, sore throat or cold, shortness of breath, cough, burning with urination, or a sore that does not heal.

Less common side effects of oxaliplatin include: constipation, fever, generalized pain, headache, and cough.

As a precaution, oxaliplatin should not be given to patients who have an allergy to platinum compounds, or to women who are or may become pregnant. Barrier methods of contraception (such as condoms) must be used while being treated with oxaliplatin, as the medication can cause fetal harm.

To reduce the common side effects associated with exposure to cold, patients taking oxaliplatin should take extra precautions to cover their skin, mouth, and nose when going outdoors in cold temperatures. Patients should not drink cold beverages, use ice cubes in drinks; or use ice packs. Additionally, gloves should be worn when touching cold objects or food from the freezer.

Angela Costello, BS

For Further Information

Abraham, J., Gulley. J. L., & Allegra, C. J. (2014). *The Bethesda handbook of clinical oncology* (4th ed.). Philadelphia, PA: Lippincott Williams & Wilkins.

Pires, I. M., Ward, T. H., & Dive, C. (2010). Oxaliplatin responses in colorectal cancer cells are modulated by CHK2 kinase inhibitors. *British Journal of Pharmacology,* 159(6): 1326-1338.

Other Resources

FDA Approval for Oxaliplatin
http://www.cancer.gov/about-cancer/treatment/drugs/fda-oxaliplatin

Eloxatin Prescribing Information
http://products.sanofi.us/eloxatin/eloxatin.html

American Cancer Society
http://www.cancer.org

CancerNet
http://www.cancer.net

Chemocare.org
http://www.chemocare.org

National Cancer Institute
http://www.cancer.gov

U.S. Food and Drug Administration
http://www.fda.gov

See also: Antineoplastics in chemotherapy; Colorectal cancer

▶ Pain Management

Category: Chemotherapy and Other Drugs

Definition: Cancer pain management is a crucial aspect of supportive care of the cancer patient and may involve medication therapy, behavioral modifications, and other lifestyle adjustments. Because pain associated with cancer results from numerous sources and manifests through multiple mechanisms, treatment options are widespread. Although pain cannot always be completely relieved, oral analgesic therapy can be successful in up to 85 percent of patients.

Cancers diagnosed or treated: Medications and other therapies that control pain symptoms are used in patients with any type of cancer; types of treatment depend on the type of pain experienced, which can be determined by the type of cancer or type of treatment (chemotherapy, radiation, surgery) used.

Subclasses of this group: Numerous classes of drugs are useful in the treatment of cancer pain, including nonopioid analgesics, opioid analgesics, tricyclic antidepressants, and anticonvulsants.

Delivery routes: These drugs may be administered orally in tablets, capsules, or solutions; topically as patches, creams, or intranasal sprays; rectally as suppositories; submucosally as lozenges; or intravenously, intramuscularly, or subcutaneously as injectable solutions and suspensions. The drugs may be administered in outpatient, inpatient, or drop-in clinic settings.

How these drugs work: Cancer pain has historically been a cause for concern in patients and caregivers alike. The treatment of pain as a whole and in cancer patients is often poorly or inadequately managed, despite numerous available treatment options. Implementation of pain management guidelines and increased awareness of health professionals about the role of pain and the importance of pain assessment in cancer therapy, however, have improved the control of many types of cancer pain.

Different types of pain require different forms of treatment. Two main types of pain include nociceptive pain—resulting from actual damage to or inflammation of a tissue or organ (visceral pain) or to bone (somatic pain)—and neuropathic pain, which results from nerve damage or compression. Any source of pain may cause acute, chronic, or breakthrough pain.

Nociceptive or neuropathic pain occurring in the cancer patient may result from various sources, all with

Common Medications for Cancer Pain

Drug Class	*Individual Drug Examples*	*Brands*	*Delivery Mode*	*Primary Pain Type Treated*
Anticonvulsants	phenytoin, valproate, carbamazepine, clonazepam	Dilantin, Depakote, Tegretol, Klonopin	Oral, injectable	Neuropathic pain
Benzodiazepines	midazolam, diazepam, alprazolam	Versed, Valium, Xanax	Oral, injectable	Neuropathic pain; muscle spasm or anxiety
Corticosteroids	dexamethasone, prednisone	Decadron, Sterapred	Oral, injectable	Somatic pain from swelling; neuropathic pain
Nonopioids	acetaminophen, aspirin, NSAIDs (e.g., ibuprofen, naproxen)	Tylenol, Motrin, Anaprox	Primarily oral	Mild-to-moderate chronic pain
Opioids	oxycodone, propoxyphene, hydrocodone, morphine, hydromorphone, meperidine, fentanyl	Percocet, Darvocet, Lorcet, Duragesic, Dilaudid, MS Contin, Vicodin	Oral, injectable, transdermal, submucosal, intrarectal	Moderate-to-severe or severe chronic pain; short-acting for breakthrough pain
Tricyclic antidepressants	amitriptyline, desipramine, nortriptyline	Elavil, Norpramin, Pamelor	Oral, injectable	Neuropathic pain; depression

differing mechanisms. Approximately 70 percent of cancer-related pain results from the tumor itself because of invasion or compression of soft tissue, bone, or nerves. Another 20 percent results from treatments such as radiation, chemotherapy, and surgical biopsy, all of which can be associated with mucositis, neuropathy, infection, and other complications.

Although many options are available to control cancer pain, pharmacologic therapy is the primary, most successful method. Other options include removal of cancer in patients whose tumor compression is the pain source; neurosurgical treatments such as epidural blocks in patients whose pain is not adequately controlled with other options; complementary therapies such as relaxation techniques, massage, and transcutaneous electrical nerve stimulation (TENS); and psychological treatments that include behavioral or lifestyle changes and support groups.

Analgesic pharmacotherapy and adjuvant medications are primarily used to control cancer pain, and 75 percent of patients experience pain severe enough to require opioid analgesia. Pain falls into many categories, which then dictate treatment options. These categories include mild-to-moderate pain, moderate-to-severe pain, breakthrough pain, and neuropathic pain. Most types of pain in cancer patients are considered chronic, with only breakthrough pain being an acute situation that requires quick-acting relief.

Mild-to-moderate pain may be relieved with nonopioid medications; aspirin, acetaminophen, and ibuprofen or other nonsteroidal anti-inflammatory drugs (NSAIDs) are the primary options. Nonopioid analgesics act primarily on the peripheral nervous system to reduce pain or inflammation at the tissue, organ, bone, or incision site. The anti-inflammatory activity of NSAIDs is useful in particular for bone pain, muscle compression, and some tissue pains from swelling.

Moderate-to-severe pain often requires opioid analgesic therapy. Drugs in the opioid class include oxycodone, propoxyphene, hydrocodone, morphine, hydromorphone, meperidine, and fentanyl. Opioids work in the central nervous system by binding to pain receptors, namely mu, kappa, and/or delta, to induce analgesia. Opioids fall into three categories of activity: pure agonists (such

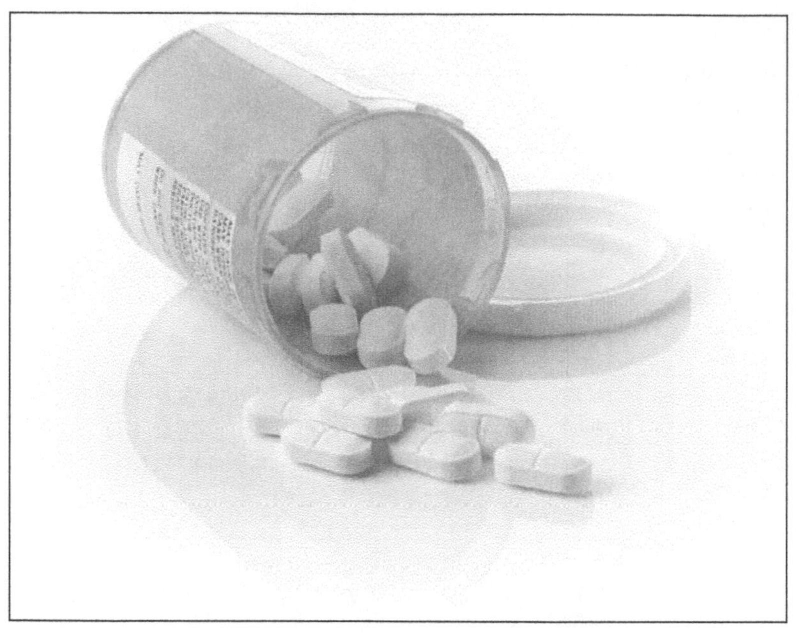

Hydrocodone (Vicodin) tablets. (iStock)

as morphine, codeine, fentanyl, hydromorphine, oxycodone, methadone), pure antagonists (such as naloxone) used to reverse opioid toxicity but without their own analgesia, and mixed or partial agonists/antagonists (such as pentazocine, butorphanol, buprenorphine) that are used in more acute settings because of limited analgesic activity. Pure receptor agonists are primarily used for the control of chronic pain. Most opioid agonists are mu or kappa receptor-selective, although individual agents may have varying amounts of activity at the two receptor subtypes and can be synergistic with each other. Because each opioid agonist interacts uniquely and to differing degrees with mu and kappa receptors, and because patient response to each drug varies, substitutions within the class should be considered before giving up on opioid therapy when pain control is incomplete.

Cancer patients often require high doses of opioids for long periods of time. Important considerations in the long-term management of pain using analgesic therapy are tolerance, withdrawal, addiction, inadequate control, and breakthrough pain. Psychological dependence, or addiction, is uncommon with the appropriate use of opiates, even when doses are increased in response to tolerance. Although the mechanisms driving opiate tolerance are unclear, dosage increases usually improve tolerance of a single agent and are limited only by side effects. Although withdrawal symptoms are possible as a result of physical dependence, tapering doses in reverse often ameliorates these concerns. Adequate control is difficult because of the highly subjective nature of pain. Patients respond differently to pain and to pain medications, and they often fail to report inadequate relief because of personal concerns about dependence or addiction. Communication between health care professionals and patients, however, often resolves this concern, and patients become comfortable with around-the-clock pain control.

Breakthrough pain, or pain that occurs despite existing pain medications, usually requires a quick-acting, short-acting secondary medication (such as immediate-release morphine tablets or submucosal fentanyl) to provide relief.

For reasons not clearly studied or understood, opioids do provide confirmed relief of peripherally mediated neuropathic pain as well. Adjuvant therapies also play a large role in the treatment of specific pain situations, including neuropathic pain. Common adjuvant drug classes used for neuropathic pain control include tricyclic antidepressants, anticonvulsants, benzodiazepines, and corticosteroids. Tricyclic antidepressants (such as amitriptyline, nortriptyline, and desimpramine) provide established analgesic effects for chronic neuropathic pain through monoamine-related pain-modulating systems in addition to and often prior to the separate relief of depressive symptoms by neurotransmitter alterations. Anticonvulsants (such as phenytoin, valproate, carbamazepine, and clonazepam) usually provide analgesia through the reduction of neuronal excitation or abnormal discharge. Benzodiazepines (such as diazepam and midazolam) have established benefits, through psychotropic and muscle-relaxant activity, in the treatment of neuropathic pain, and they reduce anxiety and associated muscle spasm. Finally, corticosteroids (such as dexamethasone) provide nonselective analgesic effects that are useful for malignant, advanced pain at long-term, low doses and for severe, unresponsive neuropathic pain at short-term, very high doses. Steroids also have nonanalgesic anti-inflammatory benefits that reduce tumor-associated swelling.

Side effects: Because of the varied treatments used to control cancer pain, side effects also differ. General concerns include breakthrough pain, medication tolerance, and withdrawal symptoms. Withdrawal symptoms vary with medication choice and length of use but include rapid breathing, yawning, perspiration, agitation, increased heart rate, muscle twitching, and loss of appetite.

Nonopioid analgesics are not associated with dependence, tolerance, or addiction, although all have a maximum analgesic dose. Select concerns with these agents include liver function damage with acetaminophen and gastrointestinal disturbances or damage with aspirin and NSAIDs.

Opioid side effects include constipation (which can be prophylactically treated with stool softeners), nausea, vomiting, pruritis, and sedation. Respiratory depression is possible in patients with decreased pulmonary function. Many side effects can limit the potential use of a particular opiate but do not rule out the entire class, because the side effects (like the analgesic effects) are linked to specific mu and kappa receptors. For example, constipation and respiratory depression are linked to mu receptor activity.

Adjuvant side effects vary drastically; overlapping toxicities are a primary concern, because adjuvant medications are often combined with each other or with opioids to provide pain relief.

Nicole M. Van Hoey, Pharm.D.

For Further Information

Ballantyne, J. C. "Opioid Analgesia: Perspectives on Right Use and Utility." *Pain Physician* 10, no. 3 (May, 2007): 479-491.

Brennan, F., D. B. Carr, and M. Cousins. "Pain Management: A Fundamental Human Right." *Anesthesia & Analgesia* 105, no. 1 (July, 2007): 205-221.

Burton, A. W., et al. "Chronic Pain in the Cancer Survivor: A New Frontier." *Pain Medicine* 8, no. 2 (March, 2007): 189-198.

Fisch, Michael J., and Allen W. Burton, eds. *Cancer Pain Management*. New York: McGraw-Hill, 2007.

Other Resources

Cancer.Net

http://www.cancer.net/portal/site/patient

See also: Acupuncture and acupressure for cancer patients; Adjuvant therapy; Antinausea medications; Bone pain; Breakthrough pain; Brief Pain Inventory (BPI); Brompton cocktail; Cordotomy; Do-Not-Resuscitate (DNR) order; End-of-life care; Hospice care; Medical marijuana; Nonsteroidal Anti-Inflammatory Drugs (NSAIDs); Opioids; Palliative treatment

▶ Palliative treatment

Category: Chemotherapy and Other Drugs

Definition: Palliative treatment is defined as active and compassionate care primarily directed toward symptom management and improving quality of life. It is targeted toward patients who are not candidates for curative cancer therapies. Because of the proliferation of supportive treatments that can extend life, palliative care can be lengthy, lasting for months to many years.

Symptom management and control: For the cancer patient, physical symptoms and discomfort may change in nature, quality, and intensity within short, unpredictable time periods, often requiring close monitoring and therapeutic modifications at regular but nonspecific time intervals. Further, possible or actual changes in mentation, functioning, and personal control may precipitate intense emotions that are unfamiliar, unwanted, and anxiety provoking. Chronicity, remissions, and exacerbations of a variety of uncomfortable symptoms; family separation; financial strain; functional limitations; and role disruptions are but a few of the issues that characterize the lives of individuals with advanced, progressive, or incurable cancer. Even for those who experience lengthy disease-free intervals, the challenge of reducing cancer's presence in their lives can be difficult, and assistance from multiple specialists is often needed. Common symptoms that are treated and controlled or relieved by palliative care interventions can include the following:

- Pain
- Difficulty breathing
- Loss of appetite and weight loss
- Fatigue
- Weakness
- Sleep problems
- Depression and anxiety
- Confusion

Palliative treatment in context: The palliative treatment experience must be examined within the context of the health care delivery system for its potential and its pitfalls to be fully understood. Treatment advances, societal attitudes, and changes in health care structure and financing have all had a dramatic impact on the delivery of palliative care and the creation of gaps between the philosophy and delivery of palliative care services. The secrecy that prevailed in the 1960's and prohibited disclosure of a cancer diagnosis by most physicians has given way to the practice of routinely imparting the particulars of diagnosis, treatment options, and prognosis. Despite this change, it has been observed that persistent cancer-related fears and negative attitudes among health care providers have led to a discrepancy between words and actions, resulting in communication of emotionally laden information in a fashion ranging from overprotective and paternalistic to blunt and matter of fact. Further, patients who are not candidates for curative treatment often find themselves without adequate information and resources to manage their abundant physical and psychosocial problems.

Discrepancies between attitude and practice have been demonstrated by clinicians who have been found to avoid clear, open discussions of topics such as prognosis and death despite consistently expressed beliefs regarding the importance of openness and honesty with all mentally competent patients. Therefore, while the prevailing attitude in health care supports disclosure of medical information and active involvement by patients in decisions that affect them, the actual behavior of health care providers reflects a more limited improvement in patient care. Clinician concerns and personal issues can affect communication with patients at key decision-making and transition points along the continuum of palliative care. The need for clinician support and access to resources is recognized as key in helping members of the palliative care team to assist patients fully, but there is much need for improvement and more resources in this area.

Psychiatric and medical comorbidity: The time during which palliative treatment is necessary has lengthened, causing an increase in the number of cases in which patients need psychiatric care alongside medical care. This phenomenon, although largely ignored, is putting inordinate stress on patients, families, professional caregivers, and the health care system at large. Psychiatric problems tend to be treated based on whether reimbursement is provided, and reimbursement occurs only when psychiatric symptoms emerge as disease states. Insurance rarely covers psychiatric interventions targeted toward symptom management and quality-of-life enhancement, although comprehensive, low-cost interventions supported by scientific evidence of their efficacy are available. Multisystem problems are generally not addressed well by the medical system, which is fragmented and oriented toward specialty care.

Because recipients of palliative cancer treatment are not candidates for curative therapies, they are faced with their own mortality and are vulnerable to intense fear and psychological distress. However, the health care system is oriented toward cure and survival, and it typically places a lower priority on treating and addressing psychosocial issues. Patients receiving palliative care are often concerned about issues such as impending death, pain or other physical discomfort that cannot be relieved, disfigurement, functional decline and increasing dependency on others, loss of mental acuity and bodily functions, and the effects of their illness on their families and friends. These patients need to be closely monitored to manage changes in symptoms and functional status and to evaluate the level of relief achieved through targeted interventions.

Ethical aspects: Care providers must be mindful that the psychological vulnerability of patients receiving palliative care may put some individuals at risk for unnecessary suffering, exploitation, and victimization based on the cure-oriented values inherent in modern health care. For example, an issue that repeatedly surfaces among patients, family members, and professional care providers pertains to the use of aggressive treatment protocols in the presence of progressive, incurable disease. Patients may seek or be recruited for participation in experimental protocols even when treatment is not expected to extend their lives. Questions of ethics and the meaning of informed consent arise in regard to the participation of terminally ill subjects in experimental protocols. Some experts question whether having a particular medical conditions or status (such as being terminally ill) diminishes full participation in the process of informed consent.

The need for health care professionals to establish structured dialogue with patients, family members, and care providers regarding treatment goals and expectations is essential. Treatment planning should take into account the fact that certain individuals with a terminal illness may respond to participation in an investigational treatment with increased hope of survival, regardless of their real chances of survival. These issues, however, become even more complex as changes in health care financing prohibit reimbursement for experimental therapies. Some people will be unable to undergo experimental therapies, and others may assume the cost of aggressive yet often medically futile treatments, creating compelling ethical issues and tensions. These are weighty issues that require active dialogue and debate. The combination of rapid medical and technological advances, diminishing ability to finance rising health care costs, growing numbers of chronically ill patients living longer periods of time, and an ever widening gap between the affluent and poor is adding to the problem.

Patients, their families, and health care providers need to separate and clarify personal values, thoughts, and emotional reactions to these delicate issues if individualized, quality palliative care is to be provided. Psychiatric consultation-liaison nurses, psychiatrists, social workers, and chaplains can be invaluable in assisting patients, family members, and staff to grapple with these issues in a meaningful and productive manner.

Dying and terminal care: Once the terminal care period has begun, it is usually not the fact of dying, but the quality of dying, that is primary for patients and families. Palliative care that continues into the terminal stage of cancer should continue to relieve physical and psychological symptoms and promote comfort and well-being until the patient dies. Often patients and families who have received palliative services in earlier stages of the illness will be more open and accepting of palliative efforts in the final stage of life. In addition, it is important that professional and family caregivers recognize that their work is emotionally draining, and they should seek guidance and support whenever possible.

Professional caregivers should target therapeutic interventions toward increasing the dying patients' sense of personal control and self-efficacy within the context of their functional decline and increased dependency. It is also therapeutic in most cases to inform patients of available resources aimed at discussing and addressing any concerns regarding death and dying. From a practical standpoint, professional caregivers may help patients by inquiring about any unfinished business, including wills and conversations with family and friends, and to provide them with the necessary support and encouragement to accomplish these final goals.

Factors including personal values, socioeconomic status, cultural background, and religious beliefs can influence patients' expectations and experiences as they approach death. For example, a stoic attitude that minimizes or negates discomfort may be related to a cultural value learned and reinforced through years of family experiences. Similarly, an extremely emotional response to routine events during the terminal phase of illness does not necessarily signal mental maladjustment but rather the person's cultural norm. Awareness of the person's cultural, religious, ethnic, and socioeconomic background is important in the process of understanding individual behaviors and limiting value judgments.

Psychiatric complications and terminal care: Delirium, depression, suicidal ideation, and severe anxiety are among the most commonly occurring psychiatric complications encountered in terminally ill cancer patients. When severe, these problems require urgent and aggressive assessment and treatment by psychiatric personnel who can initiate pharmacologic and psychotherapeutic treatment strategies. It should be stressed that psychiatric emergencies require the same rapid intervention as medical crises. In spite of the seemingly overwhelming nature of psychosocial responses in cancer patients, most of them do indeed cope effectively, and it is important to recognize that intense emotions are not one and the same as maladaptive coping.

Hospice care: Hospice care involves structured programs that offer supportive and palliative care at the end of life. The patient, family, and health care team decide when hospice care should begin, but typically patients are eligible for a hospice program when they have about six months to live. Hospice care can be home or institution based. Hospice care aims to manage physical and emotional symptoms with the overriding goal of allowing patients to live their last days with dignity and as high a quality of life as possible. Most hospice programs offer family-centered care, meaning that they involve the patient and family in decision making, which reduces distress and enhances control. A hospice team usually consists of a physician, an advanced practice nurse, a bedside nurse, nursing assistants, social workers, and chaplains. Goals of hospice treatment may include increased time of survival, symptom control, and enhanced quality of life.

Jeannie V. Pasacreta, Ph.D., A.P.R.N.

For Further Information

Barnett, Laura, ed. *When Death Enters the Therapeutic Space: Existential Perspectives in Psychotherapy and Counseling*. New York: Routledge, 2008.

Boog, Kathryn M., and Claire Tester. *A Practical Guide to Palliative Care: Finding Meaning and Purpose in Life and Death*. New York: Elsevier, 2008.

Jacobs, Léa K., ed. *Coping with Cancer*. New York: Nova Science, 2008.

Kuebler, Kim, Debra E. Heidrich, and Peg Esper. *Palliative and End of Life Care: Clinical Practice Guidelines*. 2d ed. St. Louis: Saunders/Elsevier, 2007.

Lewis, Milton J. *Medicine and Care of the Dying: A Modern History*. New York: Oxford University Press, 2007.

Lynn, Joanne, et al. *Improving Care for the End of Life: A Sourcebook for Health Care Managers and Clinicians*. 2d ed. New York: Oxford University Press, 2008.

Werth, James L., and Dean Blevins, eds. *Decision Making Near the End of Life: Issues, Development, and Future Directions*. New York: Brunner-Routledge, 2008.

Other Resources

American Academy of Hospice and Palliative Medicine
http://www.aahpm.org

American Hospice Foundation
http://www.americanhospice.org

American Pain Society
http://www.ampainsoc.org

American Psychosocial Oncology Society
http://www.apos-society.org

Americans for Better Care of the Dying
http://www.abcd-caring.org

National Palliative Care Research Center
http://www.npcrc.org

See also: Acupuncture and acupressure for cancer patients; Bone pain; Breakthrough pain; Brief Pain Inventory (BPI); Brompton cocktail; Cordotomy; Do-Not-Resuscitate (DNR) order; End-of-life care; Hospice care; Medical marijuana; Nonsteroidal Anti-Inflammatory Drugs (NSAIDs); Opioids; Pain management medications

▶ Pegfilgrastim (Neulasta)

Category: Chemotherapy and Other Drugs
Also known as: Neulasta

Definition: Long acting form of a granulocyte-colony stimulating factor (G-CSF) that is used to help stimulate the bone marrow to produce cells that can mature into neutrophils that are needed to help fight infections.

Cancers treated: Neulasta is used to treat an abnormally low white blood count (neutropenia) that has been caused by chemotherapy cancer treatment. Patients who have been diagnosed with sickle cell disorder should use extreme caution with this drug, since it may put the patient into a sickle cell crisis. Patients with chronic myeloid leukemia or myelodysplasia should not use it.

Delivery routes: Typical dose is 6 mg and is given by a subcutaneous injection. Pegfilgrastim should not be given 14 days before or 24 hours after administration of cytotoxic chemotherapy. It can also be administered using an on-body injector that is placed by the healthcare provider on last day of treatment. This on-body injector will administer an injection 24 hours after the last dose of chemotherapy.

How these drugs work: Chemotherapy can cause a decrease in the bone marrow production of white blood cells. The decrease in white blood cells, in particular neutrophils, weakens the immune system. The decrease in the neutrophil count (neutropenia) puts the patient at risk for developing life-threatening infections. Pegfilgrastim is a protein that stimulates the release of cells from the bone marrow that can then mature into neutrophils.

Side effects: The most common side effect is bone pain or muscle pain, which can be treated with acetaminophen. More uncommon side effects include shortness of breath, wheezing, and dizziness. Swelling of the mouth/tongue, racing heart, sweating, and hives can also occur. Rare side effects include rupture of the spleen or acute respiratory distress syndrome.

Katrina Green MSN, RN, OCN

For Further Information

Lambertini, M., Ferreira, A., Mastro, D. I., Danesi, R. & Pronzato, P. (2015). Pegfilgrastim for the prevention of chemotherapy-induced febrile neutropenia in patients with solid tumors. *Expert Opinion on Biological Therapy.*, 12(15): 1-19.

Weycker, D., Li, X., Barron, R., Li, Y., Reiner, M., Kartashov, A., … & Garcia, J. (2015). Risk of chemotherapy-induced febrile neutropenia with early discontinuation of pegfilgrastim prophylaxis in US clinical practice. *Supportive Care in Cancer,* doi:10.1007/s00520-015-3039-4.

Weycker, D., Li, X., Figueredo, J., Barron, R., Tzivelekis, S. & Hagiwara, M. (2015). Risk of chemotherapy-induced febrile neutropenia in cancer patients receiving pegfilgrastim prophylaxis: Does timing of administration matter? *Supportive Care in Cancer,* doi:10.1007/s00520-015-3036-7.

Xu, H., Gong, Q., Vogl, F., Reiner, M. and Page, J. (2016). Risk factors for bone pain among patients with cancer receiving myelosuppressive chemotherapy and pegfilgrastim. *Supportive Care in Cancer*, doi:10.1007/s00520-015-2834-2.

Other Resources

Neulasta website
https://www.neulasta.com/

NIH National Library of Medicine
https://www.nlm.nih.gov/medlineplus/druginfo/meds/a607038.html

See also: Chemotherapy

▶ Pemetrexed (Alimta)

Category: Chemotherapy and Other Drugs
Also known as: Almita (brand name)

Definition: Pemetrexed is a chemotherapeutic or cytostatic (anticancer) agent that belongs to the pharmacological class of antifolates and to the therapeutic class of antineoplastics or antimetabolites. It has been developed and marketed by Eli Lilly and Company. It is used as a single-agent therapy (monotherapy) or in combination with another chemotherapeutic called cisplatin.

Cancers treated: In 2004, Pemetrexed was approved by the US Food and Drug Administration for the treatment of malignant pleural mesothelioma (MPM) in combination with cisplatin if the disease is either irremovable or otherwise surgically incurable. MPM is cancer of the lining of the lungs and is caused by asbestos exposure.

In 2008, it was approved as first-line (ie, initial) therapy for use in combination with cisplatin for the treatment of locally advanced or metastatic non-squamous non-small lung cancer (NSCLC). NSCLC accounts for ca. 85% of all lung cancers. Risk factors for the disease include smoking, a person's age, or family history.

In 2009, it was approved as a maintenance monotherapy for locally advanced or metastatic NSCLC if the disease has not progressed after prior platinum-based chemotherapy, or as a second-line (ie, additional) monotherapy after prior chemotherapy.

Delivery routes: Pemetrexed is given intravenously into the patient's arm vein through a cannula (ie, a thin, short tube). It can also be given through a peripherally inserted central catheter (PICC line) inserted in the arm vein, which delivers the drug directly into a large vein in the chest. This access can be used for a prolonged period of time (several weeks or more).

How these drugs work: Anticancer drugs suppress the growth and multiplication of (cancer) cells. Antifolates are drugs that do so by blocking the actions of folic acid, a vitamin that primarily acts as a cofactor for various enzymes involved in building and repairing deoxyribonucleic acid (which carries the genetic information of a cell) and ribonucleic acid (involved in protein synthesis).

Side effects: The most common side effects of pemetrexed alone or in combination with cisplatin include: nausea, vomiting, diarrhea or constipation, pain when swallowing, low red blood cell counts that may lead to feeling tired, low white blood cells that may increase the chance for infection, low platelet counts, which may increase the chance of bleeding, redness or sores in the mouth or throat, or on the lips, loss of appetite, and rash.

Silke Haidekker, PhD, ELS

For Further Information

Hanna, N., Shepherd, F. A., Fossella, F. V., Pereira, J.R., De Marinis. F., von Pawel, J., ... Bunn, P. A. Jr. (2004). Randomized phase III trial of pemetrexed versus docetaxel in patients with non–small-cell lung cancer previously treated with chemotherapy. *Journal of Clinical Oncology* 22(9): 1589-1597.

Vogelzang, N. J., Rusthoven, J. J., Symanowski, J., Denham, C., Kaukel, E., Ruffie, P., ... Paoletti P. (2003). Phase III study of pemetrexed in combination with cisplatin versus cisplatin alone in patients with malignant pleural mesothelioma, *Journal of Clinical Oncology* 21(14): 2636-2644.

Other Resources

National Cancer Institute—Malignant Mesothelioma
http://www.cancer.gov/cancertopics/types/malignantmesothelioma

National Cancer Institute—Non-squamous non-small lung cancer
http://www.cancer.gov/types/lung

Almita Website
http://www.alimta.com

See also: Eli Lilly

▶ Photodynamic Therapy (PDT)

Category: Chemotherapy and Other Drugs
ATC code: 101XD

Definition: Photodynamic therapy (PDT) is an emerging modality for treating local precancerous and cancerous lesions of epithelial origin. The technology relies on a class of anticancer drugs called photosensitizers that become active when exposed to specific light wavelengths, usually from a laser beam. Minimally invasive, PDT is also used to treat nonmalignant diseases, particularly the ocular condition known as wet age-related macular degeneration.

Cancers treated: Esophageal cancer, lung cancer, bladder carcinoma, nonmelanoma skin cancer

Subclasses of this group: Currently, most of the clinically approved photosensitizers are porphyrins, but other drugs under clinical investigation belong to the chlorin or purpurin family.

Delivery routes: Intravenous or topical, depending on the drug's chemical structure and the type of cancer and its location

How these drugs work: The first clinical application of PDT was reported in 1903 by two German researchers, who used a topical coal tar dye called eosin in combination with visible light to treat skin cancer. The isolation of safer and more effective photosensitive dyes, called porphyrins, has propelled the field forward. Photosensitizers preferentially accumulate in abnormal tissues and cause little damage to surrounding healthy cells.

PDT is a two-part process. First, a nontoxic photosensitizer is administered to the patient. The lesion site is then exposed to light that is of a suitable wavelength to excite the photosensitive drug. Activated drug molecules initiate cytotoxic reactions that destroy tumor cells. They transfer energy to molecular oxygen, which, in turn, generates reactive oxygen species (ROS), such as singlet oxygen. These active molecular species damage deoxyribonucleic acid (DNA) and cause the oxidation of proteins and lipids. As a result, cancer cells undergo necrosis or apoptosis, the natural process of cell death. Because light needed to activate most photosensitizers cannot penetrate deeply into tissue, the therapeutic potential of PDT is limited to the treatment of local superficial tumors rather than large tumors or metastases.

Side effects: One side effect of PDT is increased sensitivity to light (sunburn-like reactions), which may last for several weeks after administration. Other side effects include constipation, irritation at the injection site, back pain, chest pain, fever, flulike syndrome, and general weakness.

Anna Binda, Ph.D.

See also: Basal cell carcinomas; Bile duct cancer; Bladder cancer; Bone cancers; Bowen disease; Cutaneous breast cancer; Esophageal cancer; Keratosis; Laser therapies; Lung cancers; Skin cancers; Squamous cell carcinomas

▶ Plant alkaloids and cancer

Category: Chemotherapy and Other Drugs
Also known as: vincas, taxanes, podophyllotoxins and camptothecans

Common Photosensitizers

Drug (Other Names)	*Brands*	*Subclass*	*Delivery Mode*	*Conditions Treated*
Aminolevulinic acid (5-aminolevulinic acid, ALA)	Levulan	Porphyrin	Topical	Actinic keratosis (precancerous skin lesion)
Methyl aminolevulinate (m-ALA)	Metvix	Porphyrin	Topical	Actinic keratosis, skin cancer
Porfimer sodium	Photofrin	Porphyrin	IV	Barrett esophagus (precancerous lesion), esophageal cancer, cervical cancer, lung cancer, stomach cancer, superficial bladder cancer
Temoporfin (meta-tetrahydroxyphenylchlorin, mTHPC)	Foscan	Chlorin	IV	Head and neck cancer

Plant alkaloid-based anticancer drug characteristics

Drug	*Classification*	*Treatment*	*Most Common Side Effects*
Etoposide (VP-16) Also called: Toposar, VePesid, Etopophos,	Plant alkaloid, Topoisomerase II inhibitor	Bladder, prostate, lung, stomach, uterine, Hodgkin's and non-Hodgkin's lymphoma, Kaposi's sarcoma, Wilm's tumor, rhabdomyosarcoma, Ewing's sarcoma, neuroblastoma, brain tumors *May be given as high dose therapy in BMT setting	Pancytopenia, hair loss, menopause, loss of fertility, nausea and vomiting, hypotension, and hypersensitivity reactions *There is a delayed risk of developing leukemia years after taking etoposide
Vincristine Also called: Oncovin, Vincasar Pfs	Plant alkaloid	Acute leukemia, Hodgkin's and non-Hodgkin's lymphoma, neuroblastoma, rhabdomyosarcoma, Ewing's sarcoma, Wilms' tumor, multiple myeloma, chronic leukemias, thyroid cancer, brain tumors	Hair loss, constipation, pancytopenia, peripheral neuropathies
Vinblastine Also called: Velban, Alkaban AQ	Plant alkaloid	Hodgkin's disease, non-Hodgkin's lymphoma, testicular, breast, lung, head and neck, bladder, Kaposi's sarcoma, T-cell lymphoma, choriocarcinoma	Pancytopenia, injection site reactions, fatigue, weakness, nausea and vomiting, poor appetite, peripheral neuropathy, constipation, diarrhea, hair loss, mouth sores, metallic taste, headache, depression, jaw pain, hypertension, shortness of breath, muscle pain
Vinorelbine Also called: Navelbine	Plant alkaloid	Non-small cell lung, breast, ovarian, Hodgkin's lymphoma	Pancytopenia, nausea and vomiting, muscle weakness, constipation
Paclitaxel Also called: Taxol, Onxal	Plant alkaloid, taxane, antimicrotubule agent	Breast, ovarian, lung, bladder, prostate, melanoma, esophageal, Kaposi's sarcoma	Pancytopenia, hair loss, pain in joints and muscles, peripheral neuropathies, nausea and vomiting, diarrhea, mouth sores, hypersensitivity reaction
Abraxane (paclitaxel protein bound)	Plant alkaloid, taxane, antimicrotubule agent	Breast cancer, non-small cell lung cancer, pancreatic cancer	Pancytopenia, hair loss, nausea, ECG changes, peripheral neuropathies, mylagias, fatigue, liver toxicity
Docetaxel Also called: Taxotere	Plant alkaloid, taxane, antimicrotubule agent	Breast cancer, non-small cell lung, stomach, head and neck, metastatic prostate. Investigated for small cell lung, ovarian, bladder, pancreatic, soft tissue sarcoma, melanoma	Neutropenia and anemia, fluid retention, peripheral neuropathies, nausea, diarrhea, mouth sores, hair loss, fatigue, infection, nail changes, hypersensitivity reactions
Camptothecin-11 Also called: Camptosar, CPT-11, Irinotecan	Plant alkaloid, topoisomerase 1 inhibitor	Metastatic colon or rectal cancer	Diarrhea, nausea and vomiting, weakness, neutropenia, anemia, hair loss, poor appetite, fever, weight loss, heartburn, swelling (of ankles/feet)
Omacetaxine Also called: Synribo	Plant alkaloid	Chronic or accelerated phase chronic myelogenous leukemia (with resistance or intolerance to Tyrosine Kinase Inhibitors)	Pancytopenia, increase uric acid, infection, diarrhea, nausea, fatigue
Topotecan Also called: Hycamtin	Plant alkaloid, topoisomerase 1 inhibitor	Ovarian (resistant disease), small cell lung cancer	Pancytopenia, nausea and vomiting, hair loss, diarrhea

Definition: Plant alkaloids are a group of chemotherapy agents that are made from a variety of different plants and are considered to be cell-cycle specific. These include: 1) Vinca alkaloids (derived from the periwinkle plant): Vincristine, Vinblastine, and Vinorelbine; 2) Taxanes (developed from the bark of the Pacific Yew tree): Paclitaxel and Docetaxel; 3) Podophyllotoxins (developed from the May apple tree): Etoposide and Teniposide; and 4) Camptothecins (derived from the Asian "Happy Tree"): Irinotecan and Topotecan.

Vinca alkaloids were developed in early 1960s, Etoposide in 1971, and taxanes have been around since 1975.

Cancers treated: Plant alkaloids treat a variety of cancers. They can be used as first- line therapy as well as for resistant disease. The dosages and exact regimens will vary based on the patient's current status and diagnosis. Please see table "Plant alkaloid-based anticancer drug characteristics" for more specific information.

Delivery routes: Most plant alkaloids are administered as an IV infusion, IV push, or by subcutaneous injection. When administering taxanes the patient may require premedications to reduce the risk of hypersensitivity reactions. These premedications may include antihistamines (H2 receptor blockers) and corticosteroids.

How These Drugs Work: These agents block the mechanisms that allow cancer cells to multiply. They are most active in the metaphase stage of cell division (mitosis). Vinca alkaloids bind to a protein called tubulin that polymerizes to form intracellular structures called "microtubules." Microtubules form the spindles that separate chromosomes during mitosis. By binding to tubulin, vinca alkaloids prevent the formation of mitotic spindles, which prevents the division of the cell. Taxanes bind to already formed microtubules and freeze them, which prevents the remodeling of these structures that is crucial for their proper function. Podophyllotoxins and camptothecans inhibit an enzyme called "topoisomerase" that unwinds tangled DNA. Without functional topoisomerase, cells cannot separate replicated chromosomes, which causes chromosome breaks, inhibits cell division, and induces cell death.

Side effects: Most common side effects that are seen with plant alkaloids are hypersensitivity reactions, peripheral neuropathies, and pancytopenia. Close monitoring for hypersensitivity reactions is necessary for those at risk to ensure that if reactions occur they are identified and treated quickly (see the included table "Plant alkaloid-based anticancer drug characteristics" for additional side effects associated with various plant alkaloids).

Katrina Green MSN, RN, OCN

For Further Information

Da Rocha, A. B., Lopes, R. M. & Schwartsmann, G. (2001). Natural products in anticancer therapy. *Current Opinion in Pharmacology*, 1(4): 364-369.

Maraldo, M., Giusti, F., Vogelius, I., Lundemann, M., van der Kaaij, M. A., Ramadan, S., … European Organisation for Research and Treatment of Cancer (EORTC) Lymphoma Group. (2015). Cardiovascular disease after treatment for Hodgkin's lymphoma: An analysis of ninc collaborative EORTC-LYSA trials. *The Lancet Haematology,* 2(11): e492-e502.

Dassonneville, L., Bonjean, K., De Pauw-Gillet, M-C., Colson, P., Houssier, C., Quetin-Leclercq, J., … Bailly, C. (1999). Stimulation of topoisomerase II-mediated DNA cleavage by three DNA-intercalating plant alkaloids: Cryptolepine, Matadine, and Serpentine. *Biochemistry*, 38(24): 7719-7726. http://pubs.acs.org/doi/abs/10.1021/bi990094t

Van Vuuren, R. J., Visagie, M. H., Theron, A. E., & Joubert, A. M. (2015). Antimitotic drugs in the treatment of cancer. *Cancer chemotherapy and pharmacology,* 6(76): 1101-1112.

Other Resources

Chemocare
www.chemocare.com

American Cancer Society
www.cancer.org

See also: Chemotherapy

▶ Plant alkaloids and terpenoids in chemotherapy

Category: Chemotherapy and Other Drugs
ATC code: 101C

Definition: Alkaloids and terpenoids are compounds derived from plants, some of which are shown to have anticancer activity and have been developed into useful chemotherapeutic agents. Subclasses of this group include vinca alkaloids, taxanes, podophyllotoxins, epipodophyllotoxins, camptothecins, ellipticine, and colchicine.

Cancers treated or prevented: Breast cancer, ovarian cancer, lung cancer, prostate cancer, lymphomas, leukemias

Delivery routes: Intravenous

How these drugs work: Plants are an important source of natural products effective in treating human cancer, with several useful chemotherapeutic agents currently on the market or in clinical trials. Specifically, many plant-derived alkaloids and terpenoids have significant anticancer properties. In addition, synthetic and semi-synthetic derivatives of alkaloid and terpenoid compounds with anticancer activity have been developed. Plants produce these compounds as secondary metabolites. These metabolites probably function as defense chemicals that inhibit cell division in invading pathogens. These same cytostatic compounds can be useful in cancer treatment by stopping the growth of cancer cells. Some examples of alkaloids and terpenoids used in chemotherapy include vinca alkaloids, podophyllotoxins, and taxanes.

Alkaloids are naturally occurring amines produced by plants and are grouped into several classifications, usually based on the metabolic pathway through which they are generated. These classifications include indole, purine, pyridine, and isoquinoline. Terpenoids are sometimes also referred to as isoprenoids and are classified according to the number of isoprene units that they contain. For example, monoterpenoids are made up of two isoprene units, whereas diterpenoids are composed of four isoprene units.

Four structural classes of plant-derived anticancer agents of alkaloid or terpenoid origin are available in the United States: vinca alkaloids, taxanes, epipodophyllotoxins, and camptothecins. These compounds work by affecting cell division and deoxyribonucleic acid (DNA) synthesis or function.

In 1947, researchers initiated the search for plant derived anticancer agents when they discovered, in laboratory experiments, that podophyllotoxins from the American mayapple (*Podophyllum peltatum*) inhibited the growth of tumor cells. The subsequent discovery of antileukemic properties of vinblastine and vincristine, bis-indole alkaloids derived from the Madagascar periwinkle (*Catharanthus roseus*), spurred broad investigations of plant-derived compounds for possible anticancer activity. *C. roseus* was found to be a storehouse of more than seventy-five alkaloids, several of which possess anticancer activity. Among other plant species that have provided clinically useful drugs are Taxus brevifolis (the source of diterpene taxol), *Ochrosia elliptica* (one of the sources of the pyridocarbazole alkaloid ellipticine), and *Camptotheca acuminata* (which contains camptothecin).

While being used to treat other conditions, the leaves of *C. roseus*, formerly *Vinca roseus*, were found to contain cytotoxic compounds. Among these compounds were two terpenoid indole alkaloids, vinblastine and vincristine, which subsequently became the first natural anticancer agents used clinically. Vinblastine and vincristine, together with a number of semi-synthetic derivatives, are collectively termed the vinca alkaloids. Although they have been in clinical usage since the 1970's, the vinca alkaloids are still extremely useful chemotherapeutic agents with well-known antimitotic activity. Vinca alkaloids work by binding specific sites on tubulin and preventing assembly of tubulin into microtubules, which are essential for cell division.

Soon after the introduction of vinblastine and vincristine, intensive chemical research was undertaken to try to develop semi-synthetic derivatives that had higher activity, lower toxicity, and broader anticancer effects. Several successful semi-synthetic derivatives were developed, including vindesine, vinorelbine, and vinflunine. Vindesine has a vincristine-like spectrum of activity and is used mainly to treat melanoma, acute lymphoblastic leukemia, and advanced non-small-cell lung cancer. Vinorelbine has reduced side effects and is now widely used in treatment of non-small-cell lung cancer and breast cancer. It has utility toward other cancers, including lymphoma and esophageal and prostate cancers, which are currently under clinical investigation. Vinflunine is a semi-synthetic fluorinated derivative of vindesine and is currently in clinical trials for treatment against various cancers, including bladder, lung, and gastric cancers.

Another class of plant alkaloids used in chemotherapy is the taxanes. Taxanes are derived from either the bark or the needles of some species of yew tree. Taxanes currently used as chemotherapeutic agents include paclitaxel and docetaxel. Paclitaxel is derived from the bark of the European yew tree (*Taxus baccata*), while docetaxel is derived from the pine needle of the Pacific yew tree (Taxus brevifolia). Paclitaxel, marketed under the name Taxol, is one of the most effective plant-derived chemotherapeutic agents. Patients with refractory ovarian cancer, metastatic breast cancer, advanced lung cancer, cancers of the head and neck, melanoma, and lymphomas respond positively to treatment with Taxol. The taxanes work by increasing the stability of microtubules, which inhibits cell division by preventing the separation of chromosomes during anaphase.

Other classes of plant alkaloids used in chemotherapy include the podophyllotoxins, camptothecins, ellipticines, and colchicine. Podophyllotoxins, or epipodophyllotoxins, are alkaloids naturally occurring in the root of the American mayapple or mandrake (*Podophyllum emodi*). Recently, a rare Himalayan mayapple (*Podophyllum hexandrum*) has also been found to contain active compounds, but this plant is endangered and consequently limited in supply. Efforts to obtain these compounds through recombinant technologies are under way. Some epipodophyllotoxin derivatives, etoposide and teniposide, are currently used in cancer treatment. Semi-synthetic derivatives such as amsacrine and etoposide phosphate also exist. Podophyllotoxins and their derivatives work by preventing cell division in tumor cells by keeping cells from entering the cell cycle and undergoing DNA replication.

Camptothecin is a quinoline alkaloid isolated from C. acuminata. Examples of camptothecins used in chemotherapy include topotecan and irinotecan. Topotecan is currently used to treat ovarian cancer, and irinotecan is currently marketed for treatment of metastatic cancer of the colon or rectum. Another compound, 9-aminocamptothecin, is also being investigated for treatment of ovarian and stomach cancers. Ellipticine is an alkaloid isolated from an evergreen tree of the Apocyanaceae family. Ellipiticine and its derivatives, including elliptinium, are promising anticancer agents and are highly effective against several types of cancer, with limited side effects. Colchicine is a tricyclic tropane alkaloid that prevents tubulin polymerization during the cell cycle. It is derived from the autumn crocus (*Colchicum autumnale*) and gloriosa lily (*Gloriosa superba*). Colchicine has been used effectively to treat chronic myelocytic leukemia, but toxic or near-toxic doses are required for therapeutic benefit. For this reason, colchicine and its analogs are primarily used as tools to study new mitotic inhibitors rather than in chemotherapy, but colchicine is used to treat gout.

The exact mechanisms of action of podophyllotoxins, camptothecins, and ellipticines remain unexplained. However, these compounds (and their derivatives) are believed to function as either type I or type II topoisomerase inhibitors (essential enzymes in cell division, DNA transcription, and DNA replication).

Side effects: Side effects of plant alkaloids and terpenoids used in chemotherapy include lowered resistance to infection, bruising or bleeding, anemia, constipation, cramps, diarrhea, nausea, peripheral neuropathy (numbness or tingling in hands or feet), headaches, tiredness, and hair loss. Mouth sores and ulcers, changes in taste, and loss of appetite can also occur. Skin rashes and allergic reactions take place less commonly.

C. J. Walsh, Ph.D.

For Further Information

Cutler, S. J., & Cutler, H. G. (2000). *Biologically Active Natural Products: Pharmaceuticals.* Boca Raton, Fla.: CRC Press. This book explores the use of plants and plant products in pharmaceutical development, including evaluation of plant extracts for anticancer treatment.

Kintzios, S. E. (2006). Terrestrial Plant-Derived Anticancer Agents and Plant Species Used in Anticancer Research. *Critical Reviews in Plant Sciences,* 25: 79-113. This is an article published in a scientific journal that reviews the literature over a 35-year period on plant-derived anticancer compounds and their potential as therapeutic agents.

Mukherjee, A. K., Basu, S., Sarkar, N., & Ghosh, A. C. (2001). Advances in Cancer Therapy with Plant Based Natural Products. *Current Medicinal Chemistry,* 8(12): 1467-1486. This is a review article that discusses anticancer properties of plants, including structure, chemistry, mechanism of action, and recent advances.

Perry, Michael C. (Ed.). (2012). *Perry's The Chemotherapy Source Book* (5th ed.). Philadelphia, PA: Wolters Kluwer Health/Lippincott Williams &; Wilkins. This book provides information on choosing chemotherapeutic agents, using combination chemotherapy, and toxicity of individual drugs. This book focuses on clinical use of chemotherapy.

Maryam, M., Rusea, G. C., Yong, S. Y., & Mohd, N. (2013). Vinca Alkaloids. *International Journal of Preventive Medicine,* 4: 1231-1235. This is a scientific article that discusses the four major vinka alkaloids currently in clinical use.

DeVita Jr., V.T., & Chu, E. (2008). A History of Cancer Chemotherapy. *Cancer Research,* 68: 8643-8653. This is a review article discussing the history of chemotherapy to treat different kinds of cancers.

Nwodo, J.N, A. Ibezim, C.V. Simoben, & Ntie-Kang, F. (2015). Natural products from African medicinal plants, Part II: Alkaloids, terpenoids, and flavonoids. *Anticancer Agents and Medicinal Chemistry,* 16(1):108-127. Describes anti-cancer activity from plant-derived compounds from African flora.

Other Resources

Cancer Backup
http://www.cancerbackup.org.uk

National Cancer Institute
http://www.cancer.gov

The Chemoth.com Website
Chemoth.com/types/vinca-alkaloids

Livestrong.com
Brogram, C. "Alkaloids Cancer Treatment." (Aug 1, 2015). www.livestrong.com/article/151562-alkaloids-cancer-treatment/

National Center for Complementary and Alternative Medicine
http://nccam.nih.gov

Drugs.com
www.drugs/com/pro/vincristine.html

See also: Antineoplastics in chemotherapy; Antioxidants; Breast cancers; Caffeine; Complementary and alternative therapies; Dietary supplements; Green tea; Herbs as antioxidants; Indoles; Leukemias; Lung cancers; Lymphomas; Nutrition and cancer prevention; Nutrition and cancer treatment; Opioids; Ovarian cancers; Prostate cancer; Stomach cancers

▶ Platinum-based anticancer drugs

Category: Chemotherapy and Other Drugs
Also known as: Cisplatin, Carboplatin, Oxaliplatin

Definition: Platinum-based anticancer drugs have a platinum molecule as their base with 4 covalent bonds. Drug makers attach other substances to the bonds to create anticancer drugs. The first platinum-based drug was cisplatin.

Cancers treated

The cancers that can be treated with platinum-based drugs are testicular, ovarian, cervical, bladder, head and neck, lung (including both small cell and non-small cell), breast, acute leukemia, colon and rectal, prostate, and lymphoma.

Delivery routes

Platinum-based drugs are administered intravenously or intra-arterially. They can also be administered directly into the abdomen. Research continues to develop a platinum-based drug that can be administered by mouth.

How these drugs work

Cisplatin has 2 chlorines and 2 ammonium molecules attached to a central platinum molecule. Cisplatin is very effective at killing cancer cells, but it has a number of toxic side effects. In order to decrease drug toxicity, 2 other platinum compounds were developed (carboplatin and oxaliplatin). To date, cisplatin, carboplatin, and oxaliplatin are the only platinum-based anticancer drugs that have been approved by the US Food and Drug Administration (FDA).

Within cancer cells, cisplatin releases the chlorine atoms, which activates the platinum atom to attach to the DNA. The platinum atom within cisplatin forms bonds with DNA at the nitrogenous base, guanine. It attaches to 2 guanines on the same or opposite strands of DNA. These interstrand and intrastrand bonds between DNA and cisplatin distort the structure of DNA and interfere with gene expression and DNA replication within cancer cells. As a result of cisplatin treatment, the cancer cells may self-destruct, or attempt to break the bonds between the guanine and cisplatin groupings.

Carboplatin has 2 diamine molecules and 2 bidentate cyclobutane dicarboxylate groups attached to the central platinum atom. Once inside cells, the bidentate cyclobutane dicarboxylate groups release the platinum atom, which then attaches to guanines, just as in the case of cisplatin. However, carboplatin is an inherently more stable compound than cisplatin, which slightly decreases its anticancer activity and side effects.

Oxaliplatin has a different action than cisplatin and carboplatin, and therefore, can be used to treat cancers that are resistant to cisplatin and carboplatin. Its action differs because of its unique chemical structure. Oxaliplatin contains 2 diaminocyclohexane groups that are shed when it binds to the DNA of cancer cells. The other compounds joined to the platinum atom are bidentate cyclobutane dicarboxylates, like carboplatin. These changes in the compounds released upon binding to DNA decrease resistance to oxaliplatin and modify the toxicity of the drug.

Because of the success of these 3 platinum drugs, researchers designed variations of platinum compounds. Several of these drugs are involved in drug testing processes. None has been approved by the FDA.

Side effects

Platinum-based drugs have a number of unpleasant side effects. They include: kidney damage (the most serious side effect of cisplatin), severe fatigue, nausea and vomiting, loss of hair, hearing damage, peripheral neuropathy, suppression of the production of blood cells (the most serious side effect of carboplatin), allergic reactions, and resistance to the drug. Oncologists are able to prevent kidney damage from cisplatin by giving intravenous fluids while it is administered. These fluids decrease the exposure of the kidneys to the drug. Peripheral neuropathy results in numbness, muscle weakness, difficulty walking, and nerve pain in the hands and feet. Oxaliplatin can cause brief muscle spasms of the larynx and the esophagus, eliciting a sensation of choking.

Christine Carroll

For Further Information

Barnard, C. F. J. (1989). Platinum anticancer agents: Twenty years of continuing development. *Platinum Metals Review*, 33(4): 162-167.

Hannon, M. J. (2007). Metal-based anticancer drugs: From a past anchored in platinum chemistry to a post-genomic future of diverse chemistry and biology. *Pure Applied Chemistry*, 79(12): 2243-2261Johnstone, T. C., Park, G. Y., & Lippard, S. J. (2014). Understanding and improving platinum anticancer drugs – phenanthriplatin. *Anticancer Research*, 34(1): 471-476.

McWhinney, S. R., Goldberg, R. M., & McLeod, H. L. (2009). Platinum neurotoxicity pharmaco-genetics. *Molecular Cancer Therapeutics*, 8(10): 10-16. http://www.ncbi.nlm.nih.gov/pmc/articles/PMC2651829/

Shah, N., & Dixon, D. S. (2009). New generation platinum agents for solid tumors. *Future Oncology*, 5(1): 33-42

Other Resources

The American Cancer Society
http://www.cancer.org

United States National Library of Medicine
https://www.nlm.nih.gov

See also: Cancer Drug development; Chemotherapy

▶ Proteasome inhibitors

Category: Chemotherapy and Other Drugs
ATC code: 101XX

Definition: Proteasome inhibitors are small-molecule drugs that target the proteasome, a large protein complex responsible for the degradation of unwanted proteins in the cell. Certain proteins are marked for proteasomal degradation by ubiquitination, the process of adding multiple ubiquitin molecules to the protein. Ubiquitinated proteins are recognized by the proteasome, allowing for the degradation of specifically targeted proteins. Cells rely on the proteasome to maintain a proper balance of particular proteins, as well as to remove damaged protein. Because the proteasome is an essential component for many cellular processes, including cell division and survival, it is an attractive target for actively growing cancer cells.

Cancers treated: Multiple myeloma, mantle cell lymphoma

Subclasses of this group: Synthetic inhibitors, natural inhibitors

Delivery routes: Intravenous (IV) injection

How these drugs work: Proteasome inhibitors are targeted therapies with specificity for the proteasome protein complex. These agents act by binding to the proteasome, impairing its ability to degrade proteins in the cell. Because degradation of excess and damaged proteins is a necessary function for normal cellular processes such as cell proliferation, these inhibitors can induce death in actively dividing malignant cells.

The only proteasome inhibitor currently approved to treat patients with cancer is bortezomib (Velcade). Bortezomib is administered by IV injection, at a recommended dosage of twice weekly for two weeks, followed by a rest period. Several cycles of this therapy may be given.

Other compounds have been discovered to have proteasome inhibitory activity, but these agents are not currently indicated for the treatment of cancers. Ritonavir is an antiretroviral drug used in human immunodeficiency virus (HIV) therapy. Preclinical studies have shown that ritonavir may have activity against brain tumor cells. Lactacystin is a natural proteasome inhibitor primarily used in laboratory settings.

Side effects: Bortezomib, the only proteasome inhibitor currently improved as an antineoplastic agent, is generally safe and well tolerated. The predominant side effects noted with bortezomib therapy are weakness, diarrhea and constipation, nausea and vomiting, and peripheral neuropathy, a tingling in the hands and feet. Additionally, myelosuppression such thrombocytopenia and neutropenia has been noted.

Lisa M. Cockrell, B.S.

See also: Antineoplastics in chemotherapy; Chemotherapy; Diarrhea; Gastrointestinal complications of cancer treatment; HIV/AIDS-related cancers; Lymphomas; Mantle Cell Lymphoma (MCL); Moles; Multiple myeloma; Myeloma; Nausea and vomiting; Neutropenia; Thrombocytopenia

▶ Radiopharmaceuticals

Category: Chemotherapy and Other Drugs
ATC code: V10

Definition: Radiopharmaceuticals are a class of therapeutic drugs that carry a radioactive isotope in trace quantities. These drugs deliver radiation to kill a targeted region of malignant cells.

Cancers treated: Various cancers metastasizing to bone tissues, especially prostate cancer and thyroid cancer, B-cell non-Hodgkin lymphoma, and polycythemia vera

Subclasses of this group: Radioisotopes of iodine, phosphorous, rhenium, samarium, strontium, and yttrium

Delivery routes: These drugs are administered intravenously, orally in capsule or liquid form, or through a direct injection to the site of cancer, on an inpatient or outpatient basis, depending on the specific drug, the type of cancer, and its location. When possible, these drugs are best delivered directly to the tumor site to limit damage to normal cells.

How these drugs work: Initially, radiopharmaceuticals were developed to diagnose various medical problems, including tumors. Using radiographic imaging, nuclear medicine specialists detect the radiation emitted by these drugs and track their activity within an organ. Since the 1980's, the role of radiopharmaceuticals has been expanded to palliation and therapy of metastatic cancers. In this case, a slightly larger amount of the radioactive isotope is used to destroy a group of cancerous cells by interfering with cell division. Instead of photons (used for imaging), the drugs emit beta particles and gamma rays that damage the machinery needed for mitosis. The radioactive isotope is attached to a carrier molecule that is capable of targeting a specific organ or group of cells. For example, radiopharmaceuticals for bone cancer therapy have a mineral-like carrier molecule taken up by bone tissues.

Radiopharmaceuticals for specific organs may have a monoclonal antibody that recognizes the cell surface receptors of certain tissue cells. Once the drug reaches its target area, the isotope emits radiation slowly over short distances. The half-life, or time required for half of the radiation to be emitted, for these drugs is two to fifty days, depending on the isotope.

In almost all cases, radiopharmaceuticals are used when chemotherapy has failed, or in conjunction with second-line chemotherapy. Radiopharmaceuticals are especially helpful in cancers that have metastasized to neighboring bones, such as prostate and thyroid cancers. Studies have shown that these drugs are valuable in palliative care for patients experiencing pain from cancerous bone tissue, resulting in better disease management and improved quality of life.

Side effects: The side effects of radiopharmaceuticals vary depending on the specific radioactive isotope, its dosage, and the individual patient's physical condition. An excessive dose of these drugs may result in toxicity that affects normal cells as well as malignant cells, which could lead to an intensification of the cancer. The most common side effect of radiopharmaceuticals, however, is a decrease in the patient's white blood cell and platelet counts. Other common side effects include black or bloody stools, coughs, fevers or chills, back or side pain, difficulty in urination, unusual bleeding or bruising, and nausea and vomiting. Less common side effects include bone pain and irregular heartbeat. Patients who take iodine 131 for thyroid cancer may also experience loss of taste and tenderness in the salivary glands and neck. Since children and older adults are particularly sensitive to radiation, they may experience more side effects during and after treatment with radiopharmaceuticals.

Bharat Burman, B.A.

For Further Information

Ballantyne, Jane C., ed. *The Massachusetts General Hospital Handbook of Pain Management.* 3d ed. Philadelphia: Lippincott Williams & Wilkins, 2006.

Leibel, Steven A., and Theodore L. Phillips, eds. *Textbook of Radiation Oncology*. 2d ed. Philadelphia: Saunders, 2004.

Common Radiopharmaceuticals Used in Cancer Therapy

Drug	*Brands*	*Delivery Mode*	*Conditions Treated*
Iodine 131 (^{131}I), sodium iodide		Oral	Thyroid cancer
Phosphorus 32 (^{32}P), sodium phosphate, chromic phosphate		Oral, IV	Polycythemia vera; bone metastases; cancers causing malignant ascites, pleural effusion, pericardial effusions, and brain cysts
Rhenium 186 (^{186}Re) HEDP		IV	Bone metastases; breast cancer
Samarium 153 (^{153}Sm) EDTMP	Quadramet	Injection	Bone metastases
Strontium 89 (^{89}Sr), strontium chloride	Metastron	Injection	Bone metastases
Yttrium 90 (^{90}Y) ibritumomab tiuxetan	Zevalin	IV	B-cell non-Hodgkin lymphoma

Parker, R. G., N. A. Janjan, and M. T. Selch. *Radiation Oncology for Cure and Palliation*. New York: Springer, 2003.

Other Resources

Radiation Oncology Online Journal
http://www.rooj.com/default.htm

Society of Radiopharmaceutical Sciences
http://www.srsweb.org

See also: Bone cancers; Chemotherapy; Imaging tests; Non-Hodgkin lymphoma; Nuclear medicine scan; Prostate cancer; Radiation oncology; Thyroid cancer; X-ray tests

▶ Ranibizumab (Lucentis)

Category: Chemotherapy and Other Drugs
Also known as: Lucentis

Definition: Ranibizumab (Lucentis, a trademark of Genentech, Inc.) is a monoclonal antibody fragment that is used to treat certain eye conditions and help prevent decreased vision and blindness. It was first approved by the US Food and Drug Administration in 2006.

Conditions treated: Ranibizumab is used to treat wet age-related macular degeneration, macular edema (swelling) caused by diabetes, diabetic retinopathy in patients with diabetic macular edema, and macular edema caused by retinal vein occlusion (a blockage in the blood vessels). It is also being tested in clinical trials as a treatment for various cancers.

Delivery routes: Ranibizumab is given by injection into the affected eye(s) by a physician in a sterile setting. The affected eye is numbed before each injection and the patient is monitored carefully before and after the injection. The patient's eye pressure is measured both before and after the medication is administered. Ranibizumab is usually given once a month or as directed by a physician. It is intended to be used in combination with other medications and lifestyle modifications to manage blood sugar, blood pressure, and cholesterol.

How this drug works: Ranibizumab works by binding to and blocking a protein called vascular endothelial growth factor A (VEGF-A). VEGF-A is believed to play a critical role in the formation of abnormal blood vessels and the hyperpermeability ("leakiness") of these blood vessels. When the abnormal blood vessels in the eye leak fluid into the macula, the fluid accumulates and the macula swells, causing blurred vision. By blocking this protein, ranibizumab may prevent damaged blood vessels from leaking fluid into the macula and also reduce swelling.

Side effects: The most common side effects of ranibizumab include increased redness in the white of the eye, eye pain, small specks in vision, and increased eye pressure. Other common side effects include nose and throat infections, headache, lung/airway infections, and nausea.

Uncommon but serious side effects that could worsen vision include infection within the eyeball (endophthalmitis), inflammation, retinal detachments, and cataracts. These conditions occurred in 0.1% of people (or 1 in 1000 people). Patients taking ranibizumab should be monitored closely for the development of the following symptoms, which should be reported to the patient's doctor immediately: redness of the eye, sensitivity to light, eye pain, or changes in vision.

Other serious, but uncommon, side effects were discovered in clinical trials. These sometimes fatal side effects included stroke, heart attack, and other problems related to blood clots.

As a precaution, ranibizumab should not be used in patients who have an infection in or around the eye or who are allergic to any of the ingredients in the medication.

Angela M. Costello, BS

For Further Information

Domalpally A., Ip, M. S., & Ehrlich, J. S. (2015). Effects of intravitreal ranibizumab on retinal hard exudate in diabetic macular edema: Findings from the RIDE and RISE phase III clinical trials. *Ophthalmology,* 122(4): 779-86.

National Institutes of Health. "NIH Study Finds Avastin and Lucentis are Equally Effective in Treating Age-Related Macular Degeneration." (2011). Retrieved at: http://www.nih.gov/news-events/news-releases/nih-study-finds-avastin-lucentis-are-equally-effective-treating-age-related-macular-degeneration

Other Resources

Lucentis
http://www.lucentis.com

American Cancer Society
http://www.cancer.org

CancerNet
http://www.cancer.net

Chemocare.org
http://www.chemocare.org

National Cancer Institute
http://www.cancer.gov

U.S. Food and Drug Administration
http://www.fda.gov

▶ Rituximab

Category: Chemotherapy and Other Drugs
Also known as: Rituxan

Definition: Rituximab is a chimeric monoclonal antibody (MoAb) directed against the B-cell-specific antigen CD20 expressed on certain cancer cells. It is considered an immunotherapy agent.

Cancers treated: Rituximab is typically used to treat B-cell non-Hodgkin lymphoma and chronic lymphocytic leukemia. Also, it is used to treat non-cancerous diagnosis such as rheumatoid arthritis, Wegener granulomatosis, and other clinical diagnosis.

Delivery routes: Rituximab is given by intravenous infusion, at a medical facility where the patient can be monitored.

How these drugs work: Rituximab attaches to a cell surface marker, CD20, on surfaces of cancerous B cells and other CD20-expressing tumors. Rituximab binding causes the immune system to recognize the tumor cell as foreign and destroy it. Rituximab binding also induces programmed cells death (apoptosis) of tumorous B-cells. When B-cells mature into antibody-producing "plasma cells," they no longer contain CD20 on their surfaces and are not affected by rituximab.

Side effects: Rituximab can cause severe side effects. Patients may be premedicated with acetaminophen and diphenhydramine in order to ameliorate potential side effects. Additionally, rituximab is typically administered slowly in order to prevent side effects. The most common side effects are infusion related and include chills and body aches. These can occur immediately or within 24 hours of the infusion. In addition, more severe reactions have been reported such as hives, facial/oral swelling, shortness of breath, difficulty breathing, weakness, dizziness, feeling faint, racing heart, and chest pain/pressure.

Rituximab can also reactivate hepatitis B. Patients with a history of hepatitis B infection require frequent monitoring during and following treatment.

Because rituximab also destroys immature B-cells, it can cause a drop in white blood cells, which can lead to serious infections.

Patients may also experience tumor lysis syndrome following the administration of rituximab.

Katrina Green MSN, RN, OCN

For Further Information

Castillo, J. J., Sa, S. D', Lunn, M. P., Minnema, M. C., Tedeschi, A., Lansigan, F., … Treon, S. P. (2015). Central nervous system involvement by Waldenström macroglobulinaemia (Bing-Neel syndrome): A multi-institutional retrospective study, *British Journal of Haematology*, doi: 10.1111/bjh.13883.

Lindorfer, M. A., Cook, E. M., Tupitza, J. C., Zent, C. S., Burack, R., de Jong, R. N., … Taylor, R. P. (2016). Real-time analysis of the detailed sequence of cellular events in mAb-mediated complement-dependent cytotoxicity of B-cell lines and of chronic lymphocytic leukemia B-cells. *Molecular Immunology*, 70: 13–23. doi: 10.1016/j.molimm.2015.12.007.

Rai, K. R. & Jain, P. (2015). Chronic lymphocytic leukemia (CLL) — then and now. *American Journal of Hematology*, doi: 10.1002/ajh.24282.

Fleury, I., Chevret, S., Pfreunschuh, M., Salles, G., Coiffer, B., van Oers, M., … Thieblemont, C. (2015). Rituximab and risk of second primary malignancies in patients with non-Hodgkin lymphoma: A systematic review and meta-analysis. *Annals of Oncology*, doi: 10.1093/annonc/mdv616.

Neves, H. & Kwok, H. F. (2015). Recent advances in the field of anti-cancer immunotherapy. *BBA Clinical*, 3: 280–288. doi: 10.1016/j.bbacli.2015.04.001.

Other Resources

NIH National Library of Medicine
https://www.nlm.nih.gov/medlineplus/druginfo/meds/a607038.html

Rituxan website
www.rituxan.com
Rituxan Prescribing Information —Genentech
http://www.gene.com/download/pdf/rituxan_prescribing.pdf

▶ Romidepsin

Category: Chemotherapy and Other Drugs
Also known as: Istodax

Definition: An anticancer drug that inhibits histone deacetylases and subsequently induces the death of tumor cells.

Cancers treated: Cutaneous and peripheral T-cell lymphomas.

Delivery routes: Injection or intravenous infusion

How this drug works: Romidepsin is a member of the histone deacetylase inhibitor (HDACI) class of anticancer drugs. HDACIs inhibit a group of enzymes called histone deacetylases (HDACs). HDACs tend to squelch gene expression by removing acetyl (CH3-COO-) groups from histone proteins.

Histone proteins form disc-like structures and DNA winds around these discs approximately 2 times to form structures known as "nucleosomes." Four different histones combine to form these discs; histone 2A (H2A), histone 2B (H2B), histone 3 (H3), and histone 4 (H4). Each nucleosome contains 2 copies of each of these different types of histones to form a protein octamer. The front part (amino-terminus) of histones contains a high concentration of positively charged amino acids, which binds the histones tightly to DNA, which is negatively charged. Nucleosomes are then wound into solenoid-type structures to form a compact DNA-protein complex known as "chromatin."

Gene expression requires that the chromatin be unwound. To accomplish this, enzymes within the nucleus of cells attach acetyl groups to lysine residues (a positively charged amino acid) in the amino termini of histones, which neutralize the positive changes in the histones and weaken their interaction with DNA. HDACs reverse this process by removing the attached acetyl groups and inducing a more compact chromatin structure upon the DNA that represses gene expression.

HDACIs are small molecules that inhibit HDACs and disrupt gene expression. However, HDACIs disrupt gene expression to a much greater degree in cancer cells than they do in normal cells. Therefore, these drugs have robust anticancer properties that tend to leave normal cells relatively unaffected.

One particular HDACI, romidepsin, is a prodrug that does not become active until the body modifies it. A member of the depsipeptide group of chemicals, romidepsin contains a disulfide bond (S-S) that becomes reduced upon interaction with enzymes in the liver. Reduction of the disulfide bond converts it into a thiol group (-SH) that binds to a zinc atom at the active site of HDAC enzymes, reversibly inhibiting them.

Romidepsin is indicated for the treatment of cutaneous T-cell lymphoma and peripheral T-cell lymphoma in patients whose treatment with other anticancer agents were unsuccessful.

Side Effects: The most common side effects are low white blood cell counts (leukopenia), low platelet counts (thrombocytopenia), infections, nausea, fatigue, vomiting, anorexia, anemia, and changes in the patient's electrocardiogram (specifically the T-wave). Patients on romidepsin can contract serious and even fatal infections, and pregnant women should not take it, since romidepsin can harm an unborn baby. Patients with advanced disease treated with romidepsin can suffer from "tumor lysis syndrome." This is a condition that results from the rapid death of large numbers of tumor cells and subsequent release of enormous quantities of cellular byproducts into the circulation that overwhelms the kidneys and disrupts the patient's metabolism.

Michael Buratovich, PhD

For Further Information

Kim, M., Thompson, L. A., Wenger, S. D., & O'Bryant, C. L. (2012). "Romidepsin: A histone deacetylase inhibitor for refractory cutaneous T-cell lymphoma." *Annals of Pharmacotherapy* 46(10):1340-1348.

Gray, Steven. (Ed.). (2015). *Epigenetic Cancer Therapy*. Waltham, MA: Academic Press.

Other Resources

Official Istodax Website
http://www.istodax.com/hcp/Default.aspx

Romidepsin Chemotherapy Drug Information
http://www.chemocare.com/chemotherapy/drug-info/romidepsin.aspx

See also: DNA methylation inhibitors

▶ Ruthenium based anticancer drug

Category: Chemotherapy and Other Drugs

Also known as: NAMI-A (Imidazolium-trans-tetrachloro(dimethylsulfoxide)imidazoleruthenium(III)); KP1019 (indazolium trans-[tetrachloridobis(1H-indazole)ruthenate(III)]); NKP1339 (the sodium salt analogue of KP1019, sodium trans-[tetrachloridobis(1H-indazole) ruthenate(III)]).

Definition: Organic compounds that contain the platinum group metal ruthenium (Ru) and show marked anticancer and antimetastatic properties.

Cancers treated: Experimental treatment of non-small cell lung carcinoma and neuroendocrine carcinoma.

Delivery routes: Intravenous.

How these drugs work: NAMI-A (New Anti-tumor Metastasis Inhibitor-A) was the first Ru-containing compound to come to clinical trials. Although NAMI-A shows little activity against primary tumors, it efficiently prevents spread of tumors (metastasis) in laboratory animals. The drug seems to enhance cancer cell adhesion, and inhibit cancer cell motility, invasiveness, and angiogenesis. NAMI-A shows no activity against tumors when given alone, but was tested in combination with gemcitabine for non-small cell lung carcinoma. In phase I/II clinical trials, NAMI-A was only moderately tolerated and was less active in patients with non-small cell lung cancer after first-line treatment than gemcitabine alone. For those reasons, the trial was prematurely terminated.

Two other closely related Ru compounds, KP1019 and its more soluble form, NKP-1339, show robust antitumor activity. These compounds accumulate around tumors because of their strong binding to blood-based proteins (such as albumin and transferrin). Once in our bodies, certain molecules (eg, ascorbic acid and glutathione) add electrons to the Ru atoms in KP1019/NKP-1339 (a type of chemical reaction known as reduction), which activates them. The activated forms of these drugs induce elevated levels of cell stress through the production of reactive oxygen species (ROS). Increased ROS induce cell cycle arrest, blockage of DNA synthesis, and induction of programmed cell death in tumor cells.

Side effects: In clinical trials, NAMI-A caused the following side effects: low white and red blood cell counts (leukopenia and anemia, respectively), nausea, vomiting, and constipation or diarrhea, inflammation of the mouth and lips (stomatitis), fatigue, liver and kidney toxicity, fever, vein inflammation (phlebitis) at the site of injection, and painful blisters on the hands and feet. Some patients also displayed allergies to the drug.

In clinical trials, NKP-1339 is typically very well tolerated but tends to convey a greenish color to the plasma, and causes fevers in some patients.

Michael Buratovich, PhD

Further Information

Amin, A., & Buratovich, M. A. (2009). New platinum and ruthenium complexes – the latest class of potential chemotherapeutic drugs – a review of new developments in the field. *Mini Reviews in Medicinal Chemistry*, 9(13): 1489-1503.

Markowska, A., Kasprzak, B., Jaszczyńska-Nowinka, K., Lubin, J., & Markowska, J. (2015). Nobel metals in oncology. *Contemporary Oncology*, 19(4): 271-275.

Trondl, R., Heffeter, P., Kowol, C. R., Jakupec, M. A., Berger, W., & Keppler, B. K. (2014). NKP-1339, the first ruthenium-based anticancer drug on the edge to clinical application. *Chemical Science* 5: 2925-2932.

Other Resources

Collerio Foundation
http://www.callerio.org/NAMI-A.htm

Dose Escalation Study of NKP-1339 to Treat Advanced Solid Tumors
https://clinicaltrials.gov/ct2/show/NCT01415297?term=Ruthenium&rank=2

▶ Stem cell cancer treatments

Category: Chemotherapy and Other Drugs
Also known as: Regenerative cell therapy; regenerative medicine

Definition: Stem cells are immature cells that can differentiate into specialized body cells. There are 2 kinds of stem cells: 1) Pluripotent stem cells, such as embryonic stem cells which are found in embryos and can differentiate into any type of adult cell type; and 2) Adult stem cells, which are found in adult organs and tissues. Adult stem cells include such examples as hematopoietic (blood-forming) stem cells, which are mainly found in bone marrow, peripheral blood, and the umbilical cord blood of newborn babies, and mesenchymal stem cells (or mesenchymal stroma cells), which are found in bone marrow, fat, muscles, liver, teeth, and many other places. Adult stem cells are multipotent, meaning they are able to differentiate into a few different cell types. For about 30 years, hematopoietic stem cell therapy has been used to treat certain cancers. This therapy, hematopoietic stem cell transplant (HSCT), uses stem cells harvested from bone marrow or umbilical cord blood. There are 2 types of HSCT procedures: autologous (AUTO) and allogeneic (ALLO) transplantations. Autologous transplants utilize cells harvested from the patient's own body. Allogeneic cells come from a healthy donor, whose array of specific cell surface proteins (ie, major histocompatibility complex proteins) closely match those of the recipient's. Since ALLO stem cells are devoid of cancer, this procedure is the one most commonly used to treat cancers.

Cancers treated: HSCT is the only widely used stem-cell therapy, and is a standard treatment for cancers: 1) that affect white blood cells or the bone marrow (leukemias, eg, acute lymphoblastic leukemia and acute myelogenous leukemia); 2) that develop in the lymphatic system (lymphomas, eg, multiple myeloma); 3) not originating in the blood system, such as neuroblastoma; and 4) for disorders of blood cell proliferation (eg, anemias). Stem cell treatments for other diseases, such as breast cancer or renal cell carcinoma are under investigation in clinical trials.

Delivery routes: In ALLO therapy, frozen stem cells are thawed and infused through an intravenous catheter into the patient's vein. In AUTO therapy, unfrozen stem cells are infused in the patient's vein.

How these drugs work: To prepare for HSCT, patients receive high doses of chemotherapy and/or radiation to treat the cancer and make room in the bone marrow for the new stem cells to grow (ablative or myeloablative therapy). The infused stem cells replace the dysfunctional blood cells in the bloodstream and stem cells in the bone marrow destroyed by chemotherapy (and radiotherapy) to create new, healthy blood cells in the bone marrow.

Side effects: ALLO transplant recipients may suffer from "graft-versus-host disease" (GVHD) in which the transplanted stem cells generate immune cells that attack the organs of the recipient. Specific anti-rejection medicines can mitigate GVHD. Because of the severe bone marrow suppression used in bone marrow transplant patients, infections are a constant threat, as is respiratory distress, low platelet and red blood cells, and organ damage. Pain resulting from mouth sores and gastrointestinal irritation is also common. Finally, graft failure is always a possibility if insufficient numbers of new stem cells engraft into the recipient's bone marrow.

Silke Haidekker, PhD, ELS

For Further Information

Knoepfler, Paul. (2013). *Stem cells: An insider's guide.* Hackensack, NJ: World Scientific.
Slack, Jonathan. (2012). *Stem cells: A very short introduction.* New York, NY: Oxford University Press.

Other Resources

The International Society for Stem Cell Research
http://www.closerlookatstemcells.org

National Cancer Institute
http://www.cancer.gov/about-cancer/treatment/types/stem-cell-transplant/stem-cell-fact-sheet

See also: Leukemia; Lymphoma; Bone Marrow transplantation

▶ Texaphyrins

Category: Chemotherapy and Other Drugs

Definition: Texaphyrins are expanded porphyrin molecules with 5 nitrogen-containing pyrrole moieties rather than the 4 found in natural porphyrin molecules. The expanded ring structure is a designed host molecule for a wide range of transition and lanthanide metal ions. By making a nearly endless number of small changes to the chemical side groups of the texaphyrin molecule or changing the metal ion captured by the texaphyrin, a wide array of potential anti-cancer molecules can be made.

Cancers treated: When the lanthanide metal gadolinium is placed in the middle of a texaphyrin host molecule, the combined compound is called Xcytrin. This molecule passed phase II clinical trials before failing to receive FDA approval at the phase III clinical trial stage for treatment of non-small cell lung cancer. Lutetium texaphyrin is uniquely designed for treatment of skin cancers and shows tremendous potential for light initiated oxygenation of cancerous tissue or photodynamic therapy.

How these drugs work: Because the basic shape of the texaphyrin molecule resembles porphyrin molecules found in blood and other biochemical systems, these molecules appear to be tolerated by the body and have a strong attraction to cancerous tissue; perhaps because the increased vasculature of cancerous tissue invites such porphyrin-containing or porphyrin-like compounds. This affinity for cancerous tissue allows the selective killing of cancers as well as the selective imaging of cancers by techniques such as MRI-contrast imaging.

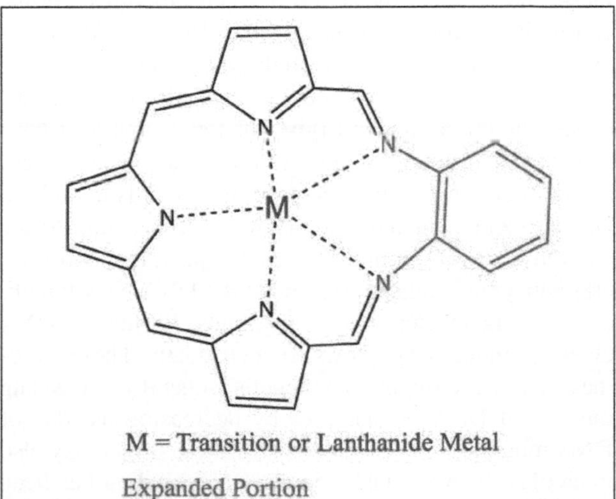

Texaphryn molecule.

Primarily, Xcytrin was shown to increase the levels of reactive oxygen species (ROS) inside cancerous tissue. Xcytrin also demonstrated the ability to inhibit natural cellular systems that target ROS. This one-two punch of Xcytrin showed great promise as a new breakthrough in chemotherapy. Even with clinical trial failure, the potential of Texaphyrin molecules is such that Pharmacyclics, a company started by chemist Jonathan Sessler and Dr. R. A. Miller, was sold to AbbVie in March 2015for $21 billion. This class of compounds clearly has great promise for helping to eliminate the scourge of cancer.

Side effects: The gadolinium and lutetium texaphyrin compounds are quite water soluble and easily administered by intravenous infusion. These compounds are eliminated by the body on a timescale measured in hours, which contributes to lower overall toxicity and a reduction in dark reactions for the lutetium texaphyrin compared to currently used PDT compounds. Yet, because these compounds have a 10:1 affinity for cancerous tissue over normal tissue, therapy is easily administered using X-rays in the case of gadolinium texaphyrin or red light as in lutetium texaphyrin.

Bruce Baldwin, PhD

For Further Information

Arambula, J. F., Preihs, C., Borthwick, D., Madga, D., & Sessler, J. L. (2011). Texaphyrins: Tumor localizing redox active expanded porphyrins. *Anticancer Agents in Medicinal Chemistry*, 11: 222-232.

Hannah, S., Lynch, V., Guldi, D. M., Gerasimchuk, N., MacDonald, C. L. B., Magda, D., & Sessler, J. L. (2002). Late first-row transition-metal complexes of texaphyrin. *Journal of the American Chemical Society*, 124: 8416-8427.

Sessler, J. L., Hemmi, G., Mody, T. D., Murai, T., Burrell, A., & Young, S. W. (1994). Texaphyrins: Synthesis and applications. *Accounts of Chemical Research*, 27: 43-50.

Sessler, J. L., Kral, V., Hoehner, M. C., Chin, O. A., & Davila, R. M. (1996). New texaphyrin-type expanded porphyrins. *Pure & Applied Chemistry*, 68: 1291-1295.

Sessler, J. L., & Miller, R. A. (2000). Texaphyrins: New drugs with diverse clinical applications in radiation and photodynamic therapy. *Biochemical Pharmacology,* 59: 733-739.

Other Resources

Company Founded by Cancer-Fighting Chemist Sold for $21 Billion.
https://cns.utexas.edu/news/company-founded-by-cancer-fighting-chemist-sold-for-21-billion

▶ Topoisomerase inhibitors

Category: Chemotherapy and Other Drugs
ATC code: 101XX, 101CB

Definition: Topoisomerase inhibitors are a group of anticancer chemotherapeutic drugs. Topoisomerases are important in changing the topology of deoxyribonucleic acid (DNA), allowing for efficient DNA replication and subsequent cell proliferation. Inhibitors of topoisomerases primarily kill tumors by interfering with DNA replication, which results in both a decrease in tumor cell division and an increase in tumor cell death. Because tumors comprise rapidly dividing cells, cancer cells are particularly susceptible to the inhibitory actions of topoisomerase inhibitors. These drugs are often administered in combination with other chemotherapy agents but may also be given as a single-agent therapy.

Cancers treated: Advanced colorectal cancer, testicular tumors, small-cell lung cancer, and acute lymphocytic leukemia; many other cancers that are refractory to first-line therapies

Subclasses of this group: Epipodophyllotoxins, camptothecin and related analogs

Delivery routes: Topoisomerase inhibitors are generally administered orally or intravenously (IV). The two main oral formulations used are either a solution or a soft gelatin capsule. Many of the topoisomerase inhibitors are not water-soluble and therefore to be administered by IV must be dissolved in a special solution of chemicals, including alcohol, polyethylene glycol, and polysorbate 80. This solution is responsible for the hypersensitivity reactions induced in some patients (less than 5 percent) following infusion, such as vasomotor changes in the gastrointestinal and pulmonary systems. Slowing the rate of infusion, as well as administration of steroids or antihistamines, can diminish these hypersensitivity reactions.

How these drugs work: As a cell prepares to undergo division, the DNA must be replicated in order to provide a copy of DNA for each of the resulting cells. Double-stranded DNA is normally tightly coiled in the nucleus of nondividing cells. The supercoiled topology of the DNA strands makes it difficult for the replication protein complexes that are necessary to copy the DNA to properly localize on the DNA strand. Therefore, to properly duplicate the DNA, it must first be "unwound," relaxing the structural topology and allowing access for the replication protein complexes. Topoisomerases are proteins located in the cell nucleus that can act to unwind the DNA. These proteins are enzymes, meaning that they have an intrinsic catalytic activity that allows them to perform a certain function in the cell. Topoisomerases relax the supercoiled DNA by making transient breaks within the DNA strand, allowing it to unwind. Once the topoisomerase cleaves the DNA and relieves the DNA topology, the enzyme then reseals the breakage.

Two types of topoisomerases have been identified, mainly differentiated by how they cleave double-stranded DNA. Type I topoisomerases alter DNA supercoiling by cleaving only one DNA strand. Type II enzymes are capable of cleaving both DNA strands. The current model of both types I and II topoisomerase activity predicts that the enzyme breaks the DNA phosphate backbone, and in an intermediate reaction step, a covalent linkage is formed between the DNA and the enzyme. For type I topoisomerases, the nicked DNA strand is then free to rotate around the unnicked strand, relieving the DNA supercoil. Type II topoisomerases relax the DNA by cleaving the entire DNA strand, inducing the passage of one DNA double-strand through a loop in another DNA double-strand. Without the action of topoisomerases, normal cell division would not be possible. However, these enzymes also play a major role in the growth of cancer cells.

Many natural compounds act to poison topoisomerases. Inhibitors to both types of topoisomerases have shown clinical activity against tumors. The primary mechanism of action of topoisomerase inhibitors is thought to be stabilization of the enzyme while it is bound to the cleaved DNA. By stabilizing this complex, the topoisomerase enzyme is unable to religate the DNA back together, resulting in cleaved DNA strands. Prolonged DNA cleavage induces apoptosis, or cell death. These drugs therefore are thought to kill cells either by increasing the rate of DNA breakage or by decreasing the rate of DNA religation. Although some of these drugs may also intercolate between DNA bases, DNA binding has been shown not to be a critical component of topoisomerase

Common Topoisomerase Inhibitors

Drug	*Brands*	*Subclass*	*Delivery Mode*	*Conditions Treated*
Etoposide, etoposide phosphate	Etopophos, VePeside (VP-16)	Epipodophyllotoxin	IV, oral	Refractory testicular tumors, small-cell lung cancer
Irinotecan hydrochloride	Camptosar (CPT-11)	Camptothecin	IV	Metastatic colon cancer, metastatic rectal cancer
Teniposide	Vumon	Epipodophyllotoxin	IV	Childhood acute lymphocytic leukemia, glioma brain tumors
Topotecan	Hycamtin	Camptothecin	IV	Refractory ovarian cancer, small-cell lung cancer, advanced cervical cancer

activity inhibition, as neither camptothecin nor etoposide binds DNA.

Two main groups of topoisomerase inhibitors are currently in clinical use, epipodophyllotoxins and camptothecin analogs. Epipodophyllotoxins, which target topoisomerase II, were synthesized in an effort to chemically improve the efficacy of the antimicrotubule drug podophyllotoxin, isolated from the mandrake plant. The epipodophyllotoxins include etoposide and teniposide. Camptothecin, an inhibitor of topoisomerase I, was discovered in an extract from the Chinese tree *Camptotheca acuminate*. The extreme side effects induced by camptothecin induced the creation of two main derivatives that cause fewer side effects, topotecan and irinotecan.

Resistance to topoisomerase inhibitors can occur through many mechanisms, including changes in the accumulation of these drugs, changes in the topoisomerase enzyme, and changes in the cellular response to the damage induced by these drugs. Because many topoisomerase inhibitors are naturally occurring substances, they are particularly susceptible to natural cellular efflux mechanisms. Cellular efflux results in a "pumping out" of the drugs, causing less total concentration of drug to be available inside the cell. By means of in vitro laboratory techniques, several cancer cell lines have been shown to display resistance to topoisomerase inhibitors. Laboratory studies have found that one mechanism of this resistance is the development of point mutations within the topoisomerase enzyme, genetic alterations that may change the target binding site where these drugs bind to the enzyme, inhibiting the ability of the drug to bind. Another way in which cells evade the effects of topoisomerase inhibitors is by increasing the expression of DNA repair enzymes, which can repair the cleavage induced by the topoisomerases.

Side effects: Topoisomerase inhibitors are generally well tolerated in most patients. The main toxicity resulting from topoisomerase inhibitors is bone marrow suppression, also known as myelosuppression. This is primarily manifested as leukopenia, or a decrease in the number of circulating white blood cells, and thrombocytopenia, a decrease in the number of blood platelets. The decrease in white blood cells increases the risk of patients developing infections, while the decrease in blood platelets may increase the risk of bleeding. Typically, the onset of myelosuppression occurs within five to seven days after the initiation of therapy, peaks within the next week, and is returned to normal approximately twenty-one to twenty-eight days after the original administration. Because of the potential seriousness of myelosuppression, patients receiving topoisomerase inhibitor therapy are required to be closely monitored by a clinician. Patients can effectively manage myelosuppression by avoiding interaction with infected people and by minimizing the risk of cuts and bruises.

Other side effects that result from drug administration mainly involve the gastrointestinal system, including diarrhea, nausea, and vomiting. Many patients often experience hair loss. These side effects can be controlled by reducing the dosage of therapy administered and by administering drugs to control the side effects, such as antinausea agents. Most of these side effects are reversible after drug therapy is stopped.

Despite the powerful effects that these drugs have in inducing tumor cell death, the use of topoisomerase inhibitors has also been linked with the development of secondary cancers in rare cases. For example, use of epipodophyllotoxins such as etoposide has been associated with an increased risk of developing secondary leukemia, at an incidence ranging from 0.7 to 3.2 percent. The reason for this increase is currently unknown.

Lisa M. Cockrell, B.S.

For Further Information

Adams, Val R., and Thomas G. Burke, eds. *Camptothecins in Cancer Therapy*. Totowa, N.J.: Humana Press, 2005.

Andoh, Toshiwo, ed. *DNA Topoisomerases in Cancer Therapy: Present and Future*. New York: Kluwer Academic/Plenum, 2003.

Kantarjian, Hagop M., et al. *The M. D. Anderson Manual of Medical Oncology*. New York: McGraw-Hill, 2006.

Kufe, Donald W., et al., eds. *Holland Frei Cancer Medicine 7*. 7th ed. Hamilton, Ont.: BC Decker, 2006.

Pratt, William B., et al. *The Anticancer Drugs*. 2d ed. New York: Oxford University Press, 1994.

Skeel, Roland T. *Handbook of Cancer Chemotherapy*. 7th ed. Philadelphia: Lippincott Williams & Wilkins, 2007.

Other Resources

American Cancer Society
http://www.cancer.org

National Cancer Institute
Drug Information Summaries
http://www.cancer.gov/cancertopics/druginfo/alphalist

See also: Acute Lymphocytic Leukemia (ALL); Antineoplastics in chemotherapy; Chemotherapy; Drug resistance and Multidrug Resistance (MDR); Infusion therapies; Leukemias; Lung cancers; Myelosuppression; Plant alkaloids and terpenoids in chemotherapy; Rectal cancer; Testicular cancer

▶ Trastuzumab (Herceptin)

Category: Chemotherapy and Other Drugs
Also known as: Herceptin, targeted therapy, Kadcyla (as a conjugate)

Definition: Trastuzumab is a humanized monoclonal antibody that blocks *HER2*, a protein that is overexpressed, or present in higher quantities, in some breast cancer cells. Trastuzumab was developed by Roche Oncology and is now marketed by Genentech in the United States and by Chugai in Japan, via Roche International in Basel, Switzerland. Trastuzumab is also available in a drug conjugate form, trastuzumab emtansine (Kadcyla), which was released by Roche.

Cancers treated: Approximately 20% of all breast cancers have higher-than-normal levels of the protein HER2 (human epidermal receptor 2). Trastuzumab works predominantly as an antineoplastic agent in these tumors, and, therefore, it is called a targeted therapy. Trastuzumab was initially approved in 1998 to treat breast cancers that overexpress the *HER2* gene, which is responsible for making more HER2 protein. In November 2006, it was approved as part of a chemotherapy combination to treat early stage breast cancer after surgery. In October 2010, trastuzumab was approved for use alone or in combination with a fluoropyrimidine and cisplatin as an initial treatment for metastatic adenocarcinomas in gastric tissue that overexpress *HER2*. In 2013, trastuzumab combined with another chemotherapy drug, DM1, was approved to treat metastatic *HER2*-positive breast cancer.

Delivery routes: Trastuzumab must be administered by a healthcare professional. Initial forms of the drug were available as standard intravenous infusions administered over 30 to 90 minutes, and these required loading doses and weight-based patient-specific maintenance doses. New in 2013, a trastuzumab subcutaneous formulation, available in some countries, is injected over only 5 minutes; the 5-ml dose contains 600 mg of drug for all patients but still requires administration in a clinical setting (not by the patient at home).

How these drugs work: Anti-HER2 targeted therapy with trastuzumab works at the cell surface to bind the HER2 receptor and block HER2 signals from increasing cell multiplication and growth. Because tumor cells in HER2-positive cancer have more HER2 receptors than normal cells, trastuzumab attaches more often to cancer cells than to normal cells. This type of targeted therapy aims to destroy cancer growth while leaving normal cells relatively untouched, which minimizes adverse effects. The HER2 blockade by trastuzumab also activates the immune system so that the body targets the tumor to destroy those cells to which the drug attaches.

Side effects: Congestive heart failure (CHF) is a dominant side effect of trastuzumab, occurring in 2% to 3% of patients (vs 1% in clinical trials). CHF is more likely when trastuzumab is given with an anthracycline, and the heart damage may be permanent. Less serious side effects, which often occur shortly after injection, include dizziness, headache, vomiting, and shortness of breath.

Nicole Van Hoey, PharmD

For Further Information

FDA. (2010). Trastuzumab (Herceptin) prescribing information. Retrieved from http://www.accessdata.fda.gov/drugsatfda_docs/label/2010/103792s5250lbl.pdf

Jackisch, C., Kim, S. B., Semiglazov, V., Melichar. B., Pivot, X. Hillenbach, C. ... Ismael, G. (2015). Subcutaneous versus intravenous formulation of trastuzumab for HER2-positive early breast cancer: updated results from the phase III HannaH study. *Annals of Oncology*, 26: 320-325.

National Cancer Institute. (2013, July 3). FDA approval for trastuzumab. Retrieved from http://www.cancer.gov/about-cancer/treatment/drugs/fda-trastuzumab#Anchor-Gastric

Roche Group Media Relations. (2013, February 22). FDA approves Roche's Kadcyla (trastuzumab emtansine), the first antibody-drug conjugate for treating HER2-postiive metastatic breast cancer. *Roche Media Release*, Retrieved from http://www.roche.com/media/store/releases/med-cor-2013-02-22.htm

Other Resources

Susan G. Komen: Trastuzumab (Herceptin)
http://ww5.komen.org/BreastCancer/Trastuzumab.html

BreastCancer.org: How Herceptin Works
http://www.breastcancer.org/treatment/targeted_therapies/herceptin/how_works?utm_medium=OBWidget&utm_source=OB

Genentech: Herceptin (trastuzumab)
http://www.gene.com/patients/medicines/herceptin

See also: Chemotherapy

▶ Tyrosine kinase inhibitors

Category: Chemotherapy and Other Drugs
ATC code: 101XE

Definition: Tyrosine kinase inhibitors are a class of antitumor drugs that act by specifically targeting tyrosine kinase enzymes. Tyrosine kinase inhibitors are particularly effective in slowing tumor growth and killing tumor cells because of the importance of these enzymes in determining cellular fate, including survival and proliferation.

Cancers treated: Chronic myeloid leukemia, gastrointestinal stromal tumors, non-small-cell lung cancer, pancreatic cancer, renal cell carcinoma, breast cancer, colorectal cancer

Subclasses of this group: Small molecule inhibitors, biologic antibody inhibitors

Delivery routes: The small molecule tyrosine kinase inhibitors are orally active and administered in a tablet form. Biologic antibody tyrosine kinase inhibitors are administered by a slow intravenous (IV) infusion, usually over the course of a few hours.

How these drugs work: Through basic scientific research, several proteins critical for cellular growth, survival, and proliferation have been identified. One of the largest classes of these proteins is known as tyrosine kinases. Kinases are enzymes, proteins that can perform a specific activity or function. Kinases act by transferring a phosphate group onto a substrate protein, a process called phosphorylation. In particular, tyrosine kinases add a phosphate group onto specific tyrosine amino acid residues in the substrate protein. Phosphorylation can perform many different functions, including activating the substrate protein through an "on-off" mechanism, inducing protein-protein interaction, and changing protein localization. The functional changes induced in the substrate protein are used in many different signaling pathways, including those important to relay growth and proliferation signals in cells.

Cells can react to many external stimuli, including circulating growth factors and hormones, through binding of these ligands to cell surface receptors. Many of these receptors are actually tyrosine kinases themselves, or signal directly to downstream tyrosine kinases after being activated. Therefore, the activity of tyrosine kinases is a critical part of the signaling required to transmit information from the outside of the cell to the cellular interior, affecting the fate of the cell. Tumor cells often hijack the normal essential function of tyrosine kinases, mutating these proteins so that they remain in a constitutive "on" state. Because the kinase activity is then unable to be halted, the signaling pathways are continuously activated, and uncontrolled cell growth and proliferation ensue.

Because of their importance in determining cellular fate, especially whether a cell will live or die, tyrosine kinases are a very attractive target for anticancer chemotherapy. There are two major categories of tyrosine kinase inhibitors, small molecule inhibitors and targeted biological therapy. The major mechanism of action of small molecule inhibitors is to inhibit the binding of adenosine triphosphate (ATP) to the kinase. Because tyrosine kinases use ATP as a source of phosphate groups to perform phosphorylation, the enzyme cannot phosphorylate substrate proteins, thereby reducing the activation of the downstream signaling pathways. The second major class of tyrosine kinase inhibitors is targeted therapy, using antibodies that are generated against the tyrosine kinase receptors that reside on the cellular surface. These antibodies mainly work by blocking the ligand-binding sites on these receptors, inhibiting the binding and thus the activation of these receptors. One of the main benefits of using tyrosine kinase inhibitors as an anticancer chemotherapy is that they can selectively target tumor cells compared to normal cells because tumor cells often develop a dependence on overactivated and overexpressed tyrosine kinases.

Side effects: The most common side effects of the oral small molecule inhibitors are nausea and vomiting, fatigue, muscle pain, fluid retention (swelling), and rash. In most cases, these symptoms can be effectively managed with medication, so that treatment can continue. The side effects caused by biologic antibody therapies are mainly induced by the actual administration of the drug. Many patients (approximately 40 percent) experience flulike symptoms, including fever, chills, muscle aches, and nausea. These side effects are generally lessened with the administration of drugs such as acetaminophen.

Lisa M. Cockrell, B.S.

For Further Information

Fabbro, Doriano, and Frank McCormick, eds. *Protein Tyrosine Kinases: From Inhibitors to Useful Drugs.* Totowa, N.J.: Humana Press, 2006.

Kantarjian, Hagop M., et al. *The M. D. Anderson Manual of Medical Oncology*. New York: McGraw-Hill, 2006.

Kufe, Donald W., et al., eds. *Holland Frei Cancer Medicine 7*. 7th ed. Hamilton, Ont.: BC Decker, 2006.

Pratt, William B., et al. *The Anticancer Drugs*. 2d ed. New York: Oxford University Press, 1994.

Skeel, Roland T. *Handbook of Cancer Chemotherapy*. 7th ed. Philadelphia: Lippincott Williams & Wilkins, 2007.

Other Resources

American Cancer Society
http://www.cancer.org

National Cancer Institute
Drug Information Summaries
http://www.cancer.gov/cancertopics/druginfo/alphalist

See also: Biological therapy; Breast cancers; Bronchial adenomas; Carcinomas; Chemotherapy; Chronic Myeloid Leukemia (CML); Gastrointestinal complications of cancer treatment; Gastrointestinal Stromal Tumors (GISTs); Infusion therapies; Leukemias; Lung cancers; Medical

Common Tyrosine Kinase Inhibitors

Drug	*Brands*	*Subclass*	*Delivery Mode*	*Conditions Treated*
Cetuximab	Erbitux	Biologic antibody therapy	IV	Metastatic colorectal cancer, head and neck cancer
Dasatinib	Sprycel	Small molecule inhibitor	Oral	Chronic myeloid leukemia, Philadelphia chromosome-positive acute lymphoblastic leukemia
Erlotinib	Tarceva	Small molecule inhibitor	Oral	Advanced non-small-cell lung cancer, advanced pancreatic cancer
Gefitinib	Iressa	Small molecule inhibitor	Oral	Advanced or metastatic non-small-cell lung cancer
Imatinib	Gleevec	Small molecule inhibitor	Oral	Philadelphia chromosome-positive chronic myeloid leukemia, gastrointestinal stromal tumor
Lapatinib	Tykerb	Small molecule inhibitor	Oral	Advanced or metastatic HER2-positive breast cancer
Sorafenib	Nexavar	Small molecule inhibitor	Oral	Advanced renal cell carcinoma
Sunitinib	Sutent	Small molecule inhibitor	Oral	Advanced renal cell carcinoma, gastrointestinal stromal tumor
Trastuzumab	Herceptin	Biologic antibody therapy	IV	HER2-positive breast cancer

oncology; Nausea and vomiting; Oncology; Pancreatic cancers; Rectal cancer

▶ Vaccines, preventive

Category: Chemotherapy and Other Drugs
ATC code: J07BC01, J07BM01, J07BM02

Definition: Vaccines are biological drugs used to induce immunity against a germ (virus or bacterium) without causing disease. After vaccination, the body's immune system develops antibodies that then kill or neutralize the germ if exposed to it. These antibodies circulate in the bloodstream. The immune response induced by a vaccine may decrease or wane over time, requiring a booster dose—some vaccines require three or more doses to provide full protection against the germ.

Vaccines may contain live germs that have been weakened so that they cannot cause disease; killed or inactivated viruses that cannot cause an infection but can stimulate antibody production; toxoids (harmless bacterial toxins) that do not cause illness but stimulate production of antibody; and parts or components of bacteria or viruses, which cannot cause disease but generate an immune response.

Cancers treated: Liver cancer, cervical cancer

Subclasses of this group: Recombinant DNA hepatitis B vaccine, plasma-derived hepatitis B vaccine, quadrivalent human papillomavirus (HPV) vaccine

Delivery routes: The hepatitis B vaccine is administered by intramuscular injection in the anterolateral thigh of infants twenty-four months of age and younger and in the deltoid muscle (shoulder) of older children, adolescents, and adults. Most people should receive three doses of the vaccine.

The HPV vaccine is also administered by intramuscular injection of 0.5 milliliter in three doses. The second and third doses should be administered two and six months after the first dose.

How these drugs work: Hepatitis B vaccine prevents hepatitis B disease and its serious consequences, such as hepatocellular carcinoma (liver cancer). The recombinant hepatitis B vaccine is made by copying the genetic sequence of a protein contained in the hepatitis B virus into a yeast cell, which is then cultured and purified. The immunization series with hepatitis B vaccines is 95 percent effective at inducing immunity.

Plasma-derived hepatitis B vaccines are made by harvesting particles of the hepatitis B surface antigen (HBsAg) from plasma of people with chronic hepatitis B infection. HBsAg is a component of the hepatitis B virus that appears in the blood before symptoms of the disease. The HBsAg particles are purified and inactivated with heat or chemicals to produce the vaccine.

Available HPV vaccines protect against two types of the virus that cause about 70 percent of cervical cancer cases—types 16 and 18. The vaccine is produced by assembling the L1 protein of HPV types 16 and 18 into virus-like-particles (VLPs). VLPs look like the virus to the immune system but do not contain deoxyribonucleic acid (DNA), so they cannot replicate and cause disease. The HPV vaccine will only protect women who have not previously been infected with HPV. The other two types included in the quadrivalent version of the vaccine—HPV 6 and HPV 11—are intended to protect against genital warts, not cancer.

The quadrivalent HPV vaccine has been tested in thousands of women sixteen to twenty-six years of age. Clinical trials showed the vaccine to be 100 percent effective in preventing cervical precancers caused by types 16 and 18 in women who had not been previously exposed to these HPV types. Also, the vaccine was almost 100 percent effective in preventing vulvar and vaginal precancers and genital warts caused by the HPV types in the vaccine.

People vaccinated against hepatitis B or HPV can still develop liver cancer or cervical cancer. Chronic hepatitis B infection is only one of many risk factors for liver cancer, and 30 percent of cervical cancer cases are caused by HPV types not included in the current HPV vaccines.

Side effects: Of those who receive the hepatitis B vaccine, 65 percent do not experience any side effects. Only 3 percent of recipients will develop pain and tenderness where the injection has been given, and between 1 and 6 percent of recipients will have a low-grade fever. Serious allergic reactions occur in less than 1 out of 10,000 vaccines given, or about 0.001 percent. Serious allergic reactions include anaphylaxis, a rapid life-threatening allergic response affecting more than one part of the body—it may also affect the whole body, causing the airway to swell, close off, and prevent the intake of oxygen.

Studies of more than 11,000 women between nine and twenty-six years of age around the world have shown that the quadrivalent HPV vaccine causes no serious side effects, but 84 percent of vaccine recipients experienced pain at the injection site. Other mild-to-moderate side effects were swelling and redness at the injection site.

Diego Pineda, M.S.

Licensed Anticancer Vaccines

Drug	*Brands*	*Subclasses*	*Delivery Mode*	*Cancers Treated*
Hepatitis B vaccine	Engerix-B, Recombivax HB, Comvax, Twinrix, Pediarix	Recombinant DNA hepatitis B vaccine, plasma-derived hepatitis B vaccine	Injection	Liver cancer
Human papillomavirus (HPV) vaccine	Gardasil, Cervarix	Quadrivalent human papillomavirus (HPV) vaccine	Injection	Cervical cancer, anogenital cancers

For Further Information

Offit, Paul A. *Vaccinated: One Man's Quest to Defeat the World's Deadliest Diseases*. New York: Collins, 2007.

Offit, Paul A., and Louis M. Bell. *Vaccines: What You Should Know*. New York: Wiley, 2003.

Plotkin, Stanley A., Walter A. Orenstein, and Paul A. Offit, eds. *Vaccines*. 5th ed. Philadelphia: Saunders/Elsevier, 2008.

Other Resources

Liver Cancer Network
http://www.livercancer.com

National Cancer Institute
Human Papillomaviruses and Cancer: Questions and Answers
http://www.cancer.gov/cancertopics/factsheet/Risk/HPV

National Network for Immunization Information
http://www.immunizationinfo.org

See also: Biological therapy; Complementary and alternative therapies; Immune response to cancer; Immunotherapy; Infectious cancers; Prevent Cancer Foundation; Prevention; Vaccines, therapeutic; Virus-related cancers

▶ Vaccines, therapeutic

Category: Chemotherapy and Other Drugs
Also known as: Biological therapy, immunotherapy

Definition: Therapeutic vaccines treat cancer by stimulating the body's natural immune system. Therapeutic vaccines contain the whole cancer cell, parts of cells, or components of the body's immune system.

Cancers treated: The Food and Drug Administration (FDA) does not currently license any therapeutic vaccines. Advanced phase III clinical trials are now in progress to evaluate vaccines against a variety of cancers.

Subclasses of this group: Whole cell vaccines, heat shock proteins, antigen/adjuvant vaccines, dendritic cell vaccines, anti-idiotype vaccines, DNA vaccines

Delivery routes: Cancer vaccines may be delivered by scarification (scratch), subcutaneous or intramuscular injection, or intranasally. The delivery route depends on the type of vaccine and cancer.

How these drugs work: The immune system is very complex and interconnected. It consists of various types of white blood cells (lymphocytes) and cytokines. The immune system is stimulated when it identifies foreign molecules known as antigens. The immune response can be either humoral (body fluids) or cellular. In the cellular process, phagocytes (macrophages and dendritic cells) engulf and digest cells and particles. The resultant fragments are attached to a molecule known as the major histocompatibility complex (MHC) and are presented on the cell surface. They are therefore known as antigen presenting cells (APCs). If helper T cells recognize the fragments as antigens, then they can either activate B cells to produce antibodies or activate cytotoxic T cells to kill the foreign invader or cancer cell directly. Another process involves natural killer (NK) cells. These cells are activated to destroy cancer cells when they recognize abnormalities on the surfaces of cells. Cytokines are soluble proteins secreted by activated immune cells. They facilitate communication and function among immune system components and enhance the immune response.

Therapeutic vaccines are used to treat existing cancers, in contrast to the traditional role of vaccines to prevent infectious diseases. The immune response is very specific, so cancer vaccines have been developed to selectively destroy cancer cells without harming normal cells. Unfortunately, the field has been fraught with disappointments over the last century. A basic problem lies with the fact that cancer cells are derived from normal cells. Success depends on the immune system recognizing very small molecular differences between normal and cancer cells. Although the immune system does respond naturally to the presence of cancer cells, this response is often weak and the cancer may be tolerated.

Cancer cells develop many methods to evade the immune system. They can hide their identity by repressing display of their antigens. They can alter their metabolism to become resistant to attacks by the immune system. They can secrete cytokines that kill lymphocytes. Cancer cells can actively suppress the activation and function of dendritic cells and T cells.

A variety of therapeutic vaccines have been developed. A key goal of the vaccines is to enhance the immune system's response to cancer antigens. Preparations include whole cell vaccines, heat shock proteins, antigen/adjuvant vaccines, dendritic cell vaccines, anti-idiotype vaccines, and DNA vaccines.

Whole cell vaccines are prepared from the patient's whole cancer cells. Whole cell vaccines do not require the identification of antigens but presumably contain the full array of cancer antigens. Unfortunately, early whole cell vaccines were not very effective. Researchers discovered that T cells are activated only when a second co-stimulatory molecule is present. Current whole cell vaccines are genetically modified to secrete cytokines or express co-stimulatory molecules.

Heat shock proteins are found in most cells and serve to repair protein structure. They are often found in excess in cancer cells. Vaccines are prepared by purifying heat shock proteins from tumor tissue removed from the patient and linking these to tumor antigen. Administration of the vaccine results in uptake and processing by APCs and a strong T-cell response.

Antigen/adjuvant vaccines are prepared by combining a known cancer antigen with a chemical known as an adjuvant, which enhances the effect of the antigen.

Dendritic cell vaccines have been found very effective. To prepare the vaccines, dendritic cells are removed from the patient, exposed to the patient's own cancer antigens in the laboratory, and grown in culture. When the resultant vaccine is injected into the patient, the T cells in the immune system are stimulated to attack the tumor cells.

Anti-idiotype vaccines have been developed for use against cancers that poorly present antigens. Antibodies that are produced in response to an antigen have unique antigen regions called idiotypes. The body can produce antibodies to these idiotypes that are called anti-idiotypes. Anti-idiotype vaccines can be prepared in the laboratory, often using synthetic monoclonal antibodies. Since these anti-idiotype vaccines appear to be like the tumor antigen, they stimulate a stronger immune response.

DNA vaccines are based on genes that code for antigen proteins. When these vaccines are administered, they are taken up by APCs. The vaccines are delivered to the APCs by means of vectors, such as modified viruses, bacteria, or synthetic polymers. Within the APCs, antigen protein is produced and presented to the T cells. This method provides a continuous supply of antigen to maintain the immune response.

Side effects: The primary concern with therapeutic vaccines is the development of autoimmune responses, although this seldom occurs. Some patients may experience a skin reaction or mild flulike symptoms.

David A. Olle, M.S.

For Further Information

Finn, Olivera J. "Cancer Vaccines: Between the Idea and the Reality." *Nature Reviews Immunology* 3, no. 8 (August, 2003): 630-641.

Greten, Tim F., and Elizabeth M. Jaffe. "Cancer Vaccines." *Journal of Clinical Oncology* 17, no. 3 (March, 1999): 1047-1060.

Orentas, Rimas, James W. Hodge, and Bryon D. Johnson, eds. *Cancer Vaccines and Tumor Immunity*. Hoboken, N.J.: Wiley-Interscience, 2008.

Weinberg, Robert A. *The Biology of Cancer*. New York: Garland Science, Taylor & Francis, 2007.

Other Resources

American Cancer Society

Cancer Vaccines

http://www.cancer.org/docroot/ETO/content/ETO_1_4X_Cancer_Vaccines_Active_Specific_Immunotherapies.asp?sitearea=ETO

National Cancer Institute

Cancer Vaccine Fact Sheet

http://www.cancer.gov/cancertopics/factsheet/cancervaccine

See also: Bacillus Calmette Guérin (BCG); Biological therapy; Chemoprevention; Complementary and alternative therapies; Cytokines; Duke Comprehensive Cancer Center; Immune response to cancer; Immunotherapy; Vaccines, preventive

▶ Vorinostat

Category: Chemotherapy and Other Drugs
Also known as: Zolinza, SAHA, suberanilohydroxamic acid, MK-0683, MSK390, N-hydroxy-N'-phenyloctanediamide; ChemID base # CID5311

Definition: Vorinostat is a small molecule that crosses the blood-brain barrier. Specifically, it is a type of cytotoxic drug called a histone deacetylase (HDAC) inhibitor. HDACs are enzymes found in the cells of all nucleated organisms. They play vital roles in numerous cell processes, including gene expression, signal transduction, cell death and survival, and cancer. Vorinostat was the first HDAC inhibitor approved to treat cancer. It functions to prevent normal histone deacetylation. This leads to a state of histone hyperacetylation, which results in cell-cycle arrest. Vorinostat is a second-generation, reversible inhibitor of HDACs. It is marketed by Merck, and synthesized in the laboratory.

Cancers treated: In October 2006, vorinostat was approved for the treatment of cutaneous T-cell lymphoma (particularly of the skin-related changes of the disease that have recurred or relapsed after 2 other systemic chemotherapy treatments). This type of aggressive T-cell lymphoma is also called Sezary syndrome and is characterized by different skin lesions. For the treatment of T-cell lymphoma, vorinostat may be taken alone or in combination with other cytotoxic or immune-modulating drugs, including interferon gamma or bexarotene.

Delivery routes: Vorinostat is taken by mouth once daily. It comes in 100-mg capsules that contain a white to light orange powder, and it is usually taken as a 400-mg dose. Daily doses may be reduced to 300 mg as often as 5 times each week for patients who poorly tolerate the full strength. Vorinostat should be taken with food.

How these drugs work: To prevent histone deacetylation, vorinostat binds to HDACs within the cell cytoplasm or nucleus. In addition to inducing apoptosis, vorinostat blocks pro-growth and pro-survival proteins in tumors. Unlike chemotherapeutic drugs that only work during one part of a cell cycle or only on cells with certain gene mutations, vorinostat inhibits HDACs found in cells at any stage of the cell cycle. Although vorinostat activity is not specific to tumor cells, HDACs may be overexpressed in tumor cells.

Side effects: Some of the most common side effects of vorinostat include fatigue, chills, anemia, and thrombocytopenia; and gastrointestinal symptoms, including dry mouth and dysgeusia. Pulmonary embolism and deep vein thrombosis have occurred at rates as high as 5%. Patients with a history of thromboembolic events should be carefully monitored while taking vorinostat. Additionally, vorinostat may increase blood sugar in up to 25% of patients. Therefore, it should be used cautiously in patients with diabetes or on antidiabetic therapy, and insulin regimens might need adjustment. Vorinostat crosses the placenta and damages the developing fetus, and, therefore, is in pregnancy category D. In animal studies, vorinostat has been associated with decreased fetal weight and numerous skeletal development impairments. It should not be used during pregnancy, nursing, or when conception or pregnancy is possible.

Nicole Van Hoey, PharmD

For Further Information

Dokmanovic, M., Clarke, C., & Marks, P. A. (2007). Histone deacetylase inhibitors: Overview and perspectives. *Molecular Cancer Research*, 5: 981-989. http://mcr.aacrjournals.org/content/5/10/981.full

Kavanaugh, S. A., White, L. A., & Kolesar, J. M. (2010). Vorinostat: A novel therapy for the treatment of cutaneous T-cell lymphoma. *American Journal of Health System Pharmacy*, 67: 793-797.

Richon, V. M. (2006). Cancer biology: Mechanism of antitumour action of vorinostat (suberoylanilide hydroxamic acid), a novel histone deacetylase inhibitor. *British Journal of Cancer*, 95: S2-S6. http://www.nature.com/bjc/journal/v95/n1s/full/6603463a.html

Other Resources

Merck.com: Zolinza (vorinostat) prescribing information
https://www.merck.com/product/usa/pi_circulars/z/zolinza/zolinza_pi.pdf

HDAC Inhibitors Base
http://www.hdacis.com

ChemoCare: Vorinostat fact sheet
http://chemocare.com/chemotherapy/drug-info/Vorinostat.aspx

UpToDate: Treatment of Sezary syndrome
http://www.uptodate.com/contents/treatment-of-sezary-syndrome

PubChem Open Chemistry Database: Vorinostat compound summary
http://pubchem.ncbi.nlm.nih.gov/compound/Vorinostat#section=Therapeutic-Uses

See also: Chemotherapy

▶ Antioxidants

Category: Complementary and Alternative Therapies; Lifestyle and Prevention

Definition: Antioxidants are a class of compounds that help prevent damage to deoxyribonucleic acid (DNA), cellular proteins, and cell membranes by combining with potentially damaging molecules called free radicals and neutralizing them. The body naturally makes many antioxidants, while others are found in fruits, vegetables, and grains. Antioxidants are also produced synthetically as dietary supplements.

Cancers treated or prevented: Antioxidants are used to treat most types of cancer, although their effectiveness is questionable. They are usually taken for cancer prevention, although the link between antioxidant consumption and cancer prevention in humans is not proven.

Delivery routes: Oral, as tablets, caplets, capsules, powder, or tea; some fruits and vegetables are high in antioxidants

How these compounds work: Free radicals are formed during normal cellular metabolism. Free radicals are compounds that are unstable because they contain an unpaired electron. This unpaired electron causes the free radical to react with other molecules in order to gain another electron, creating an electron pair and a more stable molecule. The process of gaining an electron is called oxidation. Antioxidants in the body react with free radicals and make them harmless to cells. Cells naturally make many antioxidants such as glutathione and coenzyme Q10 (ubiquinone). When the number of free radicals exceeds the antioxidants available to neutralize them, however, the body develops a condition called oxidative stress. Oxidative stress appears to make cells especially susceptible to damage.

Free radical formation and oxidation are normal processes. Oxidation and oxidative stress, however, are thought to contribute to aging, as well as to cancer, cardiovascular disease, and other chronic diseases. In the absence of adequate antioxidant compounds, free radicals most often combine with and damage DNA, cellular proteins, and molecules in cell membranes. This damage can cause gene mutations and change cellular metabolism, which may lead to cancer and other diseases. Exposure to ultraviolet (UV) light, radiation, cigarette smoke, and other known carcinogens increases the number of free radicals that are formed, suggesting another link between free radicals, oxidative stress, and cancer.

In theory, increasing the amount of antioxidants in the body should decrease the amount of damage to DNA and cells and reduce the risk of cancer. Antioxidants have been shown to prevent or slow the development of some cancers in cell cultures grown in the laboratory and in some animal studies. The results in human studies have been mixed. Despite claims by some manufacturers of antioxidant dietary supplements, no clear link between antioxidant consumption and cancer prevention or treatment has been established in humans. The role of antioxidants in the prevention and treatment of cancer is of high interest to research scientists. Many clinical trials are being conducted, and there is no cost for qualified individuals to participate in a clinical trial.

The body makes some antioxidants, but others must be acquired through diet. Common antioxidants that the body does not make include vitamins A, C, and E, carotenoids, and flavonoids. Selenium is a mineral that is not strictly an antioxidant but is essential to many antioxidant reactions and often classed with the antioxidants. Coenzyme Q10 and glutathione are antioxidants naturally produced by the body that are also manufactured sold as high-dose supplements.

Vitamin A (retinol) is a fat-soluble vitamin found in liver, egg yolks, whole milk, and dairy products made with whole milk. It is also sold as a dietary supplement and is included in most multivitamin tablets and in special antioxidant formulations such as ACE, a combination of vitamins A, C, and E. Vitamin A is essential to health, but its role in cancer prevention and treatment is unclear. All-*trans*-retinoic acid (ATRA, Vesanoid) is a pharmaceutical drug that is a derivative of vitamin A. It is successfully used to treat promyelocytic leukemia and is being studied in individuals with breast and skin cancers. To date, however, vitamin A alone has not shown the same cancer-reducing effects as ATRA.

Alpha-carotene, beta-carotene, beta-cryptoxanthin, lutein, zeaxanthin, and lycopene are all carotenoids that show antioxidant activity in laboratory tests. These compounds are found in red, yellow, and orange plants such as carrots, cantaloupe, mango, and tomato. Beta-carotene and lycopene are also sold as dietary supplements either individually or in combination with other antioxidants. In the body, carotenoids are converted into vitamin A. An examination of twenty-one studies relating lycopene consumption and prostate cancer found that men with the highest lycopene intake had a modest decrease in the incidence of prostate cancer. The role of carotenoids in cancer prevention is actively being studied.

Vitamin C (ascorbic acid) is a water-soluble vitamin found in citrus fruits. For centuries, it has been known

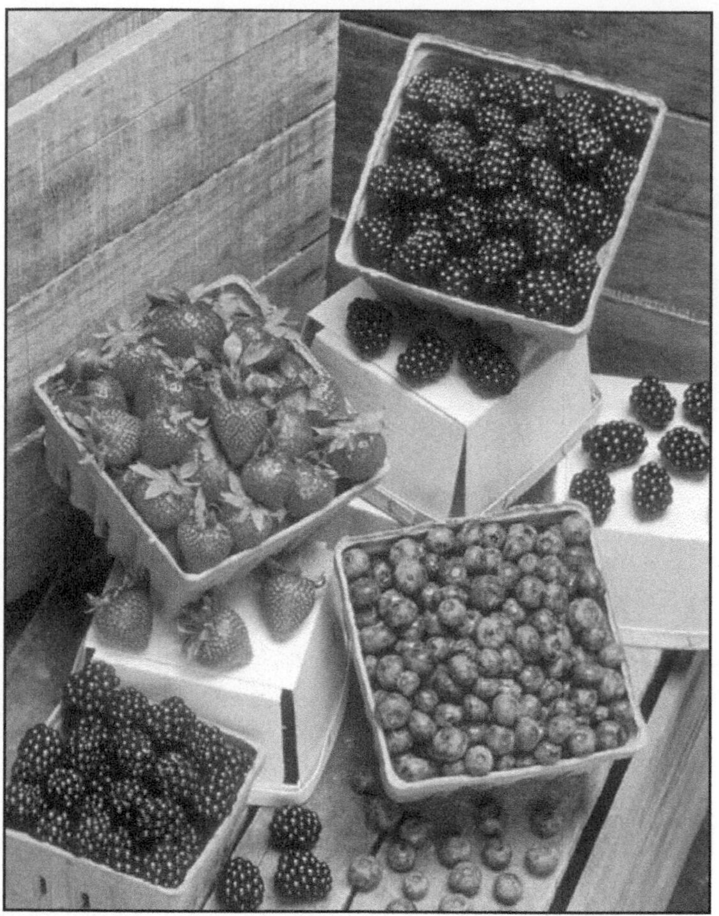

Berries contain flavonoids, a group of antioxidant compounds. (U.S. Department of Agriculture)

that vitamin C is essential for preventing the disease scurvy. Dietary supplements of vitamin C are often promoted as a preventive or treatment for the common cold, although clinical studies have not proved its effectiveness. Vitamin C has very strong antioxidant activities. Nevertheless, multiple human studies have failed to find a significant link between cancer prevention and vitamin C intake.

Vitamin E is a group of related compounds, the most active of which is alpha-tocopherol. Vitamin E is a fat-soluble vitamin with antioxidant properties. It is found in olive, sunflower, and safflower oils and in many nuts. The role of vitamin E in cancer prevention is controversial. In 2004, researchers at The Johns Hopkins University Medical School did a meta-analysis of nineteen clinical trials that included more than 136,000 individuals. This analysis showed that taking more than 400 international units (IU) of synthetic vitamin E daily increased the chance of dying by about 4 percent. This amount is less than the safe daily upper limit of 1,500 IU recommended by the United States Institute of Medicine for adults age nineteen and older. The Johns Hopkins analysis has been criticized because it did not differentiate between individuals taking different forms of vitamin E, such as the dietary supplement alpha-tocopherol acetate. This is a significant criticism because different forms of vitamin E have different activity levels in the body.

Flavonoids are a group of antioxidant compounds found primarily in brewed tea, red wine, dark chocolate, apples, berries, and citrus fruits. These compounds have antioxidant activity. Traditional Chinese medicine has promoted the health effects of green tea for centuries, and recent studies show that dark (bitter) chocolate in small quantities may promote heart health, but the role of flavonoids in cancer prevention is unclear.

Selenium is a mineral found in fish, shellfish, grains, Brazil nuts, and many vegetables that are grown in selenium-rich soils. By itself, selenium is not an antioxidant, but it plays a critical role in antioxidant activity and is often classified with the antioxidants that must be acquired through diet. Selenium deficiency has been linked to increases in colorectal, lung, and prostate cancers. Increased selenium intake in people who are not selenium deficient, however, does not decrease the risk of developing cancer. Additionally, selenium is toxic in large doses.

Coenzyme Q10 and glutathione are the main antioxidants made by the body. They are also sold as dietary supplements. Studies of individuals who supplemented their diet with synthetic coenzyme Q10 or glutathione found no evidence that these supplements protected against cancer.

Individuals who maintain a healthy weight and eat a diet low in fats and high in fruits, vegetables, and whole grains develop cancer at a lower rate than individuals who eat a more traditional American diet high in fat and low in fruits and vegetables. The American Cancer Society and the National Cancer Institute recommend that individuals meet as many of their vitamin, mineral, and antioxidant needs as possible by eating a healthy, varied diet rather than by taking dietary supplements. As of 2008, neither organization recommended the use of antioxidant supplements to treat or prevent cancer.

Side effects: In 2007, a peer-reviewed meta-analysis of antioxidant studies was published in the *Journal of the American Medical Association*. Researchers looked at the data from sixty-eight clinical trials involving 232,606 individuals. They found that taking dietary supplements of vitamin A, beta-carotene, and vitamin E increased the risk of death from all causes by 5 percent. This increase was not seen in individuals who took vitamin C dietary supplements. The study did not look at individuals who increased their intake of these antioxidants through diet.

Martiscia Davidson, A.M.

For Further Information

DeCava, Judith A. *The Real Truth About Vitamins and Antioxidants*. 2d ed. Fort Collins, Colo.: Selene River Press, 2006.

Frei, Balz, ed. *Natural Antioxidants in Human Health and Disease*. San Diego, Calif.: Academic Press, 2006.

Panglossi, Harold V., ed. *Antioxidants: New Research*. New York: Nova Science, 2006.

Quillin, Patrick. *Beating Cancer with Nutrition*. 4th ed. Tulsa, Okla.: Nutrition Times Press, 2005.

Other Resources

American Cancer Society

Antioxidants and Cancer: The Jury's Still Out
http://www.cancer.org/docroot/NWS/content/NWS_2_1x_Antioxidants_and_Cancer_The_Jurys_Still_Out.asp

MedlinePlus

Antioxidants
http://www.nlm.nih.gov/medlineplus/antioxidants.html

National Cancer Institute

Antioxidants and Cancer Prevention: Fact Sheet
http://www.cancer.gov/cancertopics/factsheet/antioxidantsprevention

See also: Beta-carotene; Bioflavonoids; Carotenoids; Chemoprevention; Coenzyme Q10; Complementary and alternative therapies; Curcumin; Dietary supplements; Essiac; Free radicals; Fruits; Garlic and allicin; Green tea; Herbs as antioxidants; Isoflavones; Lutein; Lycopene; Nutrition and cancer prevention; Phenolics; Phytoestrogens; Resveratrol; Wine and cancer

▶ Chinese medicine and cancer

Category: Complementary and Alternative Therapies
Also known as: Traditional Chinese medicine; TCM; Traditional Asian medicine

Definition: Chinese medicine, better known as traditional Chinese medicine (TCM), is a complex system of health care that focuses as much on prevention and cause as on cure. According to TCM, health depends on the balance of the mind, body, and environment, and on the flow of "chi," or energy, the vital life force. Many aspects of TCM are not recognized in Western médicine, but it is gaining credence as a potentially effective complementary treatment (treatment given along with standard therapy) for some conditions, including cancer.

Cancers treated or prevented: Because TCM addresses both prevention and treatment of disease; TCM practitioners address nearly all types of cancers. For example, treatments with some herbal cocktails (one of the main delivery routes of TCM) have shown promise for breast cancer, non-small cell lung cancer, and liver cancer. Because TCM is tailored to each patient, however, it is difficult to test using clinical trials to compare its effectiveness to conventional Western medicine. TCM practitioners measure effectiveness by looking at how the patient feels overall and at the balance of chi in the body.

Delivery routes: TCM uses 3 main pathways in preventing and treating illness: 1) Herbs alone or in combinations, usually taken in the form of a tea; 2) Acupuncture; and 3) Moving and breathing exercises, such as tai chi.

How this substance works: TCM practitioners view cancer as an "imbalance" of the whole person. Treatments address this imbalance.

Herbs and herbal combinations, many derived from folk medicine, are used to correct balance and energy flow. Four types of herbs are used in cancer prevention and treatment.

A. Anticancer herbs are used to slow tumor growth. The effectiveness of some of these herbs has been shown in laboratory experiments with animals and in a few clinical trials (although more trials are needed). Some of these herbs are the sources of chemotherapy drugs, such as indirubin, which is used to treat chronic myelogenous leukemia.

B. Immune-boosting herbs counteract the side effects of Western medical therapies and help the immune system attack the cancer.

C. Blood-vitalizing herbs are said to enhance the effectiveness of Western cancer therapies by boosting the body's natural healing process.

D. Phlegm-resolving herbs are used to treat abnormal masses, such as ovarian cysts, thyroid nodules, lymphatic swellings, and breast lumps that are not hardened; some of these masses can be malignant.

Two herbs, in particular, have shown to be effective in the treatment of certain cancers. Astragalus root is used to increase energy and improve the immune system. Researchers have found that astragalus inhibits tumor growth, blocks the spread of tumors, and reduces some of the side effects of chemotherapy on the immune system. It may also enhance the effectiveness of some chemotherapy drugs. *Oldenlandia diffusa*, known as snake needle grass in the United States, has shown promise in preventing the spread of cancer and even reversing some cancers in the laboratory and in animal studies. The herb kills cancer cells and activates the immune system to seek and destroy tumor cells.

Acupuncture is, by now, well known and accepted, at least to some degree, in the West. In treating cancers, acupuncture is used as a complementary therapy. According to TCM, acupuncture benefits cancer patients by unblocking chi, restoring energy levels to the body as a whole, and reestablishing homeostasis, or the natural balance in a healthy body.

In Western terms, acupuncture seems to stimulate certain responses in nerve cells, the pituitary gland, and parts of the brain. Nerve cells are specialized cells in the central nervous system that signal other cells to act to protect the body and prompt natural healing. When excited, the pituitary gland releases endorphins, the body's natural painkillers. And certain chemicals in the brain—notably serotonin and dopamine—are important stress reducers.

In cancer treatment, acupuncture is used to manage these common side effects of treatment:

- Pain
- Fatigue
- Nausea and vomiting
- Diarrhea and constipation
- Loss of appetite
- Weight loss
- Depression and anxiety
- Sleep disturbances
- Dry mouth

In addition, studies suggest that acupuncture may help the immune system, which is often affected by aggressive chemotherapy. Also, acupuncture can potentially reduce the need for narcotics, thereby reducing the side effects of their use. Currently, higher-quality studies on acupuncture are needed.

Tai chi is a system of exercises that combines slow, graceful, deliberate movements with mindfulness meditation and breathing techniques. Its gentle approach makes tai chi an ideal complementary treatment for cancer patients. Research has shown that the physical benefits of tai chi include enhanced immune function, heart and lung function, balance, flexibility, and strength.

But tai chi's greatest benefit for cancer patients is helping them cope with the psychological stresses of cancer. Through tai chi, patients learn to accept and deal with forces beyond their control, including the common notion of blaming oneself for one's cancer. This leads to overall improved feelings of well-being.

Side effects: Side effects of TCM treatments are mostly mild and short-lived. Side effects are usually due to unskilled practitioners rather than to the therapeutic agent.

Problems with TCM herbals include poor quality of the herbs used and herbal misidentification, which, can lead to poisoning.

The most common risks of acupuncture are infection from unsterile needles (in the United States, acupuncturists must use only sterilized needles and dispose of them after one use) and inserting a needle into the wrong spot, which can lead to soreness.

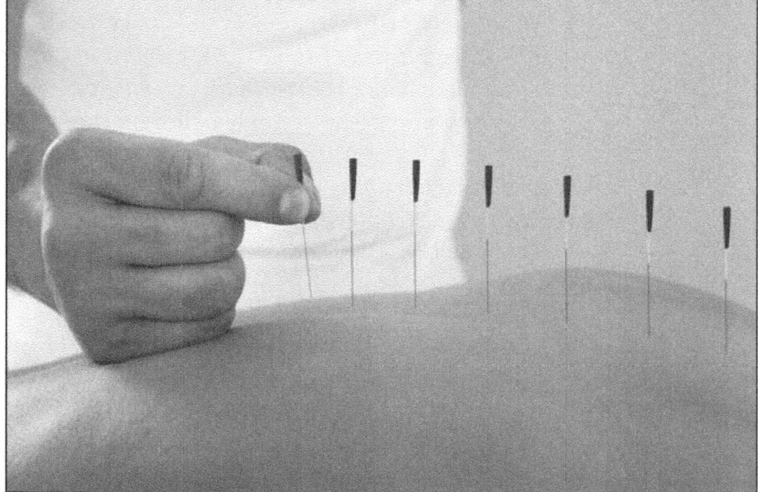

Acupuncture was originally a form of medicine practiced in ancient China, but it has now also become widely popular in the West. (iStock)

The only side effects of tai chi and other such exercises are the occasional muscle and joint pain when the patient overdoes the exercise.

Wendell Anderson, BA
Eugene, Oregon

For Further Information

Chandwani, K., Ryan, J. L., Peppone, L. J., Janelsins, M. M. Sprod, L. K., Devine, K., ...Mustian, K. M. (2012). Cancer-related stress and complementary and alternative medicine: A review. *Evidence-Based*

Complementary and Alternative Medicine, Volume 2012 (2012), Article ID 979213, 15 pages. http://dx.doi.org/10.1155/2012/979213

Konkimalla, V. B., & Efferth, T. (2008). Evidence-based Chinese medicine for cancer therapy. *Journal of Ethnopharmacology, 116*(2): 207–210.

Lu, W., Dean-Clower E., Doherty-Gilman A., & Rosenthal D. S. (2008). The value of acupuncture in cancer care. *Hematology/Oncology Clinics of North America 22*(4), 631–648.

Other Resources

Cancer Research United Kingdom
http://www.cancerresearchuk.org

American Academy of Medical Acupuncture
http://www.medicalacupuncture.org/Home.aspx

▶ Coenzyme Q10

Category: Lifestyle and Prevention; Complementary and Alternative Therapies
Also known as: Co Q 10, ubiquinone, vitamin Q 10

Definition: Coenzyme Q10 is a fat-soluble vitamin or vitamin-like substance sometimes used in cancer treatment and prevention. A vitamin is an organic compound needed in very small amounts for the body to function normally. Vitamins serve as coenzymes or precursors to coenzymes that are normally present in food or may sometimes be generated in the body. Coenzyme Q10 is produced in all bodily tissues and is present in tiny quantities in food.

Coenzyme Q10 has been shown to significantly reduce the cardiotoxicity of cancer chemotherapy drugs such as Adriamycin (doxorubicin). Studies of coenzyme Q10 used as an adjuvant to boost therapeutic outcome following standard treatment for breast cancer showed good results in a small number of patients; the studies, however, were neither randomized nor controlled.

Cancers treated or prevented: All, particularly breast cancer

Delivery routes: Orally as a pill (capsule or tablet) or intravenously (IV injection), the latter in animal studies

How this substance works: Coenzyme Q10 was first isolated from beef heart mitochondria (energy-producing structures in the cell) by Dr. Frederick Crane in 1957. A year later, Karl Folkers determined the exact structure of coenzyme Q10. Coenzymes are cofactors upon which the relatively large and complex enzymes absolutely depend in order to function. Coenzyme Q10 acts as a coenzyme for at least three mitochondrial enzymes in addition to enzymes in other areas of the cell. Mitochondrial enzymes are crucial for the production of high-energy adenosine triphosphate (ATP), upon which all cellular activities depend; coenzyme Q10 acts as a coenzyme for several of the key enzymatic energy-generating steps in the cell. It also serves as an antioxidant vital to its clinical effects. Studies in animals found that coenzyme Q10 boosts the immune system and may be helpful in fighting certain infections and cancer. Since some conventional cancer therapies such as drugs and radiation therapy destroy cancer cells by producing free radicals, researchers are trying to find out whether coenzyme Q10 in conjunction with traditional cancer treatments may affect the outcome.

Side effects: While no serious side effects have been reported with coenzyme Q10 usage, the most frequently reported side effects include insomnia, higher-than-usual levels of liver enzymes, upper abdomenal pain, sensitivity to light, irritability, headache, dizziness, heartburn, and extreme fatigue. It should be kept in mind that coenzyme Q10 is a dietary supplement; it has not been approved for use as a cancer treatment by the Food and Drug Administration (FDA) and is regulated not as a drug but as a food.

Cynthia Racer, M.A., M.P.H.

See also: Anthraquinones; Antioxidants

▶ Complementary and Alternative Therapies

Category: Complementary and Alternative Therapies
Also known as: Complementary and alternative medicine (CAM)

Definition: Complementary and alternative medicine (CAM) is defined by the National Center for Complementary and Alternative Medicine (NCCAM) as a group of diverse medical and health care systems, products, and practices not presently considered part of conventional medicine.

Differences between complementary and alternative medicine: Complementary medicine is used along with conventional medicine. Conventional medicine includes allopathic (medical doctor, M.D.) and osteopathic (doctor of osteopathy, D.O.) medicine. Allied conventional health professionals include nurses, respiratory therapists, and psychologists. Examples of complementary therapies include using aromatherapy or massage to lessen discomfort following surgery or chemotherapy.

Alternative medicine is used instead of conventional medicine. Treating cancer with the compound containing amygdalin (trademark Laetrile) in place of undergoing surgery, radiation, or chemotherapy is an example of an alternative therapy. Little reliable evidence exists for Laetrile's efficacy as a cancer drug, and the U.S. Food and Drug Administration has not approved the use of this compound for cancer treatment.

The NCCAM, part of the National Institutes of Health (NIH), defines integrative medicine as a combination of mainstream medicine and those parts of complementary and alternative medicine that have high-quality scientific evidence of safety and effectiveness.

The NIH has placed complementary and alternative medicine modalities into five major categories: alternative medical systems, biologically based therapies, manipulative and body-based methods, mind-body interventions, and energy therapies. These provide a useful framework for understanding many different therapeutic approaches to health care.

Alternative medical systems: Alternative medical systems are complete care systems, much as conventional medicine is a complete system of theory and practice. These complete systems have central philosophies, such as the healing power of nature, and use therapies in line with these philosophies. These systems include traditional Chinese medicine and other medical systems formulated outside of Western culture, such as American Indian, Tibetan, and Indian (Ayurvedic) systems, as well as homeopathic and naturopathic medicine, formulated within Western culture.

Although considered alternative medicine in the United States, traditional Chinese medicine and Ayurvedic medicine are part of the culture and heritage of China and India, respectively, and in these countries they have been practiced for millennia and coexist with conventional medicine. According to the NIH, scientific evidence supports the use of acupuncture, a technique from traditional Chinese medicine, to treat postoperative and chemotherapy-associated nausea and vomiting. Acupuncture may be useful as an adjunct for treating pain-related conditions and other maladies.

Naturopathy is a healing system initiated in Europe. It views disease as alterations in the body's natural healing processes. Naturopaths believe that the body can heal itself if it is in a healthy environment. They take a holistic approach to the body, looking at the patient's mind, body, and spirit, and use therapies such as nutrition and herbal medicine, physical medicine, hot/cold compresses, massage, lifestyle and psychological counseling, and detoxification. Scientific evidence does not support naturopathy's claims.

Homeopathy was founded by Samuel Christian Hahnemann in Germany about two hundred years ago. Hahnemann believed that effective remedies must contain substances that produce effects similar to those produced by the diseases they cured, and he called this the principle of similars. Conventional medicine uses a thought process not unlike this principle in vaccine development. Homeopathy emphasizes the careful examination of all aspects of an individual's health, including mental and emotional states, as well as distinctive physical and personality characteristics.

Homeopathy employs liquids or pills that have been diluted from the original substance to the point that sometimes no detectable trace of the original molecule may be found. The manufacturing process involves vigorous shaking between dilution steps, purportedly producing the vital essence of the substance. Homeopathy contends that the memory of the original molecule is retained after the homeopathic dilution process and that the end product is therapeutic even when the original molecule is thinned out of measurable existence. Scientific and clinical evidence of the efficacy of homeopathy is lacking.

Biologically based therapies: Biologically based therapies use natural substances such as herbs, vitamins, foods, and other dietary supplements. These substances are formulated in many ways, including tablets, capsules, gel caps, powders, teas, oils, and syrups. Although the idea of a natural substance is very attractive to many consumers, natural products can have serious side effects. Some biologically based therapies, such the use of shark cartilage or Laetrile (a compound containing amygdalin) to treat cancer, lack scientific support, while others have some scientific studies that show their efficacy.

Amygdalin is a chemical found in the pits of many fruits. In the presence of certain enzymes, Laetrile breaks down and produces cyanide, a known poison. In addition to lacking effectiveness, Laetrile creates many side effects, mostly related to cyanide poisoning, including cyanosis (bluish skin secondary to oxygen deprivation), uncoordinated walking, liver damage, low blood pressure, and droopy upper eyelids.

The essential oils used in aromatherapy are extracted from fragrant plants such as chamomile, lavender, lemon, and cedarwood. These oils are inhaled or applied to the skin. Although aromatherapy does not cure cancer, it can help patients with quality-of-life issues. Studies have shown that odors can improve mood, enhance perceptions of health, and reduce anxiety. Allergic reactions and dermatitis have been reported as side effects of aromatherapy.

The seeds of milk thistle, a plant native to Europe but also found in North and South America, have been harvested for more than two thousand years for use primarily as a treatment for liver disease. Silymarin, the chemical compound identified as the active ingredient in milk thistle seeds, is a potent antioxidant. It has been shown to help in cases of chronic hepatitis and cirrhosis, and some laboratory studies have indicated that it may increase the ability of some chemotherapeutic agents to treat cancer and decrease the drugs' toxicity. More research must be done before its true efficacy is known. Few side effects are reported regarding milk thistle.

Dietary supplements include vitamins, minerals, herbs, amino acids, enzymes, and organ tissues. Although many people take these types of compounds for health reasons, these supplements are not regulated the same way as are over-the-counter and prescription medications. Prescription medications, in particular, must go through extensive testing and clinical trials and have proven efficacy before they are allowed on the market. Dietary supplements are regulated in a manner closer to the production of salt and pepper than that of prescription medication.

Manufacturers of herbs, vitamins, minerals, and other biologically based dietary supplements follow manufacturing guidelines for the production of food. Medications require Food and Drug Administration approval before they can be placed on the market, whereas individual manufacturers of dietary supplements are responsible for the safe production of their products. The Federal Trade Commission monitors dietary supplements for accuracy in advertisement, whereas the Food and Drug Administration regulates the production of prescription medications. These differences in oversight are not usually evident to the consumer, but consumers should be aware that supplements are much different from medications.

Manipulative and body-based methods: Body-based therapies are based on movement or manipulation of body parts. Chiropractic or osteopathic manipulation and massage therapy are examples of manipulative and body-based therapies. Rolfing, reflexology, Trager bodywork, Alexander and Bowen techniques, the Feldenkrais method, and many other techniques and therapies are included in this category. The NCCAM reports that appointments with chiropractors and massage therapists represent 50 percent of all visits to complementary and alternative health practitioners.

These practices focus on the body's structural elements, such as bones and joints. Circulatory and lymphatic systems are often emphasized in manipulative and body-based practices. Some of these techniques were developed over the past two thousand years in traditional systems from China and India, whereas others, such as chiropractic and osteopathic manipulations, arose in the last 150 years. Although many practitioners are formally trained in anatomy and physiology, considerable variability exists in the education and approaches of these providers.

For example, osteopaths and chiropractors use manipulations involving rapid movements, whereas massage therapists use techniques involving slower force applications. Manipulative and body-based modalities share some principles, including the body's ability to heal itself, self-regulation by the human body, and the interdependence of parts of the human body. These characteristics, along with the laying on of hands, are attractive to some health care consumers seeking relief from various ailments. Studies have shown massage to be useful in the short-term relief of pain, anxiety, depression, fatigue, and stress in cancer patients, but there is no scientific support for claims that massage slows the growth or spread of cancer.

Mind-body interventions: Mental, emotional, spiritual, and behavioral factors affect an individual's health. Mind-body therapies focus on these powerful factors and on the interaction between mind, brain, body, and behavior. The therapies are generally based on respecting and enhancing the human capacity for self-care and individual knowledge. Techniques included in this category include hypnosis, meditation, visual imagery, biofeedback, yoga, tai chi, spirituality, support groups, and therapies tapping creative channels such as music, writing, art, or dance. Some of these therapies, such as patient support groups, have become part of integrated or even conventional medicine.

Evidence exists that a number of the mind-body therapies have been shown to help strengthen the immune system and reduce pain, anxiety, stress, and depression, thus improving the quality of life for cancer patients.

Energy therapies: Energy therapies use two major types of energy fields, biofield and bioelectromagnetic. Biofield therapies claim to manipulate energy fields surrounding and penetrating the body. These energy fields have not been adequately measured or scientifically proven. Some energy therapy techniques try to change biofields by manipulating the body or applying pressure in, on, or through these biofields. Examples include Reiki and Therapeutic Touch. Bioelectromagnetic-based techniques involve using electromagnetic fields, including pulsed, magnetic, alternating-current, or direct-current fields in unconventional manners. Their efficacy for cancer has not been proved.

Perspective and prospects: Conventional health care is disease oriented, tends toward specialty-based care, and is often used after an acute event (a major accident or illness). Allopathic and osteopathic (conventional) medicine becomes more specialty oriented as more scientific mechanisms for disease are discovered. Many people using complementary and alternative therapies are more concerned with maintaining health and optimizing defenses against disease. These people do not reject conventional health care but see conventional health care as an important part of their overall care plan, particularly for acute disease. Those who turn to complementary and alternative therapies after becoming ill typically want to optimize their chances for becoming well.

Many therapies previously considered a part of complementary or alternative medicine—such as support groups for cancer patients, hypnosis for smoking cessation, aspirin for reducing inflammation, or digitalis for heart conditions—have become part of mainstream or integrative medicine. Science does not support all modalities of complementary and alternative medicine, but it supports some aspects. The NCCAM, part of the U.S. Department of Health and Human Services, conducts and funds scientific research into nonconventional medicine in an attempt to help medical professionals and the public understand which therapies have been shown to be safe and effective.

Richard P. Capriccioso, M.D.

For Further Information

Keegan, L. *Healing with Complementary and Alternative Therapies*. Albany, N.Y.: Delmar, 2001.

Peters, David, and Anne Woodham. *Encyclopedia of Natural Healing*. London: Dorling Kindersley, 2000.

Zhang, Qunhao. "Complementary and Alternative Medicine in the United States." *Asia Pacific Biotech News* 8, no. 23 (December 1, 2004): 1274-1277.

Other Resources

MayoClinic.com
Complementary and Alternative Medicine
http://mayoclinic.com/health/alternative-medicine/PN00001

National Cancer Institute
Complementary and Alternative Medicine
http://www.cancer.gov/cancertopics/treatment/cam

National Center for Complementary and Alternative Medicine
http://nccam.nih.gov

See also: Anthraquinones; Antioxidants; Cancell; Carotenoids; Cartilage supplements; Coenzyme Q10; Curcumin; Delta-9-tetrahydrocannabinol; Dietary supplements; Electroporation therapy; Essiac; Ginseng, panax; Green tea; Herbs as antioxidants; Integrative oncology; Laetrile; Mistletoe; PC-SPES; Phenolics; Saw palmetto; Sun's soup

▶ Curcumin

Category: Complementary and Alternative Therapies
Also known as: Diferuloylmethane

Definition: Curcumin is the active principle of turmeric, which is used as a common food additive in Asian cooking. It has been used for many centuries in ancient Chinese and Ayurvedic medical treatments. Curcumin has been selected, along with other promising diet-derived compounds, for testing as a chemopreventive agent for cancer targets in the NCI Chemoprevention Drug Development Program in the United States.

Cancers treated or prevented: Supplemental treatment for chemical carcinogenesis caused by pesticides, breast cancer, metastatic melanoma, and lymphoma

Delivery routes: Oral by capsule

How this substance works: Curcumin is the active component of turmeric, a common spice found in the kitchen cabinets of Asia. Turmeric is a yellow powder obtained from the dried rhizomes of a flowering plant belonging to the ginger family. Curcumin is present in turmeric along with related yellow compounds called curcuminoids. It belongs to a chemical family of compounds known as polyphenols, which are antioxidants that destroy harmful tissue-damaging substances called free radicals.

Curcumin has been reported to possess a wide range of medicinal properties, including the ability to inhibit cancerous tumors in the breast, colon, and skin in mice, rats, guinea pigs, and hamsters. Curcumin is being investigated for the prevention of colon cancer in a phase I clinical trial at the University of Michigan sponsored by the National Cancer Institute (NCI). One study reported that it reverses the negative effects of Taxol (paclitaxel), a breast cancer drug that can cause breast cancer cells to spread. Additionally, it is being tested against multiple myeloma and advanced pancreatic cancer. Based on experimental findings, curcumin has also been postulated to enhance detoxification of carcinogens such as DDT and dioxin by blocking their access to cells.

The proposed hypothesis of the way curcumin inhibits cancerous cell growth is through its ability to block certain kinds of growth factors that are activated by chemical messengers called cytokines and kinases present in the cancer cells, sending signals to the cells to multiply. The structure of curcumin enables it to inhibit multiple kinases, thereby blocking the signals to the cells and effectively stopping the growth of certain types of cancer cells.

Side effects: Ingesting large quantities of curcumin can cause ulcers. Curcumin, when used in conjunction with anticoagulants and thrombolytic agents, could enhance their activity and increase the risk of bleeding.

Lalitha Krishnan, Ph.D.

See also: Antioxidants; Chemoprevention; Herbs as antioxidants

▶ Dietary supplements

Category: Complementary and Alternative Therapies; Lifestyle and Prevention

Definition: Dietary supplements are a broad category of materials that are defined by the U.S. Food and Drug Administration (FDA) as substances consumed in addition to a person's normal diet. Subclasses of this group are vitamins, minerals, botanicals, amino acids, enzymes, and certain animal-derived products such as bee pollen or snake venom.

Cancers treated or prevented: Dietary supplements are often taken as adjuvants to help fight many types of cancer, although their effectiveness is often anecdotal and rarely proven through rigorous clinical trials. Perhaps even more often, supplements are taken for cancer prevention or to boost the immune system.

Delivery routes: Oral in the form of tablets, caplets, capsules, powders, and liquids such as extracts and teas.

How these agents work: Worldwide in 2012, dietary supplements were a $96 billion industry. In the United States, the dietary supplement market increased from a $22 billion industry in 2007 to a $37 billion industry in 2014, with strong growth expected to continue into the 2020s. Supplements range from familiar multivitamin tablets taken by about 68 percent of Americans to unusual substances such as snake venom. Some dietary supplements such as vitamins and minerals have accepted roles in conventional medicine as well as complementary and alternative uses. Other dietary supplements, including most botanicals, are used almost exclusively in complementary and alternative medicine. Complementary medicine supplements traditional Western medical care, while alternative medicine seeks to replace traditional Western medical care.

Some dietary supplements, especially vitamins and minerals, are embraced by traditional Western medicine and play an important role in maintaining health, especially among individuals with cancer or other diseases that affect the body's metabolism. Thirteen different vitamins are essential to human health. The body cannot make these compounds; they must be obtained either from food or from dietary supplements. The fat-soluble vitamins are vitamins A, D, E, and K. The water-soluble vitamins are vitamins B_1 (thiamine), B_2 (riboflavin), B_3 (niacin), B_5 (pantothenic acid), B_6 (pyridoxine), B_7 (biotin or vitamin H), B_9 (folate or folic acid), B_{12} (cobalamin), and vitamin C. Vitamins are generally safe when taken in amounts less than the upper safe limit set by the U.S. Institute of Medicine. Megadosing (taking large quantities of vitamins) can cause serious health complications; especially megadoses of fat-soluble vitamins, which build up in the body. Minerals are inorganic compounds found in the earth that are necessary in small amounts for human health. Like vitamins, many minerals are safe and effective unless taken in megadoses.

Botanicals (herbs) are dietary supplements derived from plants. Botanicals have been used for centuries in traditional Chinese medicine, Ayurvedic or traditional Indian medicine, pre-nineteenth century Western medicine, and

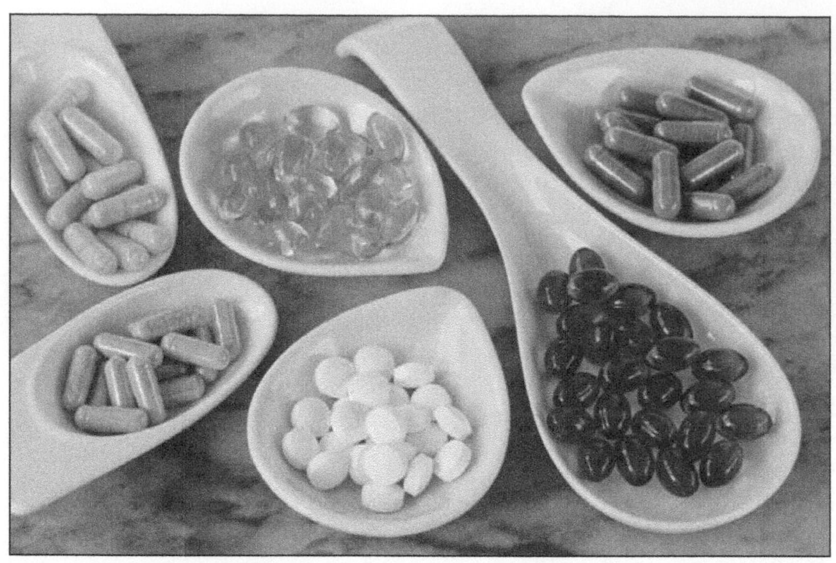

Various dietary supplements. (iStock)

and help it fight their cancer (e.g., ginseng); and to reduce specific symptoms associated with their cancer (e.g., ginger for nausea). The American Cancer Society cautions individuals with cancer to choose dietary supplements with care and with the knowledge and advice of their physician. Much misinformation and many unproved anecdotal claims about dietary supplements and cancer exist on the Internet and in some fad medicine books.

Although millions of Americans use dietary supplements daily, the safety and effectiveness of these products varies depending on the type of supplement, the purity of the manufacturing process, the dosage, the health of the individual, and the way in which the supplement interacts with other supplements and drugs. In the United States, dietary supplements are regulated under the 1994 Dietary Supplement Health and Education Act (DSHEA). This act regulates supplements as foods rather than as pharmaceutical drugs. Under the act, dietary supplement manufacturers do not need to prove that their products are either safe or effective before they are marketed. This contrasts with both over-the-counter and prescription drugs, which cannot be sold until extensive testing (clinical trials) proves them to be both safe and effective in treating specific conditions.

DSHEA limits the health claims that can be made for dietary supplements. Supplements cannot legally claim to treat or cure a particular disease. They are, however, allowed to make general claims, such as "helps build strong bones" or "helps lower cholesterol." Any structure or function claims made for dietary supplements must have on the label the exact words, "This statement has not been evaluated by the FDA. This product is not intended to diagnose, treat, cure, or prevent any disease." The packaging does not have to contain any warnings about potential side effects.

Additional FDA regulations have been added since the original 1994 law. Since 2007, all supplement manufacturers are required to report consumer complaints, including complaints of adverse reactions, ineffectiveness, and contaminated products, to the FDA. Since 2010, FDA regulations have required stronger good manufacturing practices for dietary supplements. Manufacturers must test for the identity, purity, strength, and composition of their products. These regulations are intended to help

homeopathy. The National Center for Complementary and Alternative Medicine (NCCAM) conducts rigorous investigations and clinical trials of many botanicals. Common botanicals that are claimed to treat cancer or cancer symptoms include apricot pits, foxglove (*Digitalis*), ginseng (*Panax quinquefolius*), green tea, and reishi mushrooms (*Ganoderma lucidum*). These claims have not been proved to the satisfaction of Western medicine.

Amino acids are the building blocks of proteins. Humans require twenty amino acids, twelve of which the body can produce for itself, but the rest must be obtained through diet or supplementation. Enzymes are proteins made in the body that regulate metabolic reactions. Prescription enzymes and amino acids are used in Western medicine when they replace compounds that the body is unable to make because of genetic defects. These substances are also sold as dietary supplements, some of which claim to treat cancer. Most traditional physicians do not accept these claims.

Animal-based supplements include products such as fish oil, bee pollen, and bear bile. Many of these products are used in alternative medicine and claim to prevent or treat disease. Practitioners of Western medicine generally acknowledge the benefits of some dietary supplements, such as vitamins, minerals, and fish oils, but question extreme claims.

In relation to cancer, people generally take dietary supplements for four reasons: to prevent a particular type of cancer; to meet the needs for a particular substance that they cannot acquire from diet because of their cancer (e.g., vitamin supplements); to boost the immune system consumers determine exactly what is in the supplement and to certify that it is free from contamination by bacteria, fungi, glass, pesticides, heavy metals, and nonapproved additives.

The new manufacturing regulations resulted from findings by independent laboratories and the FDA of many contaminated supplements, as well as those that contained material other that what was listed on the label or that contained less or none of the labeled ingredients. As of 2015, independent laboratory testing still finds the contents of many dietary supplements, especially those imported from Asia, do not accurately represent the composition of the supplement. Manufacturers are still not required to make any statements on the packaging about potential side effects, nor are they required to prove that a supplement is safe or effective.

Side effects: The side effects of many dietary supplements have not been studied and are unknown. Megadosing with supplements that are generally safe at lower doses, however, may cause the supplement (if fat-soluble) to build up in the body and interfere with the absorption or metabolism of other supplements or pharmaceutical drugs. Botanicals may also change the way in which other drugs or supplements act in the body by speeding up or inhibiting their actions. In addition, many natural plant substances (such as foxglove, hemlock, or ephedra) can cause dangerous or life-threatening side effects. Bee pollen can cause severe allergic reactions, since it typically contains pollen from ragweed or plants that cross-react with ragweed, such as dandelions, sunflowers, or chrysanthemums.

Finally, dependence on dietary supplements to treat cancer or any serious disease may deprive the individual of effective traditional drugs and medical care that can save or prolong life. Individuals interested in taking dietary supplements as part of their cancer treatment regimen should research information carefully and discuss their findings with their oncologist before beginning a supplement.

Tish Davidson, A.M.

For Further Information

Keum, N., & Giovannucci, E. (2014). Vitamin D supplements and cancer incidence and mortality: A meta-analysis. *British Journal of Cancer,* 111(5), 976-80. http://www.ncbi.nlm.nih.gov/pmc/articles/PMC4150260

Findings that Vitamin D supplementation does not reduce the incidence of cancer but appears to reduce mortality.

National Institutes of Health MedlinePlus

Dietary Supplements

https://www.nlm.nih.gov/medlineplus/dietarysupplements.html

A gateway site with frequently updated links to the most current news and research on dietary supplements.

National Institutes of Health Office of Dietary Supplements

Dietary Supplements: Background Information. https://ods.od.nih.gov/factsheets/DietarySupplements-HealthProfessional

An extensive explanation of what dietary supplements are, how they are regulated, and links to information sheets on individual supplements. Information also available in Spanish.

Other Resources

American Cancer Society

Dietary Supplements: What is Safe?
http://www.cancer.org/treatment/treatmentsandsideeffects/complementaryandalternativemedicine/dietarysupplements/index

National Cancer Institute

Office of Cancer Complementary and Alternative Medicine

Information for patients

http://cam.cancer.gov/health_patients.html

National Center for Complementary and Integrative Health

Cancer and Cancer Treatment
https://nccih.nih.gov/health/cancer

Quackwatch

http://quackwatch.org/

U.S. Food and Drug Administration

Dietary Supplements Overview.
http://www.cfsan.fda.gov/~dms/supplmnt.html

See also: Antioxidants; Artificial sweeteners; Beta-carotene; Bioflavonoids; Caffeine; Calcium; Carotenoids; Cartilage supplements; Chemoprevention; Chewing tobacco; Coenzyme Q10; Cruciferous vegetables; Fiber; Folic acid; Fruits; Garlic and allicin; Ginseng, panax; Glutamine; Green tea; Herbs as antioxidants; Indoles; Isoflavones; Lutein; Lycopene; Macrobiotic diet; Nutrition and cancer prevention; Nutrition and cancer treatment; Omega-3 fatty acids; PC-SPES; Phytoestrogens; Resveratrol; Saw palmetto; Soy foods; Sun's soup; Wine and cancer

▶ Electroporation therapy

Category: Procedures; Complementary and Alternative Therapies
Also known as: EPT

Definition: Electroporation therapy is a process that uses high-intensity electrical currents that increase the permeability of cell membranes and enhance the ability of cytotoxic drugs, vaccines, and genes to enter into tumor cells.

Cancers treated: Squamous cell carcinoma, basal cell carcinoma, melanoma, head and neck cancers, cutaneous and subcutaneous tumors, Kaposi sarcoma

Delivery routes: Electrical pulses are delivered directly into tumors using special devices called electroporators or applicators.

Description: Many potentially effective anticancer drugs are limited by their ability to permeate the cell membranes and gain entry into tumor cells. The lipid bilayers of cell membranes possess unique physical and biochemical properties that prevent easy entry of exogenous materials. The principle of electroporation therapy is to increase permeability of the cell membranes by pulses of intense electric current, leading to formation of transient pores in the cell membrane. Pores aid in easy uptake of cytotoxic drugs and increase the intracellular drug concentration, thereby increasing their chances of direct action on tumor cells.

An electroporator consists of a circular array of six electrode needles (as three pairs) that deliver pulses directly inside tumors and create an electric field through potential differences generated between these electrodes. Effective electroporation depends on strength and duration of the applied electric field. Optimization is required for each type of tissue and the kind of molecule being delivered (for example drug vs. deoxyribonucleic acid, or DNA). Application of short pulses of electric field results in the transient formation of pores on the cell membrane. Pores close shortly after the application of electric field is terminated, resulting in almost an entrapment of drugs or other molecules.

Electroporation therapy results in enhanced killing of cancer cells and early necrosis of tumors. Clinical trials on squamous cell carcinoma patients that incorporated a treatment regimen with the drug bleomycin (a cytotoxic drug derived from the bacterium *Streptomyces verticillus*) followed by electroporation, demonstrated complete remission in a significant proportion of patients and partial remission in others. Combination therapy with bleomycin and electroporation was more effective than either treatment alone. Bleomycin in combination with electroporation dramatically enhanced the percentage of cells killed. Among the multitudes of drugs tested in combination with electroporation, bleomycin has been proven to be the most effective. Combined therapy also increases the duration of drug retention and decreases the dose of drug needed for effective treatment.

Side effects: Minimal side effects have been observed with electroporation therapy. Some electric shocks can be experienced after administration of electric pulses.

Geetha Yadav, Ph.D.

See also: Basal cell carcinomas; Electrosurgery; Kaposi sarcoma; Melanomas; Skin cancers; Squamous cell carcinomas

▶ Gerson therapy

Category: Procedures; Complementary and Alternative Therapies
Also known as: Gerson diet, Gerson regime, Gerson method

Definition: Gerson therapy is an alternative treatment therapy developed by Max Gerson that is used to treat chronic debilitating diseases as well as cancer. This treatment involves a specialized diet, vitamin supplements, and coffee enemas that are aimed at cleansing the body, strengthening the immune system, and increasing metabolic activity.

Cancers treated: All

Why performed: The theory behind Gerson therapy is that the body needs to be detoxified frequently in order to treat a disease's underlying cause. It is theorized that people with cancer may contain levels of sodium in their bodies that are too high relative to the levels of potassium. Eating organic fruits and vegetables and taking supplements are believed to help restore a balance in the body.

Patient preparation: Patients with diabetes, brain metastases, kidney damage, and foreign bodies such as pacemakers and implants and those undergoing chemotherapy should consult a certified Gerson practitioner before beginning treatment.

Steps of the procedure: The therapy is based on maintaining a diet high in vitamins and minerals, which is achieved by consuming juices made from fresh, organic fruits and vegetables, as well as vegetarian meals. Medications are taken orally or injected.

In addition, in order to rid the body of toxins, enemas are administered. They are thought to increase bile flow, which facilitates the removal of toxins as well as the elimination of tumor and diseased tissue that is being broken down. Some items prohibited by the therapy include salt, oil, berries or nuts, coffee, drinking water, animal protein, and bottled, canned, preserved, or frozen food, as well as the use of aluminum utensils.

After the procedure: No special steps are taken following Gerson therapy.

Risks: The solutions used for enemas in Gerson therapy (such as coffee) can cause infections, dehydration, constipation, colitis, electrolyte imbalance, heart and lung problems, and even death. Some additional side effects that have been reported by those using Gerson therapy include dizziness or weakness, abdominal cramps, loss of appetite, diarrhea, aching, fever and sweating, and cold sores. The therapy can be especially problematic in women who are pregnant or breast-feeding.

Results: No conclusive scientific evidence has shown that this therapy is effective in preventing or treating cancer.

Lindsay Lewellyn, B.S.

See also: Complementary and alternative therapies; Dietary supplements; Integrative oncology; Macrobiotic diet; Nutrition and cancer treatment; Sun's soup

▶ Ginseng

Category: Complementary and Alternative Therapies
Also known as: Asian ginseng, Chinese ginseng, Korean ginseng, Oriental ginseng, red ginseng, ren shen

Definition: *Panax ginseng* C. A. Meyer, commonly known as *Panax ginseng*, is a perennial plant of Asia and northern Europe. Other types of ginseng include the related *Panax quinquefolius* (American ginseng), and Siberian ginseng, which belong to the *Eleuterococcus* genus and have different activity than *Panax* varieties. The root of *Panax ginseng* is associated with many medicinal claims, mostly encompassing energizing effects; "panax" translates as "all-healing." In Chinese medicine, *Panax ginseng* is a so-called "yang," or hot herb.

Panax ginseng is more than 5,000 years old and was first grown on the mountains of Manchuria, China. *Panax ginseng* is also native to east Russia and is cultivated currently in Korea. The mature root is the source of many active health concoctions, but the ginseng root matures only after five-six years of plant growth.

Cancers treated or prevented: Ginseng is a purported general anticarcinogenic and cell-protective agent, and it may also potentially treat chemotherapy-related side effects like cancer fatigue. Ginseng's pharmacologic claims as a general adaptogenic (or strengthening agent), include analgesia, increased mental capacity, and anti-inflammatory effects. In Western studies, ginseng use appears to have positive effects on patients' view of cancer diagnoses and symptoms. Additionally, it potentially could result in the survival of patients with breast cancer.

Delivery routes: Delivery routes include orally by capsule, tea, or powder. The standard dose is 0.5-2 grams daily of the pure, dried root, providing 4%-5% of ginsenoside content per daily dose. In the United States, the root dose is commonly formulated into capsules of up to 500 mg.

How it works: *Panax ginseng* has a history of more than two thousand years of medicinal use and has been formally studied for health claims since the 1960's. The pharmacologically active entities are a special types of saponins (sugar attached to a steroid or triterpene) called "ginsenosides" that are found in the plant root. Ginsenoside

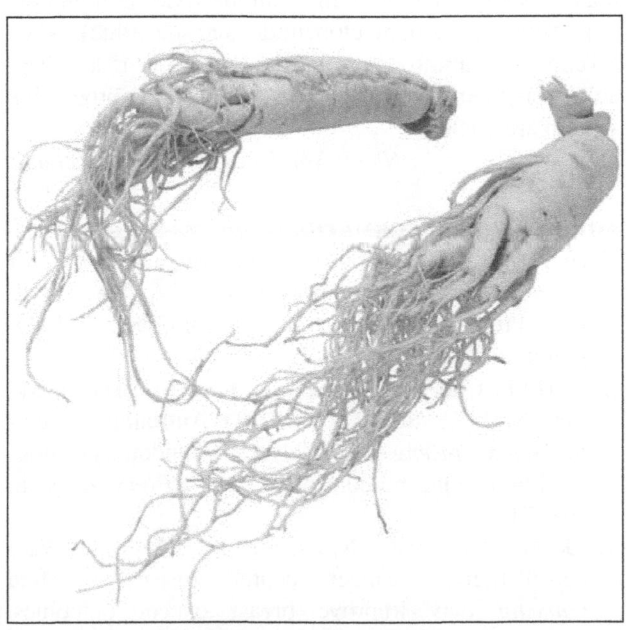

Chinese ginseng. (iStock)

content varies with species and with root age, harvest season, and preservation method, which contributes to an uneven effect of ginseng whole-root products. Dozens of ginsenosides have pharmacologic activity and more than 150 ginsenosides have been identified.

The ginsenoside RB1 appears to increases acetylcholine release and increase choline uptake; RB1 may reduce cancer proliferation by stabilizing a growth factor (IGF-1R) associated with cancer risk. Ginsenosides also competitively bind to GABA receptors *in vitro*, might increase nitric oxide in endothelial tissues, and may block part of a cancer signaling pathway (Wnt/beta-catenin).

Side effects: Toxicity, including dizziness and diarrhea, appears low with good-quality preparations, but marketed products frequently contain adulterations because of the high cost of the root. Adverse effects at high doses include increased heart rate, nausea, headache, restlessness, and trouble sleeping.

Women may experience swollen breasts and vaginal bleeding. Additionally, the safety of *Panax ginseng* during pregnancy and lactation is unknown. Ginseng should be avoided in patients with estrogenic (i.e., estrogen-receptor positive) breast cancers until more is known about the increased hormonal risks of ginseng. Estrogen concerns may relate to a root fungus or to the alcohol extraction process applied to the root rather than to ginsenosides.

Ginseng may decrease blood sugar by increasing the hypoglycemic effects of insulin, and ginseng can increase blood-clotting times. Similarly, ginseng may increase the manic-like symptoms of monoamine oxidase inhibitors (e.g., isocarboxazid, moclobemide, and selegiline). When given with imatinib, ginseng can increase the risk of hepatotoxicity. Ginseng's effects on the CYP liver processing system are unclear.

Nicole Van Hoey, PharmD, freelance

For Further Information

Chen, J., & Chen, T. (2004). *Chinese medical herbology and pharmacology*. City of Industry, CA: Art of Medicine Press. http://www.aompress.com/book_herbology/pdfs/RenShen.pdf

Kim, H-G., Cho, J-H., Yoo, S-R., Lee, J-S., Han, J-M., Lee, N-H., ... Son, C-G. (2013). Antifatigue effects of *Panax ginseng* C.A. Meyer: A randomized, double-blind, placebo-controlled trial. *PLoS One*, 8: e61271.

Vanderbilt University News. (2006, May 15). Vanderbilt-Ingram cancer center researchers find *Ginseng* may improve breast cancer outcomes. Retrieved from http://news.vanderbilt.edu/2006/03/vanderbilt-ingram-cancer-center-researchers-find-ginseng-may-improve-breast-cancer-outcomes-56874

Yun, T. K. (2001). Brief introduction of *Panax ginseng* C.A. Meyer. *Journal of Korean Medical Science*, 16: S3-S5.

Other Resources

MedicalNewsToday - Ginseng: Health Benefits and Side-Effects
http://www.medicalnewstoday.com/articles/262982.php?page=2

RxList Supplements - *Ginseng, Panax*
http://www.rxlist.com/ginseng_panax/supplements.htm

See also: Dietary supplements; Herbs as antioxidants; PC-SPES

▶ Green tea

Category: Complementary and Alternative Therapies; Lifestyle and Prevention
Also known as: *Camellia sinesis*

Definition: Green tea is a beverage made from fresh leaves of the evergreen *Camellia sinesis* plant. These leaves are rich in antioxidants, including polyphenols and flavonoids, which have been implicated in such general body health as suppressing aging, deterring food poisoning, controlling blood pressure, glucose, and cholesterol levels, and preventing cancer. One class of flavonoids,

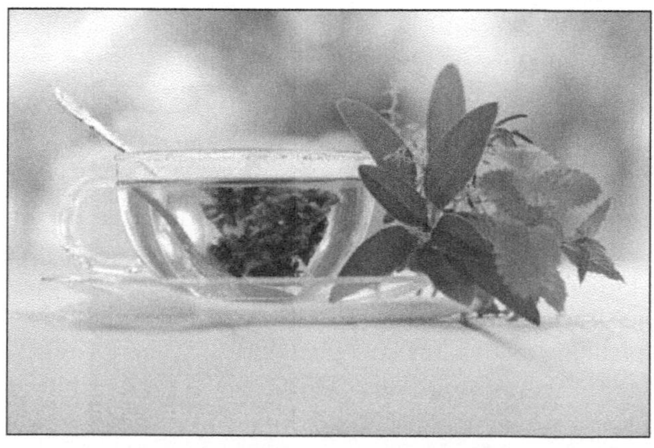

Green tea is being studied as a cancer preventative. (iStock)

the catechins, has recently become the focus of study for their anticancer potential.

Cancers treated or prevented: Implicated in both the treatment and the prevention of several cancers

Delivery routes: Most commonly oral by liquid; green tea tablets and capsules containing its main ingredients also are widely marketed

How this substance works: Green tea is currently being studied for properties that inhibit or prevent cancer. Studies have suggested relationships between green tea intake in the diet and the reduction of stomach cancer in Asians. Laboratory studies of animal subjects strongly suggest that green tea may also help reduce the incidence of a number of cancers. The cancer-fighting components of green tea are antioxidants, which provide defense against free radicals that precipitate cell dysfunction that, in turn, leads to cancer. Antioxidants in green tea include polyphenols and flavonoids such as EGCG (epigallocatechin gallate) and other catechins. EGCG binds to laminin receptors on the surface of cancer cells, thereby dramatically reducing their growth and survival. Catechins also have antioxidant properties and protect against DNA damage. These chemicals may also restrict blood flow to cancerous cells and restrict or eliminate the formation of new blood vessels, both contribute to the death of cancer cells which are unable to obtain needed nutrients for growth. Laboratory studies have also suggested that catechins may inhibit the formation and operation of specific enzyme activities that lead to cancer development.

Human studies have been much less consistent. Some studies support laboratory findings regarding green tea cancer-fighting benefits, but other studies suggest little or no benefit. Studies in China, where green tea is a staple in the diet, generally find lower incidences of cancer among tea drinkers when compared to non-tea drinkers. The National Cancer Institute (NCI), however, conducted its own study of the antitumor effects among prostate cancer patients. This study concluded that there was little to no benefit.

In response to these differing results, the Food and Drug Administration (FDA) has determined that antitumor benefits associated with green tea are not supported by current data, and suggests that further controlled studies on the connection between green tea and cancer are needed.

Side effects: Side effects from drinking large amounts of green tea in the diet are normally rare among most of the population. Green tea has high caffeine content, however, and physicians routinely warn that people with heart conditions or high blood pressure and women who are pregnant or breast-feeding should not drink green tea in excess. Some side effects of caffeine may include nausea, insomnia, frequent urination, irritability, or diarrhea. In excessive doses, caffeine can cause seizures or heart irregularities. Green tea also contains vitamin K, which can decrease the effectiveness of anticoagulant drugs.

Dwight G. Smith, Ph.D.
Updated by: Catherine J. Walsh

See also: Antioxidants; Chemoprevention; Dietary supplements; Phytoestrogens; Prevention

▶ Herbs as antioxidants

Category: Complementary and Alternative Therapies; Lifestyle and Prevention

Definition: Herbs are roots, stems, leaves, flowers, or seeds of plants used for culinary (flavoring), health (preventive and therapeutic), and other purposes. The antioxidant properties of some compounds in herbs are being investigated for their ability to prevent or fight cancer. Subclasses of this group include oregano, milk thistle, thyme, rose hips, rosemary, garlic, saw palmetto, cat's claw, and turmeric.

Cancers treated or prevented: Used in combination with standard chemotherapy for various cancers such as breast cancer, colon cancer, endometrial cancer, leukemia, and mutagenesis caused by smoking, exhaust fumes, and exposure to other carcinogens

Delivery routes: Oral in the form of capsules or powders or as decoctions (extracts) or infusions; dietary in their naturally occurring forms, such as leaves, seeds, berries, and bark; topical as oils, ointments, and tinctures.

How these agents work: Studies indicate that a plant-based diet can reduce the risk of many types of cancers. Researchers have found that many of the common herbs used as natural flavor additives to food are a very rich source of antioxidants, a class of compounds that assist in neutralizing reactive oxygen species (i.e., free radicals) and thereby preventing damage to the cells in the body. Free radicals are species generated by normal cell metabolism and by the action of environmental pollutants such as cigarette smoke and pesticides, which can cause tissue damage. The damage caused by free radicals is thought to be a precursor to degenerative diseases such as cancer. The therapeutic effect of herbs might be mediated by the high concentration of antioxidants present in them.

Many herbs are being tested in controlled studies for their anticancer properties and for supplementing standard chemotherapeutic regimens. However, there is currently very little strong evidence that herbal medicine can treat, cure, or prevent cancer, though there is evidence that herbal remedies can lessen some cancer symptoms and side effects of cancer treatments. Most of the antioxidant benefits of herbs are attributed to classes of compounds called isoflavones, polyphenols, flavonoids, lignans, and sulfur-containing compounds. These compounds act in a synergistic fashion, conferring a composite benefit greater than that of any single component.

Side effects: Using herbs in their natural form as flavor enhancers in the diet has the lowest risk of side effects compared to powders, capsules, tinctures and other forms of herbal medicine. Although herbs have great potential health benefits, it is important to exercise caution when using them in a concentrated form for the treatment of serious illnesses. Though some herbs are safe to use and do not cause noticeable side effects, other herbs can cause very serious side effects. It is important to remember that herbal medicine is a form of medicine, and should be used with the same care and caution that traditional modern medicine is used. Patients should educate themselves about these preventive therapies and consult with their physicians in order to avoid harmful interactions with standard chemotherapeutic drugs. Pregnant and lactating women should exercise special caution when using herbal remedies.

Lalitha Krishnan, Ph.D.
Updated by: Benjamin Riley

For Further Information

Booker, N.W., Pharm, D., & Zuckerman, D. (2015). Antioxidants and cancer risk: The good, the bad, and the unknown. Retrieved from http://www.stopcancerfund.org/pz-diet-habits-behaviors/antioxidants-and-cancer-risk-the-good-the-bad-and-the-unknown/

This article discusses some of the pros and cons of antioxidants using a research based approach that explores the results of both recent and less recent studies. The role of antioxidants is also briefly explained. The health benefits of antioxidant supplements as opposed to eating a diet rich in antioxidant containing foods and/or relying on antioxidants naturally produced by the body are also discussed. Also addressed is whether antioxidants are dangerous or helpful for individuals who already have cancer.

Kaefer, C.M. & Milner, J.A. (2011). Herbs and Spices in Cancer Prevention and Treatment. Boca Raton, FL: Taylor & Francis.

This source takes an in depth look at the history, usage, and applications of herbs and spices that may be useful for treating and preventing cancer. Each herb or spice is summarized individually. Beneficial properties of the herb are discussed, as well as other names for the herb or spice, it's native origin, and results and implications of studies done on the particular herb or spice discussed. The biological makeup of each individual herb or spice is also covered.

Mandal, A. (2013). What are antioxidants? Retrieved from http://www.news-medical.net/health/What-are-Antioxidants.aspx

This article defines what antioxidants are, their use and function in the body, as well as where they can naturally be found in foods. Also discussed are free radicals, their potentially harmful effects, and how antioxidants neutralize free radicals. Antioxidant deficiencies and already existing antioxidant mechanisms in the body are also briefly discussed.

Salamon, M. (2015). The truth behind three natural cancer "cures". Retrieved from https://www.mskcc.org/blog/truth-behind-three-natural-cures

This article gives an overview and analysis of some alternative therapies, and discusses a few of the pros and cons of each therapy. The possibility of using alternative therapies alongside conventional treatments as well as the increasing safety and effectiveness of conventional treatments are also discussed. In conclusion, the article mentions that because most natural therapies are not well supported by formal evidence, patients should exercise caution when considering them. It is also advocated that medical decisions, particularly decisions regarding "natural" therapies should be well researched and should be discussed with a physician.

Schulz, Volker, Hánsel, Rudolf, & Tyler, Varro E. (2001). *Rational phytotherapy*. New York, NY: Springer Science & Business Media.

One of the best references to those herbal remedies that have demonstrated pharmacological and clinical efficacy.

Other Resources

www.cancer.gov/about-cancer/treatment/cam
https://www.mskcc.org/blog/truth-behind-three-natural-cures
www.cancersupportivecare.com/herbal.html
www.mayoclinic.org/diseases-conditions/cancer/in-depth/cancer-treatment/art-20047246

http://www.cancerresearchuk.org/about-cancer/cancers-in-general/treatment/complementary-alternative/therapies/herbal-medicine

See also: Angiogenesis; Angiogenesis inhibitors; Anthraquinones; Antioxidants; Beta-carotene; Bioflavonoids; Carotenoids; Complementary and alternative therapies; Curcumin; Dietary supplements; Essiac; Free radicals; Garlic and allicin; Green tea; Isoflavones; Lutein; Lycopene; Nutrition and cancer prevention; Phenolics; Phytoestrogens; Resveratrol; Sun's soup

▶ Integrative oncology

Category: Complementary and alternative therapies
Also known as: Complementary medicine

Definition: Oncology integrative Complementary and alternative therapies Integrative oncology combines mainstream or traditional cancer care with other approaches to manage symptoms, improve quality of life, enhance wellness, and improve the efficacy of treatment. It integrates the best of conventional cancer treatment with care emphasizing the mind-body-spirit connection to provide a multidisciplinary approach to managing disease. Alternative medicine, by definition, is used to replace traditional treatment and should not be confused with complementary or integrative medicine.

The patient population: Patients receiving cancer therapy encounter a challenging treatment period that lasts for an extended period of time, often years. Side effects of therapy are significant and can include nausea, vomiting, pain, limits on mobility, fatigue, and other symptoms often difficult to manage with traditional medicine. Surveys have reported that at least 20 to almost 100 percent of cancer patients use some type of complementary therapy, with or without their physicians' knowledge, in an attempt to manage the side effects of their treatment and symptoms of their disease.

Perceived benefits: Multiple studies report that complementary and alternative medicine (CAM) can provide benefits to the well-being of the patient. There are some scientific reports that document the benefits of complementary and alternative medicine, but anecdotal reports of benefits are often accepted when complementary medicine is used in conjunction with traditional medicine. The barrier of proof with alternative therapies is higher although some have been used for many years in non-Western societies. Psychosocial interventions are an integral part of any cancer patient's care. Mind-body-spirit therapies enhance mood, reduce anxiety, decrease depression, and improve coping skills, as reported in multiple studies. Pain reduction, managing conditioned nausea and vomiting, and control of other physical symptoms are also attributed to mind-body-spirit techniques practiced by the patient on a routine basis.

Types of CAM therapies: The Office of Cancer Complementary and Integrative Health of the National Cancer Institute devotes time and resources to investigating the scientific validity and impact of complementary and alternative medicine in cancer care. Alternative medicine techniques are often based on theories generated apart from and earlier than conventional Western medicine. Some of the techniques come from Asia, including acupuncture, Ayurveda, and traditional Chinese and Tibetan medicines; others are of Western origin, including homeopathy and naturopathy. Energy therapies are based on the use of energy fields purported to surround and penetrate the human body, but to date there is no scientific evidence that these fields exist. Reiki therapy, therapeutic touch, and qi gong are examples of energy therapies. Electromagnetic therapies include pulsed electromagnetic fields and magnet therapy. Exercise therapies such as tai chi, yoga, walking, and gentle workouts all contribute to the feeling of well-being in cancer patients and are often recommended. Massage therapy, reflexology, osteopathy, and chiropractic medicine are based on manipulating body parts. All manipulation must be appropriate to the physical condition of the patient, but gentle massage and reflexology often create a feeling similar to that created by exercise if that option is limited by the patient's condition.

The most common mind-body-spirit interventions are related to learned techniques that are practiced by the patient to provide benefits related to the control of side effects of care. Meditation, relaxation therapy, guided imagery, self-hypnosis, and biofeedback, when routinely practiced, may control pain, nausea, vomiting, anxiety, and other symptoms. Participation in support groups, art therapy classes, music therapy, dance therapy, journaling, and aromatherapy programs provides potential symptom management and social interaction contributing to a feeling of well-being. Spiritual therapies are receiving greater attention, with spiritual healing and intercessory prayer as central components.

Nutritional, pharmacological, and biologic treatments have varying levels of scientific support but are frequently used by patients. Nutritional counseling, macrobiotic and vegetarian diets, dietary supplements, vitamins, and minerals are routinely accepted in complementary medicine, although evidence for the efficacy of such things remains elusive. Off-label drug use and natural products, such as shark cartilage and Laetrile (an amygdalin compound), have had varying levels of success in symptom management and are scientifically unproven as either primary or adjuvant treatments.

Future of integrative oncology: Integrative oncology is rapidly becoming an important part of cancer therapy. However, complementary and alternative medicine therapies, like other therapies, must be scientifically evaluated for safety and efficacy. Although many complementary therapies do not interfere with traditional therapies, there is still the threat of an inappropriate interaction with prescribed therapies. An increasing number of physicians and facilities are offering complementary and alternative medicine therapies as a part of their patients' care, but patients should still inform their health care practitioner of any complementary and alternative medicine therapies used at the same time that they are undergoing therapy.

Patricia Stanfill Edens, R.N., Ph.D., FACHE
Updated by: Richard P. Capriccioso, M.D.

For Further Information

Abrams, D. I., & Weil, A. (Eds.). (2014). *Integrative Oncology* (2nd ed.). New York: Oxford University Press. https://global.oup.com/academic/product/integrative-oncology-9780199329724?cc=us&lang=en&#

Davies, A. A., Davey Smith, G., Harbord, R., Bekkering, G. E., Sterne, J. A., Beynon, R., & Thomas, S. Nutritional interventions and outcome in patients with cancer or preinvasive lesions: Systematic review. *Journal of the National Cancer Institute*, 98, 961-963. http://www.ncbi.nlm.nih.gov/pubmed/16849679

National Institutes of Health (2009). Acupuncture from ancient practice to modern science. *NIH Medline Plus*, 4(1), 18. https://www.nlm.nih.gov/medlineplus/magazine/issues/winter09/articles/winter09pg18.html

Other Resources

American Cancer Society
Complementary and alternative therapies for advanced cancer
http://www.cancer.org/treatment/understandingyourdiagnosis/advancedcancer/advanced-cancer-cam

National Cancer Institute
Thinking About Complementary and Alternative Medicine.
http://www.cancer.gov/cancertopics/thinking-about-CAM/allpages

National Center for Complementary and Integrative Health
https://nccih.nih.gov

Quackwatch: Your Guide to Quackery, Health Fraud, and Intelligent Decisions
http://www.quackwatch.com/

See also: Aids and devices for cancer patients; Cancer care team; Caregivers and caregiving; Case management; Complementary and alternative therapies; Counseling for cancer patients and survivors; Dietary supplements; Duke Comprehensive Cancer Center; Home health services; Hospice care; Living with cancer; Occupational therapy; Oncology social worker; Palliative treatment; Personality and cancer; Psychosocial aspects of cancer; Stress management; Support groups

► Mistletoe

Category: Complementary and alternative therapies
Also known as: *Viscum album Lorantaceae*, all heal

Definition: European and American varieties of mistletoe are semiparasitic, woody evergreen plants with white berries that grow on deciduous trees. Mistletoe has a long history of use in Europe and Asia as a medicinal cure-all, and the species *Viscum album Lorantaceae* in particular has been studied for the treatment of multiple types of cancer.

Cancers treated or prevented: Breast, pancreatic, and other cancers

Delivery routes: Intrauscular, subcutaneous, or intravenous (IV) injection of water-based or water-and-alcohol-based extracts

How this substance works: American and European mistletoe plants both contain toxins that provide pharmacologic effects on multiple organ systems. The *Viscum album* species is the primary one used medicinally and

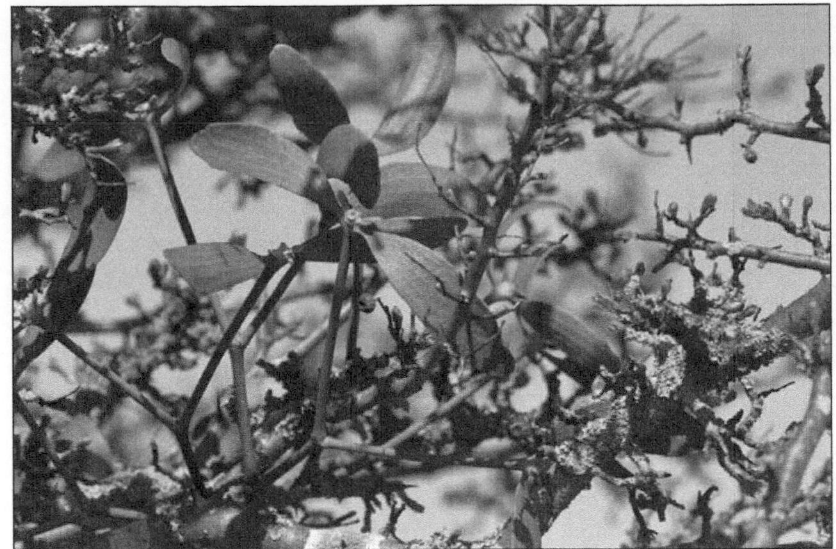

Mistletoe. (iStock)

provides activity via four viscotoxins, three distinct lectins (MI1-3), and the specific lectin viscumin. These toxins are found in the main standardized product Iscador, available in Europe and Asia but not in the United States. The cytotoxic viscotoxins and lectins provide the plant's potential direct anticancer activity by inhibiting protein synthesis in cancer cells and by inducing programmed cancer cell death, respectively.

Immunomodulation is another possible mechanism of cancer treatment and of chemotherapy side effect control. Mistletoe extract may increase white blood cell counts, protect deoxyribonucleic acid (DNA) in white blood cells exposed to damaging chemotherapy, and stimulate cellular secretions of cytokines, including tumor necrosis factor (TNF)-alpha, interleukin (IL)-1, and IL-6, from white blood cells. Increased natural killer cell activity has also been noted in breast cancer patients administered a single intravenous dose of standardized mistletoe preparation.

Varying effects have been observed with different extracts, doses, and types of cancer. Clinical trials have been conducted in Europe, but evidence supporting mistletoe's immune-boosting effect does not yet support the concept that enhanced immunity will help the body fight cancer cells.

Side effects: Mistletoe leaves and berries are poisonous to ingest and may cause nausea, vomiting, and diarrhea leading to dehydration; decreased heart rate and increased blood pressure, with possible vasoconstriction and cardiac arrest; delirium and hallucinations; and seizures. Gastric emptying is suggested after ingestion of more than three berries or more than two leaves.

Few side effects have been reported, however, with medicinal use of the mistletoe extract. Common side effects observed with extract administration include injection site reactions, headache, fever and chills, and some cases of anaphylactic shock or allergic reaction. Mistletoe is a uterine stimulant and should be avoided during pregnancy and lactation.

Nicole M. Van Hoey, Pharm.D.

See also: Breast cancers; Complementary and alternative therapies; Pancreatic cancers

▶ Motion sickness devices

Category: Complementary and alternative therapies
Also known as: ReliefBand, Sea-Band stimulators, BioBands

Definition: Nausea relief wristbands are economical devices that may decrease the nausea associated with cancer treatments such as chemotherapy and radiation therapy. Though these devices are not scientifically proven effective, many patients report relief of nausea when wearing a relief band on the wrist.

Delivery routes: Motion sickness relief bands are worn on the wrist and are available over the counter at pharmacies and drugstores.

Cancers treated: One common and disturbing side effect of cancer treatments, such as chemotherapy or radiation, is nausea and vomiting. These therapies are used as treatment for nearly all cancers.

Why used: Cancer patients who are receiving chemotherapy may feel a queasy feeling in the stomach (nausea), which can trigger vomiting, the forceful elimination of food or contents from the stomach. An estimated 70 to 89 percent of chemotherapy patients have this side effect. As many as 50 percent of cancer patients delay therapy because of fear of nausea and vomiting. Cancer patients who are receiving radiation therapy may experience a similar feeling of nausea that can lead to vomiting. Successful cancer treatment with chemotherapy or radiation depends on the patient's ability to tolerate this side effect.

How these bands work: These bands are usually made of a soft, elastic material that clings to the wrist. When a cancer patient puts on a motion sickness relief band, a small bead embedded in the band applies acupressure by pressing down on the neiguan, or P6, acupressure point. When this point on the median nerves of the inner wrist is stimulated, the trigger for nausea is suppressed.

Risks and results: Acupressure wristbands offer a cost-efficient and drug-free way to manage nausea and vomiting during cancer treatment. The therapy is safe for all ages, from children to older adults, as well as for pregnant and nursing women. The only risk is that they will not work for all people. However, the cost to try this therapy is minimal and does not require a doctor's prescription.

Marylane Wade Koch, M.S.N., R.N.

See also: Acupuncture and acupressure for cancer patients; Adjuvant therapy; Chemotherapy; Cobalt 60 radiation; Complementary and alternative therapies; Nausea and vomiting

▶ PC-SPES

Category: Complementary and alternative therapies
Also known as: PC-CARE, Ponicidin

Definition: PC-SPES is a mixture of eight herbs marketed as a dietary supplement for prostate health and as a complementary and alternative medicine (CAM) for prostate cancer. It should not be confused with SPES, a different product.

Cancers treated or prevented: Prostate cancer

Delivery routes: Oral by capsule

How this substance works: PC-SPES (a name derived from the initials for "prostate cancer" and the Latin word for "hope," *spes*) is a dietary supplement alleged to support prostate health and limit the growth of prostate cancer. The ingredients include eight herbs used in traditional Chinese medicine: Baikal skullcap (*Scutellaria baicalensis*), licorice (*Glycyrrhiza glabra L.* or *Glycyrrhiza uralensis*), reishi mushroom (*Ganoderma lucidum*), isatis (*Isatis indigotica*), ginseng (*Panax ginseng* or *Panax pseudoginseng var. notoginseng*), chrysanthemum flowers (*Dendranthema morifolium*), *Rabdosia rubescens* (*Isodon rubescens*), and saw palmetto (*Serenoa repens*). In the 1990's, PC-SPES showed promise both in preventing cell damage and in limiting tumor growth in cases of prostate cancer.

Between 1997 and 2002, PC-SPES was marketed in the United States as a dietary supplement; it therefore did not need to meet the U.S. Food and Drug Administration (FDA) standards for drug safety and efficacy and did not require a prescription. In early studies in which cancer cells from rats were mixed with PC-SPES, the mixture limited the growth of the tumor cells. When testing revealed, however, that some forms of PC-SPES illegally contained warfarin (a blood thinner), diethylstilbestrol (DES, a hormonal therapy for prostate cancer), and indomethacin (an anti-inflammatory), PC-SPES was taken off the market. Forms of PC-SPES without these drugs remain on the market but are unstandardized.

How PC-SPES may work without the prescription drugs is unknown but is being studied. The herbs contain plant estrogens (phytoestrogens) that may be effective in limiting the action of testosterone, the male hormone that contributes to tumor growth. Patients respond to PC-SPES similarly to those responding to estrogen therapy using DES. The National Center for Complementary and Alternative Medicine (NCCAM) is conducting studies on drug-free forms of PC-SPES to determine its efficacy, and clinical trials may be planned once a standard formula is established.

Side effects: Users of PC-SPES have noted side effects including breast swelling and tenderness, loss of libido, impotence (erectile dysfunction), and, less frequently, blood clots in the legs and diarrhea. PC-SPES may also have interactions with drugs, including anticancer drugs.

Christina J. Moose, M.A.

See also: Cartilage supplements; Chemoprevention; Complementary and alternative therapies; Dietary supplements; Diethylstilbestrol (DES); Gerson therapy; Herbs as antioxidants; Lutein; Lycopene; Nutrition and cancer prevention; Nutrition and cancer treatment; Prostate cancer; Saw palmetto; Sun's soup

▶ Phenolics

Category: Complementary and alternative therapies
ATC code: D08AE
Also known as: Phenols

Definition: Phenolics are a class of compounds grouped together because of their chemical structure; they are aromatic compounds (containing benzene rings), usually with hydroxyl groups. Their function varies, however, and they may have a protective role against many cancers. Subclasses of this group are benzenediols, capsaicinoids, monolignols, and phenol ethers.

Cancers treated or prevented: Primarily breast cancer

Delivery routes: Oral in diet, pills, or capsules

How these compounds work: Phenolic acids have become the topic of much study for their protective role against many cancers. Examples of phenolics include gallic acids, curcumin, and ferulic acids. Found in abundance in many plants, phenolics in even low concentrations decrease cell proliferation, which makes them critically important in the shrinkage of cancer cells and concurrent reduction in size of tumors. Though the exact mechanisms by which phenolics work as antiproliferative substances in the treatment of cancer is unclear, a diet consisting of many fruits and vegetables seems to play an important role in cancer prevention and aids in cancer treatment by reducing tumor size and spread.

Proposed mechanisms by which these phenolic acids function include antioxidant effects, steroid receptor binding, direct interaction with intracellular elements and signaling systems, and aryl hydrocarbon receptor (AhR) binding and modification of subsequent pathways. Polyphenols and phenolic acids are rich in antioxidants, which reduce the concentration of harmful free radicals in the human body. Binding to receptor sites and inhibiting particular enzymes inhibits cell growth and prevents the inflammatory response of surrounding healthy tissues. As a result of their oxidation-reduction properties, they efficiently inactivate oxyl radicals and repair amino acid and deoxyribonucleic acid (DNA) base radicals. Phenols also induce apoptosis (scheduled cell death) and restrict the formation of new blood vessels. This active mechanism of phenolics is an important feature, since both growth and metastasis of a tumor depends heavily on angiogenesis (blood vessel formation) to provide oxygen and nutrients to the growing tumor cells.

Numerous laboratory studies have shown that phenolic acids inhibit the growth of cancerous cell in vitro. Unfortunately, studies performed in vivo do not show such clear benefits. Much of this may be attributable to differences in lifestyle or genetics. One promising study, however, showed that individuals who were prescribed low doses of aspirin had a decreased risk of developing colon cancer. The main metabolite of aspirin is a phenolic acid called salicylic acid. Salicylic acid is also found in plants, where it exists as a protective hormone. Its presence in fruits and vegetables may explain their oncoprotective role when made a staple in the human diet. Many more studies are currently being conducted on this matter.

Side effects: There are no known side effects of phenolics in the diet, but phenolics can be toxic at excessive levels for those who have phenol sulfotransferase (PST) deficiency, a disease that results from a difficulty in processing phenols into useful or at least nonharmful substances. In this case, phenols in the diet should be reduced or an agent used to facilitate processing.

Dwight G. Smith, Ph.D.

See also: Angiogenesis; Antioxidants; Beta-carotene; Bioflavonoids; Breast cancer in children and adolescents; Breast cancer in men; Breast cancer in pregnant women; Breast cancers; Calcium; Carotenoids; Chemoprevention; Clinical Breast Exam (CBE); Coenzyme Q10; Complementary and alternative therapies; Cruciferous vegetables; Curcumin; Dietary supplements; Essiac; Free radicals; Fruits; Garlic and allicin; Glutamine; Green tea; Herbs as antioxidants; Isoflavones; Lutein; Lycopene; Nutrition and cancer prevention; Phytoestrogens; Resveratrol; Wine and cancer

▶ Saw palmetto

Category: Complementary and Alternative Therapies; Lifestyle and Prevention
Also known as: *Serenoa repens*, *Sabal serrulatum*, Permixon

Definition: Saw palmetto, or *Serenoa repens*, is a small fan palm native to the Atlantic and Gulf coastal plains that can be found as far inland as southern Arkansas. The olive-sized fruit of this plant is enriched with fatty acids and phytosterols, and its extracts have been the subject of research for the treatment of certain cancers, especially prostate cancer.

Cancer treated or prevented: Prostate cancer

Delivery route: Oral by capsule

How this substance works: Used as an herbal supplement, saw palmetto is considered to be safe, effective, and relatively inexpensive. It enjoys widespread use in the United States but is also popular in Germany and France for the treatment of prostate disorders.

Saw palmetto inhibits 5-alpha-reductase, an enzyme that converts testosterone into its most potent form, dihydrotestosterone (DHT). Its effects have been compared to Proscar (finasteride), which is a prescription drug that results in the shrinkage of an enlarged prostate, a condition called benign prostatic hyperplasia (BPH). While studies of the efficacy of saw palmetto are somewhat inconsistent, it largely lacks the adverse side effects of Proscar, such as decreased libido and gastrointestinal irritation. The most studied form is Permixon, which is made by using hexane as a solvent in the extraction process of the sterols and fatty acids found in the dried fruits of the saw palmetto berry. Other mixtures include ethanol, methanol, or less commonly nettle root or pumpkin seed oils. Although the extract is much studied, it is not fully understood which are its active components, but phytosterols and fatty acids seem to be the most proficient at treating symptoms.

Similarly, the mechanism by which saw palmetto actually works is yet unclear. Some suggest that it acts as an anti-inflammatory, blocks the chemical conversion of testosterone to DHT, or promotes prostate epithelial involution. Whichever is correct, studies have shown that saw palmetto relieves symptoms caused by prostate disorders, including decreased urine stream and flow, post-voidance dribbling, overflow incontinence, and excessive retention of urine in the bladder. Relief of prostate swelling aids a return to sexual function, which also contributes to the popular use of saw palmetto among older men.

Not all studies agree on the therapeutic efficacy of saw palmetto; a double-blind, randomized study by Dr. Stephen Bent of the University of California, San Francisco, and his coworkers that was funded by the National Institutes of Health (NIH) and the National Center for Complementary and Alternative Medicine (NCCAM) found that saw palmetto was no more effective in reducing symptoms associated with BPH than a placebo. This raises the question of whether it is a medically useful substance.

Overall, the Moores Cancer Center of the Medical Center of the University of California, San Diego, states that "this treatment modality is thought to manage symptoms of cancer, side effects from conventional therapies and/or control pain." Researchers warn, however, that saw palmetto should be used as a supplement to cancer treatment, not in place of standard therapy.

Side effects: Almost all patients reported that adverse side effects were mild and infrequent, differing little from those reported after placebo use. Some reports indicate that saw palmetto can cause gastrointestinal distress, but this can largely be alleviated by taking saw palmetto with food.

Dwight G. Smith, Ph.D.

See also: Complementary and alternative therapies; Fruits; Herbs as antioxidants; Nonsteroidal Anti-Inflammatory Drugs (NSAIDs); PC-SPES; Prostate cancer

▶ Sun's soup

Category: Complementary and Alternative Therapies; Lifestyle and Prevention
Also known as: Selected Vegetables (SV)

Definition: Sun's soup is a nutritional supplement consisting of plant nutrients containing phytochemicals believed to enhance immune properties and disease prevention.

Cancers treated or prevented: Cancerous tumors; effectiveness not scientifically verified

Delivery routes: Oral by diet

How this agent works: Sun's soup is believed to boost the immune system, although how it works and whether it is effective are considered unverified scientifically.

In the late 1980's, Dr. Alexander Shihkaung Sun (1939-2006), a Taiwanese American biochemist with a Ph.D. from the University of California, Berkeley, investigated the use of specific foodstuffs, mainly shiitake mushrooms, mung beans, and Chinese herbs associated with reinforcing immune systems, to aid his mother after she became ill with lung cancer. Affiliated professionally with Mount Sinai Medical Center and the Yale University School of Medicine, Sun chose ingredients with phytochemicals that Asian physicians had incorporated into treatments.

Sun freeze-dried his concoction, which he initially called Selected Vegetables (SV), as a supplement to medical treatments to extend the life spans of patients with cancerous tumors. In the early 1990's, he conducted trials with mice to assess the impact of SV on tumors. He then tested SV in humans, focusing on patients diagnosed with non-small-cell lung cancer, who orally consumed one ounce of hydrated SV powder daily and a control group who did not ingest SV. Everyone in the trial simultaneously received chemotherapy, radiation, or surgery. Sun revised his recipe for a frozen version, which included soy and legumes, and conducted a second clinical study for sixty months in which patients ate ten ounces of Sun's soup every day.

Applying for a U.S. patent, Sun sought protection of his recipe to mitigate cancerous conditions and received a patent on August 1, 1995. Sun, who established the Connecticut Institute for Aging and Cancer, summarized his results with colleagues in two *Nutrition and Cancer* articles published in 1999 and 2001. He hypothesized that some aspect of SV battled cancer and extended lives but did not address or control for the impact of chemotherapy. Sun's testing was flawed because of the limited number of subjects, most of whom volunteered, knowing about his soup's anticancer possibilities and not representing a random test group. Also, the freeze-dried powder and frozen soup thawed for consumption in the two trials differed chemically. Researchers acknowledged that Sun's soup needed more scientific trials before definitive results regarding its ability to impede cancer could be determined.

Sun stated that his mother was free of cancerous growths fifteen years after he created his first soup, crediting it for her health. Founding Sun Farm Soup Company at Milford, Connecticut, Sun oversaw the production of Sun's soup for commercial sale.

The anticancer benefits of Sun's soup remain scientifically unproven. The U.S. Food and Drug Administration (FDA) does not endorse Sun's soup because it is advertised as a supplement, and by law the FDA does not regulate supplements in the stringent way that it does drugs.

Side effects: There are no known side effects to ingesting Sun's soup, other than a bloated sensation felt by those who participated in Sun's early studies. Later study participants who ingested a frozen, rather than the earlier freeze-dried, formulation of SV did not report bloating.

Elizabeth D. Schafer, Ph.D.

See also: Bronchial adenomas; Cancell; Chemotherapy; Cobalt 60 radiation; Complementary and alternative therapies; Herbs as antioxidants; Lung cancers; Nutrition and cancer prevention; Nutrition and cancer treatment

▶ Artificial sweeteners

Category: Lifestyle and Prevention
Also known as: Aspartame, saccharin

Definition: Artificial sweeteners are nonnutritive chemical substances that have virtually no or very low caloric value and are used as substitutes in food products for natural sweeteners such as sugar and honey. Artificial sweeteners are commonly used for controlling weight and insulin levels.

Government-approved artificial sweeteners: Artificial sweeteners are nonnutritive in nature since they provide no calories or energy to the body. There are five artificial sweeteners—aspartame (NutraSweet, Equal), saccharin (Sweet'N Low, Sweet Twin, Necta Sweet), acesulfame K (Sunnet, Sweet One), neotame, and sucralose (Splenda)—approved for use in the United States by the U.S. Food and Drug Administration (FDA). Two artificial sweeteners that the FDA has not approved are alitame and cyclamate.

Aspartame is two hundred times sweeter than sugar and was approved for use as a general-purpose sweetener in all foods and drinks in 1996. Saccharin is two hundred to seven hundred times sweeter than sugar. It is used as a tabletop sweetener and in soft drinks and chewing gum. Acesulfame K was first approved by the FDA as a tabletop sweetener and is about two hundred times sweeter than sugar. Neotame, which is about seven thousand to fourteen thousand times sweeter than sugar, was approved in 2002 as a general-purpose sweetener in a wide variety of food products. Sucralose is the only artificial sweetener that has three chlorine atoms in its chemical structure and is six hundred times sweeter than sugar. It was approved in 1998 for use in food products, such as beverages, chewing gum, and frozen desserts. Sucralose was approved by the FDA as a general-purpose sweetener in all foods in 1999.

Metabolism: Sucrose, the chemical entity in natural table sugar, binds to special receptor proteins in the taste buds. This binding initiates a cascade of events that finally results in a signal sent to the brain that causes the sensation of sweet taste. Additionally, sugar is a carbohydrate that is metabolized by the body to provide calories. Artificial sweeteners have a greater affinity for the receptor proteins and work by binding two hundred to fourteen hundred times more strongly to the receptor proteins than sucrose. As a result of their stronger binding capacity, the artificial sweeteners are needed in much lower quantities than sugar to produce the same degree of sweetness.

The artificial sweeteners are either excreted by the body or converted to by-products with little or no caloric output. Saccharin, sucralose, and acesulfame K are excreted unchanged by the body and do not provide any calories. The enzymes in the body hydrolyze neotame and produce methanol as a by-product. Aspartame is broken down in the body to produce methanol and the amino acids aspartic acid and phenylalanine and very few calories compared with sugar. Methanol is further degraded to formaldehyde in the body. Both methanol and formaldehyde are toxic to human beings at high doses. People with the genetic disease phenylketonuria (PKU) lack the enzyme that breaks down phenylalanine. Because phenylalanine is produced as a by-product of aspartame digestion, people with PKU should not ingest aspartame. Foods containing aspartame must carry a label warning consumers with PKU that the product is a source of phenylalanine.

Cancer risk: Questions regarding the risk of cancer associated with the consumption of artificial sweeteners arose when early studies indicated that saccharin caused bladder cancer in test animals. Subsequent epidemiological studies of groups of people did not find a definitive correlation between saccharin use and bladder cancer. There are two more controversial reports on the correlation between aspartame use and cancer. One study found more lymphomas and leukemias in rats fed very high doses of aspartame while the other study did not find a link between aspartame use and cancer.

Artificial sweeteners are regulated by the Food and Drug Administration. Before artificial sweeteners can be launched in the U.S. market, the FDA reviews numerous safety studies conducted with them, including the studies that assess their potential cancer risk. The reviews have not conclusively demonstrated any strong positive correlation between various cancers and artificial sweetener use. Studies continue to be conducted, and the FDA will continue to review and evaluate the results.

Artificial sweeteners are beneficial for people with diabetes and for people on weight-loss plans. The effects of their long-term use on weight-maintenance and cancer risk are controversial because they are not clearly understood. In the light of insufficient experimental data and all the controversy swirling around the use of artificial sweeteners, moderation should be the watchword for everyone using them.

Lalitha Krishnan, Ph.D.

For Further Information

Abegaz, E. M. "Aspartame Not Linked to Cancer." *Environmental Health Perspectives* 115, no. 1 (January, 2007): A16-17.

Gallus, S., et al. "Artificial Sweeteners and Cancer Risk in a Network of Case-Control Studies." *Annals of Oncology* 18, no. 1 (January, 2007): 40-44.

Lim, U., et al. "Consumption of Aspartame-Containing Beverages and Incidence of Hematopoietic and Brain Malignancies." *Cancer Epidemiology Biomarkers and Prevention* 15 (September, 2006): 1654-1659.

Soffritti, Morando, et al. "First Experimental Demonstration of the Multi-potential Carcinogenic Effects of Aspartame Administered in the Feed to Sprague-Dawley Rats." *Environmental Health Perspectives* 114, no. 3 (March, 2006): 379-385.

Other Resources

Green Facts
http://www.greenfacts.org/en/aspartame/artificial-sweeteners.htm

MayoClinic.com
Artificial Sweeteners: A Safe Alternative to Sugar
http://www.mayoclinic.com/health/diabetes-diet/NU00592

National Cancer Institute
Artificial Sweeteners and Cancer: Questions and Answers
http://www.cancer.gov/cancertopics/factsheet/Risk/artificial-sweeteners

See also: Dietary supplements; Nutrition and cancer prevention; Obesity-associated cancers; Weight loss

▶ Beta-carotene

Category: Lifestyle and Prevention
ATC code: A11CA02
Also known as: A-Caro-25, betacarotene, carotene, carotenoid, Lumitene, retinal, retinol

Definition: Beta-carotene is a member of a family of nutrients called carotenoids, which are found in many red, orange, yellow, and green fruits and vegetables (such as carrots, sweet potatoes, squash, spinach, apricots, and broccoli). The body converts beta-carotene into vitamin A, which plays a role in vision, bone development, cell division, and cell differentiation.

Cancers treated or prevented: Studies have found that a diet high in fruits and vegetables containing beta-carotene reduces the risk of certain types of cancer, including those of the prostate and lung. Researchers believe that beta-carotene and other antioxidants in fruits and vegetables work together to lower cancer risk.

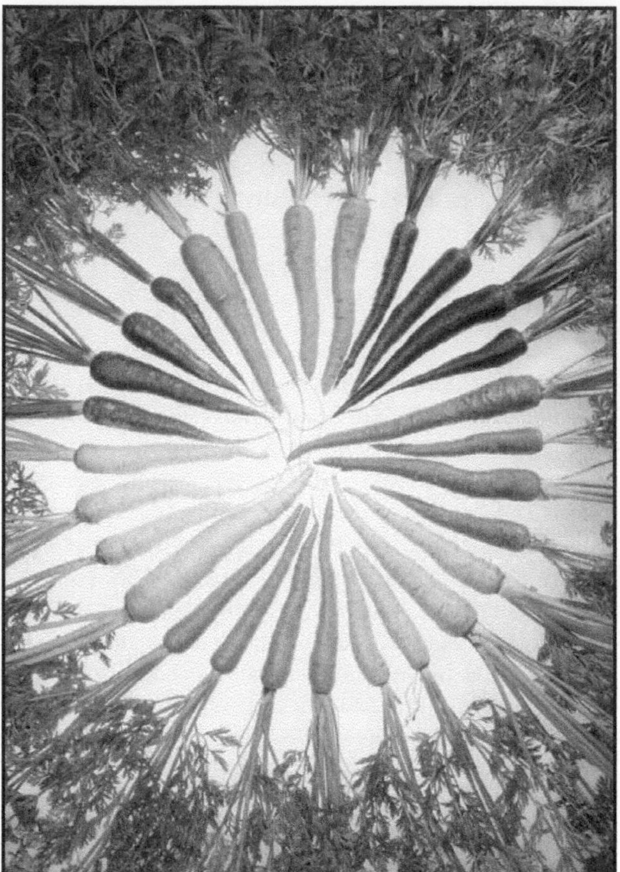

Carrots contain beta-carotene, among other nutrients. (U.S. Department of Agriculture)

It was thought that beta-carotene supplements might reduce the risk of certain cancers, especially lung cancer, but there is no evidence of any cancer preventive benefit when beta-carotene is taken alone in supplement form. In fact, studies have found that smokers and people who have been exposed to asbestos who take beta-carotene supplements have a significantly higher risk of developing lung cancer and of dying from their cancer than those who do not take the supplements. In addition, the National Cancer Institute's Prostate, Lung, Colorectal, and Ovarian Cancer Screening Trial (1992-2001) found that men with the highest levels of beta-carotene in their blood were at increased risk for developing more aggressive and deadly prostate cancer.

Delivery routes: Oral in capsule and tablet forms. Eating five servings of fruits and vegetables daily provides 6 to 8 milligrams of beta-carotene.

How this substance works: Beta-carotene is an antioxidant. It protects cells and deoxyribonucleic acid (DNA) from damage caused by unstable molecules called free radicals, which are produced during metabolic processes as cells burn up oxygen for energy. Free radicals are believed to contribute to cancer and other diseases. Vitamin A, which the body produces from beta-carotene, helps prevent the uncontrolled cell growth that occurs with cancer.

Side effects: Beta-carotene may increase the risk of lung cancer or prostate cancer in people who smoke or drink alcohol heavily or who have been exposed to asbestos. It also may increase the risk of more aggressive prostate cancers. In high doses, beta-carotene may interact with some types of chemotherapy drugs or radiation.

Stephanie Watson, B.S.

See also: Antioxidants; Carotenoids; Chemoprevention; Free radicals; Fruits; Nutrition and cancer prevention; Stomach cancers

▶ Bioflavonoids

Category: Lifestyle and Prevention
Also known as: Flavonoids

Definition: Flavonoids are the most common plant phenolic compounds. Their basic chemical structure consists of two benzene rings linked by a chain of three carbon atoms that can itself form a heterocyclic ring with oxygen. Variations of this chemical theme give rise to thousands of different bioflavonoids, which can be grouped in several families. Six families include bioflavonoids particularly common in the diet: flavonols, flavanols, flavonones (or flavanones), isoflavones, flavones, and anthocyanidines. Examples of bioflavonoids from each of these families are quercetin, cathechin, hesperitin, genistein, apigenin, and cyanidine, respectively. Most of the plant bioflavonoids occur as glycosides, that is, they have a sugar attached.

Nutrition: The principal food sources of bioflavonoids are apples, celery, onions, green and black tea, citrus fruits, berries, soy, red wine, and cocoa. Although bioflavonoids are resistant to heat, certain food manipulations, such as the peeling of fruits or boiling, can cause some loss of their content or bioavailability. After the sugar moiety is removed by enzymes of the gastrointestinal tract, a variable portion of the ingested bioflavonoids is readily absorbed. The absorbed bioflavonoids are metabolized in the liver by conjugation with other chemical groups (for example, glucuronic acid, sulfate, or methyl groups) and converted to smaller compounds.

Bioflavonoids and cancer: Numerous studies in experimental models, both in vivo and in vitro, have suggested that bioflavonoids have anticarcinogenic potential. As effective antioxidants, they prevent mutagenesis and tumor promotion by protecting deoxyribonucleic acid (DNA) and proteins from oxidative damage. By acting on signal transduction pathways that control the cell cycle, bioflavonoids inhibit proliferation and stimulate apoptosis, that is, programmed death, of human cancer cells. Cell cycle-related actions performed by bioflavonoids include suppressing nuclear factor kappa B activation, inhibiting mitogen-activated protein kinases, and blocking epidermal growth factor signaling. Bioflavonoids also stimulate detoxifying enzymes, such as cytochrome P450, which convert carcinogens into water-soluble compounds that can be eliminated from the body. In addition, they inhibit inflammation and angiogenesis.

There is also strong scientific evidence that diets rich in fruits and vegetables protect against various forms of cancer. Some epidemiological studies have shown significant associations between high consumption of bioflavonoids and a reduced risk of certain forms of cancer, such as lung, rectal, and prostate cancers. However, several other epidemiological studies have failed to find such significant associations. Although bioflavonoids are gaining increasing acceptance as cancer-preventing agents, more consistent epidemiological data is needed before issuing specific public health guidelines.

Reyniel Cruz-Aguado, Ph.D.

See also: Antioxidants; Beta-carotene; Carotenoids; Chemoprevention; Coenzyme Q10; Complementary and alternative therapies; Curcumin; Dietary supplements; Essiac; Free radicals; Fruits; Garlic and allicin; Green tea; Herbs as antioxidants; Isoflavones; Lutein; Lycopene; Nutrition and cancer prevention; Phenolics; Phytoestrogens; Resveratrol; Wine and cancer

▶ Calcium

Category: Lifestyle and Prevention
Also known as: Calcium carbonate, calcium citrate, calcium phosphate

Definition: Calcium is the most abundant mineral in the body. About 1 percent of calcium is found circulating in the blood, while the remaining 99 percent is stored in bones and teeth. Calcium must be obtained from the diet. It is found primarily in dairy products and is sold as a dietary supplement.

Cancers treated or prevented: Colorectal cancer, breast cancer

Delivery routes: Oral tablet

How this substance works: Circulating levels of calcium help control metabolic events such as muscle contraction and nerve impulse transmission. In healthy people, the amount of calcium in the blood is kept within narrow limits by hormonal regulation. Calcium also helps to build strong bones and delay bone loss caused by aging (osteoporosis). The United States Office of Internal Medicine has established a maximum safe intake level for calcium of 2,500 milligrams per day for persons over one year of age.

Animal studies and several human observational and research studies have found that increased intake of calcium is protective against the development of colorectal cancer. The reason for this protective effect is not understood, and not all studies have found calcium to be protective against colorectal cancer. In 2007, the Women's Health Initiative study of more than 36,000 women aged fifty to seventy-nine found no effect of calcium on the development of colorectal cancer. More research must be done on the relationship between cancer and calcium in different age and gender groups before drawing any firm conclusions.

Animal studies have also suggested that calcium may protect against breast cancer. In 2007, a peer-reviewed study of 10,500 premenopausal women found that when the intakes of calcium and vitamin D were simultaneously increased for an extended period, the risk of developing breast cancer was reduced by almost one-third. This effect was not seen in postmenopausal women. Clinical trials examining the relationship between cancer and calcium are under way; information is available at http:// www .clinicaltrials.gov.

Side effects: Complicating the situation with calcium is evidence that increasing calcium intake in men in amounts ranging from 600 to 2,000 milligrams or more per day may increase the risk of developing prostate cancer. This is not, however, a consistent finding, and more rigorous studies need to be done.

Many tumors that invade bone release stored calcium and cause the blood level of calcium to increase independent of dietary intake. This condition, called hypercalcemia, is the most common life-threatening metabolic disorder associated with cancer.

Martiscia Davidson, A.M.

See also: Bone scan; Breast cancers; Caffeine; Calcifications of the breast; Cartilage supplements; Chemoprevention; Colon polyps; Colorectal cancer; Ductogram; Fiber; Gastrointestinal cancers; Hypercalcemia; Kidney cancer; Microcalcifications; Nutrition and cancer prevention; Polyps

▶ Cancer vaccines

Category: Lifestyle and Prevention
Also known as: Biological Response Modifiers

Definition: Cancer vaccines work by stimulating or restoring the ability of the host's immune system to fight infections and disease either as preventive/prophylactic or treatment/therapeutic vaccines.

Cancer treated or prevented: FDA-approved vaccines Gardasil® and Cervarix® protect against infection by human papillomavirus (HPV) types 16 and 18, which cause approximately 70% of cervical cancer worldwide. HPV types 16 and/or 18 cause some vaginal, vulvar, anal, penile, and oropharyngeal cancers.

Gardasil® is used in females ages 9 to 26 to prevent cervical cancer and some vulvar and vaginal cancers. It is also used to prevent anal cancer and precancerous anal lesions in males and females ages 9 to 26. Cervarix® is used in females ages 9 to 25 to prevent cervical cancer and may provide partial protection against additional HPV types that can cause cancer.

The Hepatitis B Virus (HBV) infection can lead to liver cancer. The FDA-approved HBV vaccine (1981) was the first successful cancer vaccine. Most US children are vaccinated shortly after birth.

Delivery routes: Most cancer vaccines are delivered by intramuscular or subcutaneous injection.

How these compounds work: Cancer vaccines activate and direct B cells and killer T cells to recognize and act against specific types of cancer. They introduce one or more antigens, proteins, or another type of molecule found on the surface of or inside a cell, into the body to stimulate a specific immune response.

The immune system recognizes microbes as potential threats because they carry foreign "non-self" antigens. Normal cells have antigens identifying them as "self." Self-antigens tell the immune system that normal cells are not a threat.

Cancer cells can carry both self-antigens and cancer-associated antigens. The cancer-associated antigens mark the cancer cells as abnormal or foreign and cause immune cells like B-cells and killer T-cells to attack. Cancer vaccines are based on antigens and are relatively easy to recognize as foreign by the immune system.

Side effects: Cancer vaccines have safety profiles comparable to those of traditional vaccines with side effects varying among vaccine formulations and persons.

Common side effects include inflammation at injection site, including redness, pain, swelling, warming of the skin, itchiness, and occasionally a rash. Less common side effects consist of flu-like symptoms, fever, chills, weakness, dizziness, nausea or vomiting, muscle ache, fatigue, headache, and blood pressure or occasional breathing concerns. More serious side effects may include asthma, appendicitis, pelvic inflammatory disease, and certain autoimmune diseases, including arthritis and systemic lupus erythematosus. Rare life-threatening adverse effects include severe hypersensitivity (allergic) reactions to specific vaccine ingredients.

Robert Koch, DNSc, RN

For Further Information

Delamarre, L, Mellman, I. & Yadav, M. (2015). Neo approaches to cancer vaccines. *Science*, 348(6236): 760-761.

Dotinga, R. (2014, April 16). Cancer "vaccine" for advanced disease passes early hurdle. *Health Day Reporter.* Retrieved from http://consumer.healthday.com/cancer-information-5/mis-cancer-news-102/cancer-vaccine-for-advanced-disease-passes-early-hurdle-686863.html

Dreifus, C. (2014, March 3). Arming the immune system against cancer. *The New York Times*, pp. D2. Retrieved from http://www.nytimes.com/2015/03/03/science/arming-the-immune-system-against-cancer.html

McNeil, D. G. (2014, April 1). Expansion in use of cancer vaccine. *The New York Times,* pp. D5. Retrieved from http://www.nytimes.com/2014/04/01/health/an-expansion-in-use-of-cancer-vaccine.html?_r=0

Pollack, A. (2003, August 19). Theories vary on cancer vaccines. *The New York Times*. Retrieved from http://www.nytimes.com/2003/08/19/health/theories-vary-on-cancer-vaccines.html

Other Resources

National Cancer Institute
Cancer Vaccines
http://www.cancer.gov/

CancerNet
What are Cancer Vaccines?
http://www.cancer.net/navigating-cancer-care/how-cancer-treated/immunotherapy-and-vaccines/what-are-cancer-vaccines

History of Vaccines
Cancer Vaccines and Immunotherapy
http://www.historyofvaccines.org/

▶ Carotenoids

Category: Lifestyle and Prevention
Also known as: Carotenes (alpha-carotene, beta-carotene)

Definition: Carotenoids are chemical substances found in yellow, orange, and red fruits as well as dark green, leafy vegetables. They are rich in antioxidants, and some studies suggest that inclusion of carotenoids in diets sharply reduces the risks of a variety of cancers. Other studies warn that they may actually promote cancer when taken in pill or capsule form, especially in smokers or former smokers.

Cancers treated or prevented: May reduce risk of prostate, breast, lung, cervical, colon, stomach, rectal, ovarian, oral, pharyngeal, bladder, and other cancers

Delivery routes: Oral in diet, tablet, or capsule

How these compounds work: Carotenoids are chemicals produced by plants best known for their reddish and yellowish colors, as in the reds of a tomato or carrot. Carotenoids reduce the risk and incidence of cancer by acting as antioxidants, binding with and thereby reducing the amount of free radicals in the human body. Free radicals (which act as oxidants) are unstable molecules that lack a sufficient number of electrons. In their quest to become stable, they can wreak havoc on genetic material and proteins, disrupting cell molecules and chemical processes and making cells more susceptible to cancer. Antioxidants eliminate many of these cell-harming free radicals, in theory reducing the predisposition of cells to become cancerous. Studies have also suggested that carotenoids in the diet can inhibit cancer development by stimulating the manufacture of detoxifying enzymes and inhibiting the proliferation of cancer cells by the regulation of communication between cancer cells.

The mechanism by which carotenoids may affect or prevent cancerous cells is unknown. Lycopene and beta-carotene are the two most widely studied carotenoids, though there are at least six hundred known carotenoids in all. Researchers have shown in the laboratory that small concentrations of alpha- or beta-carotene severely hindered the growth and spread of neuroblastoma cells. The *N-myc* gene exists in all cells and codes for proteins that stimulate cell growth. Usually, this gene is dormant unless the cell becomes damaged or receives signals to activate cellular growth. Carotenoids inhibit this gene activity, causing a decrease in activation or complete inactivation of this gene in cancerous cells.

Most—but not all—studies show an inverse relationship between serum levels of carotenoids and cancer incidence, but others show no affiliation and still others even show that high levels of certain carotenoids such as 3-carotene may increase the risk of certain types of cancers. All, however, agree that the antioxidant role of carotenoids reduces the concentration of harmful oxidants, and many more studies are being conducted that may better control for lifestyle differences, age, gender, and genetic predisposition. It remains the consensus among researchers and physicians that regardless of the study outcomes, carotenoids are most likely beneficial and play some role in cancer prevention.

Side effects: Although no specific side effects are known, consumption of large amounts of 3-carotene may increase the risk of lung cancer, especially in smokers. As stated in the *Wellness Guide to Dietary Supplements* (produced by the *Berkeley Wellness Letter*, available online at http://www.wellnessletter.com/):

> Don't assume that beta carotene or other antioxidants in supplement form are beneficial, or even harmless. Don't take beta carotene pills, particularly if you've ever been a smoker. Beta carotene is plentiful in vegetables and fruits, and is safe and beneficial when consumed from such foods.

Dwight G. Smith, Ph.D.

See also: Antioxidants; Beta-carotene; Chemoprevention; Fruits; Nutrition and cancer prevention; Stomach cancers

▶ Coffee and cancer

Category: Lifestyle and Prevention
Also known as: Coffee consumption and cancer

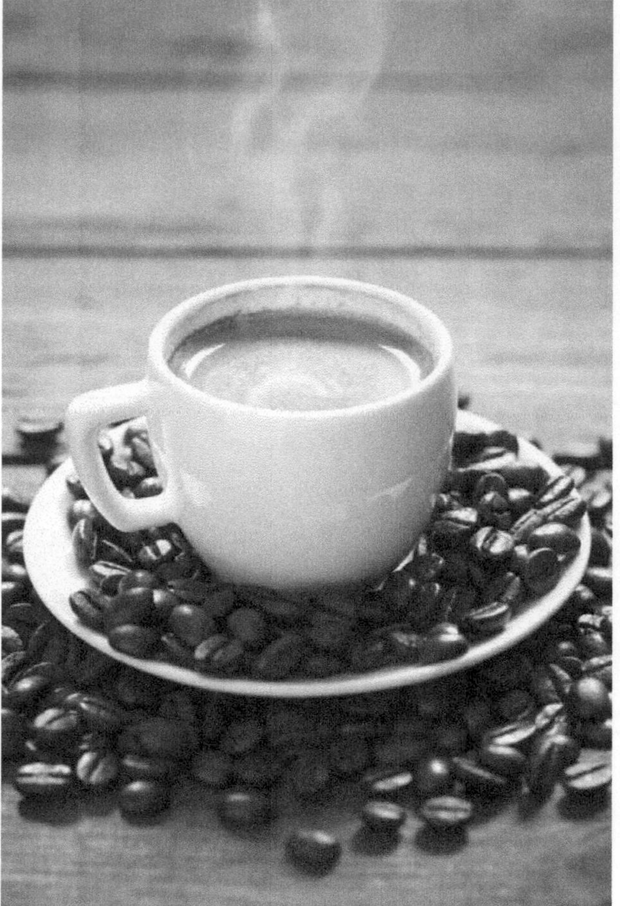

(iStock)

Definition: A globally consumed beverage derived from the coffee bean, which is the pit of the coffee cherry that grows on the coffee tree. Coffee consumption predates the 15th century with legend placing its discovery in Ethiopia and later cultivation in the Arabian Peninsula.

Cancer treated or prevented: Thousands of studies have been conducted to evaluate the relationship of coffee and cancer. A 1980s study suggested a causal relationship between drinking coffee and pancreatic cancer. Yet the majority of recent studies link drinking coffee on a regular basis to a reduced risk of cancers such as endometrial cancer, lethal prostate and prostate cancer reoccurrence or progression, colon cancer, aggressive breast cancer and breast cancer in postmenopausal women, breast cancer recurrence, malignant cutaneous melanoma, glioma, pharyngeal and oropharyngeal cancer, and hepatocellular liver cancer.

Delivery routes: Coffee is usually consumed orally as a hot or cold drink. People drink coffee black or with additives like cream, sugar or sweeteners, and/or flavorings. The studies on coffee and cancer generally suggest that one needs to drink 2 to 5 cups per day to reduce risk of cancer.

How these compounds work: The coffee bean has about 1000 natural compounds. Among these are antioxidant phytochemicals that can help combat disease. Specific compounds in coffee that may provide reduced risk of cancer are chlorogenic acid, quinic acid, cafestol and kahweol in unfiltered coffee, and caffeine. N-methylpyridinium, created in the coffee bean during the roasting process, may make the naturally occurring antioxidants even more powerful. Some studies specifically differentiate the value of caffeinated versus non-caffeinated coffee and the risk of cancer.

Side effects: Coffee contains caffeine, a natural central nervous system stimulant, which can disrupt sleep and cause insomnia if taken close to bedtime. It can increase anxiety and agitation, elevate the blood pressure, cause headaches, and stimulate rapid or irregular heartbeats. Long-term use of coffee has been associated with gastrointestinal disturbances such as nausea, ulcers, acidity, IBS, and acid reflux. Drinking coffee can affect mineral absorption such as iron or magnesium. The potentially carcinogenic acrylamide may appear when coffee is roasted at high temperatures.

Marylane Wade Koch, MSN, RN

For Further Information

Cancer Network Editors. (2015). Coffee and Cancer Risk. *Cancer Network: Home of the Journal Oncology*. http://www.cancernetwork.com/articles/coffee-and-cancer-risk

Doheny, K. (2015).Coffee May Lower Endometrial Cancer Risk. *WebMD News from Health Day*. http://www.webmd.com/cancer/news/20150206/coffee-linked-to-possible-lower-endometrial-cancer-risk

Mozes, A. (2015). Can Coffee Lower Risk of Colon Cancer's Return? *WebMD News from Health Day*. http://www.webmd.com/colorectal-cancer/news/20150817/can-coffee-lower-risk-of-colon-cancers-return

Schmeck, Jr. H.M. (1981). Study Links Coffee Use to Pancreas Cancer. *The New York Times*. http://www.nytimes.com/1981/03/12/us/study-links-coffee-use-to-pancreas-cancer.html

Zelman, K.M. (2008). The Buzz on Coffee. *WebMD*. http://www.webmd.com/diet/the-buzz-on-coffee

Other Resources

Coffee: Beyond the Buzz. *National Geographic*. http://www.nationalgeographic.com/coffee/ax/frame.html

Coffee and Health
http://www.cancernetwork.com/articles/coffee-and-cancer-risk

National Coffee Association USA (NCA, Est. 1911).
http://www.ncausa.org/Coffee-Health

Vanderbilt University Institute for Coffee Studies. (Est. 1999).
http://vanderbilt.edu/ics/

See also: Caffeine

▶ Cruciferous vegetables

Category: Lifestyle and Prevention
Also known as: *Brassicaceae* family, glucosinolates, isothiocyanates, indole-3-carbinol

Definition: Cruciferous vegetables are edible plants from the *Brassicaceae* family that include broccoli, cauliflower, brussels sprouts, cabbage, arugula, watercress, bok choy, turnip and mustard greens, kale, kohlrabi, turnips, rutabagas, and radishes. Cruciferous vegetables contain a variety of healthful substances such as vitamin C, selenium, fiber, and sulfur-containing compounds called glucosinolates. The sulfur compounds give cruciferous vegetables their pungent taste and aroma.

Cancers treated or prevented: Colorectal cancer, lung cancer, prostate cancer

Delivery routes: Oral by diet

How these compounds work: Cruciferous vegetables are rich sources of glucosinolate compounds, which may be the source of their cancer-fighting effects. When the vegetables are chopped or chewed, bioactive hydrolysis products of glucosinolates, such as isothiocyanates and indole-3-carbinol, are formed. These compounds may help prevent certain cancers by eliminating dietary carcinogens from the body or by preventing normal cells from becoming cancerous. Cooking or boiling cruciferous vegetables decreases the amount and bioavailability of glucosinolates, so raw vegetables provide much higher levels of the compounds than do cooked vegetables.

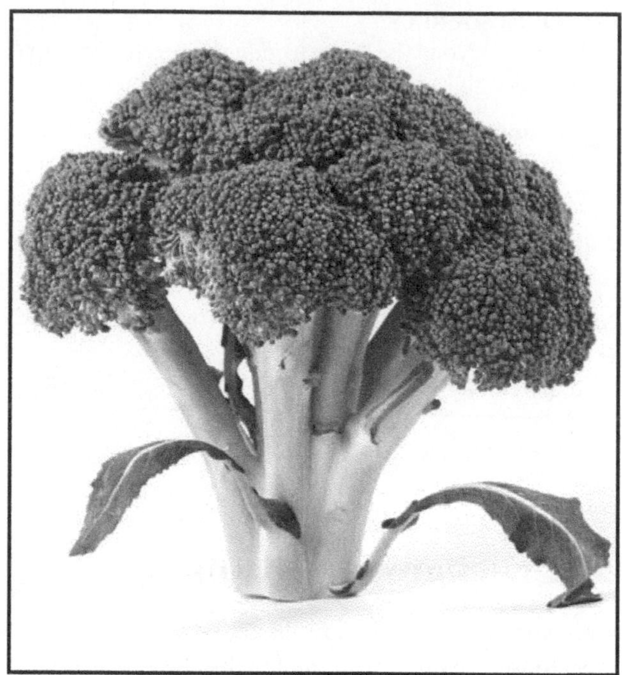

Cruciferous vegetables such as broccoli are rich sources of glucosinolate compounds, which may be the source of their cancerfighting effects. (iStock)

Higher intakes of cruciferous vegetables have been linked to a lower risk of lung, prostate, and colorectal cancer in epidemiological studies. Current evidence is limited, however, and the effects are not consistent. In addition, it is not clear whether the beneficial effects of cruciferous vegetables come from the glucosinolate compounds or from other phytochemicals that act synergetically. Genetic variability may influence the effects of cruciferous vegetables on cancer risk. For example, individuals may vary in their capacity to absorb, metabolize, and eliminate glucosinolate compounds from the body. Thus, genetic differences that affect how long these compounds or their metabolites remain in the body may influence how protective they are against cancer. The National Cancer Institute recommends the daily consumption of five to nine servings of fruits and vegetables; human epidemiological studies suggest five weekly servings of cruciferous vegetables are beneficial.

Side effects: Very high intakes of cruciferous vegetables may cause hypothyroidism. In addition, some of the isolated metabolites of glucosinolates in cruciferous vegetables, such as indole-3-carbinol, have produced mixed results in animal studies. For example, depending on when the compound is administered or the length of exposure, indole-3-carbinol can prevent or promote the development of cancer in animals. These studies highlight the disadvantages of isolating potentially beneficial compounds from food, as isolated compounds may produce unwanted effects, and the synergy of many compounds may be critical in cancer prevention.

Linda Hart, M.S., M.A.

See also: Beta-carotene; Chemoprevention; Folic acid; Indoles; Lutein; Nutrition and cancer prevention; Polyps; Prevention; Stomach cancers; Thyroid cancer

▶ Esophageal speech

Category: Lifestyle and Prevention; Social and Personal Issues

Definition: Esophageal speech, also called esophageal voice, is speech produced by swallowing air and forcing it out again through the esophagus. Patients who have had their larynx, or voice box, removed because of cancer have to practice esophageal speech to communicate verbally.

Anatomy and physiology: The larynx (voice box) is a 2-inch (5-centimeter, or cm), tube-shaped organ in the neck toward the front of the body between the pharynx (throat) and the trachea (windpipe). The larynx is part of the body's respiratory (breathing) system. One of its main functions is to protect the airway to the lungs from food or drink "going down the wrong tube." The pharynx is a hollow tube about 5 inches (12 cm) long that starts behind the nose and ends at the top of the trachea and esophagus. The trachea, also part of the respiratory system, connects the larynx to the lungs. The esophagus is a muscular tube that connects the mouth and pharynx to the stomach. It lies between the trachea and the spine. The esophagus is part of the digestive system. When food is chewed and swallowed, the esophagus contracts to push the food down into the stomach, where digestion takes place.

Briefly, the human speech process begins when air streams from the lungs and passes over the vocal folds (vocal cords) in the larynx. The steady airstream causes the vocal folds to vibrate, which produces sound waves. The sound waves are then shaped and modified by the pharynx, tongue, lips, palate, and teeth to produce intelligible speech sounds.

Throat cancer: Throat cancer—also called vocal cord cancer, laryngeal cancer, and cancer of the glottis—strikes the vocal folds, larynx, or other areas of the throat.

It appears as a malignant tumor in almost any part of the throat. Although a person's genes may contribute to the development of throat cancer, the most common cause is smoking. Excessive alcohol use also increases the risk of developing throat cancer. Throat cancer occurs most often in adults older than the age of fifty and in men ten times more often than in women.

In the early stages, doctors can successfully treat throat cancer with radiation therapy or chemotherapy or a combination of the two. Following such treatments, most patients are able to keep their larynx and speak more or less normally. In the later stages of the disease, the most common treatment is surgery to remove the larynx along with the cancerous tumor. When a patient needs surgery, the type of operation depends on the size and exact location of the tumor. Surgeons may remove part of the larynx (partial laryngectomy) or the entire larynx (total laryngectomy).

Speaking after a laryngectomy: Patients without a voice box must learn to speak all over again. Several methods and a number of medical devices are available to help patients recover their ability to speak. One of the most common techniques is esophageal speech. With esophageal speech, the patient learns to take air into the mouth and swallow it or force it into the esophagus and then trap the air by locking the tongue to the roof of the mouth. The air is now in the digestive system, not in the respiratory system as normal. The patient then forces the air through the esophagus and back up into the mouth, much like a controlled belch. This causes the air to vibrate, along with the walls of the esophagus and the throat, and produce a low-pitched sound that becomes the patient's voice. The patient then shapes the voiced sound into recognizable words, as normal speakers do, with the tongue, lips, palate, and teeth. The esophageal voice emits a low-pitched guttural, croaking, sometimes soft and barely audible sound that many listeners find difficult to understand.

Because they must learn to train parts of their body for a new purpose, many patients find esophageal speech more difficult than speech they might produce with special medical devices. On the plus side, esophageal speech costs patients less than some other techniques because it does not require special equipment.

Living without a larynx: People who have had their larynx removed are known as laryngectomees. They must contend with more than learning to speak a new way. When the larynx is taken out, it leaves an opening in the neck called a tracheostoma, or stoma, for short. Patients cough, sneeze, and breathe through the stoma. They become neck breathers. The trachea is exposed through the stoma, so they need to take special care of the stoma. They have to keep it clean and moist. They have to cover it when showering and shaving. They usually have to avoid activities such as swimming or water skiing. They have to watch for a buildup of dried mucus, a substance that lubricates and moistens the esophagus. They must be especially careful of coughing and sneezing, which can expel large amounts of phlegm, a mucus of the respiratory system. They must eat much more slowly. They also must cope with the changes in their physical appearance.

Wendell Anderson, B.A.

For Further Information

Lazaroff, M. *The Complete Idiot's Guide to Anatomy and Physiology*. Indianapolis, Ind.: Alpha Books, 2004.

Prosek, R., and L. Vreeland. "The Intelligibility of Time-Domain-Edited Esophageal Speech." *Journal of Speech, Language, and Hearing Research* 44, no. 3 (2001): 525-534.

Thomas, J., and R. Keith. *Looking Forward: The Speech and Swallowing Guidebook for People with Cancer of the Larynx or Tongue*. New York: Thieme, 2005.

Other Resources

American Cancer Society

Speech After Laryngectomy

http://www.cancer.org/docroot/MBC/content/MBC_3_2X_Speech_After_Laryngectomy.asp?sitearea=MBC

WebWhispers

http://www.webwhispers.org

See also: Cordectomy; Electrolarynx; Laryngeal cancer; Laryngeal nerve palsy; Laryngectomy; Laryngoscopy; Parathyroid cancer; Throat cancer; Tracheostomy; Upper Gastrointestinal (GI) series

▶ Exercise and cancer

Category: Lifestyle and Prevention

Definition: Regular exercise has been found to reduce cancer risk and mortality. The more time a person spends in occupational or leisure activities requiring physical exertion, the lower their risk of cancer. For those who have cancer, regular exercise has been shown to improve recovery and help manage the side effects of treatments.

Physical Activity Recommendations for Healthy Adults from the Centers for Disease Control and Prevention

Aerobic or Cardio Activity

Option 1: 30 minutes (minimum) of moderate-intensity exercise most days of the week

- Walking, moderate to brisk pace (3-4.5 mph) on level surface
- Bicycling 5-9 mph, level terrain
- Yoga
- Ballroom dancing
- Tennis, doubles
- Golf, wheeling clubs and walking
- Shooting baskets
- Swimming recreationally
- Horseback riding
- Gardening and yard work
- Moderate housework (scrubbing the floor on all fours, carrying out trash)
- Hand washing and waxing a car
- Walking, running, or climbing when playing with children
- Walking while pushing or pulling a child in a stroller
- Option 2: 20 minutes (minimum) of vigorous-intensity exercise 3 days a week
- Jogging or running
- Walking briskly up a hill
- Roller skating or in-line skating briskly
- Bicycling more than 10 mph or on uphill terrain
- Karate, judo
- Jumping rope
- Stair climber machine at fast pace
- Professional or energetic ballroom dancing
- Tennis, singles
- Competitive sports such as football, basketball, soccer
- Ice skating quickly or speed skating
- Swimming laps
- Heavy yard work or gardening (felling trees, digging ditches)
- Racewalking or jogging while pushing a sports stroller

Strength Building Activity

2 days a week

- Weight lifting, 6 to 8 exercises, with 8 to 12 repetitions per exercise

Protective effects of exercise: Many studies have found an inverse relationship between exercise and many types of cancer, however, exactly how exercise protects individuals against various cancers is difficult to determine. A number of logical theories have been presented.

Regular exercise positively affects the blood by lowering glucose and insulin levels and improving white blood cell function. Hormonal changes include an increase in steroid hormones from the adrenal cortex and improvements in the insulin effects on cancer-fighting T cells. Exercise is also believed to improve vitamin C metabolism. All of these effects could protect the body from cancer.

A more complex area in which benefits are likely is cell division, which is rapid in cancers. Exercise increases anti-inflammatory cytokines, which decrease cell division. It also produces beneficial effects in preventing the activation of cancer genetic material called oncogenes. Another effect is the promotion of interferon production, which decreases viral reproduction. By decreasing cell reproduction, exercise may slow cancer growth.

Rehabilitation effects of exercise: The main goal of exercise for those who have cancer is to maintain or improve the physical capabilities of the body, resulting in an improved quality of life during and after treatment. No obvious effects of exercise on the immune system of cancer patients have been identified at this time. Some of the immediate effects of exercise on the cancer patient are decreased nausea and lessened symptoms of fatigue.

Part of the goal of exercise for cancer patients is to protect them from other health problems. Exercise helps them maintain healthy weights by decreasing fat but also decreasing the loss of muscle due to inactivity and treatments. Exercise increases blood flow throughout the body, reducing blood clot formation, particularly in the legs. Longer-term health risks such as osteoporosis (loss of bone) and cardiovascular disease are lowered by regular exercise.

Psychological benefits can also be obtained by cancer patients who exercise. Decreased anxiety and depression and improved self-esteem have been found. The ability to be more independent and do normal daily activities can contribute to this improved psychological state. With all of these potential benefits, cancer patients are advised to participate in exercise programs with individualized exercise prescriptions.

Exercise prescription and cancer: Cancer patients must check with their physicians before beginning an exercise program. It has been generally recommended that patients first complete a supervised exercise assessment to determine which types of exercise can be done safely. However, if exercise testing is a barrier to starting the exercise program it is acceptable to start a light-intensity program without an exercise test. Exercise assessments usually include a graded exercise test with evaluations of strength and flexibility. The graded exercise test is conducted on a treadmill or stationary bicycle, paying close attention to symptoms and fatigue. This should not be a maximal test to exhaustion but rather a submax test.

The information obtained from the medical assessment and exercise test (if done) are used to complete an exercise prescription. Mode, frequency, intensity, duration, and progression are considered. The type of exercise recommended includes aerobic activities that work the large muscle groups such as walking and cycling with moderate resistance training and stretching.

It is recommended that cancer patients exercise aerobically three to five times per week. In cases in which patients have low levels of conditioning, shorter sessions are attempted every day. Cancer patients' ability to tolerate exercise varies widely. Most are advised to exercise aerobically at a lower intensity than the general population. For healthy people, the typical heart rate range considered desirable for exercise is 70 to 85 percent of maximum heart rate, whereas in cancer patients, it is 60 to 70 percent of maximum heart rate. For cancer survivors who are undergoing treatment the heart rate may be less reliable for monitoring exercise intensity. Therefore rating of perceived exertion (RPE) is often advised instead. The RPE is a scale from 6 to 20 used by patients to indicate how hard they are exercising. Patients should exercise at an RPE of 12 to 16. The recommended duration of the exercise session is twenty to thirty continuous minutes. However, many cancer patients may not be able to exercise that long. In these cases, the patients can space out the twenty to thirty minutes with periodic rest intervals. The goal is gradually to shorten the length and frequency of rest periods until the patient can complete the exercise session without stopping. No matter what duration the patient can tolerate the ultimate goal is to accumulate 150 minutes of moderate-intensity exercise per week or 75 minutes of vigorous-intensity exercise per week. This is the same recommendation as for the healthy population.

Resistance training two to three times per week and daily flexibility exercises are also recommended. Resistance training should use weights, machines or weight-bearing exercises. About ten different exercises should be done at least one time with eight to twelve repetitions each. Moderate-intensity is recommended by using lighter weights. Flexibility exercises must be selected with movement limitations from cancer treatment in mind and include all major muscle groups.

In the healthy population, people progress by gradually increasing intensity, duration, or frequency. This may not be possible for cancer patients because of treatments that may cause regression. Therefore periodic modifications in the exercise program may need to be made which may include reducing the level of exercise.

Several precautions are advised for cancer patients. Treatments frequently lower blood counts, resulting in increased risk for infections, anemia, and bleeding. Blood counts are monitored during treatment and used to determine appropriate exercise times. Patients are advised to stop exercise during periods of low blood counts. Sodium and potassium levels can decrease with excessive vomiting. This decrease can lead to other health complications, and exercise should be avoided during these times. Treatments can also cause severe fatigue. When patients are fatigued, less intense exercise, or a break in exercise, is appropriate.

For cancer patients, lifting heavy weights and exercising on uneven floors that can affect balance are not advised. Conditions that warrant contacting a physician are swollen ankles; unexplained weight loss; shortness of breath with low-level activity; or exercise-induced nausea, vomiting, or unrelieved pain. Dizziness or blurred vision that does not go away with rest needs immediate attention from a physician. By paying attention to these safety measures, cancer patients can exercise safely and effectively.

The more people exert themselves physically, whether as part of work or leisure, the lower their risk of cancer.

Exercise, cancer, and fatigue: Cancer treatments such as chemotherapy and radiation cause fatigue in most patients. Incorporating exercise into the treatment gives the expectation of greater fatigue and less willingness to participate. However, appropriate, low-level aerobic exercise can actually decrease fatigue. Strategies exist to improve exercise adherence during cancer treatments.

One important factor is rest. Physical activity and rest must be balanced so there is no interference with nighttime sleep. This is best accomplished with a regular daily routine in which exercise takes place during times when the patient feels best. Reducing stress with regular relaxation techniques is helpful, along with a balanced diet that includes adequate protein. Getting plenty of fresh air, such as exercising outside, is beneficial as well.

Perspective and prospects: Although much progress is being made in the fight against cancer, it continues to be one of the major health problems. New drugs and other treatments to force cancer into remission will be developed, giving more hope to cancer patients. However, lifestyle interventions involving exercise, nutrition, and stress management can also be used to help treat and minimize treatment side effects. At the least, lifestyle interventions will improve the quality of life for cancer patients.

The correlation between cancer prevention and exercise has not been investigated to the same extent as exercise and cardiovascular disease. The cardiovascular benefits of exercise were found many years ago, and many studies have been conducted to determine the best exercise practices. As more research is conducted, the mechanisms for decreasing cancer risk will become more evident and the specific types of exercises associated with both prevention and treatment of specific cancers will be identified. This will give health professionals more options for fighting cancer and improving the quality of life for cancer survivors.

In the meantime, cancer patients can participate in appropriate exercise programs that include **moderate**-intensity aerobic **and resistance training** activities **with flexibility exercises**. Health care professionals as well as exercise leaders and trainers need to be continually updated about cancer and the benefits of exercise as additional information is found. Cancer is a challenging disease and all strategies must be used to reduce risk and improve outcomes.

Bradley R. A. Wilson, Ph.D.

For Further Information

American College of Sports Medicine. *ACSM's Guide to Exercise and Cancer Survivorship.* Champaign, IL: Human Kinetics, 2012.

American College of Sports Medicine. *ACSM's Guidelines for Exercise Testing and Prescription.* Baltimore: Wolters Kluwer/Lippincott Williams and Wilkins, 2014. (pp 264-273)

McTiernan, Anne, Julie Gralow, and Lisa Talbott. *Breast Fitness: An Optimal Exercise and Health Plan for Reducing Your Risk of Breast Cancer.* New York: St. Martin's Press, 2014.

Michaels, Carol and Maria Drozda. *Exercises for Cancer Survivors.* Victoria, BC:FriesenPress, 2013.

Smith, William, Keneth Adler, and Jo Brielyn. *Exercises for Cancer Wellness: Restoring Energy and Vitality While Fighting Fatigue.* Hobart, NY:Hatherleigh Press, 2016.

Other Resources

American Cancer Society

ACS Guidelines on Nutrition and Physical Activity for Cancer Prevention

http://www.cancer.org/healthy/eathealthygetactive/acsguidelinesonnutritionphysicalactivityforcancerprevention/

Exercises After Breast Surgery

http://www.cancer.org/cancer/breastcancer/moreinformation/exercises-after-breast-surgery

Physical Activity and the Cancer Patient

http://www.cancer.org/treatment/survivorshipduringandaftertreatment/stayingactive/physical-activity-and-the-cancer-patient

National Cancer Institute

Physical Activity and Cancer

http://www.cancer.gov/about-cancer/causes-prevention/risk/obesity/physical-activity-fact-sheet

See also: Aging and cancer; Anxiety; Chemoprevention; Dietary supplements; Fiber; Macrobiotic diet; Nutrition and cancer prevention; Prevention; Self-image and body image; Smoking cessation; Stress management

▶ Fiber

Category: Lifestyle and Prevention

Definition: Fiber is a natural structural chemical component of plants responsible for strength and architectural form. Examples of plant fiber include cellulose, hemicellulose, pectins, and lignins. Most plant fiber is difficult to digest and absorb because it is chemically complex and insoluble. Dietary fiber functions to clean out the digestive tract and move waste quickly through the intestines.

Cancers treated or prevented: Colorectal cancers, spastic bowel syndrome

Delivery routes: Fruits, vegetables, leafy greens, grains, or oral supplements as tablets or liquid form

How this substance works: Fiber in diets helps maintain optimal movement of food and wastes through the lower human digestive tract. Fiber helps cleanse the intestinal tract and colon, preventing the formation of pockets of residue. There are two basic types of dietary fiber, insoluble fiber and soluble fiber. Water-soluble fiber absorbs water in the intestines and via enzymatic activity mixes food into a gel on which intestinal enzymes work. Conversely, insoluble fiber is the more valuable in reducing risk of cancer as it is considerably more difficult to digest; thus carcinogens and toxins in the food are not released in the presence of the metabolically active cells of the intestinal lining but rather pass harmlessly out of the body. It

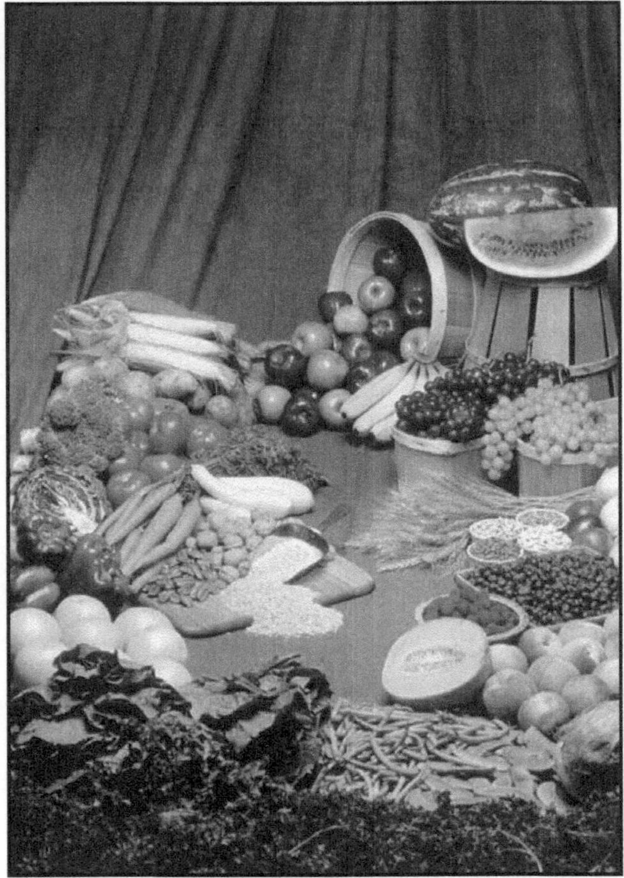

A diet rich in fiber from complex carbohydrates—grain, fruit, and vegetables—may reduce the risk of cancer. (U.S. Department of Agriculture)

follows that the less time carcinogens are in contact with the intestinal walls, the lower the risk of cancer should be because of decreased exposure to carcinogens carried in food and food wastes.

Insoluble fiber is sometimes referred to as the "scrub brush" for the human internal digestive tract because it "scrubs" the intestines clean as it passes through the small intestine and colon. This type of fiber acts to absorb many times its own weight in water, which softens the waste in the intestine and facilitates motion through the body, thereby decreasing irritation, constipation, and blockage.

Research has shown that fiber increases peristalsis, the involuntary muscular contractions of the digestive system. Regular and efficient peristalsis resulting from increased bulk in soft stools decreases the period of time that toxins are in contact with intestinal tissue. Fiber may also bind to carcinogens, lessening their proximity to internal cells. Water absorbed by fiber dilutes toxins, rendering them less harmful and decreasing the risk of cancer. Fiber can also help absorb intestinal acids such as bile, hydrochloric acid, and other irritants that may predispose cells to disease. Fiber can promote intestinal health by encouraging the growth of beneficial bacteria while discouraging the growth of harmful bacteria. A high-fiber diet may also reduce the incidence of diverticulosis and irritable bowel syndrome, both implicated in intestinal cancer.

Human studies suggesting an inverse relationship between insoluble dietary fiber intake and colorectal cancer incidence remain inconclusive because of the complexity of the disease. Many other factors, including heredity and lifestyle, play a role in the appearance of disease. An overwhelming majority of the long-term cohort studies, however, have pointed to dietary fiber as a means of reducing the risk for colorectal cancer.

Side effects: Some studies also show that excessive amounts of fiber may interfere with the absorption of certain minerals such as calcium, copper, iron, magnesium, selenium, and zinc. Excessive dietary fiber may also lead to constipation and occasional blockage. The frequency and intensity of both of these negative side affects can be reduced with the use of softening agents such as psyllium.

Dwight G. Smith, Ph.D.

See also: Chemoprevention; Colonoscopy and virtual colonoscopy; Colorectal cancer; Cruciferous vegetables; Diarrhea; Diverticulosis and diverticulitis; Fruits; Gastrointestinal cancers; Gastrointestinal complications of cancer treatment; Hemorrhoids; Laxatives; Nutrition and cancer prevention; Nutrition and cancer treatment; Polyps; Premalignancies; Prevention; Risks for cancer; Stomach cancers

▶ Folic acid

Category: Lifestyle and Prevention
Also known as: Folate, pteroylglutamic acid

Definition: Folate is a water-soluble B vitamin found naturally in foods such as lentils, green leafy vegetables, broccoli, cereals, citrus fruits, and liver. It is an essential cofactor for deoxyribonucleic acid (DNA) synthesis and replication and is necessary for the production of normal red blood cells. Folic acid is the synthetic, oxidized form used in commercial vitamin supplements and food fortification.

Cancers treated or prevented: Colorectal cancer, breast cancer

Delivery routes: Natural dietary sources, fortified foods, oral supplements

How this substance works: Folate is an essential cofactor in the de novo synthesis of purines and thymidylate and therefore plays a role in DNA synthesis, replication, stability, and repair. Evidence suggests that folate deficiency can lead to DNA damage and is associated with macrocytic anemia, neural tube defects, and cancer. In 1998, the U.S. Food and Drug Administration (FDA) began requiring the fortification of all flour and cereal grains with folic acid. These products are thus a major source of folic acid in the U.S. population. Large epidemiological studies that followed subjects for many years have found that higher dietary intake of folate and folic acid supplementation decreased the risk of colon and breast cancer. A possible explanation for its protective effect is that folate prevents DNA damage that may lead to the development of cancer.

Side effects: Research results on the benefits of folate in preventing cancer are inconsistent. Despite population studies showing positive effects of higher folate intake, studies in animals and humans also have shown that folic acid supplementation increased the risk of breast cancer and the development of colon polyps. These mixed results suggest that folate has a dual role in the development of cancer. In normal tissues, folate appears to suppress the development of cancer, presumably by preventing mutations. Once early lesions or tumors have developed, however, folate appears to promote their progression in colorectal and breast cancers. In these cases, folic acid may provide a source of nucleotides for rapidly proliferating tissues, including tumors. Indeed, antifolate drugs are sometimes used in the treatment of cancer. Thus, the timing, dose, and form of folate appear to be critical in whether this substance prevents or actually promotes certain types of cancers. For these reasons, the National Institutes of Health (NIH) do not currently recommend folic acid supplements to reduce the risk of cancer.

Linda Hart, M.S., M.A.

See also: Anemia; Antimetabolites in chemotherapy; Antineoplastics in chemotherapy; Antioxidants; Colon polyps; Dietary supplements; Free radicals; Fruits; Mesothelioma; Myelofibrosis

▶ Fruits

Category: Lifestyle and Prevention

Definition: In terms of nutrition, cancer prevention, and botanically, a fruit is the ripened ovary of an angiosperm (flowering plant). In the human diet, fruit generally refers to sweet and fleshy parts of certain plants. Examples of fruits include cherries, peaches, plums, apples, strawberries, and oranges.

How phytochemicals work: Fruits contain many phytochemicals that are believed to have an inverse relationship to cancer incidence or at least act as a protective agent against cancer-causing substances in the human body. Some of these chemicals believed to be active include allium compounds, carotenoids, coumarins, dietary fiber, dithiolthiones, flavonoids, folic acid, endole-3-carbinol, inositol hexaphosphate, isoflavones, isothiocyanates, D-limonene, phytosterols, protease inhibitors, saponins, selenium, and vitamins, especially vitamins C and E.

Carotenoids, including alpha- and beta-carotene, lutein, and lycopene, are found in yellow and orange vegetables and fruits, and act as antioxidants to maintain the functioning of the immune system. Antioxidants bind free radicals in the human body, which are unstable molecules that lack a sufficient number of electrons and can damage genetic material and proteins. This disrupts cell molecules and chemical processes, making cells more susceptible to cancer. When the amount and availability of free radicals in cells and tissues is decreased, the likelihood of cells becoming cancerous is similarly decreased. Studies have also suggested that carotenoids stimulate the manufacture of detoxifying enzymes and increase the formation of "gap junctions" between cells. Gap junctions are common pores between cells that allow the passage of small molecules, ions, and metabolites, and the formation of gap junctions between cancer cells and normal cells inhibit cancer cell proliferation and invasion. Ascorbic acid, or vitamin C, functions in a similar manner and can be found in citrus fruits and strawberries. Folic acid (also found in citrus fruits) is involved in the synthesis, repair, and function of deoxyribonucleic acid (DNA), while dietary fiber encourages peristalsis and, in turn, the elimination of harmful wastes and estrogens.

How fruits help: Overall, the benefits of moderate fruit intake in the diet include cell differentiation (which decreases cell proliferation), antioxidant potential, increase in activity of naturally protective enzymes, lower estrogen levels, and enhanced immune function.

Research shows a mixed relationship between cancer prevention and fruit consumption. In the past, total cancer risk was reported to decrease by at least 12 percent in populations that received adequate amounts of fruit per the dietary guidelines of the U.S. Department of Health and Human Services and the U.S. Department of Agriculture. However, in recent years, professionals have changed their views on the relationship between fruit consumption and cancer, based on new research. Although increased fruit and vegetable consumption tends to have a positive relationship on overall health, its preventative effect on certain types of cancer is statistically minimal. It is important to note, however, that this may be due to the inconsistent reporting of fruit intake and quality of fruits consumed. Nevertheless, fruits are still considered an important part of a healthy diet.

Side effects: Excessive consumption of fruit may cause gastrointestinal discomfort in some individuals and could increase the incidence or extent of diarrhea in others. Eating too much fruit or consuming fruit with high sugar content, such as grapes, ripe bananas, and mangos can also raise blood sugar levels. This may cause adverse health affects in patients with diabetes, insulin resistance, or polycystic ovarian syndrome (PCOS).

Dwight G. Smith, Ph.D.
Updated by: Gina Riley, Ph.D.

For Further Information

Boffetta, P., Couto, E., Wichmann, J., Ferrari, P., Trichopoulos, D., Bueno-de-Mesquita, H. B., … Trichopoulou, A. (2010). Fruit and vegetable intake and overall cancer risk in the European Prospective Investigation into Cancer and Nutrition (EPIC). *Journal of the National Cancer Institute,* 102, 529-537.

Researchers reviewed data on almost 500,000 people enrolled in a longitudinal large scale study on cancer and nutrition in Europe. Results showed that eating a recommended (200g) of fruit per day decreased cancer risk slightly by 3% in females only, concluding a minimal benefit in terms of cancer prevention.

Produce for Better Health Foundation. (2011). Fruits, vegetables, and health: A scientific overview. Retrieved from http://www.pbhfoundation.org/pdfs/about/res/pbh_res/PBH_Health_Benefit_Review.pdf.

Provides a meta analytic report (from research published between 2006 – 2011) on data regarding the effect of fruits and vegetables on health. Discusses the overall benefits of a diet rich in fruits and vegetables, and reviews data on the effects of fruits and vegetables on specific diseases and disorders, including cancer. Relays mixed results regarding the effect of fruit on the prevention and progression of different types of cancers.

Wang, M., Qin, S., Zhang, T., Song. X., & Zhang, S. (2015). The effect of fruit and vegetable intake on the development of lung cancer: A meta analysis of 32 publications and 20,414 cases. *European Journal of Clinical Nutrition,* 69, 1184–1192.

A meta analytic study on the effect of fruits and vegetables on rates of lung cancer. Results indicated that increased intake of fruits and vegetables may have a protective effect on lung cancer, especially in females. However, the authors note that further study in this area is needed, as it is difficult to isolate the effects of fruit and vegetables from other variables.

Other Resources

Anticancer: A New Way of Life
http://www.anticancerbook.com/

Dana Farber Cancer Institute: Sugar and Cancer Cells
http://www.dana-farber.org/Health-Library/Sugar-and-Cancer-Cells.aspx

Harvard T.H. Chan School of Public Health: The Nutrition Source
http://www.hsph.harvard.edu/nutritionsource/what-should-you-eat/vegetables-and-fruits/

See also: Antioxidants; Beta-carotene; Bioflavonoids; Carotenoids; Chemoprevention; Coenzyme Q10; Dietary supplements; Fiber; Folic acid; Free radicals; Herbs as antioxidants; Isoflavones; Lutein; Lycopene; Macrobiotic diet; Nutrition and cancer prevention; Phytoestrogens; Prevention; Resveratrol; Saw palmetto; Sun's soup; Wine and cancer

▶ Garlic and allicin

Category: Lifestyle and Prevention
Also known as: *Allium sativum*

Definition: Garlic (*Allium sativum*) is a nontoxic plant bulb in the *Allium* genus, which includes onions, leeks, and shallots. Allicin, a chemical created by enzymes when garlic is processed, produces garlic's odor and taste.

Cancers treated or prevented: Gastric (stomach) cancer, colon cancer, breast cancer, prostate cancer, throat cancer

Delivery routes: Oral ingestion by pill or in food

How this compound works: Historically, humans have consumed garlic for medicinal purposes to soothe digestive and circulatory problems. Aware of nutritional

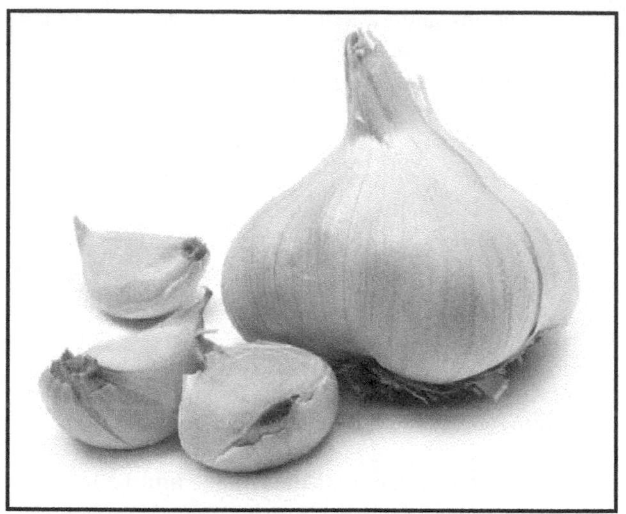

Garlic has been studied for cancer prevention and treatment.

strategies to prevent and control diseases, scientists initiated cancer research exploring garlic and its allyl sulfur components in the mid-twentieth century. Researchers identified allicin as garlic's most significant chemical that could fight cancer. Allicin is created as the enzyme alliinase reacts with alliin when garlic bulbs are sliced or crushed. Scientists hypothesized that biochemical processes in garlic which boost distribution of antioxidants might prevent cancerous cells from forming and increasing.

Studies regarding use of garlic and allicin for cancer prevention and treatment have given rise to both skepticism and optimism. In 1990, the National Cancer Institute (NCI) studied the potential use of allium vegetables, including garlic, for stomach cancer. That year, researchers attended the First World Congress on the Health Significance of Garlic in Washington, D.C. Despite some scientists' suggestion that garlic and its allyl sulfur components could prevent or inhibit malignancies, experts emphasized that garlic's anticancer effectiveness had not been scientifically proven.

By the early twenty-first century, international researchers had published several thousand scientific journal articles discussing allium plants. Studies focused on garlic's effect on gastric, colon, breast, prostate, and throat cancers. Investigators achieved promising laboratory results regarding allicin use in mice. At the Weizmann Institute of Science at Rehovot, Israel, scientists delivered alliinase and alliin to malignant tumors, where they produced allicin that entered and destroyed those cells. When researchers combined allicin with rituximab, an anticancer drug, they found that this mixture killed 95 percent of cancerous cells in mice.

In October, 2006, the *University of California, Berkeley Wellness Letter* noted that the cancer-fighting properties of garlic and allicin remained uncertain because tests had been limited to animal subjects and cell cultures and were inconclusive. That newsletter discounted previous studies as presenting minimal evidence, stressing that clinical scientific trials using humans were necessary to declare definitively anticancer properties expressed by garlic and allicin.

Although garlic and allicin have not been scientifically shown to cure cancer in humans, they contribute to healthy diets. People with cancer often consume garlic to strengthen their immune systems and receive other health benefits relevant to cholesterol and heart concerns. Garlic can be consumed raw, cooked, or in synthetic formats, providing people varying amounts and versions of allyl sulfur compounds.

Side effects: Garlic, when ingested regularly as part of diet, may cause halitosis and body odors. These effects are mitigated by taking it in pill form. Some people develop gas, bloating, diarrhea, or heartburn when taking garlic, which can be mitigated by taking enteric-coated supplements. Finally, because garlic and allicin can increase prothrombin time (PT), a measure of how long it takes for blood to form clots, people taking blood thinners such as warfarin (Coumadin) and anyone about to undergo surgery should consult their physicians before taking these substances.

Elizabeth D. Schafer, Ph.D.

See also: Fruits; Herbs as antioxidants; Nutrition and cancer prevention; Phytoestrogens; Prevention

▶ Indoles

Category: Lifestyle and Prevention

Definition: Dietary indoles are a family of organic phytonutrients found in plants that work with natural nutrients to protect against disease.

Cancers treated or prevented: May provide some protection from certain types of cancer, especially hormone-related cancers (such as prostate, breast, thyroid, and cervical cancer) as well as colon cancer

Delivery routes: Oral ingestion through diet

How these compounds work: Cruciferous vegetables (named for cross-shaped pattern on the underside of the stalk) contain the phytonutrients indole-2-carbonal (13C) and sulforaphane. The mechanism by which dietary indoles protect against cancer is unclear. One theory is that dietary indoles contain phytonutrients that work as estrogen blockers. Researchers believe that the positive effect of dietary indoles may be related to improving the estrogen ratio of harmful estrogen to good or helpful estrogen. Indoles seem to lessen the effects, or rid the body, of the estrogen hormone and positively affect the estrogen metabolite balance. Research studies have demonstrated that dietary indoles participate in many biochemical processes in the human body and may increase the production of anticancer enzymes to improve the body's natural ability to fight cancer.

Dietary indoles can be found in *Brassica* or cruciferous vegetables such as cauliflower, brussels sprouts, cabbage, broccoli, bok choy, kale, and watercress, as well as collard, turnip, and mustard greens. These vegetables can be prepared in a variety of ways, including raw, added to salads, boiled, steamed, stir-fried, braised, or fermented as in sauerkraut or pickled cabbage.

Some people avoid cabbage, as the cooking process releases a strong and somewhat unpleasant odor as a result of the sulfur compounds. To minimize the odor, the cabbage can be shredded so that it cooks faster and a large pan can be used with the cabbage submerged in a large amount of water. The sulfur will dissolve into the water and minimize release into the air. The cabbage should be cooked only until tender, as overcooking contributes to the odor. Also, covering it immediately contains the smell.

Cooking cabbage in a large amount of water can diffuse its strong taste and smell. However, steaming or quick cooking it in smaller amounts of water better retains its nutrients.

Consuming naturally occurring dietary indoles is preferred, but cruciferous vegetable extract supplements may provide some benefit as well. They are available at reputable health food stores.

Side effects: It is unclear whether indoles cause side effects when taken in higher doses.

Marylane Wade Koch, M.S.N., R.N.

For Further Information

Cruciferous Vegetables and Cancer Prevention. National Cancer Institute. Retrieved from http://www.cancer.gov/about-cancer/causes-prevention/risk/diet/cruciferous-vegetables-fact-sheet

Higdon, J. (Spring/Summer 2006). Cruciferous Vegetables and Cancer Risk. *The Linus Pauling Institute Research Newsletter*. pp. 7-9. Retrieved from http://lpi.oregonstate.edu/files/pdf/newsletters/ss06.pdf

The International Agency for Research on Cancer (2004). *Cruciferous Vegetables, Isothiocyanates and Indoles (IARC Handbooks of Cancer Prevention) 1st Edition.* Washington, DC: International Agency for Research on Cancer Press, WHO office.

See also: Antimetabolites in chemotherapy; Carcinomas; Chemoprevention; Cruciferous vegetables; 5-Hydroxyindoleacetic Acid (5HIAA) test; Mantle Cell Lymphoma (MCL); Mucosa-Associated Lymphoid Tissue (MALT) lymphomas; Multiple myeloma; Non-Hodgkin lymphoma; Plant alkaloids and terpenoids in chemotherapy; Tumor markers; Watchful waiting

▶ Isoflavones

Category: Lifestyle and Prevention
Also known as: Phytoestrogens

Definition: Isoflavones are a subclass of plant chemicals known as flavonoids (also referred to as bioflavonoids in the media). The beneficial effects attributed to isoflavones have encouraged nutritional supplement manufacturers to purify and market isoflavones derived from soybeans. Most of these purported benefits, however, are based on epidemiological or laboratory animal studies. More definitive conclusions with regard to human health await the results of long-term clinical trials.

Cancers treated or prevented: Breast, prostate, and endometrial cancers, although no conclusive evidence exists

Delivery routes: Oral by diet, pill, or capsule

How these compounds work: Isoflavones occur in foods bound to sugar in the form of glycosides. After ingestion, the glycosides are digested in the small intestine with the help of bacteria, releasing the active isoflavones. The isoflavones are absorbed and bound to plasma proteins for transport in the blood. There are two forms of estrogen receptors. Alpha receptors are predominantly found in reproductive tissue (uterus, breast, and ovaries), while beta receptors are predominant in other tissues. Isoflavones bind with greatest affinity to beta receptors, while the estrogen hormone principally targets the alpha receptor. When isoflavones bind to estrogen receptors in the breast, endometrium, or prostate (in place of estrogen), they may help prevent cancer by inhibiting activation of the receptor and the resultant growth-signaling process.

Isoflavones are found naturally in legume plants. Soybeans contain the isoflavones genistein and daidzein, which are the most common active isoflavones in human foods. They are also known as phytoestrogens, since they are similar in structure to estrogen hormones produced in the human body and demonstrate weak estrogenic activity.

Many claims have been made regarding beneficial actions of isoflavones. This may be attributable to the binding of isoflavones to beta receptors in various tissues to enhance the estrogen effect. One study evaluated the results of nineteen clinical trials with isoflavones and found that isoflavones had a negligible effect on cardiovascular risk factors. Likewise, isoflavones did not appear to be beneficial in reducing flushing or bone loss in postmenopausal women.

Epidemiological (population) studies indicate that Asians, who consume a traditional diet high in soy products, have a much lower incidence of breast and prostate cancer than do Western peoples. Studies have suggested that long-term exposure to high levels of estrogen may increase the risk of women developing breast or endometrial cancer. The lifetime consumption of isoflavones may provide protection for Asian women. Very few clinical trials, however, have been conducted to support this idea.

Side effects: Some studies have indicated that the protective effect of hormone therapies for cancer, such as tamoxifen or other antiestrogenic drugs, may be abrogated by use of isoflavones. Those undergoing hormone therapies should consult their physician about the use of isoflavones.

David A. Olle, M.S.

See also: Antioxidants; Bioflavonoids; Chemoprevention; Dietary supplements; Fruits; Herbs as antioxidants; Nutrition and cancer prevention; Phytoestrogens; Soy foods

▶ Lutein

Category: Lifestyle and Prevention
Also known as: Xanthophyll, non-provitamin A carotenoid

Definition: Lutein is a yellow pigment and micronutrient found in some vegetables, fruits, and eggs, and also in the human retina. It is best known as a carotenoid, a plant phytochemical thought to have antioxidant properties that protect against cell-damaging molecules known as free radicals.

Cancers treated or prevented: Prostate, breast, colon, lung, and ovarian cancers

Delivery routes: Oral via food or dietary supplements. The most significant food sources for lutein are broccoli, brussels sprouts, collards, kale, peas, pumpkin, spinach, turnip, mustard and dandelion greens, summer and winter squash, and sweet yellow corn. Egg yolks contain a more quickly absorbed form of lutein. Lutein absorption is increased from the intestine when combined with a dietary fat source, such as oil or margarine.

How this substance works: Lutein is chemically similar to the micronutrient zeaxanthin, and they often work together to provide protective benefits. Lutein, also known as a non-provitamin A carotenoid, cannot convert into vitamin A when needed by the body. Most studies find that lutein protects the eyes from disease, such as age-related macular degeneration and cataracts. Some studies find lutein effective against cancer because it decreases the growth of blood vessels to cancerous tumors, increases cancer cell destruction, and improves cell deoxyribonucleic acid (DNA) repair. Overall study results are mixed, however, with one study showing lutein reduced prostate cancer by 25 percent (and as much as 32 percent when combined with the carotenoid lycopene) and another showing an increase in stomach cancer. In general, most studies find that lutein provides some protection against breast, colon, lung, ovarian, and prostate cancers. The dosage and safety of lutein dietary supplements are still unknown. Doses of lutein up to 20 milligrams per day have been determined to be safe. Consuming lutein from food sources is advised, however, because of its interaction with other compounds found within these foods.

Side effects: Caution is advised for individuals with allergies or sensitivities to eggs or lutein-containing vegetables. In general, no toxicities or drug interactions have been reported with lutein from food sources. Caution, especially in pregnant or lactating women, should be used with lutein supplements because the risks are still unknown.

Alice C. Richer, R.D., M.B.A., L.D.

See also: Amenorrhea; Antiandrogens; Antioxidants; Carotenoids; Complementary and alternative therapies; Craniopharyngiomas; Dietary supplements; Free radicals; Fruits; Lycopene; Nutrition and cancer prevention; Pituitary tumors

▶ Lycopene

Category: Lifestyle and Prevention
Also known as: Non-provitamin A carotonoid

Definition: Lycopene is the red pigment in some fruits and vegetables that gives them their colorful appearance. It is best known as a carotenoid, a plant-produced phytochemical well known for its antioxidant properties.

Cancers treated or prevented: Prostate, lung, and stomach cancers

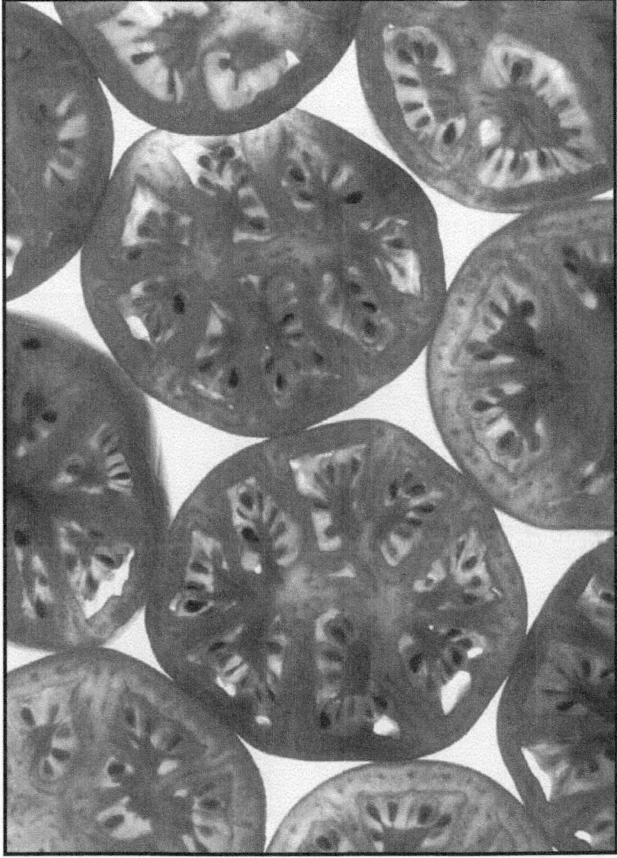

Tomatoes are a major source of lycopene. (U.S. Department of Agriculture)

Delivery routes: Oral via food or dietary supplements. The most common food sources for lycopene are tomatoes and tomato products. Other significant food sources are apricots, guava, watermelon, papaya, and pink grapefruit. Processed tomatoes and tomato products provide more available lycopene than raw forms. The absorption of lycopene is increased when combined with a dietary fat source, such as the oil used in preparing pizza or tomato sauce.

How this substance works: Lycopene is believed to act as an antioxidant, blocking the destructive action of cell-damaging molecules known as free radicals. Also known as a non-provitamin A carotenoid, it cannot convert into vitamin A in the body, like some other carotenoids, when needed. Lycopene is fat-soluble; thus it is stored in the body and broken down in the intestine for use. Because of this, including dietary fat with a lycopene source increases its absorption. Lycopene is believed to play a role in preventing many diseases, such as cancer, heart disease, and macular degeneration, and it may slow the progression of some cancers. Some studies show the strongest protective evidence against lung, stomach, and prostate cancers. Other nutrients and compounds in fruits and vegetables are thought to combine with lycopene, however, and this synergy may actually be responsible for the protective benefits seen in these studies. The dosage and safety of dietary lycopene supplements are still unknown. Many studies have found positive benefits from consuming lycopene from fruit and vegetable sources, rather than dietary supplements, with no known safety issues.

Side effects: Caution is advised for individuals with allergies or sensitivities to tomatoes and tomato products or to fruits, vegetables, and dietary supplements that include lycopene. The high level of acid in tomatoes may irritate stomach disorders. While there is some belief that lycopene could decrease the side effects of radiation and chemotherapy, it may also decrease their effectiveness. As a rule, lycopene dietary supplements should be avoided during cancer treatment. Lycopene from food sources, however, has not been found to interfere with treatment. Some drugs may also decrease lycopene absorption.

Alice C. Richer, R.D., M.B.A., L.D.

See also: Antioxidants; Carotenoids; Chemoprevention; Complementary and alternative therapies; Dietary supplements; Free radicals; Fruits; Lutein; Nutrition and cancer prevention

▶ Nutrition and cancer prevention

Category: Lifestyle and Prevention

Definition: Everyday eating habits are increasingly associated with cancer incidence, prevention, and management. According to the National Cancer Institute, 80 percent of cancers are caused by environmental factors that are within people's control. It is estimated that the types of foods people eat directly cause 35 to 50 percent of environmental cancers. Studies show that diet and lifestyle changes can prevent and reduce the risk and recurrence of most cancers.

Epidemiology: As a rule, the human immune system is able to stop carcinogens from damaging cells within the body. However, sometimes cell deoxyribonucleic acid (DNA) is attacked and altered, causing cancer cells to begin to develop and multiply. Studies show that most cancers can be prevented through lifestyle choices (a healthful diet, avoidance of tobacco and excessive alcohol use, and adequate physical activity) and changes in the environment. Strong associations link diet to some cancers, but many other factors contribute as well. Genetics, infectious agents, some viruses, and exposure to radiation, chemicals, and some carcinogenic substances in the air, water, and soil also play a role. The American Cancer Society reported that 23.1 percent of deaths in the United States in 2004 were due to cancer.

Nutrition risk factors: Studies find populations that eat a diet rich in fatty foods, especially animal fats, have higher rates of cancer than populations that eat a plant-based diet high in whole grains, vegetables, fruits, and legumes. Increased death rates from breast, prostate, and colon cancers are associated with high-fat diets. Higher rates of cancer have also been linked with the consumption of low-fiber diets and excessive alcohol.

Being overweight or obese is also strongly linked with cancer. Overweight people are more likely to develop breast (postmenopausal women), colon, endometrial, esophageal, and kidney cancers. Obese individuals are also at risk for developing cervical, gallbladder, ovarian, pancreatic, thyroid, and colorectal cancers; Hodgkin disease; multiple myeloma; and aggressive forms of prostate cancer. These findings are of particular concern as westernized societies are experiencing increasing rates of obesity.

Excessive alcohol intake, defined as more than two drinks per day for men and more than one drink per day for women (one serving equals 5 ounces of wine, 12 ounces of beer, or 1.5 ounces of liquor), is clearly associated with cancers of the mouth, throat, larynx, esophagus, liver, and breast.

No known nutrition factors are associated with brain cancer, leukemia, and lymphoma. However, some cancers related to diet may result in secondary tumors or metastatic disease in these areas.

Research findings: A number of different food compounds, minerals, and vitamins are thought to protect against some cancers. Some of those that have become well known are antioxidants, carotenoids, and phytochemicals, substances or nutrients found in foods. Antioxidants include vitamins C and E and the mineral selenium; carotenoids include lycopene, lutein, and beta-carotene; and phytochemicals include a number of plant-based compounds, such as resveratrol (found in red wine), catechin (found in teas), and allium (found in garlic). The use of dietary supplements containing these substances has

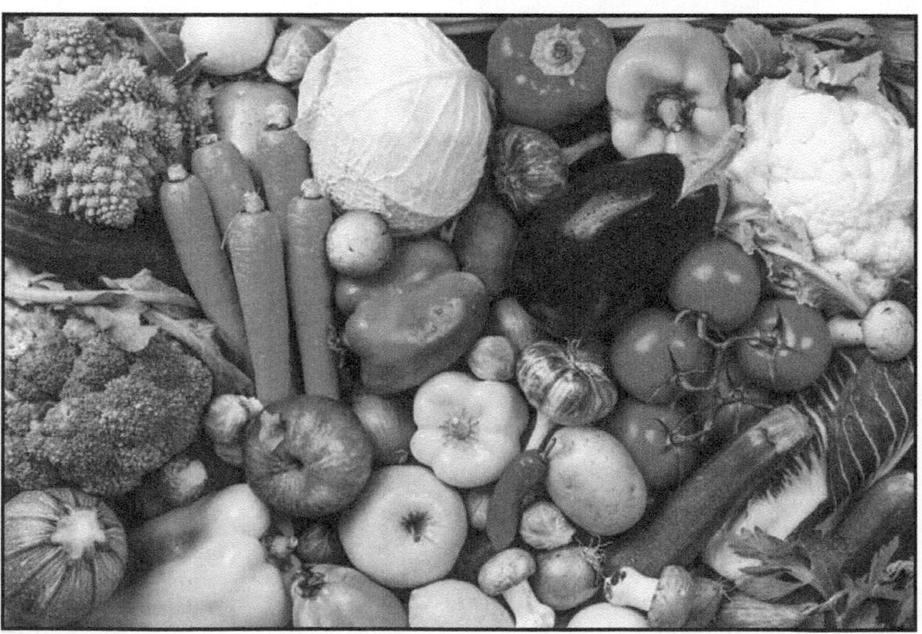

Vegetables are an important part of a cancer-prevention diet. (iStock)

A Healthful Diet

The U.S. Department of Agriculture, in its *Dietary Guidelines for Americans*, 2005, gave these broad guidelines for a diet that would be healthful for most Americans.

- Centers on fruits, vegetables, whole grains, nonfat or low-fat dairy products.
- Contains some lean meats, poultry, fish, beans, eggs, and nuts.
- Has minimal amounts of saturated fats, trans fats, cholesterol, salt, and added sugar.

increased dramatically in the United States because of the popular belief that they prevent aging and illness.

Research shows that antioxidants, carotenoids, and phytochemicals do have some protective effects against free radicals, which are cell-damaging molecules arising from normal biological functions and the environment. Free radical cell destruction is believed to cause aging and many diseases in humans. However, although some studies show benefits from including antioxidants, carotenoids, and phytochemicals in the diet, other studies actually show that they cause harm. In two studies in which high doses of beta-carotene supplements were taken to prevent lung cancer, former cigarette smokers experienced increased lung cancer death. However, when beta-carotene was consumed via food sources (not supplements), cancer risk was reduced.

Coffee, aspartame, saccharin, and sugar have been suspected of causing cancer, but studies have not conclusively linked them to cancer. An increased cancer risk has been associated, however, with the consumption of highly salted, preserved, or smoked meats and those cooked at high temperatures (fried, broiled, and grilled). Many experts recommend limiting consumption of these types of meats.

Studies regarding concerns over the effects of bioengineered and irradiated foods, fish contaminated with mercury, food additives, fluoride in dental products and water, and pesticide residue on foods have not shown any increased risk for cancer. There is no evidence to date that distinguishes organic foods from conventional foods in terms of a cancer risk. However, some studies have shown that the phytochemical content of organic fruits and vegetables may be higher than that of conventionally grown crops. This finding leads some to think that this might convey some level of protection against cancer.

Soy, calcium, and vitamin D are thought by some to help prevent cancers. Soy is an excellent source of protein and phytochemicals, but very little data supports the premise that soy lowers the risk of cancer. Soy contains compounds called phytoestrogens (plant estrogens), which closely resemble the hormone estrogen and may actually increase the risk of estrogen-responsive cancers, such as breast and endometrial cancers. It may also reduce the effectiveness of tamoxifen drug treatments. Therefore, some researchers recommend that soy foods and products containing soy isoflavones should be limited to two servings per day and that dietary soy supplements should be avoided. Patients taking tamoxifen should avoid all soy products. The connection between soy and cancer, however, remains unclear.

Calcium has been associated with a lower incidence of colorectal cancers, but there is also evidence that calcium supplements may increase prostate cancers, especially the aggressive form. Because of this, calcium recommendations remain at 1,000 milligrams per day for people between the ages of nineteen and fifty and 1,200 milligrams per day for people older than fifty. Nonfat or low-fat dairy sources of calcium and some leafy green vegetables are preferable to supplements as sources of calcium. Vitamin D is also increasingly thought to protect against colon, prostate, and breast cancer. The existing recommendations for intake of vitamin D, between 200 and 600 International Units (IU) daily, may not be sufficient to provide protection against cancers, especially for those living in northern climates, the elderly, people with dark skin, and exclusively breastfed babies. However, more research is needed before these recommendations can be changed. In the meantime, many researchers suggest exposing the skin (without sunscreen) to sunlight for 15 minutes every day and balancing the diet to include foods fortified with vitamin D.

Many more studies need to be done to verify diet and cancer connections, but the best way for people to lower their cancer risk appears to be eating a balanced, low-fat diet that includes a variety of fruits and vegetables daily.

Dietary recommendations: Research points to a number of dietary recommendations that should be followed to lower the risk for developing cancer or having it recur. The following recommendations are from the American Cancer Society:

- Maintain a healthy weight throughout life: People are advised to lose weight if they are overweight or obese, avoid excessive weight gain, and balance food intake with physical activity.
- Adopt a physically active lifestyle: Adults are advised to exercise at least 30 minutes a day (ideally 45 to 60 minutes a day), five or more days of the week. Children and

adolescents are advised to exercise at least 60 minutes per day, five or more days per week.

• Eat a healthy diet, with an emphasis on plant sources: People are advised to eat five or more servings of vegetables and fruits every day, choose whole grains, and include legumes for protein. Also, they are to limit intake of processed and refined foods, sugars, red meat, and processed meats. A simple way to make sure the diet has the right emphasis is to fill one-fourth of the plate with a protein source, one-fourth with whole grains, and one-half with colorful vegetables. One serving of fruit is one-half cup of canned fruit, three-quarters cup of 100 percent juice, or a small to medium-sized piece of fresh fruit. One serving of vegetables is one-half cup of cooked or one cup of raw vegetables.

• Limit consumption of alcoholic beverages: Women should not exceed one drink per day, and men, two drinks per day.

Alice C. Richer, R.D., M.B.A., L.D.

For Further Information

American Institute for Cancer Research. *Diet and Health Recommendations for Cancer Prevention: Healthy Living and Lower Cancer Risk*. Washington, D.C.: Author, 2006.

Awad, Atif B., and Peter G. Bradford, eds. *Nutrition and Cancer Prevention*. Boca Raton, Fla.: CRC, Taylor & Francis, 2006.

Kushi, Lawrence H., et al. "American Cancer Society Guidelines on Nutrition and Physical Activity for Cancer Prevention." *Cancer: A Cancer Journal for Clinicians* 56 (2006): 254-281.

McTiernan, Anne, ed. *Cancer Prevention and Management Through Exercise and Weight Control*. Boca Raton, Fla.: Taylor & Francis, 2006.

Other Resources

American Institute of Cancer Research

Recommendations for Cancer Prevention

http://www.aicr.org/site/PageServer?pagename=dc_home_guides

The Cancer Project

Cancer Prevention and Survival

http://www.cancerproject.org/survival/cancer_facts/factors.php

National Cancer Institute

Cancer Prevention Overview

http://www.cancer.gov/cancertopics/pdq/prevention/overview/healthprofessional

Prevent Cancer Foundation

http://www.preventcancer.org

See also: Aflatoxins; Alcohol, alcoholism, and cancer; Antioxidants; Beta-carotene; Bioflavonoids; Calcium; Carotenoids; Cartilage supplements; Chemoprevention; Coenzyme Q10; Complementary and alternative therapies; Cruciferous vegetables; Dietary supplements; Fiber; Folic acid; Fruits; Garlic and allicin; Ginseng, panax; Green tea; Herbs as antioxidants; Indoles; Isoflavones; Lutein; Lycopene; Macrobiotic diet; Nutrition and cancer treatment; Obesity-associated cancers; Omega-3 fatty acids; Phytoestrogens; Poverty and cancer; Prevention; Resveratrol; Saw palmetto; Soy foods; Sun's soup; Wine and cancer

▶ Nutrition and cancer treatment

Category: Lifestyle and Prevention

Definition: Cancer treatments often affect people differently, and side effects can range from minor to severe. Eating well and following good nutrition habits before and during treatment help maintain strength, prevent body tissue breakdown, rebuild tissues, defend against infection, cope with side effects, and make some treatments more effective.

Cancer treatments: There are five main treatments used to fight cancer: surgery, radiation therapy, chemotherapy, hormone therapy, and immunotherapy. Surgery is used to remove tumors and cancer cells that have not spread to surrounding body tissues. It is often combined with other treatment methods. After surgery, the protein content and number of calories in the diet need to be increased to assist in wound healing and the recovery process. Eating healthfully following surgery also helps the patient feel better by maintaining strength, energy, and a stable weight while maintaining the body's stores of nutrients. Good nutrition is essential for the healing process, to decrease risk of infection, and to increase tolerance to side effects from other treatments used. Any surgery involving the gastrointestinal tract must be carefully monitored, as it can lead to malnutrition.

Radiation therapy directs radiation at the affected body area, preventing cancer cells from multiplying and spreading. Although healthy tissue is affected along with the cancer cells, it usually recovers after treatment ends.

Effects of Cancer Treatments on Nutrition

Treatment	*Common Nutrition Problems*	*Nutrition-Related Side Effects*
Surgery	May slow digestion; affect proper function of mouth, throat, stomach; increase healing and recovery needs	• May be unable to eat normally and require liquid nutrition • Chewing, swallowing, digestion functions may be impaired
Radiation therapy	Affects healthy tissues and may affect digestive system	Head, neck, chest, breast cancer treatments may cause: • dry or sore mouth • difficulty swallowing • changes in food taste • dental problems • phlegm production Stomach or pelvis cancer treatments may cause: • nausea, vomiting • diarrhea • cramps, bloating
Chemotherapy	May affect the digestive system and desire or ability to eat	• nausea, vomiting • loss of appetite • diarrhea • constipation • sore mouth or throat • weight gain or loss • changes in food taste
Hormonal therapy	May affect ability and desire to eat	• nausea, vomiting • diarrhea • sore or dry mouth • severe weight loss • changes in food taste • fatigue, muscle aches, fever
Immunotherapy	May increase appetite and how the body handles fluid	• change in appetite • fluid retention

Radiation can be used alone or combined with other treatments. Treatments are usually given five days a week and last from two to nine weeks. Nutrition side effects depend on the length of treatment and the area to which the radiation is directed.

Chemotherapy requires the use of strong drugs to disrupt the cancer cells' ability to grow and multiply. Chemotherapy drugs are either taken orally or injected and may be used alone or combined with other treatments. Chemotherapy affects the entire body, not just the cancer site. As a result, healthy tissue is affected. The digestive tract is very susceptible to side effects from this treatment.

Hormone therapy uses drugs to block hormone production by the body. Hormones that influence the growth of some cancers, such as breast and prostate cancers, are targeted. Hormone therapy can also involve the removal of hormone-producing organs, which is thought to end or slow tumor growth by removing the source of the hormones on which these tumors thrive. Hormone therapy can affect the ability and desire to eat.

Immunotherapy, also called biological therapy, enlists the body's immune system to stimulate natural defenses to help fight the offending cancer. It can be used alone but is usually combined with other therapies. This type of therapy can affect fluid retention and may actually increase the appetite.

Nutrition suggestions during treatment: Eating a healthy diet is very important during treatment. This often requires that patients plan ahead, enlist the help of family and friends, and be ready to try different foods and preparation techniques. When experiencing nutrition-related

Tips for Managing Nutritional Side Effects of Treatment

Side Effect	*Suggestions for Managing Effect*
Constipation	• Eat high-fiber foods (whole grains, fresh fruits and vegetables) • Add unprocessed wheat bran to foods • Get daily exercise • Drink a hot beverage about one-half hour before usual time for bowel movement • Discuss fiber supplements with doctor
Diarrhea	• Avoid: beans, onions, strong spices greasy, fried, and fatty foods raw vegetables, fruits, nuts high-fiber vegetables (broccoli, corn, beans, cabbage, cauliflower, peas) alcohol dairy only if it increases diarrhea very cold or hot liquids/foods • Try: rice or noodles hot wheat cereal well-cooked eggs bananas pureed or soft-cooked vegetables canned/cooked fruits (no skin) white bread skinless chicken/turkey soft or ground beef fish mashed potatoes clear liquid diet during first 24 hours • Eat foods high in sodium and potassium (bananas, peaches, apricot nectar, potatoes)
Difficulty swallowing	• Take deep breaths before swallowing • Exhale or cough after swallowing • Try thick liquids or gelatin • Mash foods to thin or pureed consistency • Drink room-temperature fluids between meals • Use a straw or spoon to eat • Avoid very hot or cold foods • Work with a speech therapist on safe swallowing techniques
Dry mouth	• Avoid: salty or tart foods and beverages • Try: ice pops, sugar-free gum, hard candy, thick nectars sip water every few minutes • Discuss products that protect your mouth with doctor or dentist
Food aversion	• Avoid favorite foods until treatment over
Mouth or throat pain, tooth decay	• Avoid: citrus fruit and juices spicy and salty foods rough and dry foods hot spices alcohol • Try: bananas, applesauce, watermelon, canned fruits peach, pear, and apricot nectars cottage cheese, yogurt, and milkshakes mashed potatoes macaroni and cheese custards, puddings, gelatin scrambled eggs hot cooked cereals pureed or mashed vegetables and meats foods cooked until tender and then cut up or pureed stews and casseroles • Mix food with margarine, gravy, or sauces • Use a straw to drink liquids • Eat foods and drink liquids cold or at room temperature

(continued)

Tips for Managing Nutritional Side Effects of Treatment *(continued)*

Side Effect	*Suggestions for Managing Effect*
Nausea	• Avoid: fatty, greasy, fried, spicy foods sweets (candy, cake, and so on) foods with strong odors or warm or strong-smelling rooms • Try: toast, crackers, pretzels yogurt sherbet, ice pops angel food cake canned fruits skinless chicken (baked or broiled) hot cooked cereals clear liquids (apple juice, broth) ice chips • Eat small amounts often and slowly • Sip cool or chilled liquids throughout the day, except at meals • Eat room temperature or cool foods • Do not eat favorite foods • Always sit upright when eating • Rest after meals for at least one hour • Eat dry toast or crackers before getting up if nauseated in the morning • Wear loose-fitting clothes • Do not eat 1-2 hours before treatment • Keep track of which foods cause nausea • Eat biggest meal of the day when hungry • Discuss antinausea medications with doctor
Taste changes	• Choose and eat foods that look and smell good • Try different foods • Marinate meats, fish, poultry, or try different spices • Try tart foods • Eat foods at room temperature • Maintain good oral hygiene
Vomiting	• Do not drink or eat while vomiting • Sit upright after vomiting for at least an hour • When feeling better, try small amounts of clear liquid, such as apple juice, flat ginger ale, or room temperature broth, drinking 1 teaspoon every 10 minutes as tolerated, gradually increasing to 2 tablespoons every 30 minutes • When able to tolerate clear liquids without vomiting, increase to full liquids (hot wheat cereal, ice cream, broth, gelatin, milk, custard, pudding, and so on)
Weight gain, fluid retention	• Avoid salty foods, add less salt to foods • Drink at least 3-4 glasses of water daily and when thirsty • Exercise as much as is realistic • Meet with a registered dietitian
Weight loss, poor appetite	• Maintain normal activities as much as possible • Do not hurry meals and stay calm when eating • Eat whenever hungry • Keep nutritious snacks available • Try new foods or restaurants • Eat favorite foods • Use candlelight or favorite music at mealtimes, or change timing of meals • Meet with a registered dietitian

side effects during active treatment, patients are advised to eat foods and liquids that are well tolerated. All patients undergoing treatment should be encouraged to drink plenty of fluids throughout the day and visit with a registered dietitian to ensure proper eating habits.

Alice C. Richer, R.D., M.B.A., L.D.

For Further Information

Bloch, Abby, et al., eds. *Eating Well, Staying Well During and After Cancer*. Atlanta: American Cancer Society, 2004.

Elliott, Laura, Laura L. Molseed, and Paula Davis McCallum, eds. *The Clinical Guide to Oncology Nutrition*. 2d ed. Chicago: American Dietetic Association, 2006.

Keane, Maureen, and Daniella Chace. *What to Eat If You Have Cancer: Healing Foods That Boost Your Immune System*. 2d ed. New York: McGraw-Hill, 2007.

Other Resources

American Cancer Society
Handling the Side Effects of Treatment
http://www.cancer.org/docroot/MBC/MBC_6_1_what_to_do_about_side_effects.asp

American Institute of Cancer Research
Nutritional Effects of Cancer Treatment
http://www.aicr.org/site/PageServer?pagename= dc_cr_treatment#nutrition

National Cancer Institute
Eating Hints for Cancer Patients: Before, During, and After Treatment
http://www.cancer.gov/cancertopics/eatinghints/page3

See also: Anthraquinones; Antioxidants; Cancell; Carotenoids; Cartilage supplements; Coenzyme Q10; Complementary and alternative therapies; Curcumin; Delta-9-tetrahydrocannabinol; Dietary supplements; Electroporation therapy; Essiac; Gerson therapy; Ginseng, panax; Green tea; Herbs as antioxidants; Integrative oncology; Laetrile; Mistletoe; PC-SPES; Phenolics; Saw palmetto; Sun's soup

▶ Omega-3 fatty acids

Category: Lifestyle and Prevention
Also known as: Polyunsaturated fatty acids (PUFAs)

Definition: Omega-3 fatty acids are essential polyunsaturated fats that must be obtained from food, particularly cold-water fish, fish oil, flaxseeds, soybeans, walnuts, green leafy vegetables, and canola oil. Three forms of omega-3 fatty acids exist: alpha-linolenic acid (ALA), eicosapentaenoic acid (EPA), and docosahexaenoic acid (DHA).

Cancers treated or prevented: Colon cancer, breast cancer, prostate cancer, pancreatic cancer

Delivery routes: Oral by food, capsule, or liquid

How this substance works: Omega-3 fatty acids are highly concentrated in the brain and appear to play an important role in cognitive and behavioral functions, as well as normal growth and development. Research indicates that these acids are important in numerous physiological functions, particularly muscle contraction and relaxation, movement of calcium and other material into and out of cells, regulation of blood clotting, and secretion of substances including hormones and digestive enzymes. They also play a role in controlling cell division and fertility, indicating their possible importance in protection against certain types of cancer. Omega-3 fatty acids seem to reduce inflammation and retard tumor growth. On the other hand, omega-6 fatty acids, which are found in sunflower oil, safflower oil, and most saturated fats and vegetable oils, promote inflammation and feed tumor growth. An appropriate balance between omega-3 and omega-6 fatty acids is necessary to promote good health.

Some research indicates that omega-3 fatty acids help to prevent certain chronic diseases, including heart disease and some cancers. EPA appears to be important in cancer prevention by affecting the production of cytokines and the tumor necrosis factor (TNF). Other research indicates that omega-3 fatty acids may play an adverse role in treating some cancers. If the latter is true, then these acids still play an indirect role in cancer prevention if cold-water fish, such as salmon, halibut, and tuna, are substituted for red and processed meats, which are known to increase the risk of colon and prostate cancers.

Side effects: The consumption of omega-3 fatty acids and cancer incidence have had unfavorable associations in some case studies. One study on skin cancer and another on lung cancer showed that these fatty acids increased the risk for developing these cancers. A study on prostate cancer showed that ALA increased its risk, while EPA and DHA reduced the risk. More specific case studies need to be conducted in order to build a significant statistical database.

Alvin K. Benson, Ph.D.

See also: Alopecia; Chemoprevention; Dietary supplements; Thyroid cancer

▶ Phytoestrogens

Category: Lifestyle and Prevention
Also known as: Soy isoflavones (genistein, daidzein, glycitein, formononetin), lignans (secoisolariciresinol, matairesinol, pinoresinol, lariciresinol), coumestans (coumestrol) Plant estrogens

Definition: Phytoestrogens are naturally occurring, estrogen-like chemicals found in many plants. There are three basic categories of phytoestrogens: isoflavones, lignans, and coumestans. They come primarily from food sources.

Cancers treated or prevented: May mitigate breast, prostate, uterine, and possibly lung and colon cancers

Delivery routes: Oral through diet, pill, or capsule

How these compounds work: Phytoestrogens have been touted as natural substances that help prevent certain types of cancer, especially hormone-related cancers such as breast, prostate, and uterine cancer. Phytoestrogens can provide hormonal modulation, which naturally regulates hormones. Though not conclusive, some studies demonstrate that phytoestrogens may also provide some protection against lung and colon cancers.

Phytoestrogens can be absorbed into the body chemistry either to act as estrogens at low levels or to block the estrogen effect at high levels. These substances can mimic a weak estrogen to stimulate or to inhibit the growth of cells. Research has shown that increased exposure to certain hormones can increase the risk of cancer. Phytoestrogens appear to protect the body from hormones that can produce cancer.

The best sources of phytoestrogens occur naturally in plants. More than three hundred foods contain phytoestrogens. The most common ones are whole grains such as oats, wheat, and corn; edible seeds such as flax and sesame; legumes such as lentils, soybeans, sprouts, black beans, and chickpeas; vegetables such as leafy greens, fennel, celery, asparagus, carrots, parsley, and seaweed; fruits such as oranges, bananas, and strawberries; olive, safflower, and pumpkin oils; nuts such as pistachios, chestnuts, and walnuts; and other sources such as garlic, onions, and red wine. Soy products such as tofu (bean curd), soy milk, tempeh, and soy yogurt are well-known sources of isoflavone phytoestrogens. Certain herbs also contain phytoestrogens, such as red clover, green tea, hops, alfalfa, licorice, citrus peel, and flax seeds; herbal teas are considered longevity tonic.

Phytoestrogens are also marketed in pill and capsule form as food supplements. The U.S. Food and Drug Administration (FDA) does not regulate food supplements for safety and effectiveness; these supplements are not recommended, as their safety has not been established and could increase the incidence of cancer.

Phytoestrogens consumed in food are generally considered safe when taken in moderate amounts. Though some research studies have shown that phytoestrogens may protect against cancer, others dispute this effect. Some physicians think that consuming phytoestrogens in food may be safer for breast cancer patients than the estrogen medications used in post-menopausal hormone replacement therapy. More studies are needed to fully assess the effect of phytoestrogens on the body chemistry.

Side effects: Patients taking hormone therapies for cancer, such as tamoxifen or other antiestrogenic drugs, should seek the advice of their health care providers before taking supplementation of phytoestrogens, as these phytonutrients may interfere with drug therapy.

Marylane Wade Koch, M.S.N., R.N.

Further Information

Flaxseeds and breast cancer. *Oncology Nutrition*. Retrieved from https://www.oncologynutrition.org/erfc/hot-topics/flaxseeds-and-breast-cancer/

Post-menopausal hormone therapy after breast cancer. American Cancer Society. Retrieved from http://www.cancer.org/cancer/breastcancer/detailedguide/breast-cancer-after-post-menopausal-therapy

Food Sources of Phytoestrogens

Phytoestrogen content of foods, from highest to lowest combined isoflavones (genistein, daidzein, glycitein, formononetin), lignans (secoisolariciresinol, matairesinol, pinoresinol, lariciresinol), and coumestan (coumestrol), in micrograms per 100 grams.

Food	*mcg/100g*	*Food*	*mcg/100g*
Flax seeds	379,380.0	Dried dates	329.5
Soy beans	103,920.0	Sunflower seeds	216.0
Tofu	27,150.1	Chestnuts	210.2
Soy yogurt	10,275.0	Olive oil	180.7
Sesame seeds	8,008.1	Almonds	131.1
Flax bread	7,540.0	Green beans	105.8
Multigrain bread	4,798.7	Peanuts	34.5
Soy milk	2,957.2	Onions	32.0
Hummus	993.0	Blueberries	17.5
Garlic	603.6	Corn	9.0
Mung bean sprouts	495.1	Coffee, regular	6.3
Dried apricots	444.5	Watermelon	2.9
Alfalfa sprouts	441.4	Milk, cow	1.2

Phytoestrogen: Foods high in phytoestrogens and health benefits (2014, June 7). *Cholesterol and Fat Data Base.* Retrieved from http://www.dietaryfiberfood.com/phytoestrogen-hormones/phytoestrogen-food-sources.php

See also: Antioxidants; Beta-carotene; Bioflavonoids; Breast cancers; Calcium; Carotenoids; Chemoprevention; Coenzyme Q10; Complementary and alternative therapies; Cruciferous vegetables; Curcumin; Dietary supplements; Essiac; Free radicals; Fruits; Garlic and allicin; Glutamine; Green tea; Herbs as antioxidants; Isoflavones; Lutein; Lycopene; Macrobiotic diet; Nutrition and cancer prevention; PC-SPES; Phenolics; Prevention; Prostate cancer; Resveratrol; Soy foods; Uterine cancer; Wine and cancer

▶ Prevention

Category: Lifestyle and Prevention

Definition: Prevention of cancer can be defined as reducing cancer mortality by reducing the incidence of cancer.

Cancer in the United States: In 2015, the National Cancer Institute issued a report entitled, "The Annual Report to the Nation on the Status of Cancer, 1975-2011." This report documented that the overall death rates for the most common cancers (such as breast, lung, colorectal, and prostate) had declined and survival rates for cancer patients were rising. The overall incidence of cancer for men had decreased, the incidence for women had stabilized, and incidence for youth increased. However, the incidence of cancers such as thyroid, kidney, liver, oral/orophangeal, and uterine had increased. Cancer remained the second leading cause of death in the United States. In 2013 more than two and a half million Americans had lost their lives to cancer.

Lowering the number of cases of cancer is a multifaceted process of avoiding exposures to known carcinogens, modifying lifestyle habits, and taking active steps to enhance the body's immune system. Although behaviors that help people avoid developing cancer (such as not smoking and lessening consumption of unhealthy fat and alcohol) are on the rise in the United States, more needs to be done. Prevention generally falls into the categories of lifestyle, chemoprevention (use of vitamins and medicines), preventive surgery, screening, and environment. Prevention of cancer is an active process in which all Americans need to involve themselves to reduce their lifetime chance of cancer.

Research suggests that as much as one-third of all cancer can be prevented with lifestyle changes in daily living. Every day, each person makes choices that could increase or reduce their likelihood of developing cancer. No knowledge or program can prevent cancer on its own: People must make responsible choices and integrate them into their lifestyle. The American Institute for Cancer Research (AICR) suggests common cancers could be prevented by following the AICR guidelines including eating a healthy diet, participating in regular physical activity, and maintaining a healthy weight.

Nutrition: Nutrition cancer prevention and is a key part of cancer prevention. Much has been researched and written about the importance of nutrition. Although the relationship between diet and cancer is complex, numerous studies show that nutrition can make a difference in preventing cancer. The American Cancer Society promotes eating five to seven or more servings of fruits and vegetables each day as the single most important step people can take to prevent cancer. People can achieve this goal by eating vegetables and fruits at each meal and for snacks. Strawberries, raspberries, blueberries, and blackberries have cancer-fighting chemicals, as do citrus fruits such as oranges and grapefruit. Certain phytonutrients in vegetables, such as the indoles found in broccoli and cabbage, can help protect against cancer, especially hormone-related cancers. Generally the more color the vegetable has, the healthier and more protective it is. The likelihood of developing colon cancer and other gastrointestinal cancers may be decreased by eating dark green and yellow vegetables. Fruits and vegetables in their whole or natural form (fresh, frozen, dried, or canned) are more protective than supplements with dried extracts.

The nutritional aspect of prevention includes other foods besides fruits and vegetables. The use of whole-grain breads and cereals adds fiber to the diet. High-fiber diets increase motility of food through the colon and are thought to protect against colon cancer. Meat consumption has been associated with colon and prostate cancer, and eating less meat may be accomplished by choosing beans as a protein source. Some experts think other foods protect against cancer, such as garlic, onions, soybeans, and ginger. Herbal teas such as red clover or green tea have also demonstrated promise in studies on cancer prevention.

How food is cooked can affect the nutrients or introduce carcinogens into the body. For example, meat protein cooked at high temperatures produces toxic substances. Studies have linked colorectal adenomas to red meat cooked at high temperatures. Processed meats and bacon contain carcinogens. Boiling vegetables can release nutrients into the water, so steaming is preferred to preserve the vitamins.

Studies have looked at the possibility of food preservatives and additives being carcinogenic, but the studies have not been conclusive. Foods are treated with chemicals to improve taste, increase shelf life, and allow them to be transported long distances in trucks. More than 3,000 preservatives and additives are used in the U.S. food supply system. Some experts say that formaldehyde, a suspected carcinogen, is either contained in or released by some food preservatives and constitutes a hazard to humans; however, this has not been proven. Some people have chosen to minimize their exposure to additives and preservatives by eating more food in the raw state and purchasing organic foods and milk.

Exercise: Physical activity and exercise can help protect against developing certain cancers of the breast, colon, and prostate. The Centers for Disease Control and Prevention (CDC) recommend that adults have two types of exercise: aerobic and muscle-strengthening. The CDC guidelines for aerobic exercise for adults include 150 minutes of moderately intense aerobic exercise (for example, walking at a brisk pace) or 75 minutes of vigorous aerobic exercise (for example, racewalking, jogging, or running) or a mixture of each of these each week. This can be done in increments of at least 10 minutes throughout the week. Muscle-strengthening is recommended two or more days a week to include all major muscle groups such as legs, hips, back, abdomen, chest, shoulders, and arms. Muscle-strengthening works well with repetition of 8 to 12 times per set with increasing level of weights. This recommendation complements the need to decrease the epidemic of obesity in the United States, as obesity is associated with increased risk of developing cancers of the colon and rectum, breast, prostate, kidney, and uterus (endometrium).

Alcohol: Alcohol and alcoholism is associated with increased risk of mouth, esophagus (throat), larynx (voice box), and liver cancer. The amount of alcohol consumed affects the risk of cancer. Men are advised to have no more than two drinks per day and women no more than one drink per day (one drink is defined as 12 ounces of beer, 5 ounces of wine, or 1.5 ounces of 80-proof liquor). Women who drink are at increased risk for breast cancer. When smoking is combined with excessive alcohol consumption, the risk is compounded. Excessive alcohol consumption can result in liver damage that affects the body's ability to excrete toxins and can effect cancer treatment. Wine is associated with an increased risk of upper digestive tract cancers in heavy users. However, some studies have shown that moderate consumption of red wine, which contains phytochemicals, may convey some cancer-fighting benefits.

Tobacco: Smoking and use of tobacco products is a choice made by many Americans. Smoking produces known carcinogens that can result in lung cancer as well as cancer of the upper respiratory tract (throat, mouth, and windpipe). Secondhand smoke (smoke in the environment that is inhaled by nonsmokers) can affect people's health. As a result, many states and cities have banned smoking in restaurants or require them to have nonsmoking sections. Many states and cities also ban smoking in workplaces, bars, public buildings, and public gathering places. Though smoking overall is declining and death rates from lung cancer in men are declining, death rates from lung cancer in women have continued to rise.

Other methods of cancer prevention: Chemoprevention is a term that describes the use of natural or synthetic substances to avert cancer. Methods include the use of cancer-fighting nutrients (such as phytoestrogens) in food, herbs, and supplements that are believed to help prevent cancer. Medications such as tamoxifen or raloxifene to reduce the incidence of breast cancer, and vaccines such as the human papillomavirus (HPV) vaccine can prevent cervical cancer.

Preventive (prophylactic) surgery may be useful in some cases for patients at high risk for cancer. Preventive procedures include removal of the breast (mastectomy), ovaries, and fallopian tubes.

Cancer Screening, a key part of cancer prevention, is covered by many insurance companies, including Medicare. Coverage may include mammograms for breast cancer, colorectal cancer diagnostic tests (such as a colonoscopy), digital rectal exam or prostate-specific antigen (PSA) tests for prostate cancer, and Pap smears for cervical cancer. Early detection and treatment is one reason that cancer survival rates are rising.

Protective clothing and gear can help reduce the cancer risk from environmental hazards. Examples of cancer-causing substances that can be introduced into the workplace include silica from cement, wood dust, lacquers, wood finishes, paints, glues, solvents, asphalt, and pesticides. Wearing an appropriate mask and using proper ventilation can help decrease exposure to these toxins. Using the provided safeguards when taking (or giving) X-rays in a hospital or at a dental office can decrease exposure to harmful radiation that can cause cancer. Those working outdoors and exposed to the sun's ultraviolet

(UV) rays can minimize their risk of skin cancer by staying out of the sun in midday, using sunscreen, and wearing protective clothing and hats.

Cancer prevention requires vigilance on the part of each individual as well as businesses and the government. However, prevention is the best way to "treat" cancer and can save many lives.

Marylane Wade Koch, M.S.N., R.N.

For Further Information

Cancer Prevention: Putting It Together. American Institute for Cancer Research Retrieved from http://www.aicr.org/reduce-your-cancer-risk/cancer-prevention/?referrer=https://www.google.com/

2008 Physical Activity Guidelines for Americans. Centers for Disease Control and Prevention. Retrieved from http://www.cdc.gov/physicalactivity/downloads/pa_fact_sheet_adults.pdf

The Annual Report to the Nation on the Status of Cancer, 1975-2011. National Cancer Institute. Retrieved from http://www.cancer.gov/research/progress/annual-report-nation

Fast Stats Deaths: Final Data for 2013 Table 10. Centers for Disease Control and Prevention. Retrieved from http://www.cdc.gov/nchs/data/nvsr/nvsr64/nvsr64_02.pdf

Verona, Verne. (2001). *Nature's cancer fighting foods.* New York: Prentice Hall.

Other Resources

American Institute for Cancer Research
http://www.aicr.org

Breast Cancer Prevention.com
http://www.breastcancerprevention.org

Cancer Index
Cancer Screening and Prevention.
http://www.cancerindex.org/clinks4p.htm

The Community Guide to Preventive Services
http://www.thecommunityguide.org/

Prevent Cancer Foundation
http://www.preventcancer.org

Smokefree.gov
http://www.smokefree.gov

World Health Organization
Cancer Prevention.
http://www.who.int/cancer/prevention/en

See also: Cancer care team; Carcinogens, known; Carcinogens, reasonably anticipated; Chemoprevention; Childhood cancers; Exercise and cancer; Fiber; Fruits; Garlic and allicin; Green tea; Infusion therapies; Nutrition and cancer prevention; Obesity-associated cancers; Pesticides and the food chain; Relationships; Smoking cessation; Sunscreens; Tobacco-related cancers; Wine and cancer

▶ Resveratrol

Category: Lifestyle and Prevention
Also known as: *trans*-3,4',5-trihydroxystilbene, polyphenolic, stilbene, piceid

Definition: Resveratrol is a compound manufactured by plants in response to stress, injury, fungal infections, and ultraviolet radiation. These polyphenolic compounds, which belong to the stilbene chemical classification, are also known as stilbenes. Resveratrol has become synonymous with cancer prevention and is thought to have protective antioxidant, anti-inflammatory, cardio and neuro-protective, and anti-carcinogenic properties.

Cancers treated: Resveratrol can be used to treat the following cancers: leukemia, lung, multiple myeloma, pancreatic, prostate, and skin cancers.

Delivery routes: Resveratrol can be delivered orally via food and dietary supplements. Significant food sources of resveratrol are red grapes, red wine, berries in the species *Vaccinum* (bilberries, blueberries, and cranberries), peanuts, and peanut butter.

How this substance works: Resveratrol is a stilbene compound manufactured by some plants as a defense mechanism. It is primarily found in red grape skins. The amount of resveratrol found in grapes is dependent on the geographic location and exposure to fungal infections of the plant, as well as the fermentation process used to extract it. Resveratrol animal studies find it can inhibit cancer cell growth and may prevent or treat cancers. Positive benefits have also been found for those with coronary heart disease, glucose and lipid metabolic disorders, and neurodegenerative diseases. Resveratrol is rapidly metabolized and eliminated, thus bioavailability is low in humans. For this reason, blood levels of resveratrol may not reach the protective levels that have been observed in the lab setting and it may only provide limited health benefits to humans. Recommended doses for resveratrol have yet to be determined.

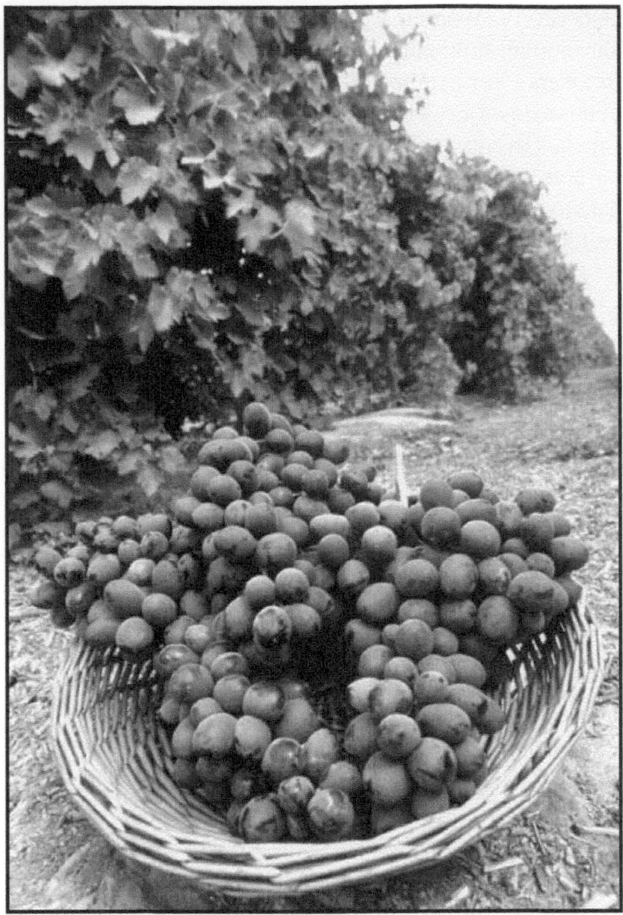

Red grapes are a good source of resveratrol, thought to have cancer-preventing properties. (U.S. Department of Agriculture)

Side effects: Caution is advised for individuals with food allergies or sensitivities to resveratrol containing foods. There have been no reported toxic or severe side effects. However, mild to moderate gastrointestinal side effects may occur. Individuals with estrogen-sensitive cancers (breast, ovarian, uterine) are advised to avoid resveratrol supplements because of its estrogen like chemical structure. Individuals taking anticoagulant, anti-platelet, or non-steroidal anti-inflammatory medications should also avoid resveratrol supplements as high doses may increase risk of bleeding. Unsafe intake of alcohol should be avoided, as this may increase the risk of cancer as well as other health risks. Additionally, Resveratrol may reduce the metabolic clearance of drugs due to its inhibition of cytochrome P3A4 (CYP3A4) enzyme activity.

Alice Richer, RDN, MBA, LD

For Further Information

Linus Pauling Institute. (2015, June 11). Resveratrol. *Micronutrient Information Center.* Retrieved from http://lpi.oregonstate.edu/mic/dietary-factors/phytochemicals/resveratrol

WebMD. (2014, July 14). *Resveratrol Supplements.* Retrieved from http://www.webmd.com/heart-disease/resveratrol-supplements

Sinha, D., Sarkar, N., Biswas, J., & Bishayee, A. (2016). Resveratrol for breast cancer prevention and therapy: Preclinical evidence and molecular mechanisms. *Seminars in Cancer Biology,* doi: 10.1016/j.semcancer.2015.11.00.

Other Resources

Linus Pauling Institute
http://lpi.oregonstate.edu/mic/dietary-factors/phytochemicals/resveratrol

WebMed
http://www.webmd.com/heart-disease/resveratrol-supplements

PubMed
http://www.ncbi.nlm.nih.gov/pubmed/?term=resveratrrol

See also: Antioxidants; Beta-carotene; Bioflavonoids; Calcium; Carotenoids; Chemoprevention; Coenzyme Q10; Complementary and alternative therapies; Cruciferous vegetables; Curcumin; Dietary supplements; Essiac; Free radicals; Fruits; Garlic and allicin; Glutamine; Green tea; Herbs as antioxidants; Isoflavones; Lutein; Lycopene; Nonsteroidal Anti-Inflammatory Drugs (NSAIDs); Nutrition and cancer prevention; Phenolics; Phytoestrogens; Wine and cancer

▶ Risks for cancer

Category: Lifestyle and Prevention

Definition: Risk is defined as the probability that exposure to a hazard will result in a negative outcome, such as the occurrence of cancer. Although cancer is one of the most feared diseases in the modern world, the majority of cancer risks can be reduced through simple lifestyle choices.

Concepts of risk: There are several concepts of risk. Absolute risk is defined as the probability that an event will occur over a defined period. Age-specific lifetime risk estimates are a type of absolute risk. For example, a woman may have a cumulative 30 percent lifetime risk of breast cancer but only have a 5 percent chance of developing the disease in the next five years. Risk is frequently described in epidemiological studies (studies of population-wide patterns of disease) using a ratio known as a relative risk (RR), which compares the incidence of disease in people who have a certain risk factor, such as family history, to those who do not have the risk factor (control group). Many studies of cancer risk factors have found higher or lower relative risks that are so slight that they could be the result of random chance. These are referred to as statistically insignificant. When assessing risk, it is also important to know the effect size, rather than just a percentage increase in risk. For example, an increase in risk from 1 to 2 percent is a much less significant finding than an increase in risk from 20 to 40 percent, yet both increases in risk could be reported in the media as a 50 percent increase in risk.

Risk perception: Risk means different things to different people. Experts often see risk differently from the average person, because experts tend to evaluate risk based on statistics and technical information. The average person, however, may judge risks based on technical information and many other factors, such as how familiar the risk is, whether the risk can be controlled, the catastrophic potential of the outcome, and the voluntariness of the exposure. Men and women also tend to perceive risk very differently, which may be related to how much power individuals feel they have over their exposure to hazards. Many people are willing to tolerate a higher level of risk from activities seen as beneficial or enjoyable, such as smoking and drinking. The perceived risk goes down as the perceived benefit goes up.

Because cancer is so common, represents such a burden on society, and is a highly dreaded disease, public health researchers are very interested in understanding risk factors for cancer. One of the most important messages coming out of this research since the early 1980's is that the majority of risks for cancer can be mitigated through lifestyle changes.

Tobacco use: Tobacco use is responsible for about one-third of all cancer deaths. The use of tobacco not only greatly increases the risk for lung cancer but also appears to influence the risk for cancer of the larynx, oral cavity, esophagus, bladder, kidney, pancreas, stomach, and cervix. Women who smoke are at a higher risk of developing lung cancer than male smokers, as are heavy smokers—for example, a person who smokes forty cigarettes a day for twenty years is at higher risk than one who smokes twenty a day for forty years. No matter how long or how much a person has used tobacco, it is never too late to quit: The risk of cancer begins to decrease as soon as tobacco use stops.

Cigars and pipes are often seen as less harmful than cigarettes. However, even if cigar and pipe smokers do not inhale, they are at increased risk for cancer of the oral cavity and lungs. Pipe smokers also are at increased risk for lip cancers in areas where the pipe stem rests. Using chewing tobacco and dry snuff increases the risk of cancer in the cheek, gums, and lips.

Diet and obesity and overweight: Poor diet, overweight, and obesity are responsible for about 30 percent of cancer deaths. Diets low in vegetables, fruits, whole grains, and beans and high in animal protein and fat have been convincingly linked to higher risk for many cancers, including those of the colon, rectum, stomach, and esophagus. However, the link between diet and breast cancer risk is unclear. Some researchers have found associations with fat intake and increased risk, while others have not. Similarly, while fiber intake was once thought to protect against colon cancer, the evidence now is inconclusive.

High fat intake is a major risk factor for cancers. In the large, well-known Nurses' Health Study, which followed more than 87,000 women for up to twenty-four years, researchers compared the occurrence of breast cancers in women who ate the most animal fat to women who ate the lowest amount and found a statistically significant relative risk of 1.33 (33 percent increased risk). Plant fats, such as those from avocados and walnuts, do not appear to increase the risk of cancer.

Processed meats, such as bacon, hot dogs, and sausage, may be particularly risky to eat. In a study that followed nearly 200,000 men and women for seven years, people who consumed the most processed meats increased their risk of pancreatic cancer by 68 percent over those who consumed few or no meat products. Other studies have shown increased risk of stomach and colorectal cancers associated with eating processed meats, pork, and red meat. Preparing meat at high temperatures (for example, grilling or using a wok) can create higher levels of cancer-causing substances in the meat. These studies suggest that eating red meat, processed meats, and pork should be limited to two to three times a week at most, particularly in childhood, when eating habits are being established.

A poor diet increases the risk of overweight and obesity, which are responsible for about 10 percent of cancer deaths in men and 15 percent in women. Researchers have identified three major ways that excess weight—especially in the midsection—may increase cancer risk. One is that body fat secretes substances that seem to promote inflammation throughout the body, increasing the chance of deoxyribonucleic acid (DNA) damage that allows cancer to start. The second is that being overweight can lead to higher blood levels of insulin and insulin-related growth factors, which promote the development of some cancers. Third, excess body fat also changes the levels of several reproductive hormones, such as estrogen and testosterone.

Preventing weight gain is best, but losing excess body fat also seems to lower cancer risk. In the Nurses' Health Study, postmenopausal women who lost 22 pounds or more and kept it off had a 30 percent lower breast cancer risk than postmenopausal women who did not lose weight. Another major study, the Iowa Women's Health Study, followed more than 33,000 women for up to fifteen years. Women who lost weight after menopause had a 23 percent lower risk of breast cancer compared with women who gained weight throughout adulthood. Women who began to lose weight before menopause reduced their risk even more. Losing weight benefits men as well: Among almost 70,000 men in the Cancer Prevention Study II, those who lost at least 11 pounds over a ten-year period had a 16 to 17 percent overall lower risk of prostate cancer and 42 percent lower risk of aggressive forms of prostate cancer.

Lack of exercise: Sedentary lifestyles are responsible for an estimated 5 percent of cancer deaths. Since regular physical activity helps prevent obesity, an indirect association between physical activity and cancer risk has been hypothesized for some time. The understanding that activity level itself is directly linked to cancer risk is new in the last several years. Physical activity changes the body's levels of hormones, insulin, and other growth factors, improves the immune system, and has an anti-inflammatory effect, all of which may help prevent cancer.

Studies consistently show that after controlling for weight, colon cancer risk drops 40 to 50 percent with exercise. Similarly, regular moderate exercise may reduce risk of breast cancer 30 to 40 percent, with greater benefits after menopause. Exercise may also independently lower the risk of prostate, lung, endometrial, ovarian, and kidney cancers, although confirming studies are needed.

Environmental hazards: Environmental hazards that increase the risk of cancer include radon, asbestos, certain chemicals (such as pesticides), and aflatoxins. Environmental hazards, combined, are blamed for about 7 percent of cancer deaths. Many of these hazards are related to occupational exposure. For example, people who work with herbicides are at increased risk of lymphoma, and construction workers are at higher risk of lung cancer from asbestos. Asbestos exposure is also related to an increased laryngeal cancer incidence, and exposure to cement dust raises the risk for pharyngeal cancer. Radon, a naturally occurring radioactive material, is known to increase the risk of lung cancer among underground miners exposed to high levels. Household levels of radon exposure have not been shown to increase lung cancer risk.

Aflatoxins are naturally occurring toxins produced by certain species of fungus, which are found on foods such as corn, peanuts, various other nuts, and cottonseed. High-level aflatoxin exposure is a risk factor for liver cancer, and infection with hepatitis B increases this risk. Food-borne aflatoxin exposure is most common in Africa, China, and Southeast Asia.

The average American is very concerned about carcinogens, and believes that the current risk from potentially carcinogenic chemicals, such as pesticides or cleaning agents, is unacceptably high. Up to 70 percent of Americans say they try to avoid contact with chemicals and chemical products in everyday life. Although it is not possible to know for sure, the best guess is that about 2 to 3 percent of cancer deaths are caused by carcinogenic chemicals.

Genetics: About 5 to 10 percent of cancer deaths are related to genetic factors and factors present at birth. A family history of any cancer raises a person's risk, but the increase varies by type of cancer. Breast-ovarian cancer syndrome results from mutations in the *BRCA1* or *BRCA2* gene. People with this mutation have an 80 to 90 percent lifetime risk of breast cancer and a 20 to 60 percent chance of developing ovarian cancer. Men with this syndrome have an elevated risk of prostate cancer, and both sexes are at increased risk of melanoma and pancreatic cancer. Hereditary forms of colon cancer, melanoma, pancreatic cancer, and brain cancers are also known.

Both low and high birth weight have both been identified as risk factors for testicular cancer. Among men, but not women, being relatively short at birth is associated with increased risk of colorectal cancer in adulthood. Because studies that follow people from birth for sixty to eighty years are expensive and logistically difficult, very little research has been done on other possible risk factors that are present at birth.

Viral and bacterial infections: About 5 percent of cancer deaths are related to viral infections. Several different types of infections raise a person's cancer risk. For example, people infected with one of the viruses that cause hepatitis are more susceptible to liver cancer and lymphoma. Chronic infection with *Helicobacter pylori*, a bacterium that lives on the lining of the stomach, increases risk for stomach cancer and lymphoma. Human immunodeficiency virus (HIV) and Epstein-Barr virus are linked to lymphoma as well. People with inflammatory bowel disease have above-average rates of colon cancer. Cervical and anal cancers are associated with the human papillomavirus (HPV). The risk is greater for people who have chronic, untreated infections, so screening for viruses to catch them early is important in preventing cancer.

Alcohol: Alcohol use is associated with increased risk for mouth, esophageal, laryngeal, pharyngeal, breast, and liver cancers. About 3 percent of cancer deaths are related to alcohol consumption. Alcohol may increase cancer risk in several ways: It may reduce the body's ability to absorb vitamins, raise the level of hormones in the body, or suppress the immune system. There may be some association with diet as well, since heavy drinkers tend to have poorer diets than abstainers. All types of alcohol—beer, wine, and liquor—increase risk equally.

People who drink more than three drinks a day are at the highest risk. One study says that for the average woman, having just one drink a day increases the lifetime risk of breast cancer from 1 in 8 (12.5 percent) to about 1 in 7 (about 14.25 percent). Moderate alcohol intake (two drinks a day for men and one a day for women) may have cardiovascular benefits for men over age fifty and women over age sixty that outweigh the increased risk of cancer, although people who do not drink should not start in the hope of gaining cardiovascular benefits.

Screening: Although screening does not, by itself, prevent cancer, it does reduce the risk of advanced or late-stage cancer. The earlier a case of cancer is detected, the better the chances of survival. There are simple screening tests for many common cancers, including breast, prostate, ovarian, colorectal, and oral.

Lisa M. Lines, M.P.H.

For Further Information

Colditz, Graham A., and Cynthia J. Stein. *Handbook of Cancer Risk Assessment and Prevention*. Boston: Jones and Bartlett, 2004.

Pensiero, Laura, Michael Osborne, and Susan Oliviera. *The Strang Cancer Prevention Center Cookbook: A Complete Nutrition and Lifestyle Plan to Dramatically Lower Your Cancer Risk*. New York: McGraw-Hill, 2004.

Ropeik, D., and G. M. Gray. *Risk: A Practical Guide for Deciding What's Really Safe and What's Dangerous in the World Around You*. Boston: Houghton Mifflin, 2002.

Slovic, P. *The Perception of Risk*. London: Earthscan, 2000.

Other Resources

American Cancer Society
Who Is at Risk?
http://www.cancer.org/docroot/WHO/WHO_0.asp

American Institute for Cancer Research
Recommendations for Cancer Prevention
http://www.aicr.org/site/PageServer?pagename= dc_home_guides

Siteman Cancer Center, Washington University School of Medicine
Your Disease Risk
http://www.yourdiseaserisk.wustl.edu/

See also: Air pollution; Asbestos; Cancer education; Carcinogens, known; Carcinogens, reasonably anticipated; Cell phones; Chewing tobacco; Cigarettes and cigars; Developing nations and cancer; Dioxins; Family history and risk assessment; Genetics of cancer; Geography and cancer; Native North Americans and cancer; Obesity-associated cancers; Occupational exposures and cancer; Pesticides and the food chain; Plasticizers; Prevent Cancer Foundation; Radon; *Report on Carcinogens* (RoC); Tobacco-related cancers

▶ Screening for cancer

Category: Procedures; Lifestyle and Prevention
Also known as: Testing, cancer detection

Definition: Screening tests are tests or procedures that can detect the presence of a specific cancer in persons who are not experiencing any symptoms.

Cancers diagnosed: The most common cancer screenings detect breast, cervical, colorectal, and prostate cancer. Some require a blood test, while others require more extensive screening procedures.

Why performed: The purpose of screening tests is to allow early identification of cancer and prevent the progression of any existing cancer. Screening and early detection can save human lives, minimize the trauma of cancer illness, and conserve limited health care resources spent on costly cancer therapies.

People participate in screenings for various reasons. Sometimes they see screening as a preventive measure, and sometimes they undergo screening because they are at high risk for a cancer. Often health-conscious people participate in routine cancer screenings, and their health insurance pays the bill. Medicare (health insurance for older adults and the disabled) Part B covers certain key preventive cancer screening tests such as colorectal screening, mammograms, Pap smears and pelvic examinations, and prostate cancer screenings within certain parameters.

Screening for cancer offers many advantages for the public. Screening can save the life of someone who may have died without early intervention. When cancer is discovered, treatment can be started immediately and decrease the possibility of radical surgery or therapy. Early intervention also results in lower health care costs. A primary advantage is that the person who receives negative (benign) results has peace of mind that, at that point in time, cancer is not present. This is reassuring for anyone but especially for someone with a family history of cancer or who has other high risks for cancer.

However, the disadvantage of screening is that some false negatives may occur so the person does not believe there is a problem even when symptoms surface. Conversely, "false positives" can cause undue anxiety until further tests confirm there is no cancer. Sometimes the screening finds a cancer that is not treatable or is so advanced that the screening does not alter the negative outcome for the person. Another disadvantage is that borderline reports from cancer screenings can result in excessive testing and associated costs.

Breast self-exam (BSE): Breast cancer can be detected through several screening tests. One is palpation of the breast tissue through a monthly breast self-examination (BSE). Palpation is a noninvasive way to examine and screen for abnormalities in the breast such as cysts, lumps, or thickening. The patient can be taught to do an examination of her breasts each month and note visual or palpable changes in the breasts.

Patient preparation. The patient should stand unclothed from the waist up and view her breasts in a mirror. The best time to complete an examination is a few days after the completion of the menses, when swelling and tenderness are lessened.

Steps of the procedure. A breast self-examination is a five-step process:

- The woman observes her breasts in the mirror, with her hands on her hips, for any visual changes in color, shape, and size. She looks for dimpling, swelling, or puckering of the skin as well as changes in the nipples or redness or rash on the breast.
- She raises her arms over her head and observes the same as above.
- She gently squeezes the nipples and observes for any liquid or discharge. (None should be present unless the woman is breast-feeding.)
- She lies down and examines each breast with the opposite hand in a circular pattern, starting at the nipple and working outward. She palpates all breast tissue from the collarbone to the abdomen and from the armpit to the cleavage area.
- She palpates the breast again in a sitting or standing position in the same pattern. Some women find that the examination is best completed when the skin is wet and slippery, such as in the shower.

After the procedure. The woman should record any observation and the date of each examination in a journal to be sure that it is completed monthly, preferably after the menses. This simple screening can detect early changes in the woman's breasts.

Risks. None.

Results. The woman makes an appointment with her health care provider if abnormalities are noted. She should schedule her annual examination with the health care provider, which includes a clinical breast exam (CBE).

Mammograms: A screening mammogram uses X rays to detect breast cancer. Mammography offers a noninvasive way to screen the breasts for cancer. A screening mammogram is useful when a woman has no history of problems with her breasts. Two X-ray views are taken of each breast. Scheduling the mammogram a week after the menses can decrease the patient's discomfort, as

Two Grading Systems for Sarcomas

American Joint Committee (AJC)
- G1 Low-grade
- G2 Moderately differentiated
- G3 Poorly differentiated

Musculoskeletal Tumor Society (MTS)
- G1 Well-differentiated
- G2 High-grade

hormonal soreness or tenderness is less at that time. An annual screening mammogram is recommended primarily for women over the age of forty. A screening mammogram can detect suspicious areas that may be breast cancer long before a mass can be palpated.

Patient preparation. The patient should avoid use of powders, deodorant, or lotion before the mammogram, since particles from these products can be viewed as abnormalities on the X ray. The patient completes paperwork such as her history, last menses, risk factors, childbearing, surgeries, implants, birth control, hormone therapy, or any problems. The patient undresses from the waist up and wears an examination gown into the X-ray room. The patient can expect the X rays to take about a half hour.

Steps of the procedure. The patient stands in front of the X-ray machine. A radiology technician exposes one breast at a time and places it on a film holder; the breast is compressed for a few seconds between the holder and a plastic paddle to take the X ray. Good compression is necessary for accurate X rays. Next the patient moves her side toward the machine, and the breast is compressed from the side. The X ray is repeated.

After the procedure. A radiologist reads the X ray either immediately or at a later time, depending on the facility's availability to the radiologist.

Risks. The risk of radiation exposure through a screening mammogram is considered minimal. Most authorities agree that the benefit of screening for breast cancer outweighs the risk of low-dose radiation.

Results. Screening mammograms do not detect breast cancer 100 percent accurately. A normal result means that the mammogram detects no abnormalities, though a cancer can be hidden in dense breast tissue. Screening mammograms may be read as borderline, which may suggest that further testing (such as a diagnostic mammogram, ultrasound, or biopsy) is indicated to confirm the diagnosis of breast cancer.

Pap smear: The Pap smear is a screening test to detect changes in the cervix that may lead to cervical cancer in women. Early detection can increase the chance of successful treatment. All women need this screening examination, including sexually active women over the age of eighteen and those at risk for cervical cancer, such as women who had a previous abnormal pap smear. This test is usually performed during the woman's annual gynecological exam.

Patient preparation. The woman should avoid douching or using any vaginal medications within forty-eight hours of the test. For accurate results, she should avoid intercourse within twenty-four hours of the screening. Optimal time for a Pap smear is at midcycle of the menses; a Pap smear cannot be performed during the menses. The woman should empty her bladder before the test to decrease discomfort.

Steps of the procedure. The Pap smear does not take long to perform. The patient lies on her back with her knees bent and her feet slightly apart. The health care provider will lubricate a speculum (an instrument that holds the walls of the vagina apart) and place it into the vagina. The patient will feel pressure as the provider swabs the cervix for a sample to examine. The sample is swabbed on a glass slide and sprayed with preservative. The slide is sent to the lab for microscopic examination for abnormal cells.

After the procedure. There are usually no side effects of this test. The lab results will be sent to the patient.

Risks. One risk is a false positive, which would lead to further testing, or a false negative, which might cause the person to ignore other warning signs of cervical cancer.

Results. Results are categorized as negative if no abnormal cells are seen. The patient usually receives a written notification of the results. Patients need to seek further testing from their health care provider for abnormalities.

Fecal occult blood, sigmoidoscopy, colonscopy: Colon cancer is the third leading cause of cancer death in the United States today. The first screening test for colon cancer is the fecal occult blood sample. This test detects blood in the stool. The next screening is a sigmoidoscopy or colonoscopy. Regular rectal and colon screening is advised in persons over fifty years of age and in those at high risk. This includes a fecal test annually, a sigmoidoscopy every five years, and a colonoscopy every ten years after age fifty-five.

Patient preparation. Certain medications (aspirin and aspirin products, ibuprofen products, iron tablets, and vitamin supplements) should be avoided for a week before screening. Prescribed medications can usually be taken, but the physician should be consulted. A sigmoidoscopy or colonoscopy requires preparation of the bowel. The exact preparation used may vary by provider preference, but these preparations usually include a diet of clear liquids for twenty-four hours prior to the test as well as a liquid laxative about two to four hours before the examination.

Steps of the procedure. Both a sigmoidoscopy and colonoscopy require the insertion of a rigid or flexible tube that contains a lens and a light into the colon. The provider can visualize the rectum, lower colon (or sigmoid colon), or upper colon.

After the procedure. Patients may need someone to drive them home after this test, especially if they have sedation. The patient can experience some soreness and mild cramping due to the air that was injected into the colon for the test, but this condition improves as the air is passed. No other aftercare is required.

Risks. A slight risk of bleeding is possible, especially when the patient has decreased clotting capacity. A perforated (torn) colon is a serious but rare complication following a sigmoidoscopy or colonoscopy.

Results. A normal result is one where the colon walls are smooth and without polyps, inflammation, or tumors. An abnormal result would be present when the colon shows precancerous polyps or tumors. A biopsy and surgical removal of the polyps or tumors would be scheduled.

Digital rectal exam (DRE) and prostate-specific antigen (PSA) blood test: Prostate cancer is the second leading cause of death in men sixty-five years of age or older. By the age of fifty, men should have screening tests for prostate cancer; in high-risk men, screening should start at the age of forty-five. The main screening tests for prostate cancer are digital rectal exam (DRE) and the prostate-specific antigen (PSA) blood test. The prostate is the male reproductive organ located under the bladder and in front of the rectum.

Patient preparation. No special preparation is required.

Steps of the procedure. For the digital rectal exam, the patient is dressed in an examination gown and placed in a relaxed position (such as lying on his side or resting over an exam table) with the rectum accessible. The doctor inserts a well-lubricated, gloved finger into the rectum and feels the size of the prostate.

After the procedure. No residual patient discomfort occurs.

Risks. None.

Results. If abnormal results are reported from either the digital rectal exam or prostate-specific antigen test, the patient will need further testing to confirm a cancer diagnosis.

Marylane Wade Koch, M.S.N., R.N.

For Further Information

Finkel, Madelon L. *Understanding the Mammography Controversy: Science, Politics, and Breast Cancer Screening*. Westport, Conn.: Praeger, 2005.

Miller, Anthony B., ed. *Advances in Cancer Screening*. Boston: Kluwer Academic, 1996.

Querna, Elizabeth. "Breast Cancer Screening: What Is the Best Way to Find Out If You Have the Disease?" *U.S. News & World Report*, September 9, 2004.

Other Resources

Centers for Disease Control
National Breast and Cervical Cancer Early Detection Program
http://www.cdc.gov/cancer/nbccedp/about.htm

MayoClinic.com
Prostate Cancer Screening: Should You Get a PSA test?
http://www.mayoclinic.com/health/prostate-cancer/HQ01273

National Cancer Institute
Screening and Testing to Detect Cancer
http://www.cancer.gov/cancertopics/screening

See also: Biopsy; Bone scan; Brain scan; Breast Self-Examination (BSE); Breast ultrasound; Clinical Breast Exam (CBE); Colorectal cancer screening; Complete Blood Count (CBC); Core needle biopsy; Genetic testing; Imaging tests; Magnetic Resonance imaging (MRI); Mammography; Nuclear medicine scan; Pap test; Positron Emission Tomography (PET); Radionuclide scan; Testicular Self-Eexamination (TSE); Ultrasound tests; Urinalysis; X-ray tests

▶ Smoking cessation

Category: Lifestyle and Prevention

Definition: Smoking cessation is the stopping of the smoking of cigarettes, cigars, or pipes. Most smokers are physically addicted to nicotine and psychologically addicted to the habit.

The depth of the problem: About 21 percent of adults in the United States (45.1 million people) are smokers. In 2006, the number of cigarettes consumed totaled 371 billion. The use of tobacco products varies with gender, age, and ethnic background. According to the Centers for Disease Control, in 2006 more men smoked (23.9 percent) than women (18.0 percent). Smoking was more common among adults between the ages of eighteen and forty-four (23.7 percent) and forty-five to sixty-four (21.8 percent) than among those age sixty-five and older (10.2 percent). Overall smoking rates are highest among American Indians and Alaska Natives (32 percent), non-Hispanic whites (21.9 percent), and those identifying as black (23 percent).

Each year, an estimated 438,000 people in the United States die prematurely from smoking or exposure to secondhand smoke, and another 8.6 million suffer from serious smoking-related illnesses, including cancer, heart disease, and lung disease. Cancer was among the first diseases causally linked to smoking, and cigarette smoking is the primary cause of cancer mortality in the United States (responsible for at least 30 percent of all cancer deaths). Smoking is the leading risk factor for lung cancer.

Smoking cessation is a difficult challenge that involves overcoming both physical and psychological dependence. Most smokers are addicted to nicotine, a psychoactive drug naturally found in tobacco products that produces dependence and makes quitting difficult. In addition, smoking becomes a routine or habit that can be hard to break, especially when it is as a coping mechanism for stress or anxiety. Cessation is difficult and may require multiple attempts. Users commonly relapse because of withdrawal symptoms and mental dependence. Cigarette cravings are usually the worst during the first two to three days of smoking cessation.

How to Quit Smoking

Get ready.

- Set a date to quit smoking.
- Get rid of all tobacco products, ashtrays, and lighters at home, in your car, and at work.
- Do not let people smoke around you.

Get medicine.

- Talk to a doctor or pharmacist.
- Choose nonprescription aids such as nicotine gum, patches, or lozenges.
- Or choose prescription aids such as a nicotine inhaler or nasal spray, buproprion hydrochloride, or varenicline tartrate.

Get help.

- Tell your friends and family that you are quitting and enlist their support.
- Ask a health care provider, such as a doctor or nurse, for help.
- Get help from your state's quitline or other supportive group.

Stay quit.

- If you start smoking again, set a new quit date.
- Avoid alcohol and smokers.
- Eat a balanced, healthful diet, and exercise.
- Stay positive that you can quit.

Sources: Agency for Healthcare Research and Quality; U.S. Department of Health and Human Services

Quit and relapse rates: An estimated 46.5 million American adults are former smokers, and more than half of all living adults who ever smoked have quit. In addition, approximately 70 percent of current U.S. adult smokers and 62 percent of high school age smokers report that they would like to quit. In 2005, an estimated 42.5 percent of adult smokers and 54.6 percent of high school students had attempted to quit smoking during the preceding twelve months.

However, not all smokers are successful in their attempts to stop smoking, and many try several times before they are able to quit. Less than 10 percent of smokers who attempt to quit on their own have long-term success. The majority of smokers cite symptoms of withdrawal and cravings as the main reasons for smoking relapse. Most relapses occur within three months of quitting. Smoking-cessation aids can increase the chances of success.

Although research findings conflict, some studies suggest that women are less successful than men in their attempts to quit smoking. Success in quitting seems to increase with higher levels of education. Motivation to quit smoking also increases success rates.

Health benefits of cessation: Smoking cessation leads to almost immediate health benefits for people with and without smoking-related diseases. For example, almost immediately after quitting, people experience improved circulation, decreased blood pressure and pulse rates, and increased body temperature in the hands and feet. In addition, cessation also leads to an almost immediate improvement in such respiratory symptoms as coughing, wheezing, and shortness of breath. Carbon monoxide and nicotine levels in the body rapidly decrease.

In the long term, the health benefits of smoking cessation can be substantial. Smoking cessation greatly reduces the risk of premature death by reducing the risk of smoking-related diseases. Even former smokers live longer than those who continue to smoke. Smoking cessation lowers the risk of developing and dying from lung cancer, other types of cancer, and other diseases (such as heart disease, stroke, and emphysema). The risk of developing cancer declines with the number of years of smoking cessation. For example, about ten years after quitting, a former smoker's risk of dying from lung cancer is 30 to 50 percent less than the risk faced by those who continue to smoke. Additional benefits include an improved sense of taste and smell and increased lung funtion. Women who stop smoking before or during pregnancy reduce their risk of having miscarriages and having babies that are small or have low birth weights.

Although cessation is beneficial at all ages, the earlier a person stops smoking, the greater the health benefits.

Smoking cessation methods: Smoking cessation is a two-step process that includes overcoming the physical dependence on nicotine and breaking the smoking habit. Methods used to increase smoking cessation rates include medications, counseling, support groups, behavioral therapies, and alternative therapies such as hypnotism and acupuncture.

Medications that have proven to be effective in treating tobacco dependence include nicotine replacement therapies (NRTs) and non-nicotine treatments, such as bupropion hydrochloride (Zyban) and varenicline tartrate (Chantrix). NRTs are designed to provide users with small amounts of nicotine that help reduce the craving for cigarettes and relieve the withdrawal symptoms associated with smoking cessation, making it easier to quit. Some are available over the counter without a doctor's prescription. Although they contain some nicotine, NRTs are not as bad as smoking because they do not contain the toxins and carcinogens found in tobacco products. Types of NRTs include gums, inhalers, nasal sprays, lozenges, and patches. Although these treatments have been shown to be safe and effective when used as directed, smokers should talk with their health care providers before beginning any smoking cessation medication.

Nicotine gum (such as Nicorette) was the first pharmacologic smoking cessation aid approved by the U.S. Food and Drug Association (FDA). First approved in 1984, it is available over the counter. The recommended treatment is typically ten to fifteen pieces of gum per day for twelve weeks.

Available only by prescription, the nicotine inhaler (Nicotrol) is a plastic cylinder that looks like a cigarette and has a cartridge that delivers nicotine. Each cartridge delivers up to four hundred puffs. The maximum recommended dosage is sixteen cartridges a day for up to twelve weeks. Side effects include mouth and throat irritation.

Nicotine nasal sprays are dispensed from pumps similar to over-the-counter decongestant sprays. The nicotine is rapidly absorbed through the nasal membranes and quickly reaches the bloodstream. A usual dose is two sprays, one in each nostril. The maximum recommended dosage is forty total doses per day. Side effects include nose and throat irritation.

Nicotine patches (such as Nicoderm) release a constant amount of nicotine into the body throughout the day. Most patches are replaced daily, and treatment periods typically range from six to ten weeks. They come in different shapes and sizes and are available over the counter or by prescription. Side effects of nicotine patches include skin irritation, dizziness, headache, and nausea and vomiting.

In 2002, the first and only over-the-counter nicotine lozenge was introduced to the market. It comes in the form of a hard candy and slowly releases nicotine as it dissolves in the mouth. Treatment typically consists of up to twenty lozenges per day for twelve weeks. The most common side effects are sore teeth and gums, indigestion, and throat irritation.

Available only by prescription, bupropion hydrochloride (Zyban) was approved by the FDA as a smoking cessation aid in 1997. Unlike with NRTs, treatment with bupropion begins while the user is still smoking—specifically, one week before the quit date—and continues for seven to twelve weeks. Length of treatment is individualized. Common side effects include insomnia, dry mouth, and dizziness.

The prescription drug varenicline tartrate (Chantrix) was approved in 2006 for smoking cessation. Typically, this nicotine-free tablet is taken twice daily for twelve weeks. Common side effects include headache, nausea and vomiting, gas, insomnia, and change in taste perception.

Symptoms of smoking withdrawal: Smokers who try to quit may face physical and psychological symptoms of withdrawal. Physically, the body reacts to the absence of nicotine. Symptoms of withdrawal include dizziness, depression, irritability, anxiety, sleep disturbances, headaches, difficulty concentrating, drowsiness, and increased appetite. They typically start within a few hours of the last cigarette and peak about two to three days later. Mentally, the smoker must break the habit of coping with stress by smoking.

Jaime Stockslager Buss, M.S.P.H., ELS

For Further Information

Aldrich, Matthew. *Stop Smoking*. Chicago: Contemporary Books, 2006.

Centers for Disease Control and Prevention. *Targeting Tobacco Use: The Nation's Leading Cause of Death, 2005*. Bethesda, Md.: Author, 2005.

DeNelsky, Garland Y. *Stop Smoking Now! The Rewarding Journey to a Smoke-Free Life*. Cleveland, Ohio: Cleveland Clinic Press, 2007.

Perkins, Kenneth A., Cynthia A. Conklin, and Michele D. Levine. *Cognitive-Behavioral Therapy for Smoking Cessation: A Practical Guidebook to the Most Effective Treatments.* New York: Routledge, 2008.

U.S. Department of Health and Human Services. *The Health Benefits of Smoking Cessation: A Report of the Surgeon General.* Washington, D.C.: Author, 1990.

Other Resources

American Cancer Society
Tobacco and Cancer
http://www.cancer.org/docroot/PED/PED_10.asp

American Lung Association
Quit Smoking
http://www.lungusa.org/site/c.dvLUK9O0E/b.33484/

Nicotine Anonymous
http://www.nicotine-anonymous.org

Smokefree.gov
http://www.smokefree.gov

See also: American Cancer Society (ACS); Chewing tobacco; Cigarettes and cigars; Coughing; Dry mouth; Family history and risk assessment; Geography and cancer; Medical marijuana; Occupational exposures and cancer; Personality and cancer; Pneumonia; Pregnancy and cancer; Prevent Cancer Foundation; Prevention; Psycho-oncology; Psychosocial aspects of cancer; Statistics of cancer; Tobacco-related cancers

▶ Soy foods

Category: Lifestyle and Prevention

Definition: Soy foods or foods made from soybeans include tofu, tempeh, edamame, miso, and soymilk. Soy foods are an excellent source of protein and contain a number of substances that are being studied for the prevention of cancer.

Background: Since the late 1990's, researchers have conducted thousands of studies on the links between diet and cancer. Epidemiological studies (studies of population-wide patterns of disease) show that many cancers are less common in Asian than in Western countries. The Japanese breast cancer mortality rate, for instance, is only one-fourth that of the women with breast cancer in the United States. Unfortunately, these types of studies are hard to interpret because they cannot account for many potential confounding factors. For example, the average person in Asia may have a more active lifestyle than a typical Westerner.

Although it is not completely clear what factors are responsible for the lower rates of cancer in these countries, many researchers have focused on the potential influence of diet on cancer risks and outcomes. There are many differences between a traditional Asian diet and a modern Western diet, such as the amount of vegetables and fruits, processed foods, meat, fish, and whole grains consumed. However, one thing that is very common in traditional Asian cuisine and historically absent from the typical Western diet is soy foods. However, this may be changing—in the year 2000, more than 25 percent of Americans reported consuming soy products at least once a week. In addition, high-dose soy protein and isoflavone supplements are being marketed in the United States to healthy people to prevent cancer.

How these compounds work: Soy products contain a number of anticarcinogenic (anticancer) compounds, including phytosterols and isoflavones. The two primary isoflavones in soybeans are genistein and daidzein. The National Cancer Institute classifies genistein (the main soybean isoflavone) as a key anticancer agent. Isoflavones act as weak estrogens, with less than 0.1 percent of the activity of estradiol (the main naturally occurring form of estrogen in humans). Isoflavones may act like antiestrogens in the body, because they can bind with the body's estrogen receptors and block some of the body's own estrogens. For cancers that have a hormonal basis, such as breast and prostate, this estrogen blocking could help reduce a person's cancer risk.

Research issues: About six hundred soy-related studies a year are published in the medical literature. There are three basic kinds of studies that have been conducted on the link between soy and cancer: population, animal, and laboratory. With population studies, there are always concerns about the accuracy of the methods used. For instance, food frequency questionnaires depend on study participants to remember what they ate over days, weeks, or even months. In addition, many of these studies have been conducted in small groups of people, so even when there is an apparent association, the link is often not statistically significant.

Animal studies have shown many potential benefits (and some risks) of soy consumption, but there is controversy over how applicable these results are to humans, because animal biology, anatomy, and physiology are not

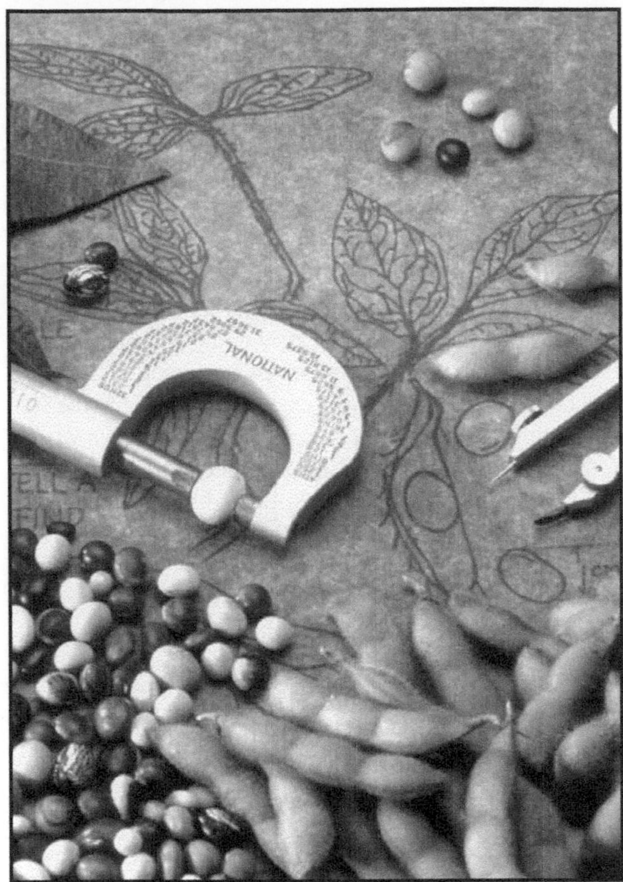

Genistein, the main isoflavone in soybeans, is classified as a key anticancer agent by the National Cancer Institute. (U.S. Department of Agriculture)

the same as those of humans. Laboratory studies, such as those that use cultured human cells to investigate the biochemical response of specific human tissues to elements found in soy, can be similarly controversial because they cannot take into account the complexity of the whole human body and its systems.

Possible risks: Although there have been more than one hundred published studies that suggest possible harm from eating soy, most are lab and animal studies, and this research represents only about 1 to 2 percent of all soy research published. One of the more prominently reported studies dealt with the interaction between soy compounds and drugs to treat breast cancer. One soy compound (genistein) was shown to decrease the effects of tamoxifen, a common breast cancer treatment, while another compound (daidzein) was shown to enhance tamoxifen's effects. There is currently no consensus on whether high levels of soy foods are appropriate for current or former breast cancer patients. In addition, animal studies have found that soy (in supplement form or highly processed isolated proteins) can promote tumor growth under some circumstances, and one study showed that high levels of soy food intake are associated with an increased risk of bladder cancer, although this was based on sixty-one cases and depended on a food-frequency questionnaire.

Possible benefits: Soy foods have been shown in many human and animal studies to be associated with statistically significant reductions in prostate, colorectal, breast, endometrial, and stomach cancer risk. Soy seems to have a particularly strong protective effect against prostate cancer. In fact, on a calorie-for-calorie basis, soy foods protect against prostate cancer at least four times more than any other dietary factor.

The best estimate is that those who eat the most soy have a 30 percent lower risk of developing colorectal cancer than those who eat the least. Regarding stomach cancer, intake of at least 10 grams per day of unfermented soy foods such as tofu may result in lower risk, but there is some question about whether these results reflect other factors, such as fruit and vegetable consumption.

As for breast cancer, modest reductions in risk have been shown for some groups of women, but most of the medical research suggests that soy intake protects against breast cancer mainly if consumed in childhood and adolescence. Postmenopausal women seem to receive little, if any, reduction in breast cancer risk. More research is needed for the effects of soy foods on cancer risk to be fully understood.

Lisa M. Lines, M.P.H.

For Further Information

Badger, T. M., M. J. Ronis, R. C. Simmen, and F. A. Simmen. "Soy Protein Isolate and Protection Against Cancer." *Journal of the American College of Nutrition* 24, no. 2 (April, 2005): 146S-149S.

Sun, C. L., et al. "Dietary Soy and Increased Risk of Bladder Cancer: The Singapore Chinese Health Study." *Cancer Epidemiology: Biomarkers and Prevention* 11, no. 12 (December, 2002): 1674-1677.

Trock, B. J., L. Hilakivi-Clarke, and R. Clarke. "Meta-analysis of Soy Intake and Breast Cancer Risk." *Journal of the National Cancer Institute* 98, no. 7 (April 5, 2006): 459-471.

Wu, A. H., D. Yang, and M. C. Pike. "A Meta-analysis of Soyfoods and Risk of Stomach Cancer: The Problem of Potential Confounders." *Cancer Epidemiology: Biomarkers and Prevention* 9, no. 10 (October, 2000): 1051-1058.

Yan, L., and E. L. Spitznagel. "Meta-analysis of Soy Food and Risk of Prostate Cancer in Men." *International*

Journal of Cancer 117, no. 4 (November 20, 2005): 667-669.

Other Resources

American Cancer Society
Soybean page
http://www.cancer.org/docroot/ETO/content/ETO_5_3X_Soybean.asp?sitearea=ETO

Memorial Sloan-Kettering Cancer Center
Soy
http://www.mskcc.org/mskcc/html/69383.cfm

See also: Antiestrogens; Breast cancer in children and adolescents; Breast cancer in men; Breast cancer in pregnant women; Breast cancers; Carcinogens, known; Carcinogens, reasonably anticipated; Childhood cancers; Epidemiology of cancer; Fruits; Isoflavones; Nutrition and cancer prevention; Nutrition and cancer treatment; Omega-3 fatty acids; Phytoestrogens; Prevention; Prostate cancer; Rectal cancer; Risks for cancer

▶ Sunscreens

Category: Lifestyle and Prevention
Also known as: Avobenzone, oxybenzone, homosalate octocrylene, octinoxate, mexoryl, zinc oxide, and titanium dioxide

Definition: Sunscreens are lotions, creams, gels, or sprays that, when applied correctly, can help prevent sunburn and other kinds of skin damage from the sun's ultraviolet (UV) rays. Using sunscreen can lower a person's risk for skin cancer.

Cancers treated or prevented: Skin cancers

Delivery routes: Topical via lotions, gels, sprays, or creams

How these agents work: There are two types of Ultraviolet radiation from the sun, UVA and UVB. UVA rays damage the skin with long-term effects such as premature wrinkles and skin aging because they penetrate deep into the skin. UVB radiation causes sunburns and most likely contributes to skin cancers. Most sunscreens do not block UVA as well as they do UVB rays. It is recommended that a broad-spectrum sunscreen be used to protect against both types of UV rays.

Sunscreens contain both organic and inorganic ingredients such as avobenzone, oxybenzone, mexoryl, homosalate octocrylene, octinoxate, zinc oxide, and titanium dioxide. They work by absorbing, reflecting, or scattering UVA and UVB rays from the sun. Most sunscreens contain a combination of these ingredients, which work together to have a synergistic effect in protecting the skin.

Sunscreens have a sun protection factor (SPF) number that refers to how long the sunscreen is effective on the skin. The higher the SPF, the more sun protection the sunscreen offers. This number is only an estimate,because many additional factors such as how much and how often the sunscreen is applied, how much sunscreen is absorbed, and the person's activity (for example, sleeping in the sun, swimming, or exercising) affect how the sunscreen works.

Sunscreen works best when applied fifteen to thirty minutes before sun exposure, followed by a reapplication fifteen to thirty minutes after being out in the sun. Sunscreen then needs to be applied every two to three hours to remain effective. Reapplying sun screen products after swimming or excessive perspiring is important for adequate protection. Using a water-resistant, broad spectrum (UVA/UVB) sunscreen with an SPF of 30 or higher is recommended when one has extended outdoor activity. Most people do not apply enough sunscreen. Studies have shown that 1 ounce or 2 tablespoons is needed to cover the average body adequately.

In reality, no matter what sunscreen is used, some UV still gets through to the skin. A comprehensive approach is needed to decrease the sun's harmful effects:

- Use sunscreen with an SPF of 15 or higher every day, even on cool or cloudy days.
- Avoid the sun during the hours of 10:00 a.m. to 4:00 p.m.
- Wear a hat, UV blocking sunglasses, and long-sleeved protective clothing with a tight weave when out in the sun. Check to see if your make up and lip balm have at least a SPF of 15.
- Select a sunscreen that contains some combination of avobenzone, oxybenzone, mexoryl, homosalate, octocrylene, octinoxate, zinc oxide, and titanium dioxide. zinc oxide, and titanium dioxide products that also provide UVA protection.

Be sure to check the expiration date of the sunscreen. The shelf life usually does not extend past three years and may be less if it was exposed to extremely high temperatures.

Some believe that sunscreens can shield the skin from making Vitamin D. However, most dermatologists agree that sunscreens do not block all production of vitamin D. Discuss this with your healthcare provider to be sure you get enough vitamin D.

Side effects: Occasionally, some people develop a mild to moderate allergic reaction or rash in reaction to some of the active ingredients in sunscreens. Discontinuing that sunscreen and switching to another type usually corrects this problem.

Michelle Kasprzak, R.N., B.S.N., O.C.N.
Updated by: Marylane Wade Koch, MSN, RN.

For Further Information

FDA Sheds Light Sunscreens. U.S. Food and Drug Administration. Retrieved from http://www.fda.gov/ForConsumers/ConsumerUpdates/ucm258416.htm

NIOSH Fast Facts: Protecting Yourself from Sun Exposure. The National Institute for Safety and Health. Retrieved from http://www.cdc.gov/niosh/docs/2010-116/

The D Dilemma. Skin Cancer Foundation. Retrieved from http://www.skincancer.org/healthy-lifestyle/vitamin-d/the-d-dilemma

Other Resources

American Cancer Society
www.cancer.org

Centers for Disease Control and Prevention
Sun Safety
http://www.cdc.gov/cancer/skin/basic_info/sun-safety.htm

Skin Cancer Foundation
http://www.skincancer.org

See also: Basal cell carcinomas; Bowen disease; Carcinomas; Eyelid cancer; Lip cancers; Melanomas; Premalignancies; Prevention; Skin cancers; Squamous cell carcinomas; Sunlamps; Ultraviolet radiation and related exposures; Young adult cancers

▶ Wine and cancer

Category: Lifestyle and Prevention

Definition: Red wine is a rich source of the natural antioxidants flavonoid and resveratrol. Antioxidants protect cells from the oxidative damage caused by free radicals, which have been implicated in cancer cell development.

How red wine protects: Red wine is a rich source of active phytochemicals (plant chemicals) called polyphenols. Polyphenols are naturally found in the seeds and skins of grapes. Red wine contains more polyphenols than white wine because when white wine is made the skins are removed after the grapes are crushed. The polyphenols found in red wine are the naturally occurring antioxidants known as flavonoid and resveratrol. These antioxidants help clear cancer-causing free radicals from the body. Resveratrol also functions as an anti-inflammatory agent, inhibiting enzymes that promote tumor development and cancer cell proliferation. The flavonoid present in red wine may be especially effective against cancer during the initiation, promotion, and progression phases.

Colorectal cancer and red wine: According to a report published by the American College of Gastroenterology, consuming three or more glasses of red wine per week may reduce a person's risk of developing colorectal cancer. In a New York study that included 1,700 people who underwent routine colorectal cancer screening, 10 percent of those patients who did not drink alcohol had colorectal cancer, while only 3.4 percent of patients who routinely drank red wine had colorectal cancer.

Prostate cancer and red wine: According to a study conducted by investigators at the Fred Hutchinson Cancer Research Center, men who drank four or more glasses of wine per week reduced the risk of prostate cancer by 50 percent. Moreover, there was a 60 percent lower incidence of aggressive types of prostate cancer. Resveratrol, according to the Fred Hutchinson Cancer Research Center, may reduce circulating testosterone levels. This is important because circulating testosterone can promote prostate cancer cell growth.

Leukemia and red wine: Resveratrol has also been effective in causing apoptosis, cancer cell death, in patients with acute promyelocytic leukemia. Resveratrol works by inhibiting deoxyribonucleic acid (DNA) synthesis in the leukemia cells, which causes cell death.

Collette Bishop Hendler, R.N., M.S.

See also: Alcohol, alcoholism, and cancer; Antioxidants; Beta-carotene; Bioflavonoids; Biopsy; Breast cancers; Calcifications of the breast; Calcium; Carotenoids; Coenzyme Q10; Complementary and alternative therapies; Curcumin; Dietary supplements; Free radicals; Herbs as antioxidants; Isoflavones; Mammography; Medical marijuana; Microcalcifications; Needle localization; Nutrition and cancer prevention; Prevention; Resveratrol; Ultrasound tests